# Noise and Its Effects

# Noise and Its Effects

*Edited by*

**Linda Luxon** BSc, MB BS, FRCP

and

**Deepak Prasher** PhD

John Wiley & Sons, Ltd

**Other Wiley Editorial Offices**

John Wiley & Sons Inc., 111 River Street, Hoboken, NJ 07030, USA

Jossey-Bass, 989 Market Street, San Francisco, CA 94103-1741, USA

Wiley-VCH Verlag GmbH, Boschstr. 12, D-69469 Weinheim, Germany

John Wiley & Sons Australia Ltd, 42 McDougall Street, Milton, Queensland 4064, Australia

John Wiley & Sons (Asia) Pte Ltd, 2 Clementi Loop #02-01, Jin Xing Distripark, Singapore 129809

John Wiley & Sons Canada Ltd, 6045 Freemont Blvd Mississauga, ONT L5R 4J3

Wiley also publishes its books in a variety of electronic formats. Some content that appears in print may not
be available in electronic books.

Anniversary Logo Design: Richard J. Pacifico

**Library of Congress Cataloging-in-Publication Data**
Noice and effects / [edited by] Linda Luxon and Deepak Prasher.
p. ; cm.
Includes bibiliographical references and index.
ISBN-13: 978-1-86156-409-2 (alk. paper)
ISBN-10: 1-86156-409-0 (alk. paper)
1. Noice--Health aspects.   I. Luxon, Linda M.   II. Prasher, Deepak.
[DNLM: 1. Noice---aderse effects. 2. Hearing Loss, Noise-Induced. WV 270 N7834 2006]
QP82.2.N6N65 2006
363.74--dc22

2006028476

**A catalogue record for this book is available from the British Library**

ISBN-13 978-1-86156-409-2

# Contents

Foreword                                                                                            ix

Preface                                                                                              xi

Contributors                                                                                       xiii

**Chapter 1**    Physical characteristics of sound                                                 1
                 *RD Knight, DM Baguley*

**Chapter 2**    Measurement of noise                                                             13
                 *Paul Radomskij*

**Chapter 3**    Interactions between noise exposure and ageing:
                 peripheral and central auditory systems                                          44
                 *Sandra L McFadden, James F Willott*

**Chapter 4**    Interaction of noise-induced hearing loss
                 and ageing: epidemiological aspects                                              64
                 *Doris-Eva Bamiou, Mark E Lutman*

**Chapter 5**    Cochlear pathophysiology in response
                 to hazardous noise                                                               85
                 *Carole M Hackney, David N Furness*

**Chapter 6**    Functional changes in the central auditory
                 system after noise-induced cochlear damage                                      110
                 *RJ Salvi, J Wang, DM Caspary*

**Chapter 7**    Factors determining an individual's
                 susceptibility to noise damage                127

                 *Deepak Prasher*

**Chapter 8**    Measurement of hearing thresholds             148

                 *Stig Arlinger*

**Chapter 9**    Noise-induced hearing loss and tinnitus
                 in children – a matter of diagnostic criteria?   165

                 *KM Holgers, Å Bratthall, ML Barrenäs*

**Chapter 10**   Clinical diagnosis of noise-induced hearing loss   182

                 *Ian Colvin, Linda Luxon*

**Chapter 11**   Disability assessment in noise-induced hearing loss   232

                 *Philip H Jones*

**Chapter 12**   Tinnitus and external sounds                  258

                 *Borka Ceranic*

**Chapter 13**   The effects of blast on the ear               279

                 *Alan G Kerr*

**Chapter 14**   Interaction of noise, general medical
                 disorders and state of health with hearing    291

                 *Ulf Rosenhall*

**Chapter 15**   Methodology and value of databases:
                 an individual hearing conservation programme   312

                 *Esko Toppila, Ilmari Pykkö, Jukka Starck, Ann-Christin
                 Johnson, Martti Juhola*

**Chapter 16**   Environmental noise: a contextual public
                 health perspective                            345

                 *Peter Lercher*

**Chapter 17**   Estimating the risk of hearing impairment
                 due to impulse noise exposure                 378

                 *Guido F Smoorenburg*

**Chapter 18**    Occupational noise    **397**

*Wieslaw J Sulkowski*

**Chapter 19**    Military noise-induced hearing loss    **435**

*J Attias, AY Duvdevany, I Reshef-Haran,*
*M Zilberberg, B Nageris*

**Chapter 20**    The hazardous aspects of music    **453**

*Rosalyn A Davies*

**Chapter 21**    Organic solvent exposures and occupational
hearing loss    **477**

*Mariola Śliwińska-Kowalska,*
*Ewa Zamyslowska-Szmytke*

**Chapter 22**    Noise hazards in the medical environment    **498**

*Moshe Chaimoff, Linda M Luxon*

**Chapter 23**    Stress effects of noise    **516**

*Hartmut Ising, Barbara Kruppa*

**Chapter 24**    Stress and noise – the psychological/physiological
perspective and current limitations    **534**

*Christian Maschke, Karl Hecht*

**Chapter 25**    Noise and cognitive performance in children
and adults    **549**

*Gary W Evans, Staffan Hygge*

**Chapter 26**    Noise and sleep    **567**

*Barbara Griefahn*

**Chapter 27**    Measurements, standards and laws    **588**

*Ronald Hinchcliffe*

**Chapter 28**    Preventing hearing loss by sound conditioning    **637**

*Barbara Canlon, Xianzhi Niu*

**Chapter 29**    Industrial noise control    **650**

*Terry Bramer*

**Chapter 30**   Hearing protectors                                              **667**
                *Jukka Starck, Esko Toppila, Ilmari Pyykkö*

**Chapter 31**   Audiological rehabilitation programmes
                and the ICF                                                      **681**
                *KM Holgers ML Barrenäs,*

**Chapter 32**   Target groups in prevention of health effects
                from listening to music                                         **706**
                *B Pettersson*

**Chapter 33**   Agencies involved with noise                                   **714**
                *Dietrich H Schwela, Andrew W Smith*


Index                                                                           **751**

# Foreword

This is a unique book which aims to cover all the main human effects of noise with contributions from most of the leading authorities in the field. In the past most books on the topic have set out to cover a narrow range of noise effects or have been limited to experimental studies, often in animals. None has combined the breadth and depth of the present book, which will surely become a standard textbook in this field.

Our understanding of noise effects and their interaction with chemicals, genetic factors, age and a range of other toxic agents, as well as with general health conditions, was the subject of major advances over the last decades of the 20$^{th}$ century and the beginning of the 21$^{st}$. Even more important in the last few years has been the first, faltering, steps towards the prevention and, ultimately, treatment of noise-induced hearing loss. All these areas are comprehensively covered in the book and a comparison with the "Classical" textbooks of Salatoff, Burns and others from the mid-latter part of the 20$^{th}$ century is remarkable.

One of the contentious areas in this field in the past has been on the interaction of noise and ageing effects on hearing, a field pioneered by Douglas Robinson. This topic is usefully covered in two valuable chapters, by McFadden and Willott on animal studies and by Bamiou and Lutman, who take a broad and in-depth look at this controversial topic.

Effects of noise on children has been an area much neglected in the past and again one full of contradictory findings. Holgers and her colleagues provide a valuable critical overview of this field which will, hopefully, stimulate further studies to clarify the potentially important effects of Social Noise in this field. With changes in the degree and nature of occupational and military noise exposure in the general population, such Social Noise exposure continues to have increasing importance. However, blast injuries from indiscriminate bombing of civilian populations are, unfortunately, still often in the headlines, and the chapter by Kerr on this topic, based on his unique experience in Northern Ireland, will be particularly useful.

Overall this book will provide an important reference source for those working in Audiology, Public Health and a range of related fields and should have an important place on our bookshelves.

**Dafydd Stephens 22/2/06**

# Preface

Hearing loss is the commonest sensory disability worldwide and whilst major advances in the understanding of the mechanisms leading to hearing loss have been made and possible treatment approaches are developing, it remains imperative that personal, societal and governmental initiatives are developed to prevent known sources of auditory damage, in particular noise. In the Developed World, education and legislation have made a significant difference, although more needs to be done. However, in the Developing World with industrialisation and limited legislation, noise induced hearing loss is an increasing problem, which must be addressed more aggressively.

Against this background of continuing man made morbidity, I would like to record my indebtedness to the authors in this book whose scientific excellence has influenced my thinking and work in this field. At a personal level, I would like to acknowledge the unstinting help, instruction and kindness of Professor Ronald Hinchcliffe whose enthusiasm and knowledge in this field fired my own interest and whose regular discussions on related topics have provided insight and support over many years. I am also especially grateful to Dr Borka Ceranic, a meticulous and dedicated scientist, who has worked with me on many of the initial projects on noise induced hearing loss and whose thoughts and ideas are always illuminating. In addition, I would like to thank all the authors and publishers who have given permission for the use either directly or through adaptation of their work. Finally, I would like to dedicate my efforts to my wonderful family without whose love and support such efforts would be impossible.

**Linda M. Luxon**

Noise has become a fact of modern life around the world today but its effect on public health remains the least recognised. However, there is a growing body of research examining the health burden of noise and this volume brings its many facets to you.

**Jian Wang** MD, PhD, Associate Professor, School of Human Communication Disorders, Dalhousie University 5599 Fenwick Street, Halifax, NS B3H 1R2, Canada

**Donald M Caspary** PhD, Professor, Department of Pharmacology, Southern Illinois University Medical School, Springfield, IL 62794 9230, USA

**Deepak Prasher** PhD, Professor of Audiology, School of Audiology, UCL Ear Institute, 330 Grays Inn Road, London WC1X 8EE, UK

**Stig Arlinger** PhD, Professor, Department of Technical Audiology, Linköping University, S-581 85, Linköping, Sweden

**Kajsa-Mia Holgers** MD, BDS, PhD, Vice-President of European Federation of Audiology Societies, Department of Audiology, Sahlgrenska University Hospital, Sahlgrenska Academy, SE 413 45 - Gothenburg, Sweden

**Marie-Louise Barrenäs** Associate Professor, Göteborg Paediatric Centre (GP-GRC), Department of Paediatrics, Institute for the Health of Women and Children, University of Göteborg, S14 85, Göteborg, Sweden

**Ian B Colvin** BMedSci, BM, BS, MSc (Distinction), MRCP Specialist Registrar in Audiovestibular Medicine, Department of Neuro-otology, National Hospital for Neurology and Neurosurgery, Queen Square, London WC1N 3BG, UK

**Linda M Luxon** BSc (Hons), MB BS (Hons & Distinction), FRCP Professor of Audiological Medicine, University College London, UCL Institute of Child Health, 30 Guilford Street, London WC1N 1EH, UK

**Philip H Jones** MA, FRCS, Consultant ENT Surgeon, South Manchester University Hospitals NHS Trust; and Honorary Associate Lecturer in Clinical Otolaryngology, Victoria University of Manchester, UK

**Borka Ceranic** MD, ENT, Spec PhD, Consultant in Audiological Medicine, Department of Audiology, Lanesborough Wing, St George's Hospital, Blackshaw Road, London SW17 0QT, UK

**Alan G Kerr** OBE, FRCS, Eng FRCS, Ed (formerly Professor of Otolaryngology, Queen's University, Belfast), Consultant Otolaryngologist, Royal Group of Hospitals, Grosvenor Road, Belfast BT12 6BA, Northern Ireland

**Ulf Rosenhall** MD, PhD, Professor, Department of Audiology, Karolinska University Hospital Solna, SE 171 76 Stockholm, Sweden

**Esko Toppila** Finnish Institute of Occupational Health, Department of Physics, Helsinki, Finland

**Ilmari Pyykkö** ENT Clinic, Tampere University Hospital, Tampere, Finland

**Jukka Starck** Finnish Institute of Occupational Health, Department of Physics, Helsinki, Finland

**Ann-Christin Johnson** Department of Otolaryngology, Karolinska Hospital, Stockholm, Sweden

**Martti Juhola** Department of Computer Science, Tampere University Hospital, Tampere, Finland

**Peter Lercher** MD MPH Associate Professor, Division of Social Medicine, Department of Hygiene, Microbiology and Social Medicine, Medical University of Innsbruck, Innsbruck, Austria

**Guido F Smoorenburg** Head, Hearing Research Laboratories, Department of Otorhinolaryngology, University Medical Center, PO Box 85500, 3508 GA, Utrecht, The Netherlands

**Wieslaw J Sulkowski** MD, PhD, Professor of Otolaryngology, Audiology and Phoniatrics; Consultant, Department of Occupational Diseases, Nofer Institute of Occupational Medicine, 8 St Theresa Str, 91-348 Lodz, Poland

**Joseph Attias** DSc, Associate Professor, Department of Communication Disorders, University of Haifa, Haifer and Schneider Children's Medical Center of Israel, Petach Tikva, Kaplan Street 14, 49202, Israel

**M Zilberberg** MA, The Institute for Noise Hazards Research and EP Laboratory, IDF Medical Corps, PO Box 02149, IDF, Israel

**A Y Duvdevany**, Lieut Colonel, PhD Acoustics and EMR Radiation Section, IDF Medical Corps, PO Box 02149, IDF, Israel

**Rosalyn A Davies** MB BS, FRCP, PhD, Consultant in Audiovestibular Medicine, Department of Neuro-otology, The National Hospital for Neurology and Neurosurgery, Queen Square, London WC1N 3BG, UK

**Mariola Sliwinska-Kowalska** MD, PhD, Professor and Head of the Department of Physical Hazards, Head of the Department of Audiology and Phoniatrics, Nofer Institute of Occupational Medicine, 8 St Teresa Str, 90-950 Lodz, Poland

**Ewa Zamyslowska-Szmytke** MD, Associate Professor, Department of Audiology and Phoniatrics, Nofer Institute of Occupational Medicine, 8 St. Teresa Str, 90-950 Lodz, Poland

**Moshe Chaimoff** MD, Vestibular Service, Rabin Medical Center, Israel

**Hartmut Ising** MD, Rheinstr. 69, D-14612 Falkensee, Germany

**Barbara Kruppa** MD, Federal Environmental Agency, Institute for Water, Soil and Air Hygiene, Berlin, Germany

**Christian Maschke** Interdisciplinary Research Network for Noise and Health, Berliner Zentrum Public Health, Berlin, Germany

**Karl Hecht** Interdisciplinary Research Network for Noise and Health, Berliner Zentrum Public Health, Berlin, Germany

**Gary W Evans** PhD, Professor, Departments of Design and Environmental Analysis and of Human Development, Cornell University, Ithaca, NY 14853-4401, USA

**Staffan Hygge** PhD, Professor, Centre for Built Environment, University of Gävle, SE-801 76 Gävle, Sweden

**Barbara Griefahn** MD, Professor and Deputy Director, Institute for Occupational Physiology, University of Dortmund, Ardeystr. 67, 44139, Dortmund, Germany

**Ronald Hinchcliffe** Emeritus Professor, Department of Audiological Medicine, University College London Medical School, UK

**Barbara Canlon** PhD, Professor, Department of Physiology and Pharmacology, Karolinska Institute, 171 71 Stockholm, Sweden

**X Niu** Department of Physiology and Pharmacology, Karolinska Institutet, 171 77 Stockholm, Sweden

**T P C Bramer** BSc(Eng), Ceng MIEE, FIOA, Principal Acoustic Consultant, Acoustic Design Consultants, Hadleigh, Suffolk IP7 6BQ, UK

**Jukka Starck** Professor, and Director of the Department of Physics, Finnish Institute of Occupational Health, Topeliuksenkatu 41 a A, FI-00250 Helsinki, Finland

**Ilmari Pykkö** ENT Clinic, Tampere University Hospital, Tampere, Finland

**Marie-Louise Andersson-Barrenäs** Associate Professor, Göteborg Paediatric Centre (GP-GRC), Department of Paediatrics, Institute for the Health of Women and Children, University of Göteborg, S14 85, Göteborg, Sweden

**Kajsa-Mia Holgers** MD, BDS, PhD, Vice-President of European Federation of Audiology Societies, Department of Audiology, Sahlgrenska University Hospital, Sahlgrenska Academy, SE 413 45 - Gothenburg, Sweden

**Bo Pettersson** Principal Administrative Officer, National Board of Health and Welfare, S-106 30 Stockholm, Sweden

**Dieter Schwela** Dr rer. nat, Diplomphysiker Stockholm Environment Institute, University of York, Sally Baldwin Building, D Block, York, YO10 5DD, UK

**Andrew W Smith** BSc, MB BS, MRCP, MSc, Medical Officer, Prevention of Blindness and Deafness NMH/CHP/CPM, World Health Organisation, 20 avenue Appia, CH-1211, Geneva 27, Switzerland

# CHAPTER 1

# Physical characteristics of sound

*Noise and Its Effects:* Edited by Linda Luxon and Deepak Prasher © 2007 John Wiley & Sons Ltd.

RD KNIGHT

DM BAGULEY

## Introduction

An introduction to the physical characteristics of sound is fundamental to an understanding of noise and its effects on humans. This chapter will introduce physical concepts in acoustics using a descriptive approach, with the intention of being accessible to those without a physics background. References will be provided to allow further reading if more detailed information is required.

## What is sound?

The *Oxford English Dictionary* defines sound variously as 'a sensation caused in the air by the surrounding air or other medium', 'vibrations causing this sensation' and 'similar vibrations whether audible or not'.[1] Thus for sound to exist there must be a medium in which it can travel, a conclusion first reached by Robert Boyle (1627–91) following an experiment

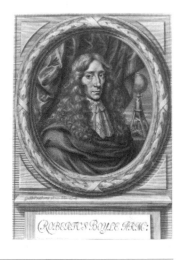

**Figure 1.1** William Faithorne's engraved portrait of Boyle, 1664 (Sutherland Collection, Ashmolean Museum, Oxford).

---

[1] Thus answering in the affirmative the question much loved by undergraduates: 'Does a tree falling in a forest make a sound if no-one is there to hear it?'

in which a vacuum that was produced surrounding a sound source abolished the sound (see Durrant and Lovrinic, 1995, for a full account).

# Aspects of sound

### Frequency, period and wavelength

In general, the *frequency* at which an event occurs is the number of times it happens per unit of time. For example, night time happens once each 24 hours, Saturday happens once a week and Christmas happens once a year. Sound waves repeat more frequently than this and their frequency is defined as the number of waves per unit of time.

When the time unit is the second (which is the convention), the unit of frequency is named as hertz (Hz). Thus one wave per second = 1 Hz.

The psychological correlate of frequency is 'pitch'. However, the terms are not interchangeable, as for example the perceived pitch of a sound may change a little with changed intensity but the frequency will stay the same. A complex waveform may also contain energy at several frequencies but still retain one single subjective pitch.

The *period* of an event is the time before that event repeats. Therefore, the greater the frequency, the smaller the period. For example, if a waveform repeats five times per second (5 Hz), the period is one-fifth of a second (200 ms).

Frequency and period can be calculated from each other:

frequency (Hz) = 1/period (seconds) and

period (seconds) = 1/frequency (Hz)

As a sound wave propagates, the distance between successive wave peaks is the *wavelength*. For a given frequency, the faster a wave is travelling the longer the wavelength will be, as the wave is more 'stretched out'. Conversely, for a given velocity, the higher the frequency the shorter the wavelength. Wavelength can be calculated from frequency and velocity as follows:

wavelength = velocity/frequency

At room temperature and normal air pressure of $1 \times 10^5$ pascals (Pa), the speed of sound in air is approximately 343 m/s; however, this varies with air pressure and temperature. For example, at 0°C the speed falls to around 331 m/s.

### Frequency and amplitude ranges of hearing

Human hearing is capable of perceiving sound waves in a wide range of frequencies. The range is commonly quoted to be from 20 Hz to 20 000 Hz (20 kHz). However, this varies from person to person and the range tends to reduce with increasing age. Hearing sensitivity is also very reduced at the extremes of the audible frequency range, so much more sound energy is required for example at 20 Hz to produce the same sensation of loudness than would be the case at a frequency of 1 kHz. This is demonstrated in Figure 1.2, where the dotted 'threshold of audibility' line gives the mean hearing threshold for the normal hearing population. The curve is lowest in the frequency region 500 Hz to 6 kHz. (The vertical scale is a decibel scale – this will be introduced in Chapter 2.)

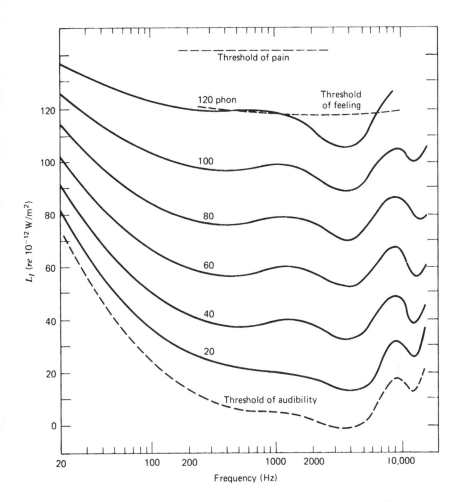

**Figure 1.2** Thresholds and free-field equal-loudness contours (phons) for pure tones presented from directly in front of the subject. (From Fundamentals of Acoustics, 3$^{rd}$ edition, Kinsler, Frey, Coppens and Sanders, New York: Wiley & Sons.)

For example, the fundamental frequency of the range of notes on a piano extends all the way from close to the bottom of the human hearing range up to about 4 kHz (but each note also contains many higher harmonic frequencies). Speech contains frequencies typically from about 200 Hz (in vowel sounds) up to 8 kHz (for example, in fricative sounds such as "s").

The range of sound-wave pressures to which the ear can respond proportionately is impressive. At a frequency of 1 kHz, a sound pressure wave of 0.00002 Pa (or 20 $\mu$Pa) is typically on the threshold of hearing. The threshold of feeling for loud sounds is around 20 Pa, although permanent hearing damage results from exposure to sounds as loud as this over a period of time. Therefore the ratio of pressures from the quietest to the loudest is 1 million!

Static air pressure, by comparison, is approximately 100 000 Pa and has natural variations of more than 20 Pa; therefore it can be seen that it is the energy contained in the sound waves rather than the static pressure that limits the dynamic range of the human ear.

**Phase**

When phase is referred to in the context of a sound wave, it is conveying the stage of a sound wave cycle at a moment in time. Phase is measured in degrees or radians, where one cycle is 360° or 2$\lambda$ radians.

By convention, phase is often defined as zero at zero displacement going positive, so, for example, the bold trace in Figure 1.3 starts at 0° and reaches 0° again (or 360°) at the centre of the chart. Without a clear reference point, there is no resolution between whole numbers of cycles of phase – in other words, we often don't know whether we are at 0°, 360° or 720°.

Phase is commonly defined as a relative quantity, for example in the figure below, the phase of the bold waveform is delayed by 0.25 of a wavelength (90° or 0.5 rad) relative to the faint curve.

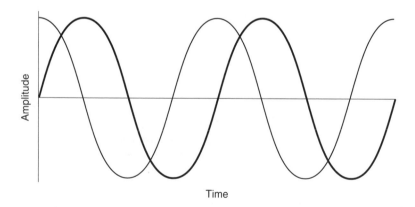

Time

Amplitude

**Figure 1.3** Illustration of two sound waves seen at one point in space over a period of time. The thin trace is 'ahead' of the bold trace by 0.25 of a cycle or 90°. (Alternatively, the bold trace may be ahead of the faint trace by three quarters of a cycle or 270°.)

The simple waveforms in the above figure each contain a single frequency and are examples of simple harmonic motion. This motion is characterized by acceleration being always towards the midpoint and proportional to the distance from the midpoint.

Usually sounds are made up of several different frequencies, leading to more complicated sound waves than those shown above. Even sounds that are perceived to have a single subjective pitch commonly contain a series of harmonics at frequencies that are multiples of the frequency at which the wave repeats (the 'fundamental' frequency). The relative phases of the harmonics are significant for the shape of the overall waveform, as shown in Figure 1.4. Determination of the frequencies at which energy is present can be determined by Fourier analysis, which is a mathematical method of analysing a waveform into the frequencies that it contains.

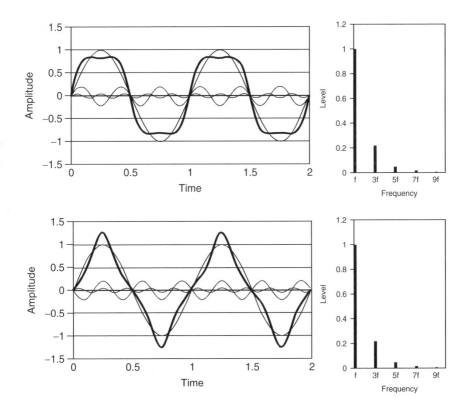

**Figure 1.4** Waveforms from a series of odd harmonics. The amplitudes of the harmonics (faint lines) (shown in the charts on the right) are the same in each example, but in the second one alternate harmonics are given a 180° phase change. This changes the wave shape (bold lines) from a square wave to a triangular wave.

Most sounds in the real world do not repeat exactly time after time. These are called aperiodic. They can be considered in two categories:

1. *Ongoing random waveforms*: laboratory examples of these include pink noise (which contains equal sound energy per octave band) and white noise (which contains equal sound energy per Hz).
2. *Clicks*: in audiology, these sounds are used widely as test signals. Of course, clicks can be repeated successively and therefore effectively become periodic but usually the time period between repeats is great enough for them to be considered as independent events in terms of the frequency content.

Interestingly, both white/pink noise and clicks contain essentially continuous and broadband frequency spectra. The way to imagine this is that both contain all frequencies jumbled up together, but in the case of a click these sounds are arranged in such a way that they cancel each other out except momentarily when the click occurs. Therefore if either of these types of sound is used as a stimulus in a hearing test, the auditory system is stimulated over a wide frequency range. Alternative stimuli such as tone pips, tone bursts and band-filtered noise can be employed to make the stimuli more frequency specific.

# Sound propagation

### Types of waveform

There are different types of propagating wave, and two common examples are called *transverse* waves and *longitudinal* waves. If displacement occurs at right angles to the direction that the wave is travelling, the wave is called a transverse wave. Surface waves on water are predominantly transverse waves, although there is also some associated forward-and-back motion because of the incompressibility of water. Another example of a transverse wave can be found on a taut string or 'slinky' spring.

If, however, the particle displacement is in the direction that the wave is travelling, the wave is called a longitudinal wave. Sound waves are longitudinal waves. Before a sound wave comes along, particles in a medium are spaced at a certain density, determined by a balancing of the atomic repulsion between air molecules. Transient pressure is applied to air (for example by a loudspeaker cone) causing molecules to move, fluctuating around their resting position. Movements of these molecules then exerts pressure on neighbouring air molecules, which in turn also move. In this way the wave is propagated (Figure 1.5).

Air molecules are continually on the move through thermal energy (Brownian motion), so sound waves are really organized movement superimposed on this underlying random movement. Air lacks the intermolecular bonds to allow transverse waves to be supported, so only longitudinal waves are possible.

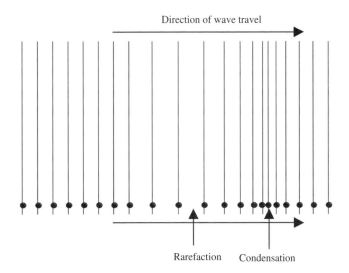

**Figure 1.5** Illustration of a longitudinal wave at an instant in time. A row of particles is shown, vertical lines are shown above each particle to aid visual clarity. Rarefaction occurs at the part of the wave cycle where the air pressure is reduced below atmospheric pressure, and condensation is the part of the cycle where pressure is increased above atmospheric pressure.

It is common to see longitudinal waves represented graphically as transverse – this is purely because of the difficulty in representing longitudinal displacement on the same axis as direction of travel of the waveform.

Other waveform types are possible, particularly in solid materials, for example torsional waves and combination types.

### Reflections

When a wave encounters a boundary, such as air next to a wall, some of the sound energy continues into the new medium and some bounces back. How much will bounce back depends on the impedance difference between the two media, as well as the angle of incidence of the wave.

The impedance of a material is essentially a measure of how much energy it takes to make particles in the material move. An abrupt impedance change results in inefficient energy transfer from one material to the next, resulting in energy being reflected.

In acoustics, a horn fitted to a loudspeaker is an example of an attempt to provide a gradual impedance transformation from the high impedance of the loudspeaker driver to the low impedance of the free air. The ideal horn shape is exponential, although most horns compromise on this for manufacturing reasons and to control directivity.

In audiology, the human middle ear is another example of an impedance transformer, transferring sound efficiently from the low impedance of free air to the higher impedance of the fluid-filled and enclosed cochlea and therefore maximizing the amount of sound energy that is passed to the cochlea.

## Standing waves

Once sound has been reflected, the reflected wave can 'interfere' with the later waves that are still approaching the reflected surface. Where two waves travelling in different directions cross each other, they both pass straight through unimpeded, but where they coexist, they add up. Therefore two wave peaks or troughs add together and result in a bigger amplitude displacement, whereas if a peak coincides with a trough they will tend to cancel each other out, resulting in a smaller amplitude wave.

This effect is observed most clearly with reflections of waves of a single frequency. At some distances from the reflecting surface, the waves are in phase and add together, whereas at other places the waves are out of phase and cancel out. The distance between adjacent maxima is half of the wavelength of the underlying sound wave (Figure 1.6).

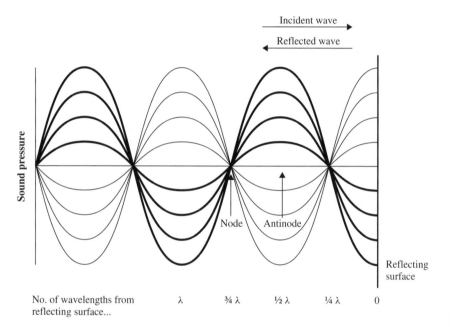

**Figure 1.6** Illustration of a standing wave. The different line thicknesses show the standing wave at different moments in time.

Note that the waves do not actually bounce off each other, but rather they add together where they coincide but then pass through each other and continue on their way unimpeded by the wave travelling in the opposite direction.

A characteristic of standing waves is that for positions where pressure is at an antinode (maximum) the particle displacement is at a node (minimum). This is because, at a pressure antinode, particles approach from both sides and then move apart again simultaneously, resulting in a pressure maximum but a minimum of particle displacement at the centre of the node.

Standing waves have the feature that the wave does not appear to be going anywhere – pressure or displacement just rises and falls without a clear sense of direction. In fact, the wave contains two waves that are propagating in opposite directions.

It is worth emphasizing here that sound is reflected by both an impedance step up and an impedance step down. Therefore sound that is propagating in a small enclosed space can be reflected by a closed end, but also by an open end because it represents an impedance step down.

In terms of pressure, there is a phase inversion at an open end of a tube but not at a closed end of a tube. This means that a tube that is open at one end and closed at the other can support resonances (sound being repeatedly reflected backwards and forwards whilst remaining in phase with itself) at a series of frequencies where the wavelength λ is 0.25L, 0.75L, 1.25L and so forth (L = tube length). This series is found, for example, in the external ear canal. A tube that has a rigid termination at both ends, or an open termination at both ends, supports resonances when λ is 0.5L, L, 1.5L, 2L and so forth (Figure 1.7).

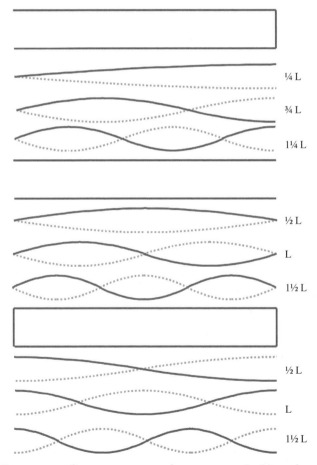

**Figure 1.7** Pressure standing wave patterns that can occur: in (a) a tube open at one end and rigidly closed at the other; (b) a tube open at both ends; and (c) a tube rigidly closed at both ends. Solid and dotted lines show the wave at different moments in time.

Note that these series are approximate as there is an end effect associated with an open end of a tube that makes the effective acoustic length slightly longer than the physical length of the tube.

These resonances can be reduced by 'damping'. This can be achieved mechanically, for example by inserting a material that inhibits the flow of air molecules but not so much that the material creates a strong reflection of its own. The effect of the 'damper' is greatest at an amplitude antinode, where the systematic movement of air molecules is greatest. Dampers are sometimes used in this way to 'smooth' the frequency response of hearing aids.

### Mechanical resonance

If a mass is connected to a rigid surface by a spring, it will exhibit a decaying oscillation at a specific frequency. This frequency is given by:

$$F_{res} = \frac{1}{2}[\frac{k}{m}]^{\frac{1}{2}}$$

where $k$ is the spring constant (stiffness) of the spring and $m$ is the mass in kilograms. If the mass is repeatedly given a push at this frequency, it will build up a large oscillation, whereas if it is driven at a significantly different frequency it will move much less. Figure 1.8 illustrates this principle.

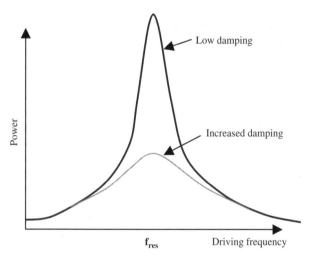

**Figure 1.8** Illustration of resonance curves of a mass–spring system. Curves are shown with a small amount of damping and with increased damping. If damping is very high, there may be no peak at all in the resonance curve.

In the real world, unwanted resonances are commonly much more complex, involving several effective springs and a few masses. Resonant behaviour can be altered by the mass or the stiffness (which would change the natural resonant frequency), changing the frequency at which the system is being driven in order to avoid the resonance, or increasing the damping in order to reduce the resonance.

## When sound goes round corners

*Directivity and diffraction*

We are quite familiar with the idea that light travels in straight lines and if an object is placed in the way of a beam of light the light does not bend around it to any great extent. However, this is not the case with sound. The reason for this is that the wavelength of sound is much longer, and the extent to which a wave will go around an object is a function of the size of the wavelength and the size of the object.

If the wavelength is small relative to the size of the object, a fairly effective shadow region will be formed behind the object. However, if the object is small compared with the wavelength, the shadow region will be filled in by waves which have bent around the corner of the obstruction. Figure 1.9 illustrates this. The same principle also happens in reverse with sound escaping through a gap in a barrier, or from a sound source (for example, loudspeaker) with a finite size – the larger the source compared with the wavelength, the more the waves will tend to be beamed straight ahead. This is why the directivity of a loudspeaker will tend to be greater at high frequencies than lower frequencies.

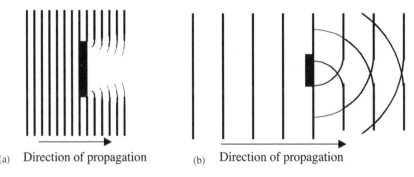

(a)  Direction of propagation     (b)  Direction of propagation

**Figure 1.9** Illustrations of diffraction: (a) small wavelength and a comparatively large obstruction – the waves predominantly continue in a straight line, leaving a shadow region; (b) large wavelength and comparatively small obstruction – the waves bend around the edges of the object, leaving no shadow region.

*Refraction*

Even without obstacles, there are factors that can bend the path of propagating sound waves. As mentioned previously, the speed of sound propagation in air depends on the air pressure and temperature. Normally air pressure reduces with height, so sound at altitude travels slower than sound at ground level. This results in propagating sound waves being bent upwards. In addition to this, air is usually colder at altitude than at ground level, also causing sound waves to bend upwards.

However, under some meteorological conditions a temperature inversion can occur, when air temperature increases with height resulting in sound waves being bent downwards.

In addition to this, wind causes sound to bend upwards when travelling up wind and downwards when travelling down wind because wind speed usually increases with height. This is the main factor behind the common perception that sound propagates better down wind than up wind.

As a result of these factors, environmental noise propagation over large distances is highly variable. Under favourable wind conditions and/or a temperature inversion, environmental noise can sometimes unexpectedly become audible over great distances from the sound source. Figure 1.10 illustrates these variable environmental factors.

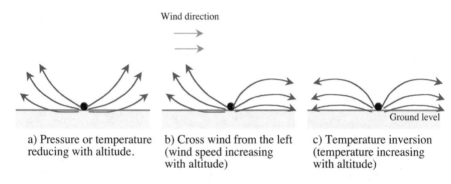

a) Pressure or temperature reducing with altitude.

b) Cross wind from the left (wind speed increasing with altitude)

c) Temperature inversion (temperature increasing with altitude)

**Figure 1.10** Curved arrows indicate direction of sound propagation from a sound source under different environmental conditions: (a) Pressure or temperature reducing with altitude; (b) Cross wind from the left (wind speed increasing with altitude); (c) Temperature inversion (temperature increasing with altitude).

# Bibliography and Further Reading

Durrant JD, Lovrinic JH (1995) Bases of Hearing Science, 3rd edn. Baltimore: Williams & Wilkins.

Gelfand SA (2001) Essentials of Audiology, 2nd edn. New York: Thième.

Kinsler LE, Frey AR, Coppens AB, Sanders JV (1982) Fundamentals of Acoustics. New York: Wiley.

Moore BCJ (1989) An Introduction to the Psychology of Hearing. San Diego: Academic Press.

Pickles JO (1988) An Introduction to the Physiology of Hearing. London: Academic Press.

Robinson DW, Dadson RS (1956) A re-determination of the equal-loudness relations for pure tones. British Journal of Applied Physics 7: 166–81.

Smith BJ, Peters RJ, Owen S (1996) Acoustics and Noise Control. Harlow: Addison Welsey Longman.

# CHAPTER 2

# Measurement of noise

*Noise and Its Effects:* Edited by Linda Luxon and Deepak Prasher © 2007
John Wiley & Sons Ltd.

PAUL RADOMSKIJ

## Introduction

Any introduction to measurement of noise should begin with a few basic definitions. What is noise / sound? In simple terms, sound may be defined as an oscillation of particles within a medium, mediated by elastic forces within the medium (Martin and Summers, 1999). More specifically, *audible* sound may be defined as sensation of hearing evoked by acoustic oscillation. International standards such as IEC-801-21-08 define noise as 'an erratic or statistically random oscillation and a disagreeable or undesired sound or other disturbance'. However, for the purposes of the Noise at Work Regulations (1989) *any* audible sound is considered as noise.

The measurement of noise, whether environmental or from a specific piece of noise-generating equipment is relatively simple if the signal is from a single source and unchanging. It becomes increasingly complicated if the signal being measured is both erratic and continually changing. How we characterise and quantify noise depends to some extent on why we want to measure it. Often it is expressed in quantities, which may predict the potential biological effects, particularly on hearing. Although it may be relatively easy to make measurements of noise in a practical sense, it is more difficult to decide what parameters you should use to quantify noise, how measurements should be taken and what type of instrumentation should be used. Entire families of terms describing noise have been established and are defined in a variety of British and International Standard documents (BS7445-1, BS3740). Indeed there are at least 200 British Standards concerned with how sound/noise is defined, how it should be measured in the environment and test codes for measurement of power emissions from specific items of noise-generating equipment. The most relevant standards, including a few examples of the standards related to specific machinery, may be found in the glossary at the end of this chapter.

The auditory effects of noise on health and hearing have been investigated for many years. These effects include permanent and/or temporary shift in hearing threshold. European commission projects such as PAN (*Protection Against Noise* concerted action) and NOPHER (*NOise Pollution Health Effects Reduction* concerted action) have and continue to promote and encourage research into noise (industrial, environmental and leisure) and reduction of ill effects arising from exposure to excessive noise. The Noise at Work Regulations 1989 list the legal duties of employers to prevent damage to hearing and legal duties of manufacturers, importers and suppliers to prevent damage to hearing. The regulations are extensive, but for the first time specified action levels when hearing protectors should be *made available* (first action level) and hearing protectors should *be worn* (second action level) by employees. It does not, however, apply to individuals exposed to excessive leisure noise. Directive 2003/10/EC issued on 6th February 2003 has introduced more stringent exposure limit values and exposure action values. The new lower exposure limits take effect in early 2006, with implementation of Control of Noise at Work Regulations 2005 and revocation of Noise at Work Act 1989 (see Table 2.1).

**Table 2.1** Exposure limit values and exposure action values

| Legislation Directives | 1st Action Level-Daily personal noise exposure of | 2nd Action Level-Daily personal noise exposure of | Peak Action Level |
|---|---|---|---|
| **Noise at Work Act 1989 (Directive 89/ 391/EEC 12th June 1989)** | $L_{EP, d}$ 85dB(A) | $L_{EP, d}$ 90dB(A) | Peak sound pressure of 200Pa |
| | **Lower Exposure Action Value** | **Upper Exposure Action Value** | **Exposure Limit Value\*** |
| **Control of Noise at Work Regulations 2005 (Directive 2003/10/EC 6th Feb. 2003)** | $L_{EX, 8h}$ 80dB(A) Peak 135dB (C) [112Pa] | $L_{EX, 8h}$ 85dB(A) Peak 137dB (C) [140Pa] | $L_{EX, 8h}$ 87dB(A) Peak 140dB (C) [200Pa] |

\*2003/10/EC action levels should not take into account attenuation provided by hearing protectors, whereas they may be in the determination of exposure limit value **Note:** $L_{EP, d}$ **corresponds to** $L_{EX, 8h}$

This chapter will describe the variety of ways in which noise may be quantified, so that the novice reader, for example, will be able to understand the difference between $L_{EP,d}$ and $L_{Aeq,T}$ dB(A). In addition the instrumentation most commonly used to measure sound (noise) will be described, as well as specific scenarios where it is important to make sound measurements. This will cover how to take basic measurements and the variables, which may affect the accuracy of these measurements, along with general problem solving. These measurements should allow scientific and quantitative analysis of noise to be made. However, obtaining a 'number' to quantify the type and nature of the noise would not automatically tell us whether the particular type of noise being analysed is more annoying to one individual or another, or indeed more damaging, but it is a start. At least it provides an indication of the degree of potential damage and/or annoyance and of course whether any action needs to be taken to prevent noise damage and comply with the Noise at Work Regulations 1989 / Control of Noise at Work Regulations 2005 or any of the other laws and statutes pertaining to noise. There will be a focus on measurements on air-borne sound (sound that is being generated and radiated from free-field loudspeakers or noise generating instruments, machinery and environmental noise). This information will provide an introduction to the measurement of noise techniques, but it is beyond the scope of this chapter to provide detailed information. The references, particularly the British and International standards listed, provide a very extensive description of methodologies and equipment that need to be employed in the measurement of noise.

## Measuring noise

Noise is variable, i.e. 'an erratic or statistically random oscillation and a disagreeable or undesired sound or other disturbance'.

The frequencies contained within the noise may be changing, as well as the level of each of these frequencies. This is what makes noise particularly difficult to quantify and to suspect measurement '*is more of an art than a science*'. If the noise level were steady or only varied slowly in terms of magnitude ($+/-$ 4dB over a few seconds – see BS5330), and frequency content, then this would usually be relatively easy to measure and quantify (for example, noise from a factory machine). Other types of noise, such as noise generated by airport activity are not steady, with the ambient noise level being interrupted by single noise events (for instance short-duration events such as engines starting up; long-duration events such as airplanes flying overhead). Measurement of such fluctuating, irregular and impulsive noise requires greater expertise.

The effects that any type of machinery and environmental noise will have on the listener will, however, ultimately depend on the overall energy received within a particular time period. This in turn will depend on:

- the average level of steady state noise;
- the level of noisy single events (noise is considered to be impulse/ impulsive noise if it is of short duration <1 s);
- the spectral content of each of the first two items;
- number of noisy single events;
- duration of noise exposure.

The parameters and units used to express noise need to take into account these factors, although sound may still be described in terms of frequency, amplitude, wavelength, particle velocity, pressure, intensity and/or power. Several parameters have been developed to help quantify the nature and level of noise; each being used for particular situations, although none would be applicable and suitable for all. The two main categories of noise measured are ambient noise and specific noise.

*Ambient noise* is composed of sound from lots of different sources, which cannot be isolated.
*Specific noise* is a component of the ambient noise, which can be isolated and measured.
*Environmental noise* is considered to be ambient although specific noise may be identifiable within it.

Measurement of specific machinery noise is either carried out in-situ and/or in anechoic chambers. This offers more flexibility, with test codes available for certain types of machinery.

**When do we need to measure noise?**

There may be scientific and/or legislative reasons for measuring noise, such as ensuring compliance with the current laws relating to noise (Noise at Work Regulations 1989/Control of Noise at Work Regulations 2005, Environmental Protection Act 1990, Noise and Statutory Nuisance Act 1993, Machinery Noise Test Codes). The Noise at Work Regulations, 1989, for example, state that noise measurements in an industrial setting may be required if there is concern that any of the action levels for noise control *(first action level 85dB(A), 2$^{nd}$ action level 90dB(A) or peak level of 200 Pascals)* are being reached or exceeded; if people need to shout or have difficulty being heard clearly by someone who is 2 meters away and/or if workers are exposed to impulse sounds e.g. jackhammers, detonators, foundry noise. Following a noise survey, ear protection zones would be set up as necessary and employees advised to take all practicable measures to reduce noise levels. From April 2006, the more stringent requirements of Control of Noise at Work Regulations 2005 should be implemented (see Table 2.1).

Noise measurements may also be made on machinery to enable prediction of noise levels in the workplace, to verify declared values and also to characterise and describe the noise being generated.

The glossary of British and International Standards related to measurement of noise provides a comprehensive, but not exclusive, list of the type of machinery and environments requiring noise measurements for *noise declaration purposes*. This declared value reflects the overall noise output of the machinery and should be one of the considerations in the option appraisal process in purchasing new equipment.

## Measurement units

The human ear is essentially a pressure detector, which can resolve changes in pressure for frequencies of sound from 20Hz to 20kHz. For this reason the magnitude of sound is usually quantified in terms of pressure. The ranges of sound pressure the ear can process are very large (20 $\mu$Pa to 200Pa) and therefore sound pressure measurements are usually expressed on a logarithmic scale.

The most basic and widespread descriptors of noise are sound pressure level (SPL) and sound intensity level (SIL). These and the derived parameters may also be expressed with different filter weightings (typically A, C or linear) and different time weightings (F-fast, S-slow or I-impulsive). For convenience in the following definitions, SPL is annotated as $L$. The format for derived parameter is $L_{XY}$, where $L$ is the sound level, X is the frequency weighting and Y is the time weighting.

### Sound pressure level

Sound pressure level (SPL in decibels) may be expressed as

$$L = 20 \log_{10}\left(\frac{p}{p_o}\right)$$

where p is root mean square sound pressure (pascals) and $p_0$, the reference pressure, 20 $\mu$Pa for air-borne sound.

This quantity may be expressed on a linear scale or weighted scale. In the latter scale, each of the frequencies comprising the sound is multiplied by a certain factor. There are several different internationally standardised weighting scales that have been developed for use, namely A, B, C, D (Figure 2.1) and recently E and SI. Environmental noise is most commonly measured using the A-weighting scale (L dBA or dB(A)). On

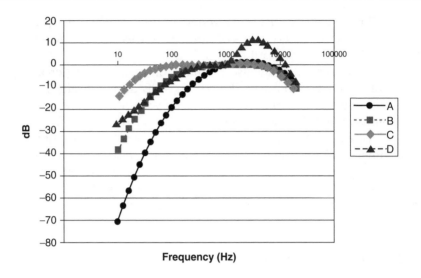

**Figure 2.1** Relative responses of different weighting scales (graphs drawn using data obtained from International Standards defining frequency weightings).

this scale the sound is weighted by an inverted equal loudness contour at low sound pressure levels thereby making corrections for the different sensitivities of the ear to the lower and higher audiometric frequencies. The 'A' frequency weighting has been found to be useable over a much wider range of sound pressure levels than the other scales, which are not therefore generally used. Control of Noise at Work Regulations 2005 specifies peak SPL measurements should be made with C–weighting. The ear's response at higher listening levels is nearly flat and so relatively 'flat' C–weighting is used to measure noise at these higher listening levels. Historically B and C–weighting were derived from the inverse of the 70 and 100 phon curves. The D-scale gives an indication of perceived loudness and has been used in aircraft noise measurements (IEC 537).

The most common terminology used to quantify noise and the nature of noise, is further described and defined in Table 2.2. Each has their own particular advantage and disadvantage depending on the objective of the measurements being made.

**Table 2.2** Noise measurement units

| Parameter | Nomenclature | Description | Application |
|-----------|--------------|-------------|-------------|
| **Sound intensity level** | $L_I$ | Sound intensity for a sound wave, may be defined as the average rate of energy flow per unit area, where the area under consideration is normal to the direction of propagation. Intensity is a vector quantity and may be measured using systems employing two microphones a fixed distance apart. It is usually expressed logarithmically as: $$L_I = 10\log_{10}\left(\frac{I}{I_o}\right)\text{dB}$$ where $I$ is measured sound intensity and $I_0$ is $10^{-12}$ W/m$^2$. | Location of sound sources (using directional qualities of vectors); measure sound intensity level of a machine in the factory. |
| **Sound power level** | $L_W$ | Sound power is the sound energy radiated by the sound source per unit time (W). $L_W$ is the sound power measured on a decibel scale and expressed using the formula | Measurement of noise emissions from instruments and machinery. |

(continued)

$$L_W = 10\log_{10}\left(\frac{W}{W_o}\right)$$

where $W_0$ is reference value of $10^{-12}$ W. ($L_{WA}$ is the A-weighted sound power level.)

This has been adapted as the basic quantity for representing environmental noise. It is a way of expressing a time-varying signal/noise. A fluctuating sound over a period of time may be represented by a continuous sound pressure level, which delivers the same amount of sound energy of a given event. $L_{Aeq,T}$ dB(A) does not represent the average A-weighted sound pressure level (SPL) but rather the integral of the SPL over a measured time period.

**Continuous equivalent sound pressure level**

$L_{Aeq,T}$ dB(A)

It is the steady state sound that has the same amount of A-weighted energy as the time-varying noise, over the same period of time T.

$$AEG_{,T} = 10\log_{10}\frac{1}{t_0}\int_{t_1}^{t_2}\frac{P_{A(t)}^{2}}{P_0^{2}}\,dt$$

where $p_{A(t)}$ is the instantaneous A-weighted sound pressure of the noise and T is measured time interval.

(continued)

It is thought to represent the same potential to damage hearing as the varying signal. $L_{Aeq}$ are used to determine the potential hearing damaging effects of noise and its annoyance potential and is used to measure railway and aircraft noise

_Alternative_: $L_{eq,T}$ dB or $L_{Leq,T}$ dB _(no reference to A-weighting - linear weighting). It is the_ <u>steady state sound</u> _that has the same amount of energy as the_ <u>time-varying noise</u>, _over the period of time T._

**Sound exposure level (SEL)**

$L_{AE}$ dB(A)

This is the A-weighted sound pressure level, which _(over 1 second)_ contains the same amount of A-weighted energy as the single event.

$$SEL = 10\log_{10}\left[ \frac{1}{t_0} \int_{t_1}^{t_2} \left( \frac{p_{A(t)}^2}{p_0^2} \right) \, dt \right]$$

where

$p_{A(t)}$ is the instantaneous A-weighted sound pressure of the noise

This is a way of expressing events of finite duration (e.g. passing lorry, train, aircraft etc). It allows different noise events to be compared simply, as for each the energy content is over 1 second, irrespective of duration of the original noise event.

(continued)

$t_0$ is reference time (e.g. 1 second) $t_1-t_2$ is the time interval, which is long enough to encompass a significant sound of the event being measured

**Personal daily noise exposure level**

$L_{EP, d}$ dB(A)

This is the steady state A-weighted sound pressure level, which (*over 8 hours*) contains the same amount of A-weighted energy received by a subject in their working day.

$$L_{EP, d} = L_{Aeq, Te} + 10\log_{10} \left( \frac{T_e}{T_o} \right)$$

where $T_e$ is the duration of the person's working day, in seconds; $T_0$ is 28,800 seconds (8 hours)

$L_{Aeq, Te}$ is the equivalent continuous A-weighted sound pressure level that represents the

This is a way of expressing the amount of acoustic energy received by the listener over an 8-hour working day. $L_{EP, d}$ is the Level of exposure of a person per day. It is equivalent continuous sound pressure level ($L_{Aeq}$) over 8 hours. It

(continued)

(continued)

| Personal weekly noise exposure level | $L_{EP,w}$ | sound the person is exposed to during their working day. $$L_{EPW} = 10\log_{10}\left(\frac{1}{5}\sum_{k=1}^{k=m} 10^{0.1(L_{EPd})k}\right)$$ | is equal to $L_{Aeq,8h}$ and was introduced in the EC Directive 86/188/EEC. |
| Daily noise exposure level | $L_{EX,\,8h}\ dB(A)$ | This is the time-weighted average of the noise exposure levels for a nominal 8-hour working day | This is a way of expressing the amount of acoustic energy received by the listener over an 8-hour working day. $L_{EX,8h}$ is the level of exposure of a person per day and covers all noise including impulsive. It was introduced in the EC Directive 2003/10/EC (equivalent to $L_{EPd}$). |
| Day-Night average sound pressure level | $L_{ADN,T}\ dB(A)$ | This is $L_{Aeq,T}\ dB(A)$ with a 10dB addition for noise measured during 10pm and 7am. | Noise at night time is generally thought to cause more annoyance hence the use and need for this weighting. (See standards relating to rating of noise.) |

| Day-Evening-Night average sound pressure level | $L_{den}$ | This is the outdoor equivalent sound level over 24 hours, with sound levels during 11pm and 7am increased by 10dB(A); and sound levels during 7pm and 11pm increased by 5dB(A). | Representative of 24-hour aircraft noise exposure at a location during the year. |
|---|---|---|---|
| Maximum A-weighted sound pressure level (peak levels) | $L_{Amax}$ or $L_{max}$ | This is simply the maximum A-weighted sound pressure level (or maximum SPL) over a specified measurement period and using FAST or SLOW time weighting. | Determine maximum SPL |
| Sound pressure percentile level | $L_{AN,T}$ | The measured noise level dB(A) is exceeded N% (percentage) of time, T.<br><br>Typically $L_{A10}$ and $L_{A90}$ are used e.g. if $L_{A10}$ (N=10%) the measured SPL is exceeded 10% of the time; $L_{A90}$ (N=90%) the measured SPL is exceeded 90% of the time. | This allows the noise levels to be smoothed.<br><br>$L_{A10,18\,hour}$–index of traffic noise 6am to midnight used as a basis for noise insulation measurements<br><br>$L_{A90,T}$–residual noise exceeded for 90% of the time T (i.e. background noise) |

# Instrumentation used to measure noise

There are essentially three main groupings for the type of equipment used to quantify noise, namely:

1. sound level meter (in its various formats);
2. personal noise exposure meters (dosimeters);
3. sound intensity analysers.

The type of instrument used would depend on the proposed application.

### Components of sound level meter

There are different types of sound level meter, Type II being the least accurate and comprehensive, with increasing accuracy in Type I. The specifications for each type are detailed in relevant standards pertaining to the instrument. Both types may be used to provide comprehensive environmental and occupational noise measurements, although a high quality microphone, of which more will be said later, is paramount to high quality measurements, irrespective of the sound level meter type.

The basic digital sound level meter *(either type I or type II)* may be used to measure steady and non-impulsive sounds, whereas the digital integrating sound level meter is used to measure time-varying noise and impulsive sounds. This type of meter for instance will automatically calculate $L_{eq}$. Sound analysers usually incorporate both elements. Both types require microphone, preamplifier, attenuator, frequency-weighting circuits, time-weighting circuits, squaring and averaging circuits, display unit and AC and DC outputs.

### *Types of microphones*

The main microphones used are typically of the condenser (capacitor) type and although expensive have stable sensitivity, considered essential

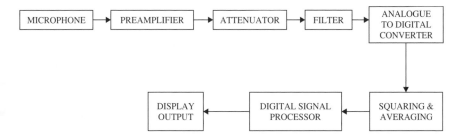

**Figure 2.2** Block diagram of sound level meter/sound analyser

for long term and accurate measurements of noise. They generate a voltage, which is dependent on the frequency and direction of the measured signal.

There are three basic types of microphone used for noise measurements as follows:

1. Free-field microphone. There is a correction factor included in calibration frequency response to take into account diffraction effects. This microphone is pointed directly at the sound source, with no obstruction between source of sound and microphone.
2. Random incidence microphone. This is used to make measurements when sound is arriving randomly from all directions.
3. Pressure microphone. This type is used in small cavities with no propagating waves (e.g. headphone calibration in artificial ear).

Each of these microphones will be defined by its sensitivity (this is the relationship between output voltage and input signal, either pressure or displacement). The frequency response of the microphone describes how this sensitivity changes with measured frequency, although ideally and usually, this should be flat over the region of interest i.e. the microphone generates the same voltage irrespective of the frequency of the signal being measured for a specific displacement of the diaphragm.

### Preamplifier

The preamplifier and amplifier will amplify the small microvolt signal generated by the microphone to millivolt level, which is then processed by the digital signal processing elements of the sound level meter. The preamplifier may sometimes contain a correction filter to take into account the microphone frequency response under different recording conditions. The frequency response of this filter would simply be the inverse of the microphone response.

### Attenuator

The full range of sound/noises measured may typically be from −10 to 140dB. Digital sound level meters have a linear operating range of at least 80dB, with regular overlapping positions covering the range specified above. Attenuators are used to increase the range of sounds that may be measured, by attenuating the output from the preamplifier. The use of attenuator improves the accuracy of measurement of very low and very high sound signals.

### Frequency weighting/filter ($^1/_3$ and $^1/_2$ octave filter, linear filter)

These are defined by internationally recognised standards, each of the frequency weightings modifying the signal accordingly. (When using a linear filter the signal is not modified.) The most commonly applied weightings are 'A' and external $^1/_3$ octave frequency bands (preferred bands centred around 16, 20, 25, 31.5, 40, 50, 63, 80, 100, 125, 160, 200, 250, 315, 400, 500, 630, 800, 1k, 1.25k, 1.6k, 2k, 2.5k, 3.15k, 4k, 5k, 6.3k, 8kHz).

## Time weighting

Three standardised detector characteristics have been defined by British/International standards.

1. F, which has a time constant 125ms;
2. S, which has a time constant 1000ms (averages out rapidly changing signal);
3. impulse time weighting, which has a time constant of 35ms. (To measure and detect impulsive/transient noise, taking into account human perception of impulsive sound. In order to hold the reading of the impulsive noise the fall time is relatively long – about 1.5s).

## Digital signal processing (frequency, level, time)

The output from the 'front end' of the analyser is digitised and the signal then processed by application software. This involves squaring and averaging the signal to establish root mean square voltages. The output from the digital signal processor is sent to a variety of devices (display, data storage etc). The application software determines how the signal is processed — which measurement parameters are activated, which frequency and time weightings are employed, and the control, starting, stopping and storage of data collection.

## Display indicator calibrated in decibels

This is simply the digital readout of the measured noise parameter. Sophisticated systems allow several parameters to be displayed simultaneously. The units will be appropriate for the parameter dB, dB(A), display of noise parameter etc. and level distribution, cumulative distribution, sound level profile and so on.

AC and DC outputs allow the measured signal to be transferred to external devices, for example, AC output to a frequency counter, and DC output to a computer or specific data storage devices (such as a tape, CD etc.).

The specification for the verification of sound level meters is detailed in BS 7580-1:1997 and for integrating sound level meters in BS 60804-2001. This is the type primarily used for the measurement of industrial noise, environmental noise (traffic, residential, industrial sites, aircraft) and the average sound pressure level around a noisy product.

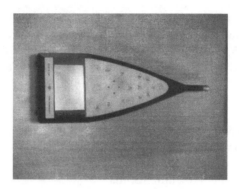

**Figure 2.3** Sound Analyser B&K 2260

## Noise Dose Meters

These are sometimes referred to as personal noise exposure meters. Noise dosimeters simply measure the A-weighted noise dose at a microphone, which should be positioned about 2 cm from the subject's ear for a specific period of time. It is used to assess occupational noise exposure and is useful in cases where individuals are moving frequently between environments with varying noise levels. It shares many features with an integrating sound level meter. The following stages lead to the noise dose measured:

- Microphone – acoustic energy converted to voltage; voltage is A-weighted (representing sound pressure);
- Voltage squared (representing sound intensity);
- Dose meter integrates the voltage squared over the exposure time T.

This provides a measure of the acoustic A-weighted energy received during the exposure time T. Using readily available conversion charts this may be converted to personal daily noise exposure level $L_{EP, d}$ dB(A). This number may then be used to determine if any of the action levels specified by the Noise at Work Regulations 1989/ Control of Noise at Work Regulations 2005 have been exceeded and so decide what type of hearing protection and/or equipment modifications may be necessary.

---

**Uses and advantages of noise exposure meters**
- Worn by the worker over the full working day
- Subject can be highly mobile
- Small, compact and user-friendly
- Microphone positioned close to the subject's body (reflections result in an increase in measured level +/–2dB(A))
- Monitor and control activity on an individual basis (i.e. keep individual exposure to below action level)
- May not be necessary to create controlled areas

**Characteristics of dosimeters**

- Sound level, maximum hold, peak hold, time-weighted average level
- Sound exposure level and Leq shown on large LCD display
- Slow, fast and impulse time weightings plus peak
- A and C frequency weightings for RMS levels plus C or linear for peak levels

These units can log noise data, which may then be downloaded to a computer for subsequent analysis. The dose data may display the percentage of allowable dose, with 100% = 85 dB(A) for an 8-hour working day, 88dB(A) for a 4-hour working day, 91dB(A) for a 2-hour working day and so on (every 3dB increase in noise reducing the working time by half with only approximately 9s exposure time allowed for noise with an intensity of 120dB(A)). Specifications for personal sound exposure meters may be found in BS EN 61252:1997, IEC 61252:1993.

**Intensity sound level meters**

A sound intensity analyser would allow computation of acoustic pressure and particle velocity and from this derive the intensity. (Intensity, I = acoustic pressure × particle velocity.) A single microphone will measure sound in terms of fluctuations in air pressure and is non-directional. A sound field, however, would be dependent on acoustic pressure and particle velocity. Using two microphones a fixed distance apart (phase matched) it would be possible to compute the sound pressure and particle velocity in the middle of the two microphones. By multiplying these together we would then get the intensity, a vector quantity. This system obviously measures the sound intensity in one direction and this is the direction of the wave travelling parallel to the axis of the microphones.

A special case of intensity measurements occurs with plane waves in which case the magnitude of sound intensity in dB will also be equal numerically to sound pressure level in dB. In this case the intensity of sound is proportional to the pressure squared ($I = p^2/\rho c$ where c = velocity of sound and $\rho$ = density of material). A plane wave is simply one in which the wave fronts are plane and parallel in all directions, the sound energy is not diverging with increasing distance from the sound source.

# Methodology of acoustic measurements

Before making any measurements of noise it is important to calibrate the measurement system using the manufacturer's recognised protocol. After describing this, the considerations required in making measurements of

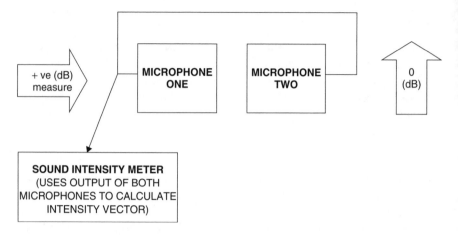

**Figure 2.4** Sound intensity meter - if direction of wave is parallel to microphone axis then probe will measure positive intensity if originated in front of microphone 1 and negative intensity if behind microphone 1; if direction is perpendicular then 0dB intensity level will be measured.

environmental noise and then machinery noises will be discussed. The description of how to reduce effect of operator and environment may be equally applicable to both these situations.

*Acoustic calibration*

Most sound level meters allow acoustic calibration to be carried out using either an external calibrator and/or an internal reference calibrator.

The internal calibration process is carried out if an external calibrator is not available. This can be problematic, as it does not take the microphone into account. For instance, with the B&K 2260, a stable, internally generated 1kHz signal is applied to the microphone preamplifier (input stage) - the calibration is adjusted according to the microphone sensitivity that has been keyed in by the user (see B&K User Manual for 2260 Analyser for further details). This obviously allows scope for human error and does not allow for any changes that may have occurred in the microphone sensitivity since its last calibration.

The preferred method is to use an external calibrator, either a pistonphone or multifrequency acoustic calibrator.

**Characteristics of acoustic calibrators**

- Pistonphone (e.g. B&K 4228) provides a stable sound source of 124dBSPL @ 250Hz (no difference in calibration level for free or random incidence fields).

- High-frequency calibrator (e.g. B&K 4231) generates 94dB or 114dB @ 1kHz. At this frequency there is a slight difference in expected measured values (approx.-0.1dB) between free-field and random incidence microphones. This type is the one typically used for 'field' measurements.
- Multi-frequency calibrators (e.g. B&K 4226) provide calibration levels at more than one level (e.g. 94dB, 104dB, 114dB) and at discrete frequencies from 31.5Hz to 16kHz (in octave steps).

Each type of calibrator provides an increasing amount of information and the choice depends ultimately on the nature of the measurements being carried out and the *permissible uncertainty* of measurements.

Whichever system is employed, the sound level meter/analyser should be calibrated prior to and after use. The calibration process changes the sensitivity of the sound level meter, so that when calibrator is on, the measured value corresponds to the nominal output of the calibrator.

**Data collection and analysis**

The sound level meter/sound analyser may be connected to data logging equipment (locally to a laptop or via remote connection to a laboratory computer). All the noise descriptive parameters may be stored using dedicated software and stored in spreadsheet format. From this point onwards it would be relatively easy to display data relevant to the particular survey.

# Scenario I – measuring environmental noise

Environmental noise consists of sound from more than one single source (ambient). The preferred instrumentation for measuring impulsive, fluctuating or cyclical environmental noise is with either an integrating sound level meter (frequency weighting A) or sound exposure meter (BS 7445-1). Sound level meters (A-weighting; time-weighting S) and data logger (A-weighting; time-weighting F) may be used, for steady or step-like variations in noise levels. The microphone should be omni-directional as the sound would be from many directions.

**Microphone locations**

After the instrument is calibrated you need to make a decision regarding where to take measurements of sound. BS7445-2 describes fully the location and number of measurement positions required. This will be dependent on the resolution required for the noise map that needs to be created, but there is some flexibility. The positions chosen may be equidistant, with greater density of measurements in places, which take into account local geographical features and shielding effects, and positions close to specific (identifiable) noise sources. An initial survey with coarse resolution may be helpful in deciding the final number and positions required. The next variable to consider is the height at which to hold the microphone. In areas with planning for new buildings, the preferred height is 3-11m, thereby reducing ground effects. In locations with lots of buildings the microphone should be at least 3.5m from any reflecting surfaces (if possible); 0.5m in front of an open window; 1 to 2m from any building façade and 1.2 to 1.5m above every floor where measurements are required.

## Measurements

The basic measurements made are equivalent continuous A-weighted sound pressure level over reference time intervals $L_{Aeq,T}$. By taking the appropriate and relevant number of measurement samples the long-term average sound level may be calculated.

## When to take measurements

The measurements should be taken at specific reference time intervals, which may be related to specific human activities on a typical day. They should reflect either the steady noise or the succession of discrete noise events. The sampling periods will affect the overall accuracy.

## Reducing effect of environment in free-field noise measurements

There are many environmental conditions that may affect the accuracy of sound measurements and so should be either eliminated, reduced or, failing this, taken into account after making the noise measurements. These are wind, humidity, temperature, ambient pressure, vibration and magnetic fields. A windshield, which may be described as being like a soft fluffy ball, positioned over the microphone, greatly reduces the effects of wind without affecting the level of ambient noise being measured. As an added bonus it can provide a certain degree of protection to the microphone from mechanical damage (for example from dust, rain and so forth). High humidity levels can be problematic, although no precautions are necessary when humidity is 90% or less. However, with higher humidity levels or perhaps when raining heavily, special outdoor microphones need to be used which have rain shields and dehumidifiers. Microphones have fairly high operating temperatures (typically −10°C to 50°C), therefore noise measurements may be made in extreme environments without difficulty. If measurements are being made in different environments leading to sudden changes in temperature, this may cause condensation on the microphone. This scenario should be avoided. Ambient pressure does not have much of an effect on microphone sensitivities, which are only changed by $+/-$ 2 dB with atmospheric changes of $+/-10\%$. Careful attention should be made when calibrating a microphone with a pistonphone, which should be supplied with correction factors for different barometric pressures. Although microphones are relatively insensitive to vibration, it should be placed on a rubber mat to help protect the sound level meter in areas of high vibration. The influence on microphones of magnetic field is negligible. Indeed measurements have been made in the high magnetic field of Magnetic Resonance Imaging Scanners, although the microphone should be used with an extension cable and the sound level meter placed well outside the 0.3mT field limit.

### Reducing effects of operator and equipment in free-field noise measurements

When making free-field measurements it is important to consider the effect of both the sound level meter and the operator on the propagating sound field. Several sound level meters have conical shaped microphone ends, which reduce diffraction errors. However, reflection from the operator errors should be minimised by using a microphone with a cable extension and tripod. If this is not possible then the sound level meter should be kept at arms length. The noise source should be unobstructed.

The rest of BS7445-2 and BS 7445-3 continues to describe the methods that should be used both to measure and describe environmental noise and, although it does not specify noise limits, it '*lays down guidelines for the specification of noise limits....*' and methods for checking '*compliance with specified noise limits*' (BS7445-3).

### Measurement report

BS7445-2 details the information that should be recorded and reported, and this should be referred to for a complete list. Concisely it should include all the noise measurements made, equipment used, microphone height and positions employed, along with qualitative (for example cloudy etc.) and quantitative (for example wind speed, humidity etc) meteorological data.

# Scenario II - measuring noise in a factory to ensure compliance with Noise at Work Act / Control of Noise at Work Regulations

The measurement of noise emission levels from machinery and environmental sources is important both to ensure compliance with existing noise legislation and to verify performance of machinery. The noise is measured with either a sound level meter and/or sound intensity meter.

## Microphone locations

The microphone location is crucial when making noise surveys and assessments. The Noise at Work Act 1989 / Control of Noise at Work Regulations 2005 provides very clear and specific instructions for obtaining noise measurements on machinery: '...*microphone should be placed in undisturbed field*'. This means that the machine operator should be absent and the measurement microphone placed where the worker's head would be positioned during normal operating procedures. If the worker needs to be in position to operate the machinery the microphone should be placed at least 4 cm away from their ear and on the side with the most noise.

## When to take noise measurements

If the aim of the procedure is to estimate the potential damage to hearing then the personal daily noise exposure level should be estimated - $L_{EP, d}$ ($L_{EX, 8h}$). It may not actually be necessary to measure the noise levels throughout the day, but simply typical periods of operation. Using noise exposure calculators (tables of data which show the time allowed for particular noise levels for $L_{EP, d}$ of 85 / 90dB(A) OR more stringent 80 / 85dB(A) - Table 2.3) it is possible to work out the $L_{EP, d}$ for the series of noise levels.

---

**Steps taken in estimating personal noise exposure**

1. Measure noise levels in dB(A)
2. Record exposure times in seconds $t_1$
3. For each noise exposure read off time T (from noise calculator) where T would be the total allowed time for measured noise to give exposure of either $L_{EP, d}$ 85 or 90dB(A) OR for Directive 2003/10/EC $L_{EX, 8h}$ 80dB(A) or $L_{EX, 8h}$ 85dB(A)
4. Calculate fraction $t_1/T_1 + t_2/T_2 + ...t_n/T_n$
5. If this is >1 the individual <u>has</u> received exposure in excess of stated level
6. For example, if subject is exposed to 85dB for 4 hours and 91dB for 1 hour and 97dB for 15 minutes, the above calculation will be as follows for $L_{EX, 8h}$ 85dB(A) = 4/8 + 1/2 + 15/30 = 1.5 (i.e. exposure greater than allowed)
7. The HSE has very useful noise calculation formulae to work out daily exposure based on noise generated by particular job processes over a particular period. http://www.hse.gov.uk/noise/calculator.htm

**Table 2.3** Simple table for noise exposure calculator (approximate times)

| $L_{EP, d}$ 80dB(A) | $L_{EP, d}$ 85dB(A)/$L_{EX, 8h}$ 85dB(A) | $L_{EP, d}$ 90dB(A) |
|---|---|---|
| 80 for 8 h | 85 for 8 h | 90 for 8 h |
| 83 for 4 h | 88 for 4 h | 93 for 4 h |
| 86 for 2 h | 91 for 2 h | 96 for 2 h |
| 89 for 1 h | 94 for 1 h | 99 for 1 h |
| 92 for 30 min | 97 for 30 min | 102 for 30 min |
| 95 for 15 min | 100 for 15 min | 105 for 15 min |
| 98 for 7 min 30 s | 103 for 7 min 30 s | 108 for 7 min 30 s |
| 119 for 3.5 s | 121 for 7 s | 120 for 28 s |

The other measurement that should be taken, if machinery is generating impact noise, is the peak sound pressure level. This is to establish if the 200 Pascal Peak Action Level is being exceeded. This should be made with a sound level meter with a rise time of at least 100 µs, using C-weighting.

**Summary of factors affecting accuracy of noise measurements and noise surveys**

- Accuracy of sound level meter (minor factor)
- Effect of scattering and reflection of sound from (a) the body and head of machine operator; (b) the person holding the sound level meter; and (c) the sound level meter (major factors)

Although noise as mentioned may be and is usually measured over short time periods over the working day, this may not accurately represent the overall noise exposure. One needs to have a sense of how the noise generation pattern changes during the day and ensure measurements reflect the times when more machines are operating, and operating at different speeds or modes.

### After a noise survey

The noise survey is the first step in the organisation of a hearing conservation programme. Possible initial outcomes include: no risks - do nothing, or create ear protection zone, or reduce machinery noise level and/or reduce worker exposure time.

### Revocation of the Noise at Work Act

A new European Directive 2003/10/EC was introduced on 6th April 2003 on *'minimum health and safety requirements regarding the exposure of workers to the risks arising from physical agents (noise)'*. New UK noise regulations should comply with these stricter standards by April 2006, essentially reducing the first and second action levels to 80 and 85dB(A) respectively. The legislation will also cover the entertainment and music industry by April 2008 and supersede the Noise at Work Act 1989. The stricter limits stated in the Control of Noise at Work Regulations 2005 are as follows:

---

**The lower exposure action values are**

(a) a daily or weekly personal noise exposure of 80 dB (A-weighted); and

(b) a peak sound pressure of 135 dB (C-weighted).

---

**The upper exposure action values are**

(a) a daily or weekly personal noise exposure of 85 dB (A-weighted); and

(b) a peak sound pressure of 137 dB (C-weighted).

---

**The exposure limit values are**

(a) a daily or weekly personal noise exposure of 87 dB (A-weighted); and

(b) a peak sound pressure of 140 dB (C-weighted).

---

# Scenario III - measuring noise emission values from equipment and machinery

The basic noise emission parameter is A-weighted sound power level. The stated noise emission for a machine or batch of machines is stated as $L_c$. The sound power level of machinery may be determined by making either sound pressure level measurements (A-weighted and/or in frequency bands) or sound intensity measurements. Again standards are available that describe the process involved in detail:

- BS3741 to BS3747 provides the methodology for determining the sound power level of machinery using sound pressure level measurements
- BS9614 parts 1 and 2 provide the methodology using sound intensity measurements.

There are two principles involved. BS3740 explains these as:

- *'Evaluation of the spatial mean-squared sound pressure built up in a highly reflective environment'* (reverberant field);

*'Evaluation of the flow of sound energy emitted by the source, with measurements using an enveloping surface'* (Free-field).

**The method employed to determine sound power level is dependent on**

- test environment (reverberant field or free-field);
- accuracy required;
- background noise;
- nature of the noise being characterised;
- instrumentation available.

Tables I and II of BS3740 describes this in detail, referring to the appropriateness of each standard in determining power levels, uncertainty of measurements and the test environment involved.

Each of the standards listed above describes:

- applicability of measurements i.e. test environment, type of noise source, size of sound source, character of noise being radiated by source. The test environments may be specially designed rooms (reverberation, anechoic, hemianechoic, hard-walled) or in-situ environments (indoors in a sufficiently reverberant field or approximate free-field; outdoors in an essentially free-field);
- measurement uncertainty ranging from precision (~10dB@1kHz), engineering (~1.5dB@1kHz) and survey (~<4dB@1kHz). The accuracy of measurements will depend on test environment and measurement equipment used;
- quantity to be measured (typically sound pressure levels, A-weighted and/or in frequency bands at specified positions);
- quantities to be determined (typically sound power levels).

Figure D1 in EN ISO3740 provides a simple flow chart on how to select the appropriate standard that should be used to determine sound power levels. The standards also describe how to validate the test environment and of course how to calculate the sound power levels from the actual measurements made. This derived parameter should be essentially independent of the environment in which it was made or the machine installation room. This is the main reason why sound power levels are used to characterise noise emitted by machinery and equipment.

BS 6805 parts 1,2,3 and 4 detail the statistical methods for determining and verifying noise emission values of machinery and equipment both for individual machines and batches of machines irrespective of whether these are produced in small or large quantities.

There are a few 'rules of thumb' that may be employed. For instance if the difference between the noise measured with machine off (background noise) and the noise measured with the machine on (specific machine and background noise) is less than 3dB the accuracy of the machine noise measurement would be unacceptable. If the difference is greater than 12dB then accuracy will not be affected by the background noise. Differences in between these values will suggest that the noise measurements will require a small correction factor.

The difficulty in perhaps choosing the correct and appropriate measurement technique is reduced for those instruments or classes of instruments that have their own noise test code. These test codes describe which methods and measurement instruments should be used, positions of work stations, operating conditions of machine under test and the technique for verifying the declared noise emission. As can be seen from the glossary the number of noise test codes is very extensive.

## Conclusions

The measurement of noise and its accurate representation depends ultimately on the correct selection and use of sound/noise-measuring equipment for the task in hand. In addition it is important to know the objective of the measurements being made, for instance: What do you want to show, illustrate or prove? What level of accuracy are you willing to accept / do you need? What measurement equipment do you have? What measurement test environment is available?

The measurement of certain types of noise is covered by measurement standards and this has tended to reduce measurement errors. For example the Noise at Work Regulations Guidance Notes 3-8 tell the user the type and accuracy of equipment to be used and how measurements should be made in an industrial setting as well at the training requirements for someone undertaking such measurements. There are many standards providing methodology and noise test codes to determine the noise emissions from noise generating machinery or equipment. Other standards tell us how to measure and describe environmental noise in detail. The validity of the statement 'noise measurement is more of an art than a science' is reduced by these measurement protocols and standards. Noise measurements made using these documents as a guide should be more standardised and less reliant on the tester's experience and underpinning knowledge on deciding why, when and how measurements should be made. The noise measurement report is a crucial part of the process and is a summary of all the relevant facts pertaining to the measurement. This should include: methodology standards and test codes utilised; details of measurement equipment used including calibration; frequency and time weightings used; background noise levels; environmental conditions; name and details of device and area being measured; microphone locations; date and time; signature and so on.

The glossary lists some of the standards applicable to noise measurements. These should be used as appropriate, but flexibility may also be necessary at times. For example, if a standard for measuring the noise emissions from a particular machine does not exist, the next most closely applicable standard should be employed.

The measurement of noise is becoming increasing relevant to the general public, not only those who work or live in 'noisy' environments, but also those in the 'new' noisy environments such as cinemas, nightclubs, restaurants. The susceptibility of individuals to annoyance by relatively low levels of noise and their unwillingness to accept it has encouraged substantial research. Effective noise measurements remain the obvious first step in a programme of noise management in both recent and traditional areas where sound measurements have been required.

# References

Hinton J How to map noise. Noise and Health Apr-June 4(15):1–5.

Babisch W (2000) Traffic noise and cardiovascular disease: epidemiological review and synthesis. Noise and Health July–Sept (8).

Martin M, Summers I (1999) Dictionary of Hearing London: Whurr.

The Control of Noise at Work Regulations 2005, ISBN 0110729846

Noise at Work Act 1989 (HSE)

Technical Documentation Modular Precision Sound Analyser Tyoe 2260 User manual BB0955-12 Revision 1995

# Addendum: Glossary of standards

Exposure limits: EU Directive 2003/10/EC
Action levels: EEC Directive 86/188/EEC (1990)
IEC-801-21-08

*The Control of Noise at Work Regulations 2005*

1. Citation and commencement
2. Interpretation
3. Application
4. Exposure limit values and action values
5. Assessment of the risk to health and safety created by exposure to noise at the workplace
6. Elimination or control of exposure to noise at the workspace.
7. Hearing protection
8. Maintenance and use of equipment
9. Health surveillance

10.   Information, instruction and training
11.   Exception certificates from hearing protection
12.   Exception certificates for emergency services
13.   Exceptions relating to the Ministry of Defence
14.   Exception outside Great Britain.
15.   Revocations, amendments and savings.

*Noise at Work Regulations 1989 – Guidance on Regulations (HSE)*

1.   Legal duties of employers to prevent damage to hearing
2.   Legal duties of designers, manufacturers, importers and suppliers to prevent damage to hearing.
3.   Equipment and procedures for noise surveys
4.   Engineering control of noise
5.   Types and selection of personal ear protectors
6.   Training for competent persons
7.   Procedures for noise testing machinery
8.   Exemption from certain requirements of the Noise at Work Regulations 1989

*Measurement equipment*

❏  Integrating-averaging sound level meters BS EN 60804:2001, IEC 60804:2000
❏  Specification for the verification of sound level meters. Comprehensive procedure BS 7580-1:1997
❏  Specification for sound level meters for the measurement of noise emitted by motor vehicles BS 3539:1986
❏  Specifications for personal sound exposure meters BS EN 61252:1997, IEC 61252:1993
❏  Instruments for measurement of aircraft noise. Performance requirements for systems to measure one-third-octave band sound pressure levels in noise certification of transport-category aircraft BS EN 61265:1995, IEC 61265:1995
❏  Specification for frequency weighting for the measurement of aircraft noise (D-weighting) BS 5721:1979, IEC 60537:1976

*Methods of rating and describing noise*

❏  Method for rating industrial noise affecting mixed residential and industrial areas BS 4142:1997
❏  Method for describing aircraft noise heard on the ground BS 5727:1979, ISO 3891:1978

## Environmental noise

❑ Description and measurement of environmental noise
Part 1: Guide to quantities and procedures BS 7445-1:1991, ISO 1996-1:1982
Part 2: Guide to acquisition of data pertinent to land use BS 7445-2:1991, ISO 1996-2:1987
Part 3: Guide to applications to noise limits BS 7445-3:1991, ISO 1996-3:1987

## Sound power levels - general

❑ Determination of sound power levels of noise sources. Guidelines for the use of basic standards BS EN ISO 3740:2001
❑ Determination of sound power levels of noise sources using sound pressure. Precision methods for reverberation rooms BS EN ISO 3741:2000
❑ Determination of sound power levels of noise sources
Part 1: Engineering methods for small movable sources in reverberant fields. Comparison for hard-walled test rooms BS EN ISO 3743-1:1995
Part 2: Engineering methods for small movable sources in reverberant fields. Methods for special reverberation test rooms BS EN ISO 3743-2:1997
❑ Determination of sound power levels of noise sources using sound pressure. Engineering method in an essentially free-field over a reflecting plane BS EN ISO 3744:1995
❑ Sound power levels of noise sources. Precision methods for determination of sound power levels for sources in anechoic and semi-anechoic rooms BS 4196-5:1981, ISO 3745-1977
❑ Determination of sound power levels of noise sources using sound pressure. Survey method using an enveloping measurement surface over a reflecting plane BS EN ISO 3746:1996
❑ Determination of sound power levels of noise sources using sound pressure. Comparison method in situ BS EN ISO 3747:2000
❑ Determination of sound power levels of noise sources using sound intensity. Measurement at discrete points  BS EN ISO 9614-1:1995
❑ Determination of sound power levels of noise sources using sound intensity. Measurement by scanning BS EN ISO 9614-2:1997
❑ Determination of sound power levels of noise sources using sound intensity. Precision method for measurement by scanning BS EN ISO 9614-3:2002

## Noise emission values - statistics

❑ Statistical methods for determining and verifying stated noise emission values of machinery and equipment

Part 1: Glossary of terms BS 6805-1:1987, EN 27574-1:1988, ISO 7574-1:1985
Part 2: Method for determining and verifying stated values for individual machines BS 6805-2:1987, EN 27574-2:1988, ISO 7574-2:1985
Part 3: Method for determining and verifying stated values for batches of machines using a simple (transition) method BS 6805-3:1987, EN 27574-3:1988, ISO 7574-3:1985
Part 4: Methods for determining and verifying stated values for batches of machines BS 6805-4:1987, EN 27574-4:1988, ISO 7574-4:1985

*Methods of noise testing - specific (examples)*

❑ Fans for general purposes. Methods of noise testing. Airborne noise emitted by small air-moving devices BS 848-2.6:2000, ISO 10302:1996
❑ Method of measurement of noise inside motor vehicles BS 6086:1981, ISO 5128-1980
❑ Airborne noise emitted by earth-moving machinery. Method of measurement of exterior noise in dynamic test conditions BS 6812-3:1991, ISO 6395:1988
❑ Chain saws. Method of measurement of airborne noise at the operator's position BS 6916-6:1988, EN 27182:1991, ISO 7182:1984
❑ Noise emitted by computer and business equipment. Method of measurement of high-frequency noise BS 7135-2:1989, EN 29295:1991, ISO 9295:1988
❑ Airborne noise emitted by woodworking machine tools. Operating conditions for woodworking machines BS 7140:1995, ISO 7960:1995
❑ Measurement of noise emitted by accelerating road vehicles. Engineering method BS ISO 362:1998
❑ Measurement of airborne sound emitted by vessels on inland waterways and harbours BS EN ISO 2922:2001

*Noise test codes*

❑ Noise emitted by machinery and equipment. Rules for the drafting and presentation of a noise test code BS EN ISO 12001:1997
❑ Test code for machine tools. Determination of the noise emission BS ISO 230-5:2000
❑ Test code for the measurement of airborne noise emitted by rotating electrical machinery BS EN ISO 1680:2000
❑ Noise test code for foundry machines and equipment BS EN 1265:1999
❑ Textile machinery. Noise test code.
  - Common requirements BS EN ISO 9902-1:2001
  - Spinning preparatory and spinning machinery BS EN ISO 9902-2:2001
  - Nonwoven machines BS EN ISO 9902-3:2001

- Yarn processing, cordage and rope manufacturing machines BS EN ISO 9902-4:2001
- Weaving and knitting preparatory machinery BS EN ISO 9902-5:2001
- Fabric manufacturing machines BS EN ISO 9902-6:2001
- Dyeing and finishing machines BS EN ISO 9902-7:2001

❑ Noise test code for fastener driving tools. Engineering method BS EN 12549:1999

❑ Liquid pumps and pump units. Noise test code. Grade 2 and grade 3 of accuracy BS EN 12639:2000

❑ Hand-held non-electric power tools. Noise measurement code. Engineering method (grade 2) BS EN ISO 15744:2002

❑ Test code for the determination of airborne acoustical noise emitted by household and similar electrical appliances. Particular requirements. Particular requirements for vacuum cleaners BS EN 60704-2-1:2001

# Interactions between noise exposure and ageing: peripheral and central auditory systems

*Noise and Its Effects:* Edited by Linda Luxon and Deepak Prasher © 2007 John Wiley & Sons Ltd.

SANDRA L MCFADDEN, JAMES F WILLOTT

## Introduction

One of the persistent questions in the field of hearing research concerns the interaction between noise exposure and ageing. Is an aged individual more susceptible to noise-induced hearing loss (NIHL) than a young individual? Conversely, does noise-induced pathology exacerbate peripheral and central changes associated with ageing? Is there a simple additive relationship between age-related hearing loss (AHL) and NIHL, or is the relationship more complex? Questions about the relationship between AHL and NIHL are particularly important to address because of their medicolegal implications. How does one separate the contributions of noise exposure and ageing in disability and compensation cases?

All questions regarding the relationship between noise exposure and ageing have been difficult to address experimentally.

**Evaluation of relationship of NIHL and AHL**
- Confounding factors such as genetic background, ototoxic drugs
- Controlled human experiments unethical
- Unknown interaction between peripheral and central auditory systems
- Knowledge based on extrapolation from animal experiments

In human populations, it is difficult or impossible to control for confounding variables such as diet, genetic background, general health, and exposure to ototoxic drugs and chemicals. Moreover, it is not possible to create permanent threshold shifts (PTSs) in humans under controlled laboratory conditions. Thus, most questions regarding interactions between noise exposure and ageing have been approached using various animal models. A number of studies have examined changes in susceptibility to acoustic trauma during development (for example, Yanz and

Abbas, 1982; Freeman et al., 1999). In this chapter, the focus is on studies that have used adult animals, particularly chinchillas, gerbils and mice, to address questions about the relationship between noise exposure and ageing. Almost all of these have focused on the peripheral auditory system – the changes that are seen in cochleae of young and aged animals after noise exposure, and how these changes are reflected in physiological measures of cochlear functioning, such as auditory brain-stem responses (ABRs), distortion product otoacoustic emissions (DPOAEs), and evoked potentials recorded from the inferior colliculus (IC-EVPs). A survey of the literature shows that surprisingly little is actually known about the relationship between noise exposure and ageing, particularly with respect to central auditory system (CAS) anatomy and physiology.

# Rodent models for studying interactions between noise exposure and ageing

Animals that have been used to study noise/ageing interactions include the long-tailed chinchilla (*Chinchilla laniger*), the Mongolian gerbil (*Meriones unguiculatus*) and various strains of mice, particularly the CBA and C57BL/6 (B6) inbred strains. Obvious advantages of using animal models include control over extraneous variables and the capability of creating PTSs under well-characterized noise exposure conditions. As the ability to translate animal research findings to humans depends on the validity of the animal as a model for the human, it is worth mentioning here some of the potential limitations of different animals for studying noise/ageing interactions.

An 'ideal animal model' would match the 'typical human' with respect to its audiogram (its range of hearing and audiometric thresholds), its onset, rate and pattern of AHL, and its susceptibility to noise damage.

## Limitations of animal models

- Range of hearing and audiometric thresholds do not match humans
- Pattern of development and configuration of AHL
- Susceptibility to NIHL

This would permit researchers to induce PTSs using acoustic exposure parameters (spectrum, level, duration) directly relevant to humans and to interpret the results unambiguously with respect to their implications for humans. Of course, none of the animal models available to us is ideal; every model falls short in all three of these criteria to some degree. It is important to recognize differences between animals and humans and consider the extent to which these differences actually limit or complicate the interpretation of research findings.

## Audiograms

The audiograms of all rodents used for auditory research are broader and shifted towards higher frequencies compared with the human audiogram. The frequency range of hearing is approximately 20–20 000 Hz for the human, 32–40 000 Hz for the chinchilla (Heffner and Heffner, 1991), 50–60 000 Hz for the gerbil (Ryan, 1976; Heffner and Masterton, 1980), and 2000–90 000 for the feral mouse (Heffner and Masterton, 1980). Furthermore, frequency is encoded over a much shorter cochlear distance in rodents. The average length of the human cochlea is 34 mm (Yost, 1995), compared with approximately 19 mm for the chinchilla (McFadden et al., 1997) and 6 mm for the mouse (Ding et al., 2001). Both the chinchilla and the gerbil have a region of maximum sensitivity close to the human, around 4 kHz (Miller, 1970; Ryan, 1976; Fay, 1988; Heffner and Heffner, 1991), whereas the mouse tends to be most sensitive to frequencies around 16 kHz (Henry, 1983). At the frequency of greatest sensitivity, behavioural thresholds are similar among the rodents, and not remarkably different from humans (Fay, 1988). Considering all these factors, it can be concluded that the chinchilla comes closest to matching the human audiometrically, followed by the gerbil, then the mouse.

## Rate and pattern of AHL

Human males develop AHL at rates of approximately 0.2–0.8 dB/year at low frequencies, and 0.8–2 dB/year at high frequencies (Pearson et al., 1995). An animal that develops AHL at a similar rate but has a short lifespan would be a poor model because it would not exhibit much, if any, hearing loss over its lifetime. On the other hand, if the same animal had a long enough lifespan to develop significant AHL, it would be impractical to use, because of the time and expense involved in raising it to 'old age'.

The chinchilla falls into the latter category. Its lifespan is 12–20 years (Bohne et al., 1990; Sun et al., 1994) – 5–10 times longer than the gerbil and mouse lifespans, and roughly 25% of the human lifespan. Anatomical studies (Bohne et al., 1990; McFadden et al., 1997) have shown that the chinchilla exhibits progressive age-related cochlear histopathology, which includes hair cell loss, degeneration of the stria vascularis and neural degeneration – pathologies also seen in humans with AHL (Willott, 1991). The chinchilla accumulates AHL at rates comparable to the human, beginning in 'middle age' (8–10 years of age). In studies of young and aged chinchillas (McFadden et al., 1997, 1998; McFadden and Campo, 1998), IC-EVP and DPOAE thresholds increased twice as fast at high frequencies as at low frequencies. IC-EVP thresholds increased by 0.8–1.1 dB/year at 0.5–4 kHz, and by approximately 2.0 dB/year at 8 and 16 kHz. DPOAE thresholds increased at rates corresponding to 1.4–1.7 dB/year at low frequencies ($f_2$ = 1.2, 2.4, 3.6 and 4.8 kHz), versus 2.3–3.2 dB/year at high frequencies ($f_2$ = 7.2, 9.6 and 12 kHz). This audiometric pattern resembles the pattern most commonly associated with human presbycusis (Pearson et al., 1995). Thus, the chinchilla is a reasonably good model of human AHL with respect to age of onset (middle age), pattern of cochlear pathology and hearing loss (base-to-apex gradient) and rate of hearing loss (less than 2–3 dB/year). Unfortunately, the long lifespan of the chinchilla makes it impractical for most research projects.

An alternative is to use an animal with a short lifespan that develops AHL at an accelerated rate compared with humans. Gerbils and mice fall into this category. One potential problem with this approach is that differences in the rate and magnitude of AHL are likely to reflect different underlying mechanisms (McFadden et al., 1998). This might have implications with regard to the suitability of gerbils and mice as models for human AHL.

Gerbils typically develop pathology of the lateral wall/stria vascularis, with little or no loss of inner hair cells (IHCs) and a maximum of 30% loss of outer hair cells (OHCs), primarily in the apical region of the cochlea (Boettcher et al., 1995). This cochlear pathology is associated with a relatively flat hearing loss from 1 to 16 kHz. There is considerable variability in the amount of AHL exhibited by individual gerbils, with some animals showing no hearing loss, and others exhibiting losses that exceed the limits of measurement, even in gerbils born and reared in a quiet vivarium where ambient noise levels are less than 40 dB (A) (Mills et al., 1990). On average, gerbils develop 30 dB of hearing loss across frequencies between 'middle age' (16–18 months of age, representing approximately half of the gerbil's lifespan) and 36–38 months of age. This translates to an average rate of 12–13 dB hearing loss/year. Thus, the gerbil is a relatively good model of human AHL with respect to age of onset (middle age), but not with respect to pattern (flat hearing loss), magnitude (approximately 30 dB hearing level or HL), or rate (12–13 dB HL/year) of loss.

Inbred mice have certain advantages because of their genetic homogeneity, thereby controlling for the effects of genetic background. Studies with various strains of mice have provided important clues regarding the genetic basis of AHL. The CBA mice, for example, show little hair cell loss until the very late stages of life, whereas B6 mice start to lose hair cells in early adulthood (around 1–2 months of age), and are essentially deaf long before the end of their 2-year lifespan (Mikaelian, 1979; Henry and Chole, 1980; Li and Borg, 1991; Willott, 1991; Spongr et al., 1997). The base-to-apex gradient of cochlear pathology in B6 mice results in hearing loss that progresses from high frequency to lower frequencies with age, at rates between 22 and 56 dB HL/year. Thus, the B6 mouse is a good model of human AHL with respect to pattern of cochlear pathology and hearing loss (base-to-apex gradient), but not with respect to age of onset (young adulthood) or rate of loss (22–56 dB HL/year).

## Gender/sex effects in AHL

Humans show clear gender differences in rate of AHL, with hearing sensitivity declining more than twice as fast in men as in women at most ages and frequencies (Pearson et al., 1995). There is considerable evidence that oestrogen can affect hearing. Thresholds and threshold shifts may be affected by the menstrual cycle in women (Swanson and Dengerink, 1988), ABR latencies are shortened during high levels of oestrogen in the menstrual cycle (Dehan and Jerger, 1990; Elkind-Hirsch et al., 1992), in postmenopausal women who were treated with hormone replacement therapy (Caruso et al., 2000) and in rats receiving hormone replacement after ovariectomy (Coleman et al., 1994). Thus, it is of interest that recent evidence indicates that B6 mice and CBA mice show sex differences in AHL (Henry, 2002, 2004; Willott and Bross, 2004). Initially, young adult B6 males and females exhibit a similar rate and pattern of genetic progressive hearing loss. However, in middle age (about 6–12 months), the period during which fertility and oestrogen function begin to decline in females, hearing of female B6 mice deteriorates more rapidly than that of males (Henry, 2002, 2004; Willott and Bross, 2004). Oestrogen receptors have been found in the rodent cochlea (Stenberg et al., 1999) providing a possible cochlear site of hormonal action for the sex/ageing effect. Numerous observations indicate that oestrogen can have neuroprotective effects (Garcia-Segura et al., 2001), suggesting the hypothesis that oestrogen has a protective role in the auditory system of young, fertile females, but that protection wanes as menopause approaches. McFadden et al. (1999, 2000b) found that chinchillas exhibit sex differences in basic hearing sensitivity and susceptibility to NIHL that parallel those reported for humans, and hypothesized that differences in oestrogen levels could underlie these sex-specific effects. Indeed, preliminary studies in our lab show that chinchillas treated with oestrogen develop less NIHL after noise exposure than their untreated counterparts (Lockwood et al., 2000). Figure 3.1 shows permanent threshold shifts caused by noise exposure in two groups of chinchillas. The group that received daily injections of oestradiol prior to exposure (group E) developed significantly less hearing loss at high frequencies than the control group that did not receive injections (group Ctr). Extending this to the present topic, one can speculate that menopause (and the loss of oestrogen's protection) could be associated with increased risk for damage by noise exposure in older women – a topic deserving of additional research.

## Susceptibility to NIHL

All animals differ from humans in the amount of damage that they sustain from a given noise exposure. Most of these differences can be explained by the transfer functions of the outer and middle ears and physical properties of the basilar membrane (Saunders and Tilney, 1982; Decory

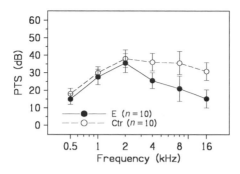

**Figure 3.1** Permanent threshold shifts (PTSs) caused by exposure to impulse noise (Lockwood et al., 2000). The groups that received daily subcutaneous injections of 17-β-oestradiol (Sigma Chemicals) dissolved in olive oil vehicle developed less PTSs than the control group that received injections of vehicle alone.

et al., 1992). For example, the resonant frequency of the human ear canal is 2–4 kHz (Hellstrom, 1995), compared with 5 kHz for the chinchilla (Saunders and Tilney, 1982), and 25 kHz for the B6 mouse (Saunders and Garfinkle, 1983). Ear canal properties result in a maximum gain at the resonant frequency of approximately 10 dB SPL for the human, 15 dB SPL for the chinchilla and 17 dB or SPL for the mouse. These differences, along with differences in the middle-ear transfer functions and the displacement patterns of the basilar membrane, will result in species-specific patterns of noise-induced cochlear damage and hearing loss from a given noise exposure.

An additional factor that is correlated with susceptibility to NIHL in humans is subject gender (McFadden and Henderson, 1999). Similar gender differences in susceptibility to NIHL have been observed in chinchillas (McFadden et al., 1999, 2000b) but not in CBA or B6 mice (Erway et al., 1996).

## Summary of species differences

Do the differences between rodents and humans matter?
- Differences between rodents and humans in audiograms and apparent susceptibility to noise may not be important from a functional point of view.
- If the differences are due simply to the transmission properties of the sound conduction pathway and not to biochemical or physiological properties of the cochlea then they are not likely to pose problems when extrapolating research findings to humans.
- From a practical point of view, however, mismatches between humans and animals make it necessary to tailor noise exposures to a given species.

- The picture may be more complicated with respect to rate and pattern of AHL because these are likely to reflect endogenous (biochemical, genetic) differences among species (McFadden et al., 1998).

# Noise/ageing interactions in the auditory periphery

Several studies have examined the issue of whether ageing influences noise-induced cochlear damage and physiological measures that reflect inner ear function. Is the aged ear more susceptible to noise? Is there an additive relationship between AHL and NIHL? Experiments using chinchillas, gerbils and mice do not provide clear or simple answers to these questions.

## Experiments with chinchillas

Sun et al. (1994) exposed eight chinchillas aged 1–3 years (young) and eight aged 9–13 years to an octave band noise (OBN) with a centre frequency of 0.5 kHz at a level of 95 dB SPL for 36 days. Prior to the exposure, the malleus and incus were removed from the left ears of the aged animals, producing a protective hearing loss of approximately 50 dB SPL; these ears were used to determine the histological effects of ageing alone. A third group of 23, young, non-exposed chinchillas served as controls for noise exposure and ageing. Cochleae were examined under the light microscope to determine the magnitude and pattern of hair cell, nerve fibre and stria vascularis degeneration. Aged control ears had a mean IHC loss of 7.4% and a mean OHC loss of 12.8%, compared with minimal losses (<1%) in non-exposed young ears. Noise-exposed aged ears had mean IHC and OHC losses of 7.8% and 20.6%, respectively, compared with IHC and OHC losses of 2.6% and 12.3%, respectively, in young exposed ears. The incidence and magnitude of focal hair cell lesions and nerve fibre degeneration increased with age and with noise exposure but there did not appear to be a significant interaction between noise exposure and ageing. Hair cell loss from noise exposure simply added to the pre-existing losses due to ageing in this experiment.

The Sun et al. (1994) results agree with findings from several studies using gerbils (for example, Schmiedt and Schulte, 1992; Mills et al., 1996) and humans (Macrae, 1971, 1991) in supporting an additive relationship between AHL and NIHL. However, many other studies using humans (Corso, 1992; Rosenhall et al., 1990), mice (Li, 1992; Li and Borg, 1993; Li et al., 1993) and gerbils (Mills et al., 1997) have suggested more complex, non-additive relationships between AHL and NIHL. Several factors could account for the discrepancies among studies, including acoustic factors (noise level, bandwidth, centre frequency or duration), the magnitude of pre-existing AHL, the actual ages of 'old' subjects, the effectiveness of the acoustic reflex pathway, or activity of the efferent olivocochlear pathway, which has been shown to attenuate NIHL in chinchillas (Zheng et al., 1997).

Studies by McFadden and colleagues (McFadden and Campo, 1998; McFadden et al., 1998) suggest that exposure level may be a particularly relevant variable. Chinchillas were exposed to 0.5 kHz OBN at a moderate level (95 dB SPL, 6 hours/day, 10 days) or a high level (106 dB SPL, 48 hours). Thresholds and response amplitudes were determined from IC-EVPs and DPOAEs before and after exposure, and cochlear histology was performed on animals exposed to high-level noise. For moderate-level exposures, there was an additive relationship between NIHL and AHL. IC-EVP and DPOAE threshold shifts of young and aged animals were equivalent, indicating that aged animals were no more susceptible to NIHL than young animals with normal hearing. By contrast, high-level noise produced two age-dependent effects. First, aged ears had greater hair cell losses than young ears, and OHC losses were greater than those predicted from the combined effects of presbycusis and noise in some frequency regions (Figure 3.2). Second, the IC-EVP amplitude functions of young animals were enhanced at high input levels after exposure, whereas those of aged animals were not (Figure 3.3). Enhancement of IC-EVPs has been observed previously in young animals after noise exposure (Salvi et al., 1990). The absence of enhancement after noise exposure in aged animals

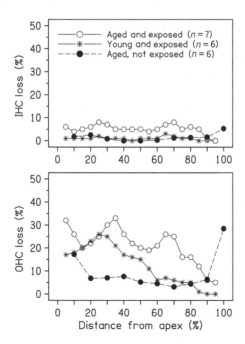

**Figure 3.2** Mean hair cell loss as a function of percentage distance from the apical end of the basilar membrane, determined from surface preparations. Top panel shows percentage inner hair cells (IHCs) missing; bottom panel shows percentage outer hair cells (OHCs) missing. (Data from McFadden et al., 1998.)

could reflect age-related alterations in the balance of excitation and inhibition in the CAS.

## Experiments with gerbils and mice

Experiments with gerbils (Mills et al., 1996, 1997) and mice (Shone et al., 1991; Miller et al., 1998) also show that the nature of the noise:age interaction changes with exposure level. When gerbils were exposed to moderate-level noise for a long period of time (a wide band noise at 85 dB (A) for 720 days), total hearing loss was simply the sum of AHL and NIHL. When gerbils were exposed to a 113 dB SPL, 3.5 kHz tone for 1 hour, however, the additivity rule significantly *over*-estimated the total loss from noise plus ageing.

Shone et al. (1991) used CBA and B6 mice to determine the influence of age and pre-existing AHL on susceptibility to NIHL. To examine the influence of ageing alone, 6-month-old CBA mice were compared with 21-month-old CBA mice. To test the influence of pre-existing AHL, 6-month-old B6 mice were compared with 6-month-old CBA mice. All of the mice were exposed to broadband noise at 101 dB SPL for 45 minutes. There were no differences in temporary threshold shifts between 6- and 21-month-old CBA mice, and neither group developed significant PTS from the exposure. Thus, age alone did not appear to increase susceptibility to NIHL. In contrast with CBA mice, B6 mice developed significant PTS (but not significant hair cell loss) from the exposure. The authors interpreted this as evidence that mice with premature presbycusis are more susceptible to NIHL than normal-hearing mice, perhaps due to 'decreased cochlear reserve' (decreased metabolic responsiveness to recover from environmental and system stress).

Miller et al. (1998) repeated the Shone et al. (1991) experiment with a higher level of noise (108 dB SPL). With the higher exposure level, 21-month-old CBA mice developed significantly greater ABR threshold shifts and hair cell losses than younger (6- and 8-month-old) CBA mice. Thus, increased susceptibility to NIHL was observed in aged CBA mice, but only when the noise level exceeded some 'critical' value.

### Conclusions from experiments with chinchillas, gerbils and mice

- Relationship between noise exposure and age may depend partly on level of the noise.
- Young and aged animals appear to be equally vulnerable to moderate-level noise.
- Aged animals may be slighly more vulnerable to high-level noise.
- Relationship between AHL and NIHL appears to be additive when exposure level is moderate and prolonged, but non-additive when the exposure level is high.

- Nature of non-additive relationship unclear — some experiments suggest sub- and some super-additive.
- Noise/age interaction may initially be additive and then change to 'blocking-like interaction' (Li, 1992) when magnitude of one or other pathological process limits additional damage.

# Noise/ageing interactions in the central auditory system

It is conceivable that intense noise exposures could have direct deleterious effects on CAS neurons (for example, by over-excitation and or excitotoxicity). However, most central effects of noise exposure are likely to be secondary to noise-induced cochlear damage that attenuates input to CAS neurons. The nature and extent of CAS pathology associated with noise-induced cochlear pathology could be influenced by the subject's age at the time of exposure. This is clearly the case for immature, developing animals.

### Central auditory effects of noise exposure

- Possible direct effect of intense noise exposure
- Probable secondary effect of cochlear damage
- Extent of change affected by age at time of exposure, chronicity of exposure and duration of survival after exposure.

Unfortunately, there are very few empirical data describing potential interactions between noise exposure and ageing on CAS anatomy or physiology in adult animals.

One of the few studies that offers a perspective on the interaction between noise exposure and ageing in the adult CAS was conducted by Willott et al. (1994). They exposed normal-hearing adult CBA/J mice to traumatic noise (broadband, 135 dB SPL for 10 minutes) at various ages, then maintained them under normal vivarium conditions for several different periods of time before evaluating changes in five regions of the cochlear nucleus (CN). Specifically, groups of mice were exposed to noise at age 2 months, euthanized at age 6 months (group 2/6); exposed at 6 months, euthanized at 11 months (group 6/11); exposed at 11 months, euthanized at 24 months (group 11/24); and exposed at 6 months, euthanized at 24 months (group 6/24). The 6/11 and 6/24 groups provided animals with the same age at induction of NIHL but different chronicity of noise-induced cochlear pathology (albeit confounded by survival age). The 6/24 and 11/24 groups provided animals with the same survival age but different chronicity (albeit confounded by age at induction of NIHL).

Non-exposed 'control' mice, aged 6–7 months (group 0/7), 11 months (group 0/11), and 24 months (group 0/24), were employed to evaluate the effects of ageing alone on CAS pathology. Varying ages at which mice were euthanized (survival ages 6, 11, and 24 months) provided information about the interaction of noise-induced cochlear damage and ageing across the adult lifespan.

The noise exposure produced substantial cochlear damage in all subject groups, with near-total obliteration of the organ of Corti and spiral ganglion cells in the middle cochlear turns. Central changes were examined in various subdivisions of the CN: the anteroventral cochlear nucleus (AVCN), the octopus cell area (OCA), and dorsal CN (DCN) layers I, II and III. In general, little or no loss of neurons was observed in any CN subdivision. However, certain CN regions of noise-exposed mice did exhibit a reduction in neuropil volume (Figure 3.4), reduction in neuron size, and increases in packing density of neurons that were complementary to reduced neuropil volume.

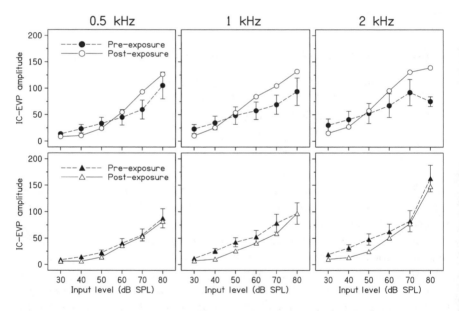

**Figure 3.3** IC-EVP amplitudes as a function of stimulus level for three stimulus frequencies (0.5, 1 and 2 kHz), before and after exposure to 106 dB noise. Top panels show amplitude functions for young animals; bottom panels show amplitude functions for aged animals. Bars show 95% confidence intervals. Note that IC-EVP amplitudes of young chinchillas are enhanced after noise exposure. No enhancement was observed in IC-EVP amplitude functions from aged animals. (Data from McFadden et al., 1998.)

The central effects of noise-induced cochlear pathology were most pronounced in CN regions that receive the heaviest direct afferent input from the cochlea (AVCN, OCA and DCN layer III). Volume of the AVCN, OCA and DCN layer III, but not DCN layers I and II, decreased in noise-exposed mice compared with similarly aged controls. With regard to neuron size, significant decreases were observed in some noise-exposed groups in the AVCN, OCA and DCN layer III, but not in DCN layers I and II. While decreased neuron size presumably contributed to reduced volume of the subdivisions, volume generally decreased to a greater degree than cell size, suggesting that reduced volume probably involved reduction of the neuropil (including degeneration of primary fibres).

To appreciate the potential interaction between noise exposure and ageing on the adult CAS, three interrelated factors are considered here: the age of the subject at the time of noise exposure, the chronicity of NIHL and the survival age of the subject.

### Age at the induction of cochlear damage

There is good evidence that, in immature, developing animals, acute, experimentally-induced cochlear damage results in significant death of CAS neurons. However, when the same peripheral damage is inflicted beyond a certain age, little or no loss of neurons occurs (Powell and Erulkar, 1962; Trune, 1982; Born and Rubel, 1985; Hashisaki and Rubel, 1989; Moore, 1990). Changes in neuron size and packing density may also be much more pronounced when peripheral damage occurs in very young animals (Coleman and O'Connor, 1979; Webster and Webster, 1979; Blatchley et al., 1983; Webster, 1983a,b, 1988; Born and Rubel, 1985; Hashisaki and Rubel, 1989).

It is not clear at what age or level of maturity this sensitivity of CAS neurons to peripheral damage completely subsides, or whether young adults are more or less vulnerable to noise-induced CAS pathology than older adults. In the study by Willott et al. (1994) there was little evidence that the age at which noise exposure occurred made any difference with respect to the severity of central changes, as is evident in Figure 3.4. This proved true even when the degree of spiral ganglion cell loss was matched across mice of different noise-exposed groups.

### Chronicity/duration of peripheral damage

Several studies have shown that cochlear damage or destruction in adult animals results in some histopathological changes in the CAS, but neuron death is not significant (Powell and Erulkar, 1962; Trune, 1982; Nordeen et al., 1983; Koitchev et al., 1986; Hashisaki and Rubel, 1989; Moore, 1990). However, these studies have not used particularly long periods of denervation (re the animal's lifespan), leaving open the possibility that *prolonged* denervation may be more deleterious to CAS cell survival. The Willott et al. (1994) study employed post-noise-exposure durations of 4, 5, 13 and 18 months (the median lifespan of CBA/J mice in their mouse

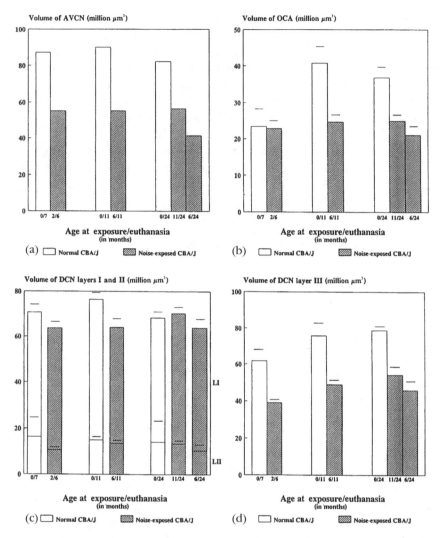

**Figure 3.4** Mean volume of the AVCN (a); OCA (b); DCN layers I and II (c); and DCN layer III (d). Horizontal bars = SEMs. In the AVCN, OCA and DCN layer III, volumes of noise-exposed groups (stippling) were less than those of controls. This was not the case for DCN layers I and II. (Figure reproduced with permission of the publisher, from Willott et al., 1994.) AVCN, anteroventral cochlear nucleus; DCN, dorsal cochlear nucleus; OCA, octopus cell area; SEM, standard error of the mean.

colony was 23.5 months). If the central changes were directly related to the duration of cochlear damage irrespective of other factors, magnitudes should have been ordered as follows: 2/6 (4 months), 6/11 (5 months), 11/24 (13 months) and 6/24 (18 months). However, most morphological measures did not differ significantly among noise-exposed groups, indicating that chronicity was not an important contributor to the observed central changes (see Figure 3.4). It can be concluded that, once the observed central changes had run their course (demonstrably here within a few months of induction of cochlear damage, but possibly much more quickly – compare Pasic and Rubel, 1989), additional periods of denervation resulted in little or no further central change (see also Morest, 1982).

**Survival age**

Even though 2-year-old CBA mice exhibit little age-related peripheral pathology (Willott and Mortenson, 1991; Spongr et al. 1997), some CAS changes are observed at this age, presumably associated with the biological ageing of the brain (Willott et al., 1987, 1992; Willott and Bross, 1990). Studies of other species also indicate that CAS changes can occur in old individuals, even when peripheral hearing loss is not great (Willott, 1991). It is evident that, in interpreting the central effects of chronic noise-induced cochlear pathology, the possible interaction with other age-related central changes must be considered. In the Willott et al. (1994) study, two groups of noise-exposed mice were allowed to reach 24 months of age. Little evidence was obtained to indicate that changes induced by peripheral damage became exaggerated in older mice (for example, groups 6/24 and 11/24 versus 2/6 or 6/11). To the contrary, some of the differences between 24-month-old control and noise-exposed mice were diminished compared with young groups. For example, neurons in groups 2/6 and 6/11 were smaller than similarly aged controls, indicating an effect of peripheral damage. In contrast, the size of neurons in 2-year-old exposed mice was very similar to that of similarly aged controls, because neuronal size decreased with age. This observation suggests that (with respect to the variables measured) processes associated with ageing did not exacerbate the effects of cochlear damage.

# Conclusions regarding central auditory effects of noise exposure

Noise-induced pathology was not exacerbated in aged animals, and early exposure to noise did not exacerbate age-related central changes. The overall findings are encouraging with regard to the potential of auditory prostheses and other therapeutic strategies for older persons who suffered NIHL as young adults.

# Conclusions

Both noise exposure and ageing produce anatomical and physiological changes in the auditory system. The peripheral pathologies associated with noise exposure and ageing have been fairly well characterized (see

Willott, 1991; Henderson et al., 1995). Central changes associated with noise exposure and ageing are currently being elucidated. For example, the study by Willott et al. (1994) found that CN volume, neuronal packing density and neuron size were affected by noise-induced cochlear damage. It is probably the case that the noise-exposed mice incurred additional central anatomical changes not revealed by the present methods (see, for example, Jean-Baptiste and Morest, 1975; Gulley et al., 1978; Morest, 1982; Morest and Bohne, 1983; Keithley and Croskrey, 1990; Jones et al., 1992) as well as alterations in physiological responses (Willott and Lu, 1982; Willott, 1986; Willott et al., 1988a,b). Yet, little cell death and only a small degree of cell shrinkage occurred.

In contrast to our knowledge about the independent effects of noise exposure and ageing on the auditory system, very little is known about potential interactions between them. However, the data reviewed here suggest two tentative conclusions. First, with respect to the peripheral auditory system, there is little evidence that ageing is associated with increased vulnerability to damage from moderate-level noise exposures. High-level noise may produce age-dependent effects, but these appear to be relatively modest. Second, there does not appear to be a strong interaction between noise exposure and ageing on CAS pathology. In the Willott et al. (1994) experiment with mice, noise exposure did not exacerbate age-related changes in the cochlear nucleus, and ageing did not influence noise-induced pathology. Taken together, the data provide an optimistic picture of resiliency of the ageing auditory system in the face of NIHL.

One question of interest for future studies concerns the aetiological mechanisms of AHL and NIHL. Is there a common genetic component underlying susceptibility to AHL and NIHL, or are different mechanisms involved? Recent studies using CBA and B6 mice have suggested that *ahl*, the recessive gene for adult-onset age-related hearing loss on chromosome 10 in B6 mice (Johnson et al., 1997), may also be responsible for increased susceptibility to NIHL (Erway et al., 1996; Davis et al., 1999). However, studies with other strains of mice suggest a dissociation between susceptibility to AHL and NIHL (McFadden et al., 2001; Yoshida et al., 2000).

# References

Blatchley BJ, Williams JE, Coleman JR (1983) Age-dependent effects of acoustic deprivation on spherical cells in the anteroventral cochlear nucleus. Experimental Neurology 80: 81–93.

Boettcher FA, Gratton MA, Schmiedt RA (1995) Effects of noise and age on the auditory system. Occupational Medicine 10: 577–91.

Bohne BA, Gruner MM, Harding GW (1990) Morphological correlates of ageing in the chinchilla cochlea. Hearing Research 48: 79–91.

Born DE, Rubel EW (1985) Afferent influences on brain stem auditory nuclei of the chicken: neuron number and size following cochlear removal. Journal of Comparative Neurology 231: 435–45.

Caruso S, Cianci A, Grasso D, Agnello C, Galvani F, Maiolino L, Serra A (2000) Auditory brainstem response in postmenopausal women treated with hormone replacement therapy: a pilot study. Menopause 7: 178–83.

Coleman JR, O'Connor P (1979) Effects of monaural and binaural sound deprivation on cell development in the anteroventral cochlear nucleus of rats. Experimental Neurology 64: 553–66.

Coleman JR, Campbell D, Cooper WA, Welsh MG, Moyer J (1994) Auditory brainstem responses after ovariectomy and estrogen replacement in rat. Hearing Research 80: 209–15.

Corso JF (1992) Support for Corso's hearing loss model. Relating ageing and noise exposure. Audiology 31: 162–7.

Crace R (1970) Morphologic alterations with age in the human cochlear nuclear complex. PhD dissertation, Ohio University.

Davis RR, Cheever, ML, Krieg EF, Erway LC (1999). Quantitative measure of genetic differences in susceptibility to noise-induced hearing loss in two strains of mice. Hearing Research 134(1-2): 9–15.

Decory L, Dancer AL, Aran JM (1992) Species differences in mechanisms of damage. In A Dancer, D Henderson, RJ Salvi, RP Hamernik (eds) Noise-Induced Hearing Loss. St Louis, MO: Mosby Year Book, pp. 73–88.

Dehan CP, Jerger J (1990) Analysis of gender differences in the auditory brainstem response. Laryngoscope 100:18–24.

Ding DL, McFadden SL, Salvi (2001) RJ Cochlear hair cell densities and inner ear staining techniques. In JF Willott (ed.) Handbook of Mouse Auditory Research: From Behavior to Molecular Biology. Boca Raton, FL: CRC Press LLC.

Elkind-Hirsch KE, Stoner WR, Stach BA, Jerger JF (1992) Estrogen influences auditory brainstem responses during the normal menstrual cycle. Hearing Research 60:143–8.

Erway LC, Shiau YW, Davis RR, Krieg EF (1996) Genetics of age-related hearing loss in mice. III. Susceptibility of inbred and F1 hybrid strains to noise-induced hearing loss. Hearing Research 93(1-2): 181–7.

Fay RR (1988) Comparative psychoacoustics. Hearing Research 34: 295–305.

Freeman S, Khvoles R, Cherny L, Sohmer H (1999) Effect of long-term noise exposure on the developing and developed ear in the rat. Audiology and Neurootology 4: 207–18.

Garcia-Segura LM, Azcoitia I, DonCarlos LL (2001) Neuroprotection by estradiol. Progress in Neurobiology 63: 29–60.

Gulley RL, Wenthold RJ, Neises G (1978) Changes in the rostral anterior ventral cochlear nucleus of the waltzing guinea pig following hair cell loss. Brain Research 158: 279–94.

Hashisaki GT, Rubel EW (1989) Effects of unilateral cochlea removal on anteroventral cochlear nucleus neurons in developing gerbils. Journal of Comparative Neurology 283: 465–73.

Heffner RS, Heffner HE (1991) Behavioral hearing range of the chinchilla. Hearing Research 52: 13–16.

Heffner H, Masterton B (1980) Hearing in glires: domestic rabbit, cotton rat, feral house mouse, and kangaroo rat. Journal of the Acoustical Society of America 68: 1584–99.

Hellstrom PA (1995) The relationship between sound transfer functions and hearing levels. Hearing Research 88: 54–60.

Henderson D, McFadden SL, Gratton MA, Spongr V (1995) Similarities and differences between noise induced and age-related hearing loss. In G Rossi (ed.) (1995) Proceedings of the International Advanced Research Workshop: 1975–1995. Man and Environmental Noise Twenty Years After. Turin: Minerva Medica.

Henry KR (1983) Ageing and audition. In JF Willott (ed.) The Auditory Psychobiology of the Mouse. Springfield, IL: Charles C Thomas, pp. 470–93.

Henry KR (2002) Sex- and age-related elevation of cochlear nerve envelope response (CNER) and auditory brainstem response (ABR) thresholds in C57BL/6 mice. Hearing Research 170: 107–15.

Henry KR (2004) Males lose hearing earlier in mouse models of late-onset age-related hearing loss; females lose hearing earlier in mouse models of early-onset hearing loss. Hearing Research 190: 141–8.

Henry KR, Chole RA (1980) Genotypic differences in behavioral, physiological and anatomical expressions of age-related hearing loss in the laboratory mouse. Audiology 19: 369–83.

Jean-Baptiste M, Morest DK (1975) Transneuronal changes in the trapezoid body following cochlear ablations in the cat. Journal of Comparative Neurology 162: 111–31.

Johnson KR, LC Erway, et al (1997). A major gene affecting age-related hearing loss in C5 7BL/6J mice. Hearing Research 114(1-2): 83–92.

Jones DR, Hutson KA, Morest DK (1992) Growth cones and structural variation of synaptic end-bulbs in the cochlear nucleus of the adult cat brain. Synapse 10: 291–309.

Keithley EM, Croskrey KL (1990) Spiral ganglion cell endings in the cochlear nucleus of young and old rats. Hearing Research 49: 169–78.

Koitchev K, Aran J-M, Ivanov E, Cazals Y (1986) Progressive degeneration in the cochlear nucleus after chemical destruction of the cochlea. Acta Oto-Laryngologica 102: 31–9.

Li HS (1992) Influence of genotype and age on acute acoustic trauma and recovery in CBA/Ca and C57BL/6J mice. Acta Oto-Laryngologica 112: 956–67.

Li HS, Borg E (1993) Auditory degeneration after acoustic trauma in two genotypes of mice. Hearing Research 68: 19–27.

Li HS, Hultcrantz M, Borg E (1993) Influence of age on noise-induced permanent threshold shifts in CBA/Ca and C57BL/6J mice. Audiology 32: 195–204.

Lockwood D, McFadden SL, Jiang H, Rosenberg L (2000) Systemic treatment with estradiol reduces noise-induced hearing loss in the chinchilla. Association for Research in Otolaryngology, Abstr. 4631.

Macrae JH (1971) Noise-induced hearing loss and presbyacusis. Audiology 10: 323–33.

Macrae JH (1991) Presbycusis and noise-induced permanent threshold shift. Journal of the Acoustical Society of America 90: 2513–16.

McFadden SL, Campo P (1998) Cubic distortion product otoacoustic emissions in young and aged chinchillas exposed to low-frequency noise. Journal of the Acoustical Society of America 104: 2290–7.

McFadden SL, Henderson D (1999) Recent advances in understanding and preventing noise-induced hearing loss. Current Opinion in Otolaryngology and Head and Neck Surgery 7: 266–73.

McFadden SL, Campo P, Quaranta N, Henderson D (1997) Age-related decline of auditory function in the chinchilla (Chinchilla laniger). Hearing Research 111: 114–26.

McFadden SL, Campo P, Ding D, Quaranta N (1998) Effects of noise on inferior colliculus evoked potentials and cochlear anatomy in young and aged chinchillas. Hearing Research 117: 81–96.

McFadden SL, Henselman LW, Zheng XY (1999) Sex differences in auditory sensitivity of chinchillas before and after exposure to impulse noise. Ear and Hearing 20: 164–74.

McFadden SL, Burkard RF, Shero M, Ding DL, Salvi RJ, Flood DG (2000a) Chronic oxidative stress does not exacerbate noise-induced hearing loss in SOD1 mice. Association for Research in Otolaryngology Abstract 217: 61.

McFadden SL, Ohlemiller KK, Ding DL, and Salvi RJ (2001) The role of superoxide dismutase in age-related and noise-induced hearing loss: Clues from Sod 1 knockout mice. In: J.F. Willott (ed.), Handbook of Mouse Auditory Research: From Behavior to Molecular Biology. Boca Raton, FL: CRC Press LLC, pp. 489–504.

McFadden SL, Zheng XY, Ding DL (2000b) Conditioning-induced protection from impulse noise in female and male chinchillas. Journal of the Acoustical Society of America 107: 2162–8.

Mikaelian DO (1979) Development and degeneration of hearing in the C57/b16 mouse: relation of electrophysiologic responses from the round window and cochlear nucleus to cochlear anatomy and behavioral responses. Laryngoscope 89: 1–15.

Miller JD (1970) Audibility curve of the chinchilla. Journal of the Acoustical Society of America 48: 513–23.

Miller JM, Dolan DF, Raphael Y, Altschuler RA (1998) Interactive effects of ageing with noise induced hearing loss. Scandanavian Audiology Supplement 48: 53–61.

Mills JH, Schmiedt RA, Kulish LF (1990) Age-related changes in auditory potentials of Mongolian gerbil. Hearing Research 46: 201–10.

Mills JH, Boettcher FA, Dubno JR, Schmiedt RA (1996) Interactions between age-related and noise-induced hearing loss. In A Axelsson, HM Borchgrevink, RP Hamernik, PA Hellstrom, D Henderson, RJ Salvi (eds) Scientific Basis of Noise-Induced Hearing Loss. New York: Thième, pp. 193–212.

Mills JH, Boettcher FA, Dubno JR (1997) Interaction of noise-induced permanent threshold shift and age-related threshold shift. Journal of the Acoustical Society of America 101: 1681–6.

Moore DR (1990) Auditory brainstem of the ferret: early cessation of developmental sensitivity of neurons in the cochlear nucleus to removal of the cochlea. Journal of Comparative Neurology 302: 810–23.

Morest DK (1982) Degeneration in the brain following exposure to noise. In RP Hamernik, D Henderson, R Salvi (1982) (eds) New Perspectives on Noise-Induced Hearing Loss. New York: Raven Press, pp. 87–93.

Morest DK, Bohne BA (1983) Noise-induced degeneration in the brain and representation of inner and outer hair cells. Hearing Research 9: 145–51.

Nordeen KS, Killackey HP, Kitzes LM (1983) Ascending projections to the inferior colliculus following unilateral cochlear ablations in the neonatal gerbil Meriones unguiculatis. Journal of Comparative Neurology 214: 144–53.

Pasic TR, Rubel EW (1989) Rapid changes in cochlear nucleus cell size following blockade of auditory nerve electrical activity in gerbils. Journal of Comparative Neurology 283: 474–80.

Pearson JD, Morrell CH, Gordon-Salant S, Brant LJ, Metter EJ, Klein LL, Fozard JL (1995) Gender differences in a longitudinal study of age-associated hearing loss. Journal of the Acoustical Society of America 97: 1196–205.

Powell TPS, Erulkar SD (1962) Transneuronal cell degeneration in the auditory relay nuclei of the cat. Journal of Anatomy 96: 249–68.

Rosenhall U, Pedersen K., Svanborg A (1990) Presbycusis and noise-induced hearing loss. Ear and Hearing 11: 257–63.

Ryan A (1976) Hearing sensitivity of the mongolian gerbil, Meriones unguiculatis. Journal of the Acoustical Society of America 59: 1222–6.

Salvi RJ, Saunders SS, Gratton MA, Arehole S, Powers N (1990) Enhanced evoked response amplitudes in the inferior colliculus of the chinchilla following acoustic trauma. Hearing Research 50: 245–57.

Saunders JC, Garfinkle TJ (1983) Peripheral anatomy and physiology I. In JF Willott (ed.) The Auditory Psychobiology of the Mouse. Springfield, IL: Charles C Thomas, pp. 131–68.

Saunders JC, Tilney LG (1982) Species differences in susceptibility to noise exposure. In RP Hamernik, D Henderson, R Salvi (eds) New Perspectives on Noise-Induced Hearing Loss. New York: Raven Press, pp. 229–48.

Schmiedt RA, Schulte BA (1992) Physiologic and histopathologic changes in quiet- and noise-aged gerbil cochleae. In A Dancer, D Henderson, RJ Salvi, RP Hamernik (eds) Noise-Induced Hearing Loss. St Louis, MO: Mosby Year Book, pp. 156–71.

Shone G, Altschuler RA, Miller JM, Nuttall AL (1991) The effect of noise exposure on the ageing ear. Hearing Research 56: 173–8.

Spongr VP, Flood DG, Frisina RD, Salvi RJ (1997) Quantitative measures of hair cell loss in CBA and C57BL/6 mice throughout their lifespans. Journal of the Acoustical Society of America 101: 3546–53.

Stenberg AE, Wang H, Sahlin L, Hultcrantz M (1999) Mapping of estrogen receptors alpha and beta in the inner ear of mouse and rat. Hearing Research 136: 29–34.

Sun JC, Bohne BA, Harding GW (1994) Is the older ear more susceptible to noise damage? Laryngoscope 104: 1251–8.

Swanson SJ, Dengerink HA (1988) Changes in pure-tone thresholds and temporary threshold shifts as a function of menstrual cycle and oral contraceptives. Journal of Speech and Hearing Research 31: 569–74.

Theopold HM (1975) Degenerative alterations in the ventral cochlear nucleus of the guinea pig after impulse noise exposure. Arch Oto-Rhino-Laryngologica 209: 247–62.

Trune DR (1982) Influence of neonatal cochlear removal on the development of mouse cochlear nucleus: 1 Number size and density of its neurons. Journal of Comparative Neurology 209: 409–24.

Webster DB (1983a) Auditory neuronal sizes after a unilateral conductive hearing loss. Experimental Neurology 79: 130–40.

Webster DB (1983b) Late onset of auditory deprivation does not affect brainstem auditory neuron soma size. Hearing Research 12: 145–7.

Webster DB (1988) Conductive hearing loss affects the growth of the cochlear nuclei over an extended period of time. Hearing Research 32: 185–92.

Webster DB, Webster M (1979) Effects of neonatal conductive hearing loss on brain stem auditory nuclei. Annals of Otology Rhinology and Laryngology 88: 684–8.

Willott JF (1986) Effects of ageing hearing loss and anatomical location on thresholds of inferior colliculus neurons in C57BL/6 and CBA mice. Journal of Neurophysiology 56: 391–408.

Willott JF (1991) Ageing and the Auditory System: Anatomy, Physiology, and Psychophysics. San Diego: Singular Publishing Group.

Willott JF, Bross LS (1990) Morphology of the octopus cell area of the cochlear nucleus in young and ageing C57BL/6J and CBA/J mice. Journal of Comparative Neurology 300: 61–81.

Willott JF, Bross LS (2004) Effects of prolonged exposure to an augmented acoustic environment on the auditory system of middle-aged C57BL/6J mice: cochlear and central histology and sex differences. Journal of Comparative Neurology 472: 358–70.

Willott JF, Lu S (1982) Noise-induced hearing loss can alter neural coding and increase excitability in the central nervous system. Science 216: 1331–2.

Willott JF, Mortenson V (1991) Age-related cochlear histopathology in C57BL/6J and CBA/J mice. Association for Research in Otolaryngology Abstracts 14: 16.

Willott JF, Jackson LM, Hunter KP (1987) A morphometric study of the anteroventral cochlear nucleus of two mouse models of presbycusis. Journal of Comparative Neurology 260: 472–506.

Willott JF, Parham K, Hunter KP (1988a) Response properties of inferior colliculus neurons in middle-aged C57BL/6J mice with presbycusis. Hearing Research 37: 15–28.

Willott JF, Parham K, Hunter KP (1988b) Response properties of inferior colliculus neurons in young and very old CBA/J mice. Hearing Research 37: 1–14.

Willott JF, Bross LS, McFadden SL (1992) Morphology of the dorsal cochlear nucleus in C57BL6J and CBA/J mice across the lifespan. Journal of Comparative Neurology 321: 666–78.

Willott JF, Bross LS, McFadden SL (1994) Morphology of the cochlear nucleus in CBA/J mice with chronic severe sensorineural cochlear pathology induced during adulthood. Hearing Research 74: 1–21.

Yanz JL, Abbas PJ (1982) Age effects in susceptibility to noise-induced hearing loss. Journal of the Acoustical Society of America 72: 1450–5.

Yoshida N, Hequembourg SJ, Atencio CA, Rosowski JJ, Liberman MC (2000) Acoustic injury in mice: 129/SvEv is exceptionally resistant to noise-induced hearing loss. Hearing Research 141: 97-106.

Yost WA (1995) Fundamentals of Hearing. San Diego, CA: Academic Press, Inc.

Zheng XY, Henderson D, Hu BH, Ding DL, McFadden SL (1997) The influence of the cochlear efferent system on chronic acoustic trauma. Hearing Research 107: 147–59.

# CHAPTER 4

# Interaction of NIHL and ageing: epidemiological aspects

*Noise and Its Effects:* Edited by Linda Luxon and Deepak Prasher © 2007 John Wiley & Sons Ltd.

DORIS-EVA BAMIOU

MARK E LUTMAN

## Introduction

It is estimated that about 11% of males and 3% of females of the UK's population will be exposed to noise cumulatively equivalent to 90 dB (A) for 50 years, and will thus be at risk of developing noise-induced hearing loss (NIHL) (Davis, 1995). However, the attribution of the hearing loss in each individual case to noise exposure, ageing or the interaction of the two, after exclusion of other possible aetiological factors, can be a challenge for the clinician. This diagnostic decision will affect not only compensation claims, in the case of occupational hearing loss, but also the prognosis that the patient is given regarding further change of his hearing thresholds over time, and the measures recommended to prevent further hearing deterioration.

The need to understand how NIHL interacts with age-related hearing loss (ARHL) also has implications for long-term planning of health services. Life expectancy is now greater than for previous generations and, since the NIHL prevalence increases with age and duration of occupational noise exposure (Palmer et al., 2002), a great deal of resources will be required in order to plan effective services for hearing loss prevention and hearing rehabilitation for a growing elderly population. But despite the fact that NIHL-associated compensation and medical costs have increased over recent years, NIHL may still be under-recognized in older individuals with a past history of noise exposure (Daniell et al., 1998), and whereas a probabilistic allocation of hearing loss to noise, ageing or other factors is possible with the use of international standards such as ISO

1999, the understanding of the interaction of NIHL and ageing that underpins these guidelines remains limited at best.

**Importance of interaction of ARHL and NIHL in Man**

- Prevalence: 11% men and 3% women in UK
- Prevalence increases with age and duration of exposure
- Demographic changes with older population
- Increased healthcare resource allocation
- Compensation claims
- Relevance and effects of environmental noise
- Relevance and effects of other ototoxic agents

# Definitions

Glorig and Nixon (1960) used the term 'socioacusis' to reflect their hypothesis that hearing loss in old age is to an extent due to noise exposure, while Kryter (1983) used the term 'nosoacusis' to describe the component of hearing loss in old age that is due to deleterious factors other than noise, such as trauma or ototoxicity. There are, indeed, reports of non-industrialized populations who maintain excellent hearing in old age (see, for example, Kapur and Patt, 1967), but these findings could also be due to genetic or other factors. Willott (1996) thus defines presbyacusis as the hearing impairment that accompanies ageing, which cannot be accounted for by genetic syndromes, pathological conditions or other insults to the auditory system, and which includes peripheral as well as central auditory deficits.

Current theories propose that the ageing process is the product of complex interactions between our genes and the environment. These theories attribute the ageing-related clinical manifestations to accumulation of unrepaired damage, for example damage/mutations of DNA, defective mitochondria, oxidative damage by free radicals (Kirkwood and Wolff, 1995), which results in deterioration of physiological functions (Khaw, 1997). As a result of these theories, strategies to address age-related changes include efforts to reduce damage, to increase protection against damage, for example by priming antioxidant defences, and to prevent loss through lack of use, for example by aiding the age- and noise-related hearing loss (Khaw, 1997).

# Audiometric and histological characteristics of NIHL versus ARHL

The clinical diagnosis of NIHL requires interpretation of audiometric findings in the light of a detailed history for noise exposure and other ototoxic factors, after consideration of potential confounders (Coles et al., 2000).

NIHL is thought to begin as an audiometric notch (threshold elevation) between 3 and 6 kHz, with relatively flat or down-sloping 2–4 kHz and flat or up-sloping 4–8 kHz, and with normal or near normal low frequencies (Cooper and Owen, 1976). It is proposed that the hearing threshold level at 3, 4 or 6 kHz should be at least 10 dB greater than the threshold at 1 or 2 kHz, after correction for earphone type (Coles et al., 2000). But while the 4-kHz notch correlates well with a history of noise exposure as ascertained by questionnaire, 6-kHz notches do not show this association (McBride and Williams, 2001). Some of the 6-kHz notches reported in the literature may be artefacts caused by a particular interaction between the TDH-39 earphones and the IEC 303 coupler (Lutman and Qasem, 1998). This raises questions regarding the clinical value of a 6-kHz notch finding. NIHL is also characterized by loss of cochlear non-linearities as reflected by loss of otoacoustic emissions (OAEs), even in the presence of normal hearing thresholds (Attias et al., 1995). In addition, there is emerging evidence that noise exposure may have long-term effects on the central auditory pathways (for example, Ryan et al., 1992; Wang et al., 2002).

Age-related hearing loss is characterized by a gradual loss of sensitivity at high frequencies. This loss is reported to be equal to 0.5–0.7 dB per year after the fourth decade in the 2- to 4-kHz range (Morrell et al., 1996). Hearing sensitivity deteriorates faster in men than in women. Thus, women have better hearing than men at frequencies above 1000 Hz, but worse hearing than men at frequencies below 1000 Hz (Jerger et al., 1993; Davis, 1995; Pearson et al., 1995). Age-related hearing loss is also associated with poor perception of speech in noise (Divenyi and Simon, 1999), while there is a negative correlation between age and transient (Quaranta et al., 2001), as well as distortion product OAE amplitudes (Oeken et al., 2000). However, other age-related effects such as age-related middle-ear alterations also seem to contribute to the OAE findings (Oeken et al., 2000). Age seems to have greater effect on hearing thresholds than on distortion product input–output function measures, consistent with a substantial strial dysfunction component of the age-related cochlear degeneration (Gates et al., 2002). In addition, ARHL is characterized by central auditory changes such as different frequency mapping in the central auditory system, impaired neural inhibition and binaural processing abnormalities that lead to increased noise masking of neural responses (Willott, 1996).

From a histopathological perspective, NIHL involves primarily loss of outer hair cells with secondary degeneration of neural fibres (Hamernik et al., 1989). Supporting and vascular cells of the cochlea also show damage after certain noise exposures (Henderson and Hamernik, 1995). The outer hair cell loss continues even after noise exposure stops, probably due to apoptosis (Hu et al., 2002), but the count of missing hair cells does not correspond closely to audiometric thresholds (Hamernik et al., 1989).

The evolution of age-related histological changes from middle to extreme old age in humans is not well understood. Schuknecht initially described four distinct types of presbyacusis: sensorineural, neural, strial and conductive (Schuknecht and Gacek, 1993), based on correlations between audiometric results and histological findings from postmortem examinations in aged patients. Other authors describe a marked loss of outer and a mild loss of inner hair cells in elderly subjects, with lengthening and thickening of stereocilia (giant stereociliary degeneration) (Figure 4.1) and with radial nerve fibre atrophy following hair cell death (Sucek et al., 1987). Most cases of ARHL appear to show a combination of Schuknecht's types rather than a discrete pattern of histological degeneration (Salvi et al., 2001).

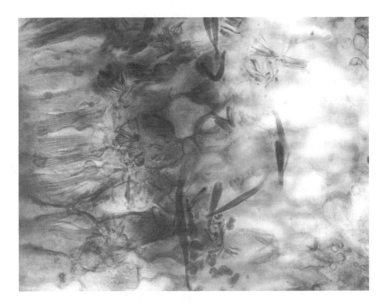

**Figure 4.1** Giant stereocilia in presbyacusis. (With many thanks to Dr Sava Sucek.)

# Apportionment of the hearing loss to noise and age

The International Organization for Standardization published ISO 1999 in 1990, in order to provide a method to estimate hearing impairment due to noise exposure, adjusted for age, in otologically normal (database A) and otologically unscreened (database B) adult populations. In ISO 1999, hearing impairment corresponds to the permanent threshold shift.

ISO 1999 assumes a predominantly additive relationship of ARHL and NIHL, as an approximation of the actual biological events. It is acknowledged that additional factors to noise and ageing may affect hearing but no effort is made to separate their effects other than provision of separate hearing normative data for an otologically normal and otologically unscreened population. The age- and noise-adjusted hearing threshold level is thus calculated as per the empirical formula:

$$H1 = H + N - \left( \frac{H \times N}{120} \right)$$

where H1 is the hearing threshold level in decibels, H is the age-related threshold level as specified by ISO 1999 in databases A and B or other databases, and N the noise-induced permanent threshold shift in decibels. The third term in the equation represents an interaction between age and noise, which has the effect of reducing the combined total below the simple additive sum. This term is small and insignificant for hearing losses less than 40 dB. Hence, for mild hearing losses, ISO 1999 can be considered to be a simple additive formula.

ISO 1999 (ISO, 1999) accepts the 'equal energy hypothesis', which stipulates that noise exposures that deliver equal acoustic energy to the ear will be equally detrimental for hearing. However, the effects of impulse noise or of the interaction of impulse noise with background continuous noise are often inconsistent with this principle (Henderson and Hamernik, 1986). Similarly, exposures to interrupted high-level noise will produce a 'toughening effect' and will result in reduced acoustic trauma compared with the equivalent uninterrupted noise (Hamernik et al., 2003). It is thus questionable whether the equal energy hypothesis can be accepted as a unifying principle for estimating the potential of a noise exposure to produce hearing loss.

The standard has been used in comparison with many experimental and epidemiological studies. For example, Macrae (1991) found that the ISO 1999 (1990) underestimated the age-related hearing deterioration at 4000 Hz in a group of war veterans who had sustained hearing loss due to wartime exposure. Conversely, Mills et al. (1997) exposed 18-month-old gerbils to 113 dB sound pressure level or SPL in one ear in order to compare ageing-only effects on hearing in the non-exposed ear and noise-plus-ageing effects on hearing in the exposed ear. They also used another group of gerbils, who were born and raised in a quiet vivarium as a control group. All animals were retested at age 36 months. The authors found that ISO 1999 over-estimated the combined effects of noise and age, and attributed this finding to both the great variability of ARHL and parameters of the noise exposure. However, another report (Boettcher, 2002) found that, when ARHL was less than NIHL, the total hearing loss in aged gerbils after noise exposure was equal to the addition of ARHL and NIHL in decibels, similar to the ISO guidelines.

Medicolegal cases of NIHL require the clinician to distinguish between possibility and probability of NIHL, with a legal criterion of 'more probable than not' (Coles et al., 2000). And while ISO 1999 should not be used to predict or assess the hearing impairment of individuals, it can be used to form probabilistic conclusions for individual cases, and forms the basis for at least two quantitative methods to do this. Dobie (1996) assumes a moderate correlation between ARHL and NIHL and bases the allocation of age-related and noise-induced hearing loss on the ratio between the median expected values of ARHL and NIHL for a given individual, by means of a five-step procedure (Figure 4.2):

1. Decide the frequencies of interest.
2. Determine whether thresholds at these frequencies exceed the ISO 1999 normal range.
3. Find the median expected ARHL from the ISO databases.
4. Find the median expected NIHL for the individual's exposure level and duration.
5. Allocate the individual's ARHL and NIHL in the same proportion as median ARHL to median NIHL from ISO 1999.

This method can be undertaken provided that the individual's audiometry is symmetrical and compatible with NIHL, when the exposure level is known and other causes of hearing loss have been excluded (Dobie, 1996). However, this allocation of hearing loss in individual cases may at times cover almost the entire probability space from 1st to 100th percentile (Mills et al., 1996).

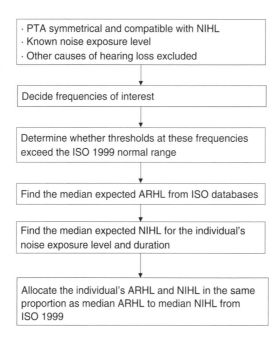

**Figure 4.2** Proposed allocation of hearing loss to age and noise (Dobie, 1996). ARHL, age-related hearing loss; NIHL, noise-induced hearing loss; PTA, pure-tone audiometry.

Coles et al. (2000) also provide guidelines for the diagnosis of NIHL for medicolegal purposes (Figure 4.3). They define NIHL on the basis of high-frequency hearing loss with a high-frequency audiometric notch after potentially dangerous noise exposure. The main parameters that they consider include the clinical picture, whether the hearing loss is compatible with the individual's age and estimated total noise exposure, other causes for hearing loss, and complicating factors such as an asymmetrical audiometric pattern or the presence of conductive or mixed hearing loss. These authors suggest that the calculation of NIHL is based on two 'anchor points' of the audiogram, usually the 1000-Hz and 8000-Hz threshold. These anchor points are then used to select, from a modified version of database A, the statistical ARHL data that best correspond to the values of the 'anchor points'. These are used to calculate the misfit values (i.e. difference between statistical values and observed thresholds) for all frequencies and thus decide whether a notch in the appropriate frequencies is present.

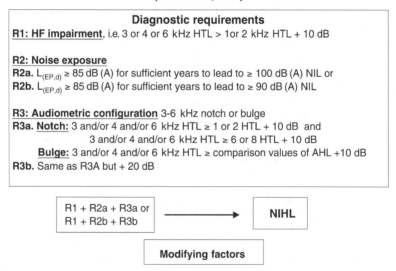

**Guidelines on diagnosis of NIHL for medicolegal purposes**
**(Coles et al., 2000)**

**Diagnostic requirements**
**R1: HF impairment**, i.e. 3 or 4 or 6 kHz HTL > 1or 2 kHz HTL + 10 dB

**R2: Noise exposure**
**R2a.** $L_{(EP,d)} \geq 85$ dB (A) for sufficient years to lead to $\geq 100$ dB (A) NIL or
**R2b.** $L_{(EP,d)} \geq 85$ dB (A) for sufficient years to lead to $\geq 90$ dB (A) NIL

**R3: Audiometric configuration** 3-6 kHz notch or bulge
**R3a. Notch:** 3 and/or 4 and/or 6 kHz HTL $\geq 1$ or 2 HTL + 10 dB  and
                       3 and/or 4 and/or 6 kHz HTL $\geq 6$ or 8 HTL + 10 dB
        **Bulge:** 3 and/or 4 and/or 6 kHz HTL $\geq$ comparison values of AHL +10 dB
**R3b.** Same as R3A but + 20 dB

R1 + R2a + R3a or                ⟶              **NIHL**
R1 + R2b + R3b

**Modifying factors**

**Figure 4.3** Guidelines on diagnosis of noise-induced hearing loss (NIHL) for medicolegal purposes (Coles et al., 2000). AHL, age-related hearing loss; HTL, hearing threshold level; NIL, noise immission level.

# Interaction of age versus noise

In practice, methods for estimation of NIHL assume an additive or predominantly additive relationship between noise and age-related hearing loss. However, this interaction may be influenced by many parameters, the significance of which is not yet well understood. In addition, this interaction cannot be defined in individuals and can at best be inferred from systematic studies that include both experimental and epidemiological approaches to these issues. Experimental studies can be tightly controlled and designed to answer specific questions in a short time but are conducted on laboratory animals; thus their results cannot be extrapolated directly to humans. Epidemiological studies, on the other hand, may supply information on human groups, but are difficult to control, with inherent limitations such as historical constraints and difficulties of ascertainment of various factors when retrospective, while they require a long-term follow-up when prospective. For these reasons, these two approaches are complementary and we will review information from both.

# Genetic mechanisms for NIHL and ARHL

Both NIHL and ARHL show a great variability. Individuals of the same age who have been exposed to the same amount of noise will vary in their degree of hearing loss, even when all other factors that may affect hearing have been controlled (for example, Davis et al., 1950; ISO, 1999). It is suggested that recognized risk factors may explain 40–60% of the variability in NIHL, and that the remaining variability is due to genetic factors (Pyykkö et al., 1989; Christensen et al., 2001). Genes may enhance or decrease susceptibility to noise or ageing, by influencing protective biochemical and metabolic mechanisms, neurotransmitter or central nervous system properties (Erway and Willott, 1996). Genes may also be the direct cause of cochlear pathology, or may influence susceptibility to ototoxic factors that have a synergistic action with noise or ageing (Erway and Willott, 1996).

### Animal data

Laboratory animals have provided valuable insight into the genetic differences in susceptibility to NIHL and ARHL and on their interaction (see Chapter 3). In mice, the CBA/Ca and C57BL/6J genetic strains have similar ARHL as humans, with auditory degeneration that begins at the high frequencies. However, the C57BL/6J strain shows a broader range of age-adjusted hearing thresholds, with hearing loss earlier in life and hearing thresholds deteriorating faster with age than the CBA/Ca strain (Shone et al., 1991; Li, 1992).

Determination of the level of the noise exposure is important when considering the age-noise interaction. Noise exposure of 101 dBSPL leads to significant permanent threshold shift in the C57BL/6J mice with early ARHL, but not in age-matched CBA/Ca (Shone et al., 1991) indicating that, at these exposure levels, mice with an ARHL are more susceptible to NIHL than age-matched subjects without ARHL. A further study found that these two strains have distinctly different dose–response curves for NIHL, in terms of offset and slope (Davis et al., 1999). Thus, C57BL/6J mice exhibit a more linear increase for permanent threshold shift for 98–113 dB noise exposure, consistent with the effects of increasing noise-induced metabolic demands on physiological mechanisms. The CBA/Ca strain have an abrupt transition in NIHL between 113 and 116 dB noise exposure, which probably reflects a structural injury of the cochlea (Davis et al., 1999). Histological examination after noise exposure at 120 dB SPL similarly showed different cochlear damage patterns in the two strains (Li, 1992). Cochlear damage in the C57BL/6J strain consisted of extensive outer hair cell (OHC) loss and all variations of damaged stereocilia, while OHC damage was less extensive in the CBA/Ca mice, where giant stereocilia were also found (Li, 1992). Despite these differences, for high level noise exposures at 120 dB SPL, the interaction between NIHL and ARHL showed the same trends in these two strains (Li, 1992). Thus in both strains, an initially additive interaction between noise and age, with the total threshold shift equal to the sum of either noise or age alone, was succeeded by a saturating interaction past a certain degree of hearing loss, in that the NIHL did not exceed the ARHL.

In a further step towards unravelling the genetics and enhancing our understanding of the interaction between NIHL and ARHL, the C57BL/6j mice were shown to be homozygous for a recessive gene *Ahl/Ahl* on chromosome 10 (Erway, 1995). It was postulated that this gene was responsible for increased susceptibility to age as well as NIHL (Erway et al., 1995). Several laboratory experiments provided further support for this hypothesis. Erway et al. (1996) produced a backcross of hybrid +/*Ahl* mice to inbred *Ahl/Ahl* mice. This backcross would be expected to produce a progeny, half of which would consist of +/*Ahl* mice, with a phenotype of normal hearing after noise exposure, and the other half of *Ahl/Ahl* mice, with a phenotype of hearing loss after noise exposure. The backcross did indeed yield the expected phenotype/genotype association in 90% of the progeny, giving support to the hypothesis that the *Ahl* recessive gene affects susceptibility to NIHL. However, Erway et al. (1996) observed a discordance of 10%, raising questions of whether other modifier genes were present within these genotypes. In a similar experiment, Davis et al. (2001) genotyped mice of the same backcrossed two inbred strains of mice, B6 mice (*Ahl/Ahl*) and CBxB6.F(1) mice (+/*Ahl*), and exposed the progeny to 110 dB SPL noise for 8 hours. Approximately half of the backcross progeny exhibited permanent threshold shift, and genotyping of these revealed a very strong association of the genetic factor within a few centimorgans of the *Ahl* gene. These findings support a role for the *Ahl* gene in both ARHL and NIHL among these strains of mice. More recent work suggested that the presence of a mitochondrial DNA mutation may worsen hearing impairment when combined with the *Ahl* gene (Johnson et al., 2001). Interestingly, the *Ahl* gene, which is responsible for ARHL in at least half of the known mice strains with this condition (Johnson et al., 2000), may be a different manifestation of the same gene as the *mdfw* gene that causes a genotype of hearing loss, head bobbing and imbalance (Zheng and Johnson, 2001). However, genetic susceptibility to ARHL may not always correspond to susceptibility to NIHL, as another genetic strain of mice with ARHL was found to be quite resistant to NIHL at a young age (Yoshida et al., 2000).

A different set of experiments assessed the relationship between mitochondrial DNA and ARHL. Seidman et al. (1997) found that the presence of the 4834-basepair (bp) deletion of mitochondrial DNA was significantly increased in Fischer rats that also had a progressive age-related hearing decline. They suggested that the 4834-bp deletion may be associated with presbyacusis, as well as with ageing. This postulate is consistent with the mitochondrial clock theory of ageing, which suggests that ageing changes are due to progressive accumulation of mitochondrial DNA damage resulting from free oxygen radicals, rendering cells deficient in terms of energy. However, it is not clear whether the mitochondrial mutation acts as a direct cause of presbyacusis, or whether the mutation is the result of the process that leads to presbyacusis. A subsequent study (Seidman et al., 2000) demonstrated that supplementing the diet of Fischer rats with the mitochondrial metabolites $\alpha$-lipoic acid and acetyl-L-carnitine led to a

**Table 4.1** Evidence from animals for a genetic basis for NIHL and ARHL

Different trends for NIHL and ARHL in different strains of mice:

|  | *CBA/Ca* | *C57BL/6J* |
| --- | --- | --- |
| Onset of ARHL | Late | Early |
| Range of ARHL | Broad | Narrow |
| ARHL deterioration | Slow | Fast |
| | | |
| 101 dB SPL N exposure | No PTS | PTS |
| 98-116 dB SPL N exposure | Abrupt transition in NIHL after 113 dB HL | Linear increase in NIHL |
| 120 dB SPL N exposure | Saturating interaction for NIHL and ARHL | Saturating interaction for NIHL and ARHL |

**C57BL/6j** mice homozygous for a recessive gene *Ahl/Ahl* on chromosome 10

**4834-bp mit DNA deletion** increased in Fischer rats with progressive ARHL

ARHL, age-related hearing loss; NIHL, noise-induced hearing loss; PTS, permanent threshold shift; SPL, sound pressure level delay of hearing loss progression that was associated with fewer mito-chondrial DNA deletions than in the non-treated controls. The authors proposed that mitochondrial metabolites protect and reverse age-related cochlear mitochondrial DNA damage and may thus improve the ability of cochlear cells to respond to energy demands.

## Human data

The genetics of ARHL and NIHL in humans are far from being unravelled. Some extrapolations from both animal and human data are possible. For example, the orthologous human chromosomal region to that of mouse chromosome 10 harbouring the age-related hearing loss (*Ahl*) gene is 10q21–q22. This region contains two human deafness loci, the DFNB12 and USH1D (OMIM, 2002). It has also been suggested that the hearing loss in DFNA5 families shows phenotypic similarities with presbyacusis (OMIM, 2002). In addition to these genes, the mitochondrial 4977-bp DNA deletion, which correspond with the 4834-bp mtDNA deletion in rats, was found in two out of three temporal bones with presbyacusis, but in none out of three temporal bones of age-matched humans without hearing loss (Seidman et al., 1996). This finding indicates that progressive accumulation of mitochondrial DNA damage due to free oxygen radicals may also play a role in ARHL in humans.

Epidemiological studies provide further support for a genetic basis of ARHL but without clarifying the mechanism. Gates et al. (2000) examined hearing in participants in a large epidemiological study, the Framingham Heart study, and in their relatives. Analysis of the audio-metric thresholds by a statistical programme for genetic epidemiology found evidence of a familial aggregation of ARHL in all parts (low, mid-dle and high frequencies) of the auditory spectrum. An estimated 35–55% of the variance of the sensory pesbyacusis and 25–42% of the variance of the strial presbyacusis phenotypes were attributable to gene effects. Familial aggregation was stronger in women than in men, which was attributed to the effects of noise exposure in the fathers, providing support for a genetic basis for ARHL in women and for a genetically acquired basis in men (Gates et al., 1999). Similar results were reported by Christensen et al. (2001), who assessed hearing diffi-culties by means of a questionnaire in twins aged 75 and older from the population-based Danish Twin Registry. Their study, which included more than 5000 subjects, reported consistently higher concordance rates, odds ratios and correlations for monozygotic than for dizygotic twin pairs in all age and sex categories, indicating heritability. Self-reported hearing difficulties were thus attributable to genetic inheritance for 40% of the variation (95%CI 19–53%), whereas environ-mental factors could account for the remaining variation (Christensen et al., 2001).

**The indications for a genetic basis for NIHL and ARHL in humans**

- The orthologous human chromosomal region to the mouse chromosomal region with the age-related hearing loss (*Ahl*) gene contains two human deafness loci: the DFNB12 and USH1D.
- The 4977-bp mtDNA deletion (corresponds to the 4834-bp mtDNA deletion in rats) in temporal bones with presbyacusis.
- Epidemiological studies suggest a familial aggregation for ARHL.
- Twin studies of ARHL show higher concordance rates, odds ratios and correlations for monozygotic than for dizygotic twins.

# The influence of acoustic factors

Acoustic factors of the noise exposure may affect the interaction between noise and ARHL. McFadden et al. (1998) examined how this interaction is affected by the level of noise exposure. They exposed aged and young chinchillas to moderate (95 dB) or high-level (106 dB) noise and measured thresholds of inferior colliculus evoked potentials up to 10 days post exposure. The authors found small but significant differences between young and aged animals exposed to 106 dB, in that aged animals had greater permanent threshold shift below 8 kHz than young animals. In addition, noise-exposed young animals had decreased inferior colliculus evoked potentials at low stimulus levels, but enhanced potentials at high stimulus levels after correcting for permanent threshold shift. The same was not observed in aged animals. Cubic distortion product otoacoustic emission (DPOAE) measurement (McFadden and Campo, 1998) showed that distortion product threshold and amplitude differences between aged and young animals were maintained after both 95 dB HL and 106 dB HL noise exposure. Histological examination of the cochleae that were harvested 30 days after exposure to 106 dB noise showed the following.

1. Outer hair cell loss was greater in aged than young ears, with little or no OHC loss in the basal region of the young cochlea but with extensive OHC loss in the 3- to 14-kHz region of the aged cochlea.
2. Noise-exposed aged cochleae had 5% more inner hair cell loss than young exposed or aged non-exposed cochleae.
3. Only aged ears showed OHC loss in rows 2 and 3.
4. Aged cochleae showed pigment clusters and patchy degeneration of the marginal layer of the stria vascularis.

The distortion product results suggest that young and aged animals do not differ in susceptibility to moderate or high-level noise and that there is an additive relationship between ARHL and NIHL. However, histological results would indicate that, although equally vulnerable to moderate noise, aged animals are more vulnerable to high-level noise than young animals. These findings could be explained by the presence of a diminished antioxidant defence system in the aged cochlea, with a reduced ability to scavenge free radicals formed after high noise exposure. There is some evidence that may give support to this hypothesis in that susceptibility to NIHL is influenced by melanin, and this has been attributed to the properties of different types of melanin to generate or neutralize radical oxygen species (Barrenas, 1997). Overall, NIHL and ARHL may be additive after prolonged exposure to moderate level noise, but the relationship may be more complex for high-level noise exposure. In terms of central auditory function, the evoked potential results in McFadden's study (1998) also indicate that NIHL affects midbrain sound-driven excitation and inhibition patterns differently in young and aged animals.

Mills et al. (1998) sought to assess how the duration parameters of the noise exposure affect the interaction between NIHL and ARHL, by experimenting on laboratory animals. They found that ISO 1999 overestimated thresholds after intense short-duration exposure. However, ISO 1999 predicted combined-effect noise- and age-related thresholds were consistent with the thresholds observed after a lifetime noise exposure, rendering some support to the additivity concept of ISO 1999. An epidemiological study (Henderson and Saunders, 1998) similarly found that the rate of growth of hearing loss over time of noise-exposed workers can be adequately predicted by the ISO 1999, even in the absence of detailed knowledge of the frequency spectrum or the level of the noise exposure.

# The influence of other factors/diseases

Several non-acoustic factors may also affect the susceptibility to both noise and ARHL. Hearing thresholds adjusted for age and noise exposure seem to be consistently worse across all frequencies in the manual versus the non-manual occupational population (Lutman and Spencer, 1991; Davis, 1995). Socioeconomic factors may therefore play a consistent role in this interaction, possibly by accounting for a collection of intrinsic health factors.

Although blood chemistry does not correlate with ARHL, serum vitamin $B_{12}$ deficiency, lower red-cell folate as well as β-adrenergic drugs and antihistamines may be an ARHL predisposing factor in women, but not in men (reviewed in Divenyi and Simon 1999). Moreover, Rosenhall et al. (1993) found a weak correlation between ARHL and smoking, alcohol abuse and trauma in a longitudinal study of a 70-year-old cohort in Sweden. However, it has also been suggested that smoking may have a preventive influence on NIHL, due to a higher melanin content of the nicotine-exposed epithelia (Hedin, 1991). In addition, it is of note that some factors that are reported to increase susceptibility to NIHL, such as high blood pressure, high cholesterol and use of analgesics, as well as smoking and shorter duration of ear-protector use, also correlate with increasing age (Pyykkö et al., 1998).

The interpretation of the influence of these factors is complicated by confounding of many other possible factors and the picture remains unclear.

# Progression of NIHL with age

Several studies indicate that, for long-term noise exposure, the pre-existence of hearing difficulties will not increase susceptibility to NIHL, while differences in hearing thresholds between noise-exposed and non-exposed subjects become much less prominent in old age. Rosenhall et al. (1990) evaluated the long-term effect of occupational noise exposure on hearing in a representative sample of the geriatric population in Gothenburg (Sweden), who were tested at 70, 75 and 79 years of age. At age 70 and 75, men who had been exposed to occupational noise for 15 years or more had significantly poorer hearing than men without noise exposure, but there was no significant difference between no noise versus noise exposure at the age of 79.

Grayson (1992) examined the association between previously existing hearing loss and the susceptibility to noise-induced permanent threshold shifts by a pair-matched case–control study. They matched cases with permanent hearing loss from the Air Force Hearing Conservation Data Registry in the USA with normal controls for noise intensity, duration of exposure and age. They found that cases with pre-existing hearing loss were no more likely than controls to develop future permanent threshold shifts at an odds ratio of 1.06.

Rösler (1994) compiled and critically evaluated the results of 11 previous separate investigations regarding the long-term progression of occupational NIHL, after controlling for methodological differences between the studies. The majority of these studies had taken place prior to the advent of hearing protection. The types of noise exposure included factories and industries such as mines, shipyards, forges, weaving mills (Figure 4.4) and others, as well as hunting and artillery. Hearing deterioration was first noted at 4–6 kHz and similar hearing thresholds between 3 and 8 kHz after 30–40 years of noise exposure were reported by nearly all the reviewed studies. However, there was a wide range of hearing thresholds at 1 and 2 kHz, which probably reflected the different types of noise exposure in the different studies. Rösler applied the ISO 1999 age-corrected hearing thresholds to the data of these studies and concluded that the noise effect on hearing is initially quite dominant, with the ageing effect just noticeable in the high frequencies. However, the ARHL and NIHL audiological patterns become more difficult to distinguish at the age of 35–40 years, whereas at ages over 45–50 years the addition to the hearing loss due to continued noise exposure will be minimal, and even less than the hearing loss component due to normal ageing. It is thus difficult to ascribe the hearing loss to either noise or ageing, when hearing thresholds exceed 50 dB.

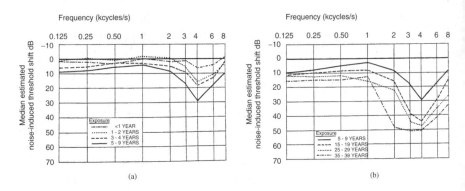

**Figure 4.4** Median estimated noise-induced threshold shift in decibels after different durations of noise exposure in jute weavers. (From Taylor et al. (1965), with many thanks to Professor William Burns.)

Henderson and Saunders (1998) assessed the rate of growth of NIHL in 500 workers randomly selected from 5000 who were compensated for hearing loss by a railroad company. The average thresholds were corrected with ISO 1999 Annex B, averaged as a function of years on the job, and the resulting curves were compared with predictions based on the ISO 1999 data. Hearing at hire was worse than ISO norms, and early NIHL was as a result under-estimated by the ISO predictions. However, the rate of growth of hearing loss after long-term exposure was consistent with that predicted from ISO 1999. A subgroup of workers with a pre-existing hearing loss when first employed showed a flatter growth of hearing loss (they acquired further hearing loss more slowly) than the rest of the group or the ISO 1999 projection. Their hearing loss growth curve was better aligned with comparable data from later years for the general population. However, there were only sufficient data to examine the evolution of hearing loss over 10–14 years on the job for hearing-impaired workers.

Gates et al. (2000) used data from longitudinal studies on hearing of the Framingham Heart study cohort in order to determine whether the mean age-adjusted auditory thresholds in male ears with evidence of noise damage show the same changes over 15 years as those in ears with no noise damage. The classification in the noise versus no noise groups was based on the presence or not of an audiometric high-frequency notch, as there was no documentation of previous noise exposure. They found that, over a 15-year span, and in people aged 58–83 years at the first hearing test and 72–95 at the second test, ears with an audiometric notch had a reduced rate of threshold change in the notch frequencies (3–6 kHz). This is consistent with the negative (saturating) interaction of ISO 1999. However, ears with a deep notch had accelerated threshold deterioration in the adjacent frequencies (2 and 8 kHz) of the notch than ears with no notch. They suggested that the effects of noise damage may continue long after noise exposure has ceased, presumably due to changes of cochlear structure or function that foster continuing deterioration of hearing sensitivity in the areas of the cochlea adjacent to those that have been damaged by noise. This type of interaction is not represented in ISO 1999, nor in any other predictive formula. However, there were several caveats in this study. A deep audiometric notch was interpreted as evidence for NIHL without documenting the noise exposure history of the subject. In addition, the authors did not establish whether noise exposure had ceased over the 15 years of the study.

# Conclusions: a conceptual model of the accumulating effects of age and noise

Current research indicates that the interaction of NIHL and ARHL is influenced at least in part by genetic factors and it is likely that more than one gene determines the susceptibility to ARHL, NIHL or both. Acoustic factors of the noise seem to affect different age groups in different ways, while the early stages of NIHL deterioration with age will have some characteristics different from ARHL in the previously normal hearing population. However, the end result in the geriatric population may well be the same, regardless of acoustic factors of the noise or the initial hearing thresholds.

A conceptual model of the accumulating effects of age and noise may thus arise from current scientific knowledge. This model would suggest that, for the initial stages of noise- and/or age-related damage, the resulting physiological changes (such as hair cell loss) will be minor and will have no effect on hearing threshold levels (HTLs). This dissociation between physiological changes and behavioural correlates is due to intrinsic redundancy, which allows for considerable damage to be sustained without affecting hearing thresholds. Eventually, the redundancy margin is exceeded and hearing thresholds start to deteriorate. The margin may be reached due to effects of age or noise or combined effects of age and noise, as each agent in isolation may be insufficient to cause any measurable hearing loss. Therefore, prior effects of either agent (with or without change in hearing thresholds) increase susceptibility to the same agent or the other agent, by removing the redundancy margin. Once this margin is lost, noise and age may be additive until a point is reached where the addition starts to saturate due to all OHCs having been lost or to the cochlear amplifier gain being reduced to zero.

The consequence of the above model is that the following pattern should be expected:

1. Superadditivity until mild loss is sustained and for mild losses.
2. Additivity for mild-to-moderate losses.
3. Less-than-complete additivity for moderate losses.

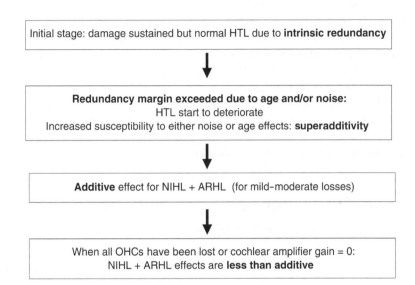

**Figure 4.5** Conceptual model of the accumulating effects of age and noise. ARHL, age-related hearing loss; HTL, hearing threshold level; NIHL, noise-induced hearing loss; OHC, outer cell hair.

This model remains to be evaluated. Some of the questions that remain unanswered include the exact genes and the mechanism that underlie ARHL and NIHL in humans, and the susceptibility to noise in the existence of various genetic conditions that affect hearing directly or indirectly. In addition, while both NIHL and ARHL are predominantly described and for medicolegal purposes quantified in terms of hearing thresholds, both forms of hearing loss have central auditory aspects, which have a major impact on the patient-reported disability. However, these central aspects are not well understood in terms of the pathophysiological mechanism, nor are they efficiently assessed by our current testing battery. Clearly, future research that targets these issues could facilitate potential pharmacological treatment or prevention of age- and noise-related hearing loss and rehabilitation of the associated disability.

# References

Attias J, Furst M, Furman V, Reshef I, Horowitz G, Bresloff I (1995) Noise-induced otoacoustic emission loss with or without hearing loss. Ear and Hearing 16: 612–18.

Barrenas ML (1997) Hair cell loss from acoustic trauma in chloroquine-treated red, black and albino guinea pigs. Audiology 36: 187–201.

Boettcher FA (2002) Susceptibility to acoustic trauma in young and aged gerbils. Journal of the Acoustical Society of America 112: 2948–55.

Christensen K, Frederiksen H, Hoffman HJ (2001) Genetic and environmental influences on self-reported reduced hearing in the old and oldest old. Journal of the American Geriatrics Society 49: 1512–17.

Coles RR, Lutman ME, Buffin JT (2000) Guidelines on the diagnosis of noise-induced hearing loss for medicolegal purposes. Clinical Otolaryngology 25: 264–73.

Cooper JC, Owen JH (1976) Audiometric profile of noise induced hearing loss. Archives of Otolaryngology 102: 148–50.

Daniell WE, Fulton-Kehoe D, Smith-Weller T, Franklin GM (1998) Occupational hearing loss in Washington state, 1984–1991: II. Morbidity and associated costs. American Journal of Industrial Medicine 33(6): 529–36.

Davis A (1995) Hearing in Adults. London: Whurr Publishers.

Davies H, Morgan CT., Hawkins JEJ, Galambos R and Smith FW (1950). Temporary deafness following exposure to loud tones and noise. Acta Otolaryngology Suppl, 88, pp. 1–56.

Davis RR, Cheever ML, Krieg EF, Erway LC (1999) Quantitative measure of genetic differences in susceptibility to noise-induced hearing loss in two strains of mice. Hearing Research 134(1–2): 9–15.

Davis RR, Newlander JK, Ling X, Cortopassi GA, Krieg EF, Erway LC (2001) Genetic basis for susceptibility to noise-induced hearing loss in mice. Hearing Research 155 (1–2): 82–90.

Divenyi PL, Simon HJ (1999) Hearing in aging: issues old and young. Current Opinion in Otolaryngology, Head and Neck Surgery 7: 282–9.

Dobie RA (1996) Estimation of occupational contribution to hearing handicap. In A Axelsson, H Borchgrevink, RP Hamernik, PA Hellstrom, RJ Salvi (eds) Scientific Basis of Noise-induced Hearing Loss. New York: Thième.

Erway LC, Willott JF (1996) Genetic susceptibility to noise induced hearing loss in mice. In A Axelsson, H Borchgrevink, RP Hamernik, PA Hellstrom, RJ Salvi (eds) Scientific Basis of Noise-induced Hearing Loss. New York: Thième.

Erway LC, Willott JF, Cook SA, Johnson KR, Davisson MT (1995) Segregation of genes for age-related hearing loss from C57Bl/6J and DBA/2J inbred mice. ARO midwinter meeting, abstract 548.

Gates GA, Couropmitree NN, Myers RH (1999) Genetic associations in age-related hearing loss. Archives of Otolaryngology, Head and Neck Surgery 125: 654–9.

Gates GA, Schmid P, Kujawa SG, Byung-ho N, D'Agostino R (2000) Longitudinal threshold changes in older men with audiometric notches. Hearing Research 141: 220–8.

Gates GA, Mills D, Nahm BH, D'Agostino R, Rubel EW (2002) Effects of age on the distortion product otoacoustic emission growth functions. Hearing Research 163(1-2): 53–60.

Glorig A, Nixon J (1960) Distributuion of hearing loss in various populations. Annals of Otology, Rhinology and Laryngology 69: 497–516.

Grayson JK (1992) Previous hearing loss and susceptibility to future permanent threshold shifts. Military Medicine 157(5): 248–9.

Hamernik RP, Patterson JH, Turrentin GA, Ahroon WA (1989) The quantitative relation between sensory cell loss and hearing thresholds. Hearing Research 38: 199–211.

Hamernik RP, Qiu W, Davis B (2003) Cochlear toughening, protection, and potentiation of noise-induced trauma by non-Gaussian noise. Journal of the Acoustical Society of America 113: 969–76.

Hedin CA (1991) Smoker's melanosis may explain the lower hearing loss and lower frequency of Parkinson's disease found among tobacco smokers – a new hypothesis. Medical Hypotheses 35: 247–9.

Henderson D, Hamernik RP (1986) Impulse noise: critical review. Journal of the Acoustical Society of America 80: 569–84.

Henderson D, Hamernik RP (1995) Biologic bases of noise-induced hearing loss. Occupational Medicine 10: 513–34.

Henderson D, Saunders SS (1998) Acquisition of noise-induced hearing loss by railway workers. Ear and Hearing 19:120–30.

Hu BH, Henderson D, Nicotera TM (2002) Involvement of apoptosis in progression of cochlear lesion following exposure to intense noise. Hearing Research 166: 62–71.

International Organization for Standardization (1990) ISO 1999. Acoustics–Determination of Occupational Noise Exposure and Estimation of Noise-induced Hearing Impairment. Geneva: ISO.

Jerger J, Chmiel R, Stach B, Spretnjak M (1993) Gender affects audiometric shape in presbyacusis. Journal of the American Academy of Audiology 4: 42–9.

Johnson KR, Zheng QY, Erway LC (2000) A major gene affecting age-related hearing loss is common to at least ten inbred strains of mice. Genomics 70: 171–80.

Johnson KR, Zheng QY, Bykhovskaya Y, Spirina O, Fischel-Ghodsian N (2001) A nuclear-mitochondrial DNA interaction affecting hearing impairment in mice. Nature and Genetics 27: 191–4.

Kapur YP, Patt AJ (1967) Hearing in Todas of South India. Archives of Otolaryngology 85: 400–6.

Khaw KT (1997) Healthy aging. British Medical Journal 315: 1090–6.

Kirkwood TBL, Wolff SP (1995) The biological basis of ageing. Age and Ageing 24: 167–71.

Kryter KD (1983) Presbyacusis, sociocusis and nosocusis. Journal of the Acoustical Society of America 1897–916.

Li HS (1992) Genetic influences on susceptibility of the auditory system to aging and environmental factors. Scandinavian Audiology Supplementum 36: 1–39.

Lutman ME, Qasem HYN (1998) A source of audiometric notches at 6 kHz. In D Prasher, LM Luxon (eds) Advances in Noise Research, Volume I. Biological Effects of Noise London: Whurr, 170–6.

Lutman ME, Spencer HS (1991) Occupational noise and demographic factors in hearing. Acta Otolaryngologica Supplementum 476: 74–84.

Macrae JH (1991) Presbyacusis and noise-induced permanent threshold shift. Journal of the Acoustical Society of America 90: 2513–16.

McBride D, Williams S (2001) Audiometric notch as a sign of noise induced hearing loss. Occupational and Environmental Medicine 58: 46–51.

McFadden SL, Campo P (1998) Cubic distortion products otoacoustic emissions in young and aged chinchillas exposed to low frequency noise. Journal of the Acoustical Society of America 104: 2290–7.

McFadden SL, Campo P, Ding D, Quaranta N (1998) Effects of noise on inferior colliculus evoked potentials and cochlear anatomy in young and aged chinchillas. Hearing Research 117(1–2): 81–96.

Mills JH, Lee FS, Dubno JR, Boettcher FA (1996) Interactions between age-related and noise-induced hearing loss. In A Axelsson, H Borchgrevink , RP Hamernik, PA Hellstrom, RJ Salvi (eds) Scientific Basis of Noise-induced Hearing Loss. New York: Thième.

Mills JH, Boettcher FA, Dubno JR (1997) Interaction of noise-induced permanent threshold shift and age-related threshold shift. Journal of the Acoustical Society of America 101: 1681–6.

Mills JH, Dubno JR, Boettcher FA (1998) Interaction of noise-induced hearing loss and presbyacusis. Scandinavian Audiology. Supplementum 48: 117–22.

Morrell CH, Gordon-Salant S, Pearson JD, Brant LJ, Fozard JL (1996) Age-and gender-specific reference ranges for hearing level and longitudinal changes in hearing level. Journal of the Acoustical Society of America 100: 1949–67.

National Statistics on line. UK Census 2001: www.statistics.gov.uk/census2001/default.asp

Oeken J, Lenk A, Bootz F (2000) Influence of age and presbyacusis on DPOAE. Acta Oto-Laryngologica 120: 396–403.

OMIM (Online Mendelian Inheritance in Man), Johns Hopkins University 2002. www.ncbi.nlm.nih.gov/entry/query.fcgi? db = OMIM.

Palmer KT, Griffin MJ, Syddall HE, Davis A, Pannett B, Coggon D (2002) Occupational exposure to noise and the attributable burden of hearing difficulties in Great Britain. Occupational and Environmental Medicine 59: 634–9.

Pearson JD, Morrell CH, Gordon-Salant S, Brandt LJ, Metter EJ, Klein LL, Fozard JL (1995) Gender differences in a longitudinal study of age-associated hearing loss. Journal of the Acoustical Society of America 97: 1196–205.

Pyykkö I, Koskimies K, Starck J, Pekkarinen J, Inaba R (1989) Risk factors in the genesis of sensory neural hearing loss in Finnish forestry workers. British Journal of Internal Medicine 46: 439–46.

Pyykkö I, Starck J, Toppila E, Kaksonen R (1998) Ageing as a major confounding factor in noise-induced hearing loss. In D Prasher, L Luxon (eds) Advances in Noise Research, Volume 1. Biological Effects of Noise. London: Whurr.

Quaranta N, Debole S, Di Girolamo N (2001) Effect of ageing on otoacoustic emissions and efferent suppression in humans. Audiology 40: 308–12.

Rosenhall U, Pedersen K, Svanborg A (1990) Presbycusis and noise-induced hearing loss. Ear and Hearing 11: 257–63.

Rosenhall U, Sixt E, Sundh V, Svanborg A (1993) Correlations between presbycusis and extrinsic noxious factors. Audiology 32: 234–43.

Rösler G (1994) Progression of hearing loss caused by occupational noise. Scandinavian Audiology 23: 13–37.

Ryan AF, Axelsson GA, Woolf NK (1992) Central auditory metabolic activity induced by intense noise exposure. Hearing Research 61(1–2): 24–30.

Salvi RJ, Ding D, Eddins AC, McFadden SL, Henderson D (2001) Age, noise and ototoxic agents. In P Hof, C Mobbs (eds) Functional Neurobiology of Aging. San Diego, CA: Academic Press.

Schuknecht HF, Gacek MR (1993) Cochlear pathology in presbycusis. Annals of Otology, Rhinology and Laryngology 102: 1–16.

Seidman MD, Bai U, Khan MJ, Murphy MP, Quirk WS, Castora FJ, Hinojosa R (1996) Association of mitochondrial DNA deletions and cochlear pathology: a molecular biologic tool. Laryngoscope 106: 777–83.

Seidman MD, Bai U, Khan MJ, Quirk WS (1997) Mitochondrial DNA Deletions Associated With Aging and Presbyacusis. Archives of Otolaryngology, Head and Neck Surgery 123:1039–45.

Seidman MD, Khan MJ, Bai U, Shirwany N, Quirk WS (2000) Biological activity of mitochondrial metabolites on aging and age-related hearing loss. American Journal of Otology 21: 161–7.

Shone G, Altschuler RA, Miller JM, Nuttall AL (1991) The effect of noise exposure on the aging ear. Hearing Research 56: 173–8.

Sucek S, Michaels L, Frohlich A (1987) Pathological changes in the organ of Corti in presbyacusis as revealed by microslicing and staining. Acta Otolaryngologica Supplementum 436: 93–102.

Taylor J, Pearson J, Mair A, Burns W (1965) Study of noise and hearing in jute weaving. Journal of the Acoustical Society of America 38: 113–20.

Wang J, Ding D, Salvi RJ (2002) Functional reorganization in chinchilla inferior colliculus associated with chronic and acute cochlear damage. Hearing Research 168(1–2): 238–49.

Willott JF (1996) Anatomic and physiologic aging: a behavioral neuroscience perspective. Journal of the American Academy of Audiology 7(3): 141–51.

Yoshida N, Hequembourg SJ, Atencio CA, Rosowski JJ, Liberman MC (2000) Acoustic injury in mice: 129/SvEv is exceptionally resistant to noise-induced hearing loss. Hearing Research 141: 97–106.

Zheng QY, Johnson KR (2001) Hearing loss associated with the modifier of deaf waddler (mdfw) locus corresponds with age-related hearing loss in 12 inbred strains of mice. Hearing Research 154: 45–53.

# CHAPTER 5

# Cochlear pathophysiology in response to hazardous noise

*Noise and Its Effects:* Edited by Linda Luxon and Deepak Prasher © 2007
John Wiley & Sons Ltd.

CAROLE M HACKNEY, DAVID N FURNESS

## Introduction

Our sense of hearing depends on the hair cells of the organ of Corti converting the mechanical vibrations set up by sound in the cochlea into neural signals that are sent to the brain along the auditory portion of the vestibulocochlear nerve. These hair cells can detect vibrations down to atomic dimensions and in young humans can respond to frequencies up to 20 kHz (see review by Fettiplace, 2002). That such a sensitive mechanism might be damaged by overstimulation is no surprise. What is more remarkable is the intensity range over which the cochlea normally operates without being damaged. Intense noise can cause temporary (TTS) and/or permanent threshold shifts (PTS) and thus hearing loss. However, the most intense sound that can be heard without damaging the ears is about 120 dB above the faintest sound that can be detected, a ratio of intensities of $10^{12}:1$ (see Moore, 1995, for further details). This great range implies that active mechanisms exist both to protect the hair cells and other cochlear structures from the effects of noise and to minimize noise-induced damage when loud sounds are heard. There are likely to be several different processes involved in protecting cochlear structures from damage; indeed, TTS may itself be a protective mechanism (Altschuler et al., 1999). Understanding these processes might lead to better strategies for preventing or reducing damage to the hair cells when accidental exposure to high-intensity sounds occurs. This is especially important because cochlear hair cells in humans like those in other mammals cannot regenerate so their destruction leads to permanent hearing loss (see review by Stone and Rubel, 2000). It has been demonstrated that a PTS involves structural modifications of the cochlear sensory epithelium with losses of the hair cells and auditory neurons in particular (Nordmann, Bohne and Harding, 2000). Under these circumstances, the effectiveness of devices such as cochlear implants that could be used to restore hearing by stimulating cochlear nerve afferents is bound to be less.

It is therefore important to understand how and why high-intensity sounds cause hair cell loss and also damage other cochlear structures. In this chapter, the cytoarchitecture of the sensory epithelium of the cochlea, the organ of Corti, and its innervation will be described and some of the effects of high-intensity noise on their integrity discussed.

## Functional anatomy of the cochlea

The mammalian cochlea consists of a coiled bone-covered canal containing the organ of Corti spiralling round a central bony axis or modiolus (Figure 5.1). At its base are two openings that are covered by flexible membranes,

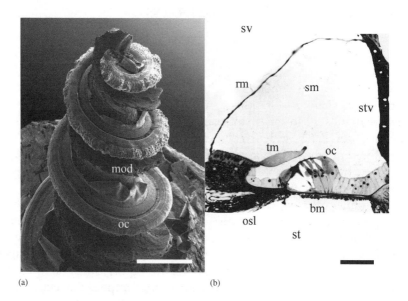

(a)                                                                         (b)

**Figure 5.1** Gross anatomy of the cochlea and cochlear partition. (a) The mammalian cochlea consists of a coiled bone-covered canal spiralling round a central bony axis or modiolus (mod). (b) The canal is divided along its length into three chambers, the scala tympani (st), scala vestibuli (sv) and scala media (sm), except at the very apex where the scala tympani and scala vestibuli are in continuity via an opening called the helicotrema. The scala media is the central chamber, its lower boundary formed by the osseous spiral lamina (osl), projecting from the modiolus, and basilar membrane (bm), its upper boundary formed by Reissner's membrane (rm) which projects obliquely from the spiral limbus on the osseus spiral lamina and its lateral wall formed by a capillary bed, the stria vascularis (stv) to either side of which the basilar membrane and Reissner's membrane attach. The organ of Corti (oc) lies on the basilar membrane with the tectorial membrane (tm) lying above its upper surface, the reticular lamina. Low-frequency sounds cause maximum deflection of the basilar membrane towards the apex of the cochlea where it is wider and more flexible and high-frequency sounds deflect it more towards the base where it is narrower and stiffer (Békésy, 1960). (Note that in (a) the stria vascularis and Reissner's membrane have been removed to show the organ of Corti.) Scale bars: (a) = 0.5 mm, (b) = 100 $\mu$m.

the oval window and the round window. The oval window membrane bears the footplate of the stapes, the last in the chain of middle-ear ossicles that deliver the vibrations set up by sound in the tympanic membrane to the fluids of the inner ear. The round window membrane conversely serves to release the pressure variations (see review by Wilson, 1987).

The organ of Corti consists of a sheet of epithelial cells that sits on the basilar membrane within the scala media (Figure 5.1b). It contains the sensory hair cells and the supporting cells that surround them (see review by Lim, 1986). The organ of Corti is divided into an inner and outer portion by one category of supporting cells, the pillar cells. The bases of these are attached to the basilar membrane and the upper portions overlap thus forming the tunnel of Corti. On the modiolar side of the tunnel is a single row of about 3500 inner hair cells (IHCs) and on the strial side are three (sometimes four) rows of about 12 000 outer hair cells (OHCs). The cell bodies of the IHCs are flask shaped whereas those of the OHCs are cylindrical. Adjacent to the IHCs are the inner phalangeal and border cells and lying between the OHCs and spiral ligament, which attaches the basilar membrane to the outer wall of the cochlea, are further supporting cells including Hensen's cells and Claudius' cells. The base of each OHC is located in a cup-shaped Deiter's cell which also extends a thin phalangeal process diagonally up between the hair cells. The heads of these phalanges, the phalanges of the outer pillar cells, and the apices of the inner pillar cells, other supporting cells and the hair cells are all connected

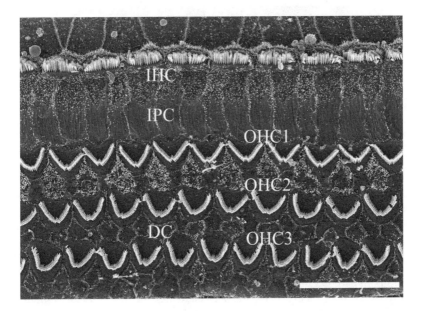

**Figure 5.2** Scanning electron micrograph of the reticular lamina showing the apices of one row of inner (IHC) and three rows of outer (OHC1–3) hair cells, inner pillar cells (IPC) and Deiter's cells (DC). Scale bar = 25 μm.

by tight junctions (Figure 5.2). This network of cell apices forms the reticular lamina, a highly impermeable barrier to the passage of ions except via the mechanotransduction channels of the hair cells when they are opened by deflection of their hair bundles (Figure 5.3). The phalangeal processes are important because if hair cells are lost through trauma caused, for example, by excessive noise, the phalanges expand rapidly to fill the gap and restore the integrity of the reticular lamina (see, for example, Ahmad, Bohne and Harding, 2003).

The upper portion of both types of hair cell contains a fibrous structure, the cuticular plate, from which project several rows of modified microvilli called stereocilia. The OHCs usually have three rows of stereocilia arranged in a pronounced V or W shape whilst the IHCs tend to have more than three rows arranged in a more linear formation (Figure 5.2).

*scala media:* 150 mM $K^+$, 1 mM $Na^+$, 0.02 mM $Ca^{++}$

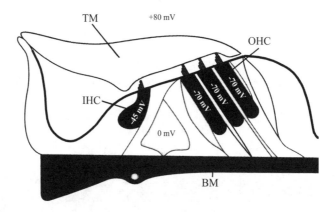

*scala tympani:* 5 mM $K^+$, 140 mM $Na^+$, 2 mM $Ca^{++}$

**Figure 5.3** Electrochemical organization of the cochlea. The reticular lamina (dark line running along hair cell and supporting cell apices) below the tectorial membrane (TM) and Reissner's membrane act as diffusion barriers, whereas the basilar membrane (BM) does not. The scala media thus provides a special ionic environment into which the stereocilia project. It contains endolymph, a fluid similar in composition to intracellular fluid in that its principal cation is $K^+$ (Johnstone and Sellick, 1972). It also contains a low concentration of $Ca^{2+}$, around 30 $\mu$mol/l in mammals (Bosher and Warren, 1978). The scala vestibuli and the scala tympani contain perilymph, a fluid that has the same composition as cerebrospinal fluid and whose principal cation is $Na^+$. The helicotrema allows free mixing of perilymph in the two outer scalae. The electrochemical differences thus established result in a potential in the scala media that is about 80 mV more positive than that of the scala tympani, whereas the inner (IHC) and outer (OHC) hair cells both have negative membrane potentials (as indicated), thus producing a large driving force for cations across the hair-cell membrane (Davis, 1958). It has been proposed that the high $K^+$ concentration and positive endolymphatic potential are due to active secretion of $K^+$ and uptake of $Na^+$ by the marginal cells of the stria vascularis (Johnstone and Sellick, 1972).

Stereocilia contain actin filaments densely packed in a paracrystalline array (Flock and Cheung, 1977) which are held in stiff bundles by various actin-bundling proteins including fimbrin. In the narrow ankle region at the base of each stereocilium, a dense rootlet runs into the cuticular plate. This is the point that the stereocilium pivots about as it is deflected towards or away from the modiolus as the basilar membrane and tectorial membrane shear past each other. It also appears to be the point where they are most likely to fracture if deflected too far as can happen when the cochlea is exposed to intense sound (Liberman, 1987) (Figure 5.4).

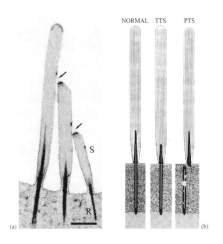

**Figure 5.4** (a) Transmission electron micrograph of the apex of a hair cell showing the stereocilia (S) arranged in three rows of decreasing height, each with a dense rootlet (R) and connected by tip links (arrows). Scale bar = 0.5 $\mu$m. (Courtesy of Y Katori. Department of Otolaryngology and Head and Neck Surgery, Tohoku University, Japan.) (b) Diagrammatic representation of the effects of temporary (TTS) and permanent (PTS) threshold shift on the structure of stereocilia and their rootlets. Note that in TTS rootlets may be shortened and in PTS they may fracture. (Adapted from Liberman (1987) and Liberman and Dodds (1987).)

The stereocilia on both IHCs and OHCs are linked together by extracellular filaments that run laterally between them. Strands also run from the apices of the shorter stereocilia to the sides of the taller stereocilia in the row behind (Figure 5.4). These strands have been called tip links and have been proposed to open cationic channels in the tips of the stereocilia as tension is placed on the links by deflections of the hair bundle towards the tallest row of stereocilia (Pickles, Comis and Osborne, 1984). This model for mechanotransduction is not the only one but it is clear that deflection of the hair bundle acts directly as a gate to the opening of the channels (see review by Hackney and Furness, 1995). The mechanotransduction channels are permeable to small cations such as sodium and potassium. Because of the difference in the concentration of potassium ions in the endolymph and perilymph (Figure 5.3), the majority of the mechanotransduction current is carried by these ions entering through the stereociliary bundle and leaving via other types of potassium channel in their basolateral membranes. However, the mechanotransduction channels are also very permeable to calcium ions (Ricci and Fettiplace, 1998) so when they are opened, calcium ions enter too. These ions play an important role in adaptation, the process that rapidly reduces the sensitivity of the hair cells when they are stimulated (see review by Fettiplace, Ricci and Hackney, 2002). Once they have entered the cell, calcium ions block the mechanotransduction channels leading to the rapid adaptation to deflection of the stereociliary bundle that is seen in recordings of the mechanotransducer current (Crawford, Evans and Fettiplace, 1989, 1991). Calcium ions are also thought to interact with cytoskeletal proteins within the stereocilia that reset the bundle position somewhat more slowly, possibly by changing tension in the links between them (Howard and Hudspeth, 1987). Controlling the level of intracellular calcium is crucial to the function of the sensory hair cells. They therefore contain calcium-buffering proteins to chelate incoming calcium (see, for example, Hackney et al., 2003) and their stereociliary membranes contain a high density of calcium pumps to remove it from the cell (Yamoah et al., 1998). They also contain calcium stores such as mitochondria and cisternae to sequester calcium ions. If these mechanisms are overwhelmed or rendered dysfunctional in any way, the hair cells become overloaded with calcium and start to die. Excessive entry of calcium through the mechanotransduction channels may occur during overstimulation of the hair cells by high-intensity sounds.

Just below the plasma membrane of the hair cells lies a layer of smooth endoplasmic reticulum or a subsurface cistern. The OHCs generally contain more stacks of cisternae than the IHCs with the longer OHCs of the cochlear apex containing the most cisternal layers (Furness and Hackney, 1990). The outer cisternal layer is connected to the plasma membrane by regularly spaced pillars lying along actin filaments that run in the gap between the two. OHCs lengthen and shorten when electrically stimulated (Brownell et al., 1985) and it has been suggested that these subsurface cisternae mediate shape changes by binding or releasing calcium as in the sarcoplasmic reticulum of muscle. However, OHCs have been observed to contract at rates that are far faster than can be accounted for by a conventional actomyosin system. Recently their lateral membranes have been discovered to contain a high concentration of a protein called prestin that changes shape rapidly in response to changes in the electric field (Zheng et al., 2000). Length or tension changes by the OHCs have been proposed to account for the narrow frequency selectivity that is observed both psychophysically and in the mechanics of the living basilar membrane. It is believed that the OHCs augment the vibrations of the basilar membrane locally by supplying extra energy to the points at which it is being stimulated by sounds. Altering the energetic contribution of the OHCs themselves may be one way in which the organ of Corti protects itself from overstimulation.

Overlying the hair cells is the tectorial membrane, an acellular gelatinous flap that projects from the spiral limbus. It is composed of three classes of collagens (types II, V and IX) interspersed with glycoproteins called tectorins (for review, see Goodyear and Richardson, 2002). The interdental cells embedded in the spiral limbus probably secrete at least some of the components of the tectorial membrane. The tectorial membrane is important because it is the relative movements of the basilar membrane and the tectorial membrane as they vibrate that ultimately stimulate the sensory hair cells. The tips of the tallest row of stereocilia appear to be embedded in the underside of the tectorial membrane as judged by the corresponding position of the imprints observed there (Figure 5.5) and the ease with which their stereociliary bundles are disturbed or damaged by removal of the tectorial membrane. There is less evidence that the IHC stereocilia are

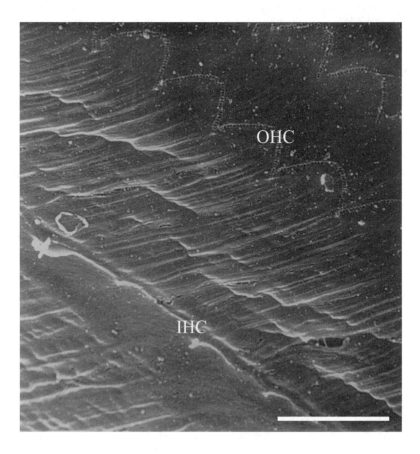

**Figure 5.5** Scanning electron micrograph of the underside of the tectorial membrane showing imprints of the outer hair cell (OHC) stereocilia and bow-shaped indentations corresponding to the position of the inner hair cell (IHC) stereocilia. Scale bar = 10 $\mu$m.

attached to the tectorial membrane although, in some species, shallow indentations are seen that may correspond with their position (Figure 5.5). In other species, it has been suggested that they may interact via Hensen's stripe, a ridge or protrusion that runs along its underside just above their bundles. It is unknown whether the properties of the tectorial membrane change during overstimulation of the cochlea but alterations in its stiffness or position would be another way in which the hair bundles could potentially be protected from damage.

## Cochlear innervation

The innervation of the two types of cochlear hair cell differs very markedly. Each IHC is contacted by up to 20 radial fibres that are the peripheral processes of sensory neurons called type I spiral ganglion cells whose cell bodies lie just within the modiolus (see review by Spoendlin, 1972). The OHCs, on the other hand, are contacted by outer spiral fibres that are the peripheral processes of type II spiral ganglion cells. Each outer spiral fibre contacts up to 10 OHCs. This innervation pattern means that the vast majority of the afferent fibres in the auditory portion of the vestibulo-cochlear nerve carry signals from IHCs rather than OHCs (Figure 5.6).

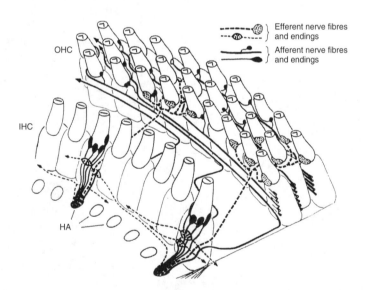

**Figure 5.6** Diagram showing the innervation of the organ of Corti. About 90% of afferent auditory nerve fibres contact inner hair cells (IHCs), with up to 20 terminating on a single hair cell (large black endings), whereas the remaining afferents branch and contact several outer hair cells (OHCs) (small black endings). In contrast, most efferents terminate on OHCs (stippled endings) with a few contacting the afferents beneath the IHCs. The nerve fibres run to and from the auditory nerve to the organ of Corti via openings in the habenula perforata (HA). (Adapted from Spoendlin (1967).)

The axons from both types of spiral ganglion cell run down the centre of the cochlea within the bony modiolus. The nerve fibres from the hair cells at the apex of the cochlea that respond best to low frequencies run in the centre of the bundle whilst those from hair cells towards the base of the cochlea that respond best to high frequencies, run down the outside. The axons of type I spiral ganglion cells from the IHCs are thicker and myelinated and are the ones from which microelectrode recordings are usually obtained. In fact, very little is known about what the unmyelinated axons of the type II spiral ganglion cells signal from the OHCs to the brain because it is so difficult to record from them. The only recordings that have been made from them suggest that they respond to very loud sounds (see Brown, 1993, for a review). Various lines of evidence suggest that the major neurotransmitter at the afferent synapse in both the IHCs and OHCs is the excitatory amino acid glutamate (see Furness and Lehre, 1997; Furness et al., 2002 for more details). In addition to carrying afferent fibres *to* the brain stem, the vestibulocochlear nerve contains efferent axons running *from* it to the cochlea.

These efferent nerve fibres come from periolivary nerve cells around the superior olivary complex and form the olivocochlear bundle. Most of the axons in the bundle contact the OHCs (see, for example, Dallos, 1992) and are the large-diameter myelinated axons of the medial olivocochlear neurons from the contralateral superior olivary complex. They form the crossed olivocochlear bundle and the tunnel radial fibres synapsing directly with the OHCs (Figure 5.6) are predominantly cholinergic. Since the electromotile response of OHCs is known to be affected by acetylcholine (Dallos et al., 1997) and changes in the level of intracellular calcium (Szönyi et al., 2001), it seems likely that the role of the tunnel radial fibres is to control their length or stiffness. The olivocochlear bundle also contains the small unmyelinated axons of lateral olivocochlear neurons from the ipsilateral superior olivary complex. These fibres innervate the type I dendrites rather than the IHCs themselves and must therefore affect the signals being sent by the IHCs postsynaptically.

In fact, only 10% or so of the axons in the cochlear nerve are efferents but they are important for auditory discrimination in noise. Stimulation of the olivocochlear bundle reduces firing in the cochlear nerve (Wiederhold and Kiang, 1970), decreasing cochlear mechanical responses to low level sound (Dolan and Nuttall, 1988; Murugasu and Russell, 1996) mainly by dampening the amplification produced by the OHCs (Dallos, 1992). In other words, sound signals in the cochlear nerve result in feedback via the olivocochlear bundle that reduces cochlear sensitivity in a frequency-specific way. This efferent feedback loop may help protect the ear from very loud sounds but takes several milliseconds to operate because several synapses are involved.

# The effects of noise on the organ of Corti

It has been known for some time that intense sound exposure induces damage occurring initially in the first row of OHCs, then in the IHCs and subsequently in the second and third row of OHCs (Saunders, Dear and Schneider, 1985).

## Causes of OHC degeneration due to noise

- mechanical damage (see, for instance, Spoendlin, 1985);
- metabolic exhaustion (see, for example, Lim and Dunn, 1979);
- ischaemia (see, for example, Hawkins 1971; Quirk and Seidman, 1995);
- generation of free oxygen radicals (see, for example, Yamane et al., 1995; Ohlemiller et al., 1999).

It has been shown previously that OHC pathology affects cochlear sensitivity, tuning and compression whilst IHC pathology primarily affects sensitivity (Liberman and Dodds, 1984). The relationship between TTS and PTS is probably dependent on the extent of the damage to the OHCs, IHCs and their innervation and whether the integrity of the reticular lamina is compromised as hair cells die. Exposure to extremely high-intensity noise (at least 130 dB SPL) is known to cause direct mechanical destruction of the sensory hair cells and supporting cells in the organ of Corti (Hamernik, Turrentine and Wright, 1984) which is probably a result of necrosis. At the extreme, as in the case of damage by impulse noise, the organ of Corti may become detached from the basilar membrane. In contrast, exposure to moderate-intensity noise initiates what appear to be apoptotic processes in the hair cells and auditory neurons which lead to cell death (Pirvola et al., 2000). In fact, in addition to swollen and misshapen hair cells with pyknotic nuclei being observed, subtler changes such as disrupted and damaged stereociliary bundles (Figure 5.7) have been found to be associated with substantial changes in auditory function (Liberman, 1987). This stereociliary disruption has been suggested to be sufficient to account for the majority of the initial acute threshold shift (Liberman and Dodds, 1987) and may initiate other processes in the hair cells that result in apoptosis.

Bohne (1976) and Hamernik and Henderson (1974) found that immediately after the noise exposure (15 minutes to several hours) when hearing loss is greatest, the area of missing OHCs is relatively small. Several days later when hearing sensitivity is recovering, the area of missing OHCs actually grows larger. This suggests that pathological changes continue post-exposure that are not just associated with the initial loss of hair cells. The extent and the type of the damage also appear to depend on cochlear location. For instance, in one study by Bohne and Harding (2000), when chinchillas were exposed to either low-frequency (0.5 kHz) or high-frequency (4 kHz) noise at 47–95 dB SPL for 2–432 days, different

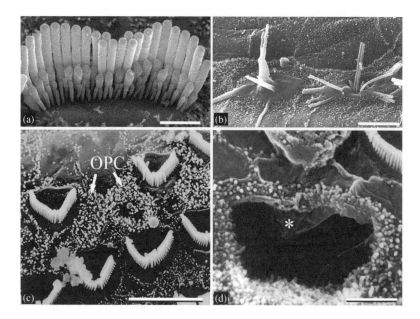

**Figure 5.7** Scanning electron micrographs showing the range of damage to the organ of Corti that can be caused by noise trauma. (a) A normal guinea-pig inner hair cell (IHC) stereociliary bundle showing the precise organization of stereocilia that is seen in an undamaged cochlea. Scale bar = 2 $\mu$m. (b) Two rat IHC bundles with disturbed and fused stereocilia as a result of noise damage caused by 130 dB SPL for 15 min at 6 kHz. (Image courtesy of M Lenoir, INSERM, Montpelier, France.) Scale bar = 5 $\mu$m. (c) A scar in the reticular lamina, formed by expanded apices of outer pillar cells (OPC) replacing a missing outer hair cell. Scale bars = 10 $\mu$m. (d) A hole in the reticular lamina, through which a Deiter's cell process is seen (*). Scale bar = 2 $\mu$m.

patterns of damage were found in different regions of the cochlea. With continued exposure to high-frequency noise, primary damage in the high-frequency region began as focal losses of OHCs. Then, a whole segment of the organ of Corti was lost along with adjacent myelinated nerve fibres. With low-frequency noise, the primary damage in the low-frequency region appeared as scattered OHC losses but the supporting cells, IHCs and nerve fibres remained intact. However, focal lesions also appeared in the basal high-frequency region of the cochlea too. These experimental findings suggest that the high-frequency region of the cochlea is particularly vulnerable to overstimulation of the cochlear partition, even if it is being overstimulated at some other location.

When damaged hair cells degenerate, they are replaced in the reticular lamina by phalangeal scars (Figure 5.7). Depending on the row to which the hair cell belongs, the phalangeal process from two to three Deiter's cells, one to two pillar cells or two inner phalangeal cells enlarge to form the scar (see review by Bohne, 1976). However, this process may not always be fast enough to prevent local mechanical damage from causing more widespread disruption of cochlear function. An in vivo tracer study of noise-induced damage to the reticular lamina recently showed that it can be breached by the rapid loss of hair cells and supporting cells (Figure 5.7) and that the api-cal membranes of the cells themselves may also be disrupted (Ahmad, Bohne and Harding, 2003). The breakdown of the permeability barrier between the scala media and scala tympani would result in the intermixing of cochlear fluids and may partly account for the continuing loss of sensory and supporting cells after the noise has terminated as suggested previously (Bohne and Harding, 2000).

**Causes of disruption of cochlear function after acoustic overstimulation**

- mechanical damage and loss of hair cells;
- breakdown of reticular lamina with intermixing of cochlear fluids;
- exposure to elevated levels of potassium with irreversible damage to OHCs;
- increases in intracellular calcium;
- excess release of excitotoxic neurotransmitters such as glutamate;
- significant decreases in OHC stiffness;
- significant decreases in stiffness of stereociliary bundles.

Exposure to elevated potassium levels depolarizes OHCs and long-term exposure causes them to contract and then to swell, and ultimately dam-ages them irreversibly (Zenner et al., 1994). If the cochlea sustains so much damage that all the sensory and supporting cells in a particular area degenerate, phalangeal scars obviously cannot form. Rather, a squamous epithelial scar replaces the missing organ of Corti and seals off the open ends of tunnel space (Ahmad, Bohne and Harding, 2003). The extent to which cochlear function recovers depends on the extent of the damage to the cochlea but the remaining auditory deficit is not tightly correlated to the total number of hair cells lost but more to the pattern of damage (see, for example, Emmerich et al., 2000).

It has been demonstrated that acoustic overstimulation results in large increases in calcium levels in the intact hearing organ (Fridburger et al., 1998) and that mechanical overstimulation of OHCs results in a signifi-cant increase in intracellular calcium levels (Fridberger and Ulfendahl, 1996). Interestingly, although overstimulation causes contraction of the organ of Corti, isolated cells do not show a length change. Exposure to impulse noise also causes a significant decrease in OHC stiffness (Chan, Sunesen and Ulfendahl, 1998) although in this case shortening of some OHCs has been seen. A calcium-induced loss of cellular stiffness has been proposed (Dallos et al., 1997) so this effect may be the result of excessive calcium entering the OHCs if their stereocilary bundles are damaged. It has also been shown that increased intracellular calcium levels block the regen-eration of tip links once they have been broken (Zhao, Yamoah and

Gillespie, 1996). It is possible that short-term but recoverable effects on hair cell function could occur if the tip links break and the mechano-transduction channels close and they are no longer opened by deflection of the bundle. However, after tip-link loss, large deflections of the bundle still appear to be able to open the channels (Meyer et al., 1998) and, in the case of continuous high-intensity noise, calcium loading of the hair cells might continue despite the breakage of the links.

Acoustic overstimulation both in vivo (Canlon et al., 1986) and in vitro (Saunders, Canlon and Flock, 1986) causes a reduction in the stiffness of stereociliary bundles. Pure-tone stimulation has been reported to change the micromechanical properties of the IHC stereocilia (Canlon et al., 1986) and ultrastructural studies have shown that noise-induced stereo-ciliary damage is associated with degeneration–depolymerization of the rootlet, which anchors stereocilia into the cuticular plate (Liberman, 1987). Such changes might result from the changes in the organization of the actin filament array that have also been noted to occur following noise damage (Saunders, Canlon and Flock, 1986). F-actin is particularly rele-vant to hearing and acoustic injury because it is a major protein of stereocilia and the cuticular plate into which they insert (Raphael et al., 1994) and a range of other cytoskeletal proteins involved in the develop-ment and subsequent function of the stereocilia is associated with the actin filaments (Frolenkov et al., 2004). In this respect, it is of interest to note the changes that have been reported in the expression of various heat shock proteins (hsps) in the hair cells after noise exposure, some of which are confined to the stereocilia (Lim et al., 1993).

Heat shock proteins are present in cells under normal conditions; they act as molecular chaperones ensuring that new or distorted proteins fold into the right shape. They are also involved in protein transport during cytoskeletal assembly and disassembly. Protein-damaging stresses result in their increased expression (Mosser et al., 2000), an adaptive change that can improve the cell's ability to tolerate normally lethal conditions. Upregulation of cochlear hsp70 after heat stress or noise exposure has been reported in the rat (Lim et al., 1993) and guinea pig (Thompson and Neely, 1992; Akizuki et al., 1995). It has also been shown that upregulation of hsps by TTS coincides with protection from a second noise exposure (Altschuler et al., 1999). A smaller protein, hsp27, has been found in the cuticular plate and lateral wall of the rat cochlea (Leonova et al., 2002). This hsp is known to bind to actin (Miron et al., 1991) which may provide a clue to one potential role of hsps in cochlear protection. Although its role as a molecular chaperone is similar to other hsps (Jakob et al., 1993), it associates specifically with F-actin filaments and controls their polymer-ization and depolymerization (Lavoie et al., 1993, 1995), a process that is likely to be ongoing in the stereocilia at all times (Schneider et al., 2002).

The protective effects of heat stress were explored by Yoshida, Kristiansen and Liberman (1999) who used a variety of treatment–trauma intervals to study the growth and decay of hsp70 gene expression in the cochlea as well as the accompanying heat stress-mediated protection. A dramatic increase in mRNA synthesis was seen by 30 minutes after heat stress, which had decayed significantly 6 hours later. The cochlear protective effects were maximal at the shortest interval tested (6 hours), were no longer statistically significant at 24 hours and had disappeared completely by 96 hours. These results, taken together with the role played by hsps in cytoskeletal stabilization, led Yoshida and colleagues to suggest that heat stress-induced stabilization of stereociliary rootlets could underlie at least some of the protective effects that are found following their expression.

Changes in gene expression induced by heat stress in particular, and stressors in general, are not restricted to changes in hsps. It is also possible, for example, that any stress including noise leads to upregulation of enzymes such as superoxide dismutase, or others involved in the control of cellular redox status, given reports of protection from acoustic injury via free-radical scavengers (Jacono et al., 1998). However, the role of enzymes associated with cellular antioxidant defence is complex; for instance, it has been found that under some circumstances, copper/zinc superoxide dismutase can actually increase noise-induced hearing loss (Endo et al., 2005). Further work is clearly needed to permit the relationship of stress, the cytoskeleton and protective effects in the cochlea to be fully understood.

## Effects of noise on cochlear innervation

Intense sound stimulation has been suggested to result in an excess release of the neurotransmitter glutamate by the IHCs, in particular, that may be responsible for the destruction of the primary auditory dendrites. Normally glutamate is removed from the synaptic cleft by a glutamate–aspartate transporter situated in the membranes of the supporting cells (Furness and Lehre, 1997). However, increases in intracellular calcium levels caused by prolonged or intense sound stimulation results in excess release of glutamate from the synapses which builds up to excitotoxic levels and produces the swelling and loss of afferent cochlear terminals (Figure 5.8). Interestingly, application of glutamate antagonists such as kynurenate during noise exposure of 130 dB SPL in guinea pigs has been reported to abolish damage to the type I afferent dendrites. It also results in a 50% reduction in the threshold shift (a 40-dB loss compared with an 80-dB loss) compared with animals whose cochleae were perfused with artificial perilymph alone (Puel et al., 1998). In addition, thresholds have been reported to recover from 80 dB to 20 dB within 2 weeks (Puel et al., 1995, 1996). The remaining hearing loss has been attributed to permanent hair cell damage but the recovery to synaptic repair, a suggestion supported by the observation of regenerated nerve fibres

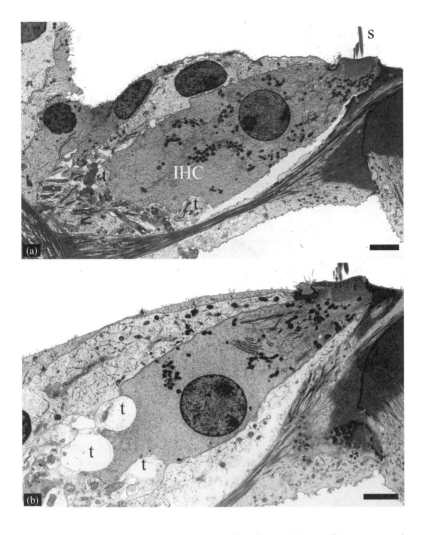

**Figure 5.8** Transmission electron micrographs of inner hair cells (IHCs) and their innervation. (a) An IHC showing the stereocilia (s) and normal nerve terminals (t). (b) An IHC with swollen nerve terminals (t) typical of excitotoxicity, a mechanism that may be common to various auditory traumas including noise damage. Scale bars = 5 $\mu$m.

after noise-induced hair cell loss in other species such as chinchillas (Strominger, Bohne and Harding, 1995).

A role for the efferent innervation in protection from acoustic stimuli has also been proposed. This suggestion has come from experiments showing that, in anaesthetized animals, electrical stimulation of the efferent pathway reduces TTS from simultaneous exposure to high-intensity sound (Rajan, 1988; Reiter and Liberman, 1995). It is also suggested by the fact that chronic surgical de-efferentation makes awake animals more vulnerable to hearing loss from high-level noise (Kujawa and Liberman, 1997). Recently, Maison et al. (2002) showed that overexpression of the α9-nicotinic acetylcholine receptor in the OHCs of transgenic mice significantly reduced acoustic injury. The transgenic mice were protected from exposures causing either TTS (caused by 8–12 kHz, 92 dB SPL followed by full recovery after 1 week) or PTS (caused by 8–12 kHz, 110 dB SPL followed by a threshold shift of 15–20 dB SPL after 1 week). This protection occurred without affecting the pre-exposure cochlear sensitivity to low or moderate levels of sound. This finding indicates the importance of the cholinergic efferent system in protecting the inner ear from noise.

## Possibilities for repair and regeneration

**Neuroprotection may be promoted by:**

- glutamate antagonists;
- anti-apoptotic agents;
- free-radical inhibitors;
- inhibitors of calpain and calcineurin;
- neurotrophic factors.

Therapeutic strategies for preventing or reducing the effects of acoustic trauma are under investigation in auditory research laboratories around the world. It has been found that different mice strains are differentially susceptible to noise exposure (Ohlemiller et al., 2000), which may provide a clue to why people differ in their vulnerability to noise. The complex structure and function of the cochlea is now being shown to be under the control of many different genes (see reviews by Steel and Kros, 2001; Frolenkov et al., 2004). Given the multifactorial effects of high-intensity noise, a range of pathological changes in response to the same traumatic stimulus is not unexpected so different susceptibilities given different genetic backgrounds are to be expected.

A better understanding is also emerging from animal experiments of the danger of being exposed to continuous but non-painful noise (see, for example, Emmerich et al., 2000), emphasizing the need to reduce our exposure to unnecessary noise and thus prevent hearing loss. Strategies for reducing susceptibility are also under investigation. An interesting phenomenon in this context is 'sound conditioning' (Canlon, 1996) in which pre-exposure to moderate levels of non-traumatic sound reduces PTS from subsequent traumatic exposures. This may be an inner ear example of the more general observation that exposure of some tissues to sublethal insults affords significant protection from subsequent, more dangerous challenges (Barbe et al., 1988; Tytell, Barbe and Brown, 1993). Other challenges for which such protective effects have been demonstrated in various tissues include hypoxia, ischaemia and chemical toxins as well the heat stress mentioned above. In addition to such direct cellular insults, psychological stressors can also induce changes in gene expression in the same 'protective' pathways induced by the direct cellular challenges (Ghoshal et al., 1998). These stress-related effects on gene expression may be mediated via changes in circulating glucocorticoid levels and their actions on glucocorticoid receptors. Direct cellular stresses, such as changes in intracellular $Ca^{2+}$, redox status or protein structure, can lead to upregulation of the same protective pathways through modulation of a variety of other transcription factors.

Acoustic exposure of the type used in sound-conditioning experiments affects cochlear blood flow (Axelsson and Vertes, 1982). It also probably changes intracellular ion concentrations and redox status and can elicit an array of psychological stress responses (Kryter, 1976), not least because such exposure usually involves some degree of physical restraint. Thus, the conditioning-mediated protective effects in the ear may involve changes in stress-induced gene expression mediated by a combination of systemic and local cellular signals. The fact that there can be unilateral protection from acoustic injury after unilateral sound conditioning (Yamasoba , Dolan and Miller, 1999) suggests, however, that conditioning-related protection cannot be completely caused by modulation of systemic stress levels. The existence of multiple mechanisms, with differing time constants for onset and decay, may explain why different authors have obtained apparently contradictory results. For example, Ryan et al. (1994) showed that protective effects of sound conditioning were absent when the trauma was presented immediately after conditioning, yet were clear cut with a treatment trauma interval of 1 week. On the other hand, Canlon and Fransson (1998) showed that a 2-hour conditioner trauma interval gave more protection than a 1-week interval. The decay of protective effects observed in the latter study is consistent with that seen in the heat stress paradigm used by Yoshida, Kristiansen and Liberman (1999) whereas the former is not. Unravelling the complexity of these stress-related responses will be essential if they are to be used safely and effectively in a clinical setting.

Once noise damage has taken place, there is a need to limit its extent and, if possible, reverse its effects. Given that apoptotic processes may be involved in hair cell death under some circumstances, it is thought that anti-apoptotic agents may be effective in reducing inner-ear damage after acoustic trauma (Pirvola et al., 2000). A neuroprotective agent called riluzole (2-amino-6-trifluoromethoxybenzothiazole) has been shown to prevent PTS and rescue cochlear hair cells from acoustic trauma (Wang et al., 2002). Riluzole appears to prevent mitochondrial damage and subsequent translocation of cytochrome $c$, a molecule known to trigger the programmed cell death pathway but the precise way in which it protects hair cells is not yet fully understood. However, it is a drug that is already in clinical use for the treatment of other neurological disorders so its usefulness in reducing or preventing ototoxic effects is being explored further.

Acoustic overstimulation increases $Ca^{2+}$ concentration in auditory hair cells. Excessive calcium entry may lead to the formation of free radicals that can trigger cell death genes (Mattson, 1996). In this context, it is interesting to note the growing evidence for the protective effects of free-radical inhibitors and anti-inflammatory agents. One molecule known to be involved in calcium-induced cellular damage is calpain so it is also interesting that leupeptin, a potent calpain inhibitor, can protect the hair cells from acoustic trauma (Wang et al., 1999). Another molecule, calcineurin, is also known to activate cell death pathways and is controlled by $Ca^{2+}$ and calmodulin. The role of calcineurin in auditory hair cell death has therefore also been investigated in guinea pigs after intense noise exposure (Minami et al., 2004). Immediately after noise exposure (4-kHz octave band, 120 dB for 5 hours), a population of hair cells exhibited calcineurin immunoreactivity at the cuticular plate, with a decreasing number of positive-stained cells on 1–3 days after exposure. By day 7, the levels of calcineurin immunoreactivity diminished to near control, non-noise-exposed values, concomitant with an increasing loss of hair cells. Staining of hair cell nuclei with propidium iodide restricted to calcineurin-immunopositive cells suggested breakdown of cell membranes symptomatic of incipient cell death. The local application of the calcineurin inhibitors, FK506 and cyclosporin A also reduced the level of threshold shift in noise-induced auditory brain-stem response and of hair cell death, indicating that calcineurin is a factor in noise-induced hearing loss. These results suggest that calcineurin inhibitors may also be of potential therapeutic value for long-term protection of the morphological integrity and function of the organ of Corti against noise trauma.

Excessive release of the excitatory amino acid neurotransmitter, glutamate, has also been implicated in noise-induced hearing loss so agents that block glutamate receptors are also under investigation as protective agents. One example is caroverine (N-methyl-D-aspartate [NMDA] and α-amino-3-hydroxy-5-methyl-4-isoazole proprionic acid [AMPA] receptor antagonist) which has been shown to protect the inner ear from excitotoxicity and to be effective in treatment of cochlear synaptic tinnitus (see, for example, Chen et al., 2003).

Other approaches involve preventing cochlear nerve fibre afferent degeneration or attempting to encourage regrowth with neurotrophins such as brain-derived neurotrophic factor and glial-line-derived neurotrophic factor and are providing encouraging results that may prove useful clinically (Shoji et al., 2000; Yagi et al., 2000). Perhaps the most exciting possibility is that of finding ways to stimulate the terminally differentiated hair cells and supporting cells of the mammalian cochlea to divide and produce replacement cells. Manipulation of genes that control the cell cycle has been shown to result in additional hair cells being produced in the mammalian cochlea (Löwenheim et al., 1999; Sage et al., 2005). However, ensuring that cell division provoked in these ways can be controlled and will not lead to tumours is crucial to the therapeutic value of such approaches. The safe delivery of genes into the human inner ear of vectors borne by viruses is also an important issue for strategies involving upregulation of growth factors or hair cell regeneration (Nakaizumi et al., 2004).

In conclusion, a wide range of strategies for preventing noise-induced hearing loss and for restoring the damaged cochlea is currently being explored, only some of which have been discussed here. Their variety is an indication of the complexity and delicacy of the inner ear and the fact that there is still much to learn about how it functions despite major advances in the last few years.

# References

Ahmad M, Bohne BA, Harding GW (2003) An *in vivo* tracer study of noise-induced damage to the reticular lamina. Hearing Research 175: 82–100.

Akizuki H, Yoshie H, Morita Y, Takahashi K, Hara A, Watanabe T et al. (1995) Nuclear transition of heat shock protein in guinea pig cochlea after hyperthermia. Hearing Research 92: 126–30.

Altschuler RA, Miller JF, Raphael R, Schacht J (1999) Strategies for protection of the inner ear from noise-induced hearing loss. In D Prasher, B Canlon (eds) Cochlear Pharmacology and Noise Trauma. London: Noise Research Network Publications, pp. 98–111.

Axelsson A, Vertes D (1982) Histological findings in cochlear vessels after noise. In RP Hamernik, D Henderson, R Salvi (eds) New Perspectives on Noise-induced Hearing Loss. New York: Raven, pp. 49–68.

Barbe MF, Tytell M, Gower DJ, Welch WJ (1988) Hyperthermia protects against light damage in the rat retina. Science 241:1817–20.

Békésy G von (1960) Experiments in Hearing. New York: McGraw-Hill.

Bohne, B (1976) Mechanisms of noise damage in the inner ear. In D Henderson, RP Hamernik, DS Dosanjh, JH Mills (eds) Effects of Noise on Hearing. New York: Raven Press, pp. 41–68.

Bohne B, Harding GW (2000) Degeneration in the cochlea after noise damage: primary versus secondary events. American Journal of Otology 21: 505–9.

Bosher SK, Warren RL (1978) Very low calcium content of cochlear endolymph, an extracellular fluid. Nature 273: 377–8.

Brown MC (1993) Anatomical and physiological studies of type I and type II spiral ganglion neurons. In M Merchán, JM Juiz, DA Godfrey, E Mugnaini (eds) The Mammalian Cochlear Nuclei: Organization and function. New York: Plenum Press, pp. 43–54.

Brownell WE, Bader CR, Bertrand D, de Ribaupierre Y (1985) Evoked mechanical responses of isolated cochlear outer hair cells. Science 227: 194–6.

Canlon B (1996) The effects of sound conditioning on the cochlea. In R Salvi, D Hendserson (eds) Auditory System Plasticity and Regeneration. New York: Thième, pp. 118–27.

Canlon B, Fransson A (1998) Reducing noise damage by using a mid-frequency sound conditioning stimulus. NeuroReport 9: 269–74.

Canlon B, Miller J, Flock Å, Borg E (1986) Pure tone overstimulation changes the micromechanical properties of inner hair cell stereocilia. Hearing Research 30: 65–72.

Chan E, Suneson A, Ulfendahl M (1998) Acoustic trauma causes reversible stiffness changes in auditory sensory cells. Neuroscience 83: 961–8.

Chen Z, Duan M, Lee H, Ruan R, Ulfendahl M (2003) Pharmacokinetics of caroverine in the inner ear and its effects on cochlear function after systemic and local administration in guinea pigs. Audiology and Neuro-Otology 8: 49–56.

Crawford AC, Evans MG, Fettiplace R (1989) Activation and adaptation of transducer currents in turtle hair cells. Journal of Physiology 419: 405–34.

Crawford AC, Evans MG, Fettiplace R (1991) The actions of calcium on the mechano-electrical transducer current of turtle hair cells. Journal of Physiology 434: 369–98.

Dallos P (1992) The active cochlea. Journal of Neuroscience 12: 4575–85.

Dallos P, He DZZ, Lin X, Sziklai I, Mehta S, Evans BN (1997) Acetylcholine, outer hair cell electromotility, and the cochlear amplifier. Journal of Neuroscience 17: 2212–26.

Davis H (1958) A mechano-electric theory of cochlear action. Annals of Otology, Rhinology and Laryngology 67: 789–601.

Dolan DF, Nuttall AL (1988) Masked cochlear whole-nerve response intensity functions altered by electrical stimulation of the crossed olivocochlear bundle. Journal of the Acoustical Society of America 83: 1081–6.

Emmerich E, Richter F, Reinhold V, Linss W (2000) Effects of industrial noise exposure on distortion product emissions (DPOAEs) and hair cell loss of the cochlea – long term experiments in awake guinea pigs. Hearing Research 148: 9–17.

Endo T, Nakagawa T, Iguchi F, Kita T, Okano T, Sha SH et al. (2005) Elevation of superoxide dismutase increases acoustic trauma from noise exposure. Free Radical Biology and Medicine 15: 492–4.

Fettiplace R (2002) The transformation of sound stimuli into electrical signals. In D Roberts (ed.) Signals and Perception: The fundamentals of human sensation. Basingstoke, New York: Palgrave & Macmillan, pp. 17–28.

Fettiplace R, Ricci AJ, Hackney CM (2001) Clues to the cochlear amplifier from the turtle ear. Trends in Neuroscience 24:169–75.

Flock Å, Cheung HC (1977) Actin filaments in sensory hairs of inner ear receptor cells. Journal of Cell Biology 75: 339–43.

Fridberger A, Ulfendahl M (1996) Acute mechanical overstimulation of isolated outer hair cells causes changes in intracellular calcium levels without shape changes. Acta Otolaryngologica 116: 17–24.

Fridberger A, Flock Å, Ulfendahl M, Flock B (1998) Acoustic overstimulation increases outer hair cell $Ca^{2+}$ concentrations and causes dynamic contractions of the hearing organ. Proceedings of the National Academy of Sciences of the USA 95: 7127–7132.

Frolenkov GI, Belyantseva IA, Friedmann, Griffith AJ (2004) Genetic insights into the morphogenesis of inner ear hair cells. Nature Reviews Genetics 5: 489–98.

Furness DN, Hackney CM (1990) Comparative ultrastructure of subsurface cisternae in inner and outer hair cells of the guinea pig cochlea. European Archives of Otorhinolaryngology 247: 12–15.

Furness DN, Lehre KP (1997) Immunocytochemical localisation of a high affinity glutamate-aspartate transporter, GLAST, in the rat and guinea-pig cochlea. European Journal of Neuroscience 8: 79–91.

Furness DN, Hulme JA, Lawton DM, Hackney CM (2002) The distribution of the glutamate/aspartate transporter, GLAST, in relation to the afferent synapses of outer hair cells in the guinea pig cochlea. Journal of the Association for Research in Otolaryngology 3: 234–47.

Ghoshal K, Wang Y, Sheridan JF, Jacob ST (1998) Metallothionein induction in response to restraint stress. Journal of Biological Chemistry 273: 27904–10.

Goodyear RJ, Richardson GP (2002) Extracellular matrices associated with the apical surfaces of sensory epithelia in the inner ear: molecular and structural diversity. Journal of Neurobiology 53: 212–27.

Hackney CM, Furness DN (1995) Mechanotransduction in vertebrate hair cells: structure and function of the stereociliary bundle. American Journal of Physiology 268 (Cell Physiol 37): C1–C13.

Hackney CM, Mahendrasingam S, Jones EMC, Fettiplace R (2003) The distribution of calcium buffering proteins in the turtle cochlea. Journal of Neuroscience 23: 4577–89.

Hamernik RP, Henderson D (1974) Impulse noise trauma. A study of histological susceptibility. Archives of Otolaryngology 99: 118–21.

Hamernik RP, Turrentine G, Wright CG (1984) Surface morphology of the inner sulcus and related epithelial cells of the cochlea following acoustic trauma. Hearing Research 16: 143–60.

Hawkins JE (1971) The role of vasoconstriction in noise-induced hearing loss. Annals of Otology, Rhinology and Laryngology 80: 903–14.

Howard J, Hudspeth AJ (1987) Mechanical relaxation of the hair bundle mediates adaptation in mechanoelectrical transduction by the bullfrog's saccular hair cell. Neuron 1: 189–99.

Jacono AA, Hu B, Kopke RD, Henderson D, Van de Water TR, Steinman HM (1998) Changes in cochlear antioxidant enzyme activity after sound conditioning and noise exposure in the chinchilla. Hearing Research 117: 31–8.

Jakob U, Gaestel M, Engel K, Buchner J (1993) Small heat shock proteins are molecular chaperones. Journal of Biological Chemistry 268: 1517–20.

Johnstone BM, Sellick PM (1972) The peripheral auditory apparatus. Quarterly Review of Biophysics 2: 1–57.

Kryter KD (1976) Extraauditory effects of noise. In D Henderson, RP Hamernik, DS Dosanjh, JH Mills (eds) Effects of Noise on Hearing. New York: Raven Press, pp. 531–46.

Kujawa SG, Liberman MC (1997) Conditioning-related protection from acoustic injury: effects of chronic de-efferentation and sham surgery. Journal of Neurophysiology 78: 3095–106.

Lavoie JN, Hickey E, Weber LA, Landry J (1993) Modulation of actin microfilament dynamics and fluid phase pinocytosis by phosphorylation of heat shock protein 27. Journal of Biological Chemistry 268: 24210–14.

Lavoie JN, Lambert H, Hickey E, Weber LA, Landry J (1995) Modulation of cellular thermoresistance and actin filament stability accompanies phosphorylation-induced changes in the oligomeric structure of heat shock protein 27. Molecular and Cellular Biology 15: 505–16.

Leonova EV, Fairfield DA, Lomax MI, Altschuler RA (2002) Constitutive expression of Hsp27 in the rat cochlea. Hearing Research 63: 61–70.

Liberman MC (1987) Chronic ultrastructural changes in acoustic trauma: serial-section reconstruction of stereocilia and cuticular plates. Hearing Research 26: 65–88.

Liberman MC, Dodds LW (1984) Single-neuron labelling and chronic cochlear pathology III. Stereocilia damage and alterations of threshold tuning curve. Hearing Research 16: 55–74.

Liberman MC, Dodds LW (1987) Acute ultrastructural changes in acoustic trauma: serial-section reconstruction of stereocilia and cuticular plates. Hearing Research 26: 45–64.

Lim DJ (1986) Functional structure of the organ of Corti. Hearing Research 22: 117–46.

Lim DJ, Dunn DE (1979) Anatomic correlates of noise induced hearing loss. Otolaryngologic Clinics of North America 12: 493–513.

Lim DJ, Melnick W (1971) Acoustic damage of the cochlea. A scanning and transmission electron microscopic observation. Archives of Otolaryngology 94: 294–305.

Lim HH, Jenkins OH, Myers MW, Miller JM, Altschuler A (1993) Detection of HSP 72 after acoustic overstimulation in the rat cochlea. Hearing Research 69: 146–50.

Löwenheim H, Furness DN, Kil J, Zinn C, Gültig K, Fero ML et al. (1999) Gene disruption of $p^{27Kip1}$ allows cell proliferation in the postnatal and adult organ of Corti. Proceedings of the National Academy of Sciences of the USA 96: 4084–8.

Maison SF, Luebke AE, Liberman MC, Zuo J (2002) Efferent protection from acoustic injury is mediated via α9-nicotinic acetylcholine receptors on outer hair cells. Journal of Neuroscience 22: 10838–46.

Mattson MP (1996) Calcium and free radicals: mediators of neurotrophic factor and excitatory transmitter-regulated developmental plasticity and cell death. Perspectives in Developmental Neurobiology 3: 79–91.

Meyer J, Furness DN, Zenner H-P, Hackney CM, Gummer AW (1998) Evidence for opening of hair-cell transducer channels after tip-link loss. Journal of Neuroscience 18: 6748–56.

Minami SB, Yamashita D, Schacht J, Miller JM (2004) Calcineurin activation contributes to noise-induced hearing loss. Journal of Neuroscience Research 78: 383–92.

Miron T, Vancompernolle K, Vandekerckhove J, Wilchek M, Geiger B (1991) A 25-kD inhibitor of actin polymerization is a low molecular mass heat shock protein. Journal of Cell Biology 114: 255–61.

Moore BCJ (1995) Perceptual Consequences of Cochlear Damage. Oxford: Oxford University Press.

Mosser DD, Caron AW, Bourget L, Meriin, AB, Sherman MY, Morimotot RI, Massie B (2000) The chaperone function of hsp70 is required for protection against stress-induced apoptosis. Molecular and Cellular Biology 20: 7146–59.

Murugasu E, Russell IJ (1996) The effect of efferent stimulation on basilar membrane displacement in the basal turn of the guinea pig cochlea. Journal of Neuroscience 16: 325–32.

Nakaizumi T, Kawamoto K, Minoda R, Raphael Y (2004) Adenovirus-mediated expression of brain-derived neurotrophic factor spiral ganglion neurons from ototoxic damage. Audiology and Neuro-Otology 9: 135–43.

Nordmann AS, Bohne BA, Harding GW (2000) Histopathological differences between temporary and permanent threshold shift. Hearing Research 139: 13–30.

Ohlemiller KK, McFadden SL, Ding D-L, Reaume AG, Hoffman EK, Scott RW et al. (1999) Targeted deletion of the cytosolic Cu/Zn-superoxide dismutase gene (SOD1) increases susceptibility to noise-induced hearing loss. Audiology and Neuro-Otology 4: 237–46.

Ohlemiller KK, Wright JS, Heidbreder AF (2000) Vulnerability to noise-induced hearing loss in 'middle-aged' and young adult mice: a dose-response approach in CBA, C57BL and BALB inbred strains. Hearing Research 149: 239–47.

Pickles JO, Comis SD, Osborne MP (1984) Cross-links between stereocilia in the guinea-pig organ of Corti and their possible relation to sensory transduction. Hearing Research 15: 103–12.

Pirvola U, Qun LX, Virkala J, Saarma M, Murukata C, Camoratta AM et al. (2000) Rescue of hearing, auditory hair cells and neurons by CEP-1347/KT7515, an inhibitor of c-Jun N-terminal kinase activation. Journal of Neuroscience 20: 43–50.

Puel JL, Safieddine S, d'Aldin C, Eybalin M, Pujol R (1995) Synaptic regeneration and functional recovery after excitotoxic injury in the guinea-pig cochlea. Compte Rendu de l'Académie des Sciences. Série III (Paris), Sciences de la Vie 318: 67–75.

Puel JL, d'Aldin C, Safieddine S, Eybalin M, Pujol R (1996) Excitotoxicity and plasticity of the IHC-auditory nerve synapse contribute to both TTS and PTS. In A Alexsson, RP Hamernik, RJ Salvi (eds) Scientific Basis of Hearing Loss. New York: Thème Medical Publishers Inc., pp. 36–42.

Puel JL, d'Aldin C, Ruel J, Pujol R (1998) Noise-induced hearing loss: current physiological investigations. In D Prasher, L Luxon (eds) (1998) Biological Effects of Noise. London: Whurr, pp. 17–21.

Quirk WS, Seidman MD (1995) Cochlear vascular changes in response to loud noise. American Journal of Otology 16: 322–5.

Rajan R (1988) Effect of electrical stimulation of the crossed olivocochlear bundle on temporary threshold shifts in auditory sensitivity. I. Dependence on electrical stimulation parameters. Journal of Neurophysiology 60: 549–68.

Raphael Y, Athey BD, Wang Y, Lee MK, Altschuler RA (1994) F-actin, tubulin and spectrin in the organ of Corti: comparative distribution in different cell types and mammalian species. Hearing Research 76: 173–87.

Reiter ER, Liberman MC (1995) Efferent-mediated protection from acoustic overexposure: relation to slow effects of olivocochlear stimulation. Journal of Neurophysiology 60: 549–68.

Ricci AJ, Fettiplace R (1998) Calcium permeation of the turtle hair cell mechanotransducer channel and its relation to the composition of endolymph. Journal of Physiology 506: 159–73.

Ryan AF, Bennett TM, Woolf NK, Axelsson A (1994) Protection from noise-induced hearing loss by prior exposure to a nontraumatic stimulus: role of the middle ear muscles. Hearing Research 72: 23–8.

Sage C, Huang M, Karimi K, Gutierrez G, Vollrath MA, Zhang DS et al. (2005) Proliferation of functional hair cells in vivo in the absence of the retinoblastoma protein. Science 307:1114–18.

Saunders JC, Dear SP, Schneider ME (1985) The anatomical consequences of acoustic injury: a review and a tutorial. Journal of the Acoustical Society of America 78: 833–60.

Saunders JC, Canlon B, Flock Å (1986) Growth of threshold shift in hair-cell stereocilia following overstimulation. Hearing Research 23: 245–55.

Schneider ME, Belyantseva IA, Azevedo RB, Kachar B (2002) Rapid renewal of auditory hair bundles. Nature 418: 837–8.

Shoji F, Miller AL, Mitchell A, Yamasoba T, Altschuler RA, Miller JM (2000) Differential protective effects of neurotrophins in the attenuation of noise-induced hair cell loss. Hearing Research 1: 134–42.

Spoendlin H (1967) The innervation of the organ of Corti. Journal of Laryngology and Otology 81: 717–38.

Spoendlin H (1972) Innervation densities of the cochlea. Acta Otolaryngologica 73: 235–48.

Spoendlin H (1985) Anatomy of cochlear innervation. American Journal of Otolaryngology 6: 453–67.

Steel KP, Kros CJ (2001) A genetic approach to understanding auditory function. Nature and Genetics 27: 143–9.

Stone JS, Rubel EW (2000) Cellular studies of auditory hair cell regeneration in birds. Proceedings of the National Academy of Sciences of the USA 97: 11714–21.

Strominger RN, Bohne BA, Harding GW (1995) Regenerated nerve fibers in the noise-damaged chinchilla cochlea are not efferent. Hearing Research 92: 52–62.

Szönyi M, He DZ, Ribari O, Sziklai I, Dallos P (2001) Intracellular calcium and outer hair cell electromotility. Brain Research 922: 65–70.

Thompson AM, Neely JG (1992) Induction of heat shock protein in interdental cells by hyperthermia. Otolaryngology, Head and Neck Surgery 107: 769–74.

Tytell M, Barbe MF, Brown IR (1993) Stress (heat shock) protein accumulation in the central nervous system. Advances in Neurology 59: 293–303.

Wang J, Ding D, Shulmann A, Stracher A, Salvi RJ (1999) Leupeptin protects sensory hair cells from acoustic trauma. NeuroReport 10: 811–16.

Wang J, Dib M, Lenoir M, Vago P, Eybalin M, Haeg A et al. (2002) Riluzole rescues cochlear sensory cells from acoustic trauma in the guinea pig. Neuroscience 111: 635–48.

Wiederhold ML, Kiang NY (1970) Effects of electric stimulation of the crossed olivocochlear bundle on single auditory-nerve fibers in the cat. Journal of the Acoustical Society of America 48: 950–65.

Wilson JP (1987) Mechanics of middle and inner ear. British Medical Bulletin 43: 821–57.

Yagi M, Kanzaki S, Kawamoto K, Shin B, Shah PP, Magal E et al. (2000) Spiral ganglion neurons protected from degeneration by GDNF gene therapy. Journal of the Association for Research in Otolaryngology 1: 315–25.

Yamane H, Nakai Y, Takayama M, Iguchi H, Nakagawa T, Kojima A (1995) Appearance of free radicals in the guinea-pig inner ear after noise-induced acoustic trauma. European Archives of Otorhinolaryngology 252: 504–8.

Yamasoba T, Dolan DF, Miller JM (1999) Acquired resistance to acoustic trauma by sound conditioning is primarily mediated by changes restricted to the cochlea not by systemic responses. Hearing Research 127: 31–40.

Yamoah EN, Lumpkin EA, Dumont RA, Smith PJ, Hudspeth AJ, Gillespie PG (1998) Plasma membrane $Ca^{2+}$-ATPase extrudes $Ca^{2+}$ from hair cell stereocilia. Journal of Neuroscience 18: 610–24.

Yoshida N, Kristiansen A, Liberman MC (1999) Heat stress and protection from permanent acoustic injury in mice. Journal of Neuroscience 19: 10116–24.

Zenner HP, Reuter G, Zimmermann U, Gitter AH, Fermin C, LePage EL (1994) Transitory endolymph leakage induced hearing loss and tinnitus: depolarization, biphasic shortening and loss of electromotility of outer hair cells. European Archives of Otorhinolaryngology 251: 143–53.

Zhao Y, Yamoah EN, Gillespie PG (1996) Regeneration of broken tip links and restoration of mechanical transduction in hair cells. Proceedings of the National Academy of Sciences of the USA 93: 15469–74.

Zheng J, Shen WX, He DZ, Long K, Madison LD, Dallos P (2000) Prestin is the motor protein of cochlear outer hair cells. Nature 405: 149–55.

# CHAPTER 6

# Functional changes in the central auditory system after noise-induced cochlear damage

*Noise and Its Effects:* Edited by Linda Luxon and Deepak Prasher © 2007 John Wiley & Sons Ltd.

RJ SALVI, J WANG, DM CASPARY

## Introduction

Noise-induced hearing loss has traditionally been considered a peripheral phenomenon because the primary lesion resides in the cochlea. Consequently, the vast majority of studies have focused on the biochemical, morphological and physiological changes in the cochlea, particularly the hair cells, cochlear ganglion neurons and stria vascularis (Salvi et al., 1982; Hamernik et al., 1984). However, in recent years, a growing body of evidence has suggested that cochlear damage, which reduces the neural output of the cochlea, can alter the structure and function of the central auditory pathway in unexpected ways (Lonsbury-Martin and Martin, 1981; Gerken, Simhadri-Sumithra and Bhat, 1986; Wang, Salvi and Powers, 1996; Illing, Horvath and Laszig, 1997; Morest, Kim and Bohne, 1997).

> Cochlear damage secondary to noise may alter the structure and function of the central auditory pathway by, for example, tonotopic reorganization or neural hyperactivity.

The notion that functional changes could arise in the central auditory pathway following cochlear damage (Robertson and Irvine, 1989; Harrison et al., 1991; Willott, Aitkin and McFadden, 1993) should not seem surprising given that similar changes occur in the somatosensory and visual system following damage to the peripheral receptors (Eysel, Gonzalez-Aguilar and Mayer, 1980, 1981; Merzenich and Kaas, 1982; Kaas et al., 1990). This chapter will focus on two striking changes that occur in the central auditory pathway following cochlear damage, specifically, tonotopic reorganization and neural hyperactivity.

# Tonotopic reorganization

One of the hallmarks of the auditory system is its precise tonotopic organization. At each level of the auditory pathway, there is an orderly mapping of frequency on to place. When the inner and outer hair cells in a segment of the cochlea are destroyed by acoustic overstimulation, the sound frequencies normally transduced by the damaged segment of the cochlea are no longer transmitted to the central auditory brain (Salvi et al., 1982). Thus, a subset of neurons in the auditory nerve and cochlear nucleus become 'silent' when they are 'cut off' from their normal inputs (Salvi et al., 1982; Kaltenbach, Czaja and Kaplan, 1992). A similar situation initially occurs in the auditory cortex (AC) (Robertson and Irvine, 1989; Willott, Aitkin and McFadden, 1993). Cortical neurons originally responsive to frequencies corresponding to the damaged region of the cochlea are initially 'silenced' by cochlear damage; however, after a few weeks of recovery, these neurons begin to respond to frequencies that are associated with frequencies just outside the damaged region of the cochlea, i.e. they shift their best frequencies to higher or lower frequencies bordering the damaged region (Figure 6.1). Similar, but less dramatic, changes in tonotopic

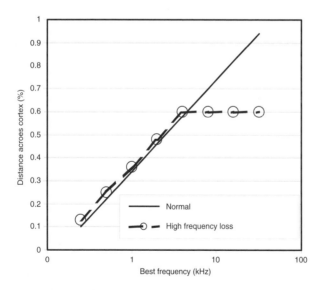

**Figure 6.1** Schematic illustrating the change in the tonotopic organization of auditory cortex in animals with a high-frequency hearing loss. Normal subjects (solid line) show a gradual increase in best frequency of cortex neurons as a function of percentage distance from the edge of the cortex. Subjects with high-frequency hearing loss (dashed line) also show a progressive increase in best frequency with distance from the edge of cortex until the edge of the hearing loss is reached, after which the best frequency remains constant. This leads to an overrepresentation of neurons with best frequencies near the edge of the hearing loss.

reorganization have been seen in the inferior colliculus (IC) following acoustic overstimulation (Salvi, Wang and Powers, 1996). The mechanisms responsible for the lesion-induced tonotopic reorganization are not fully understood.

**Proposed mechanisms responsible for lesion-induced tonotopic reorganization**

- Formation of new synaptic connections
- Anatomical remodelling
- Functional activation of pre-existing 'silent' excitatory synapses

As the tonotopic maps takes weeks or months to reorganize, it seems likely that this process involves the formation of new synaptic connections and anatomical remodelling (Darian-Smith and Gilbert, 1994; Illing, Horvath and Laszig, 1997). Alternatively, the reorganization could involve the functional activation of pre-existing excitatory synapses that extend over a broad range of best frequencies, but which may normally be silenced by surround inhibition in the intact system (Wang, Caspary and Salvi, 2000).

## Evoked response hyperactivity

The auditory nerve provides the only pathway for transmitting information from the cochlea to the central auditory system. When the cochlea is damaged by acoustic overstimulation or ototoxic drugs, the neural output of the cochlea, as reflected in the amplitude of the compound action potential (CAP), is invariably reduced (Eldredge, Mills and Bohne, 1973; Salvi, Henderson and Hamernik, 1979; Wang et al., 1997b). Thus, when the cochlea is damaged, the central auditory system receives less neural activity than a normal ear. This raises an important question, specifically, how does the central auditory system respond to sound when it receives less neural activity? To address this question, local field potentials have been recorded at different sites along the auditory pathway before and after acoustic overstimulation. For example, after a 1-hour exposure to white noise of 120 dB sound pressure level (SPL), the threshold of the CAP and the evoked response from the IC and AC increased by 20–30 dB across all three structures. As expected, the amplitude of the response from the CAP and IC decreased significantly whereas the amplitude of the AC unexpectedly increased (Popelar, Syka and Berndt, 1987). The amplitude enhancement in AC increased with exposure levels from 105 to 125 dB SPL (Syka, Rybalko and Popelar, 1994). These results suggest that the AC attempts to compensate for the decreased input from the periphery by increasing its gain.

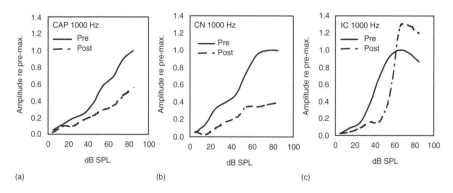

**Figure 6.2** Schematic illustrating local field potential amplitude level functions evoked with 1-kHz tone bursts from (a) the auditory nerve (compound action potential or CAP), from (b) cochlear nucleus (CN) and (c) inferior colliculus (or IC). Measurements made before (solid line) and approximately 1 day after (dashed line) the chinchillas were exposed to a 2.8-kHz tone at 105 dB SPL for 2 hours. Response amplitude from the auditory nerve (a) and cochlear nucleus (b) is depressed after the exposure. The amplitude from the inferior colliculus (c) increases rapidly with intensity and is enhanced at high sound levels. (Adapted from Salvi et al., 1992)

Several studies employing pure-tone exposures have found that the IC response amplitude increases in certain frequency regions after acoustic trauma. For example, acoustic overstimulation with a 2.8-kHz tone (105 dB SPL, 2 hours) caused a significant reduction in CAP amplitude and a 20-dB threshold shift at 1 kHz, a frequency just below the exposure frequency (Salvi et al., 1992) (Figure 6.2a). Measurements obtained from the cochlear nucleus (CN), the first relay station beyond the auditory nerve, also showed a significant amplitude reduction and an elevation of threshold similar to that seen in the auditory nerve (Figure 6.2b). Evoked response input/output functions measured from the IC, one of the major binaural relay nuclei in the auditory midbrain (Figure 6.2c) showed a threshold shift of approximately 25 dB and amplitude reduction at low sound levels. However, at suprathreshold intensities, the IC response amplitude increased at an abnormally rapid rate (recruitment-like behaviour) and the maximum response amplitude was larger than before the exposure. Some IC amplitude enhancements similar to this have been observed after other types of acute acoustic trauma (Gerken, Simhadri-Sumithra and Bhat, 1986; Szczepaniak and Moller, 1996a, 1996b; Caspary et al., 2005).

**How does the central auditory nervous system respond to sound when it receives less neural activity due to acoustic overstimulation?**

Possible answers from animal experiments:

- Cortical tonotopic reorganization
- The auditory cortex increases its gain

- IC demonstrates 'recruitment' like activity at suprathreshold intensities of auditory stimulation
- Loss of lateral inhibition from higher frequencies in the IC giving rise to amplitude enhancement at frequencies below the maximum hearing loss

Previous studies involving high-level (105 dB SPL), long-duration exposures (5 days) at 2.8 kHz have found that the amplitude enhancement in the IC occurs at frequencies below the maximum hearing loss (4 kHz) as schematized in Figure 6.3a. For example, the maximum response amplitude at 0.5 kHz, where there was no hearing loss, increased significantly as schematized in Figure 6.3b. By contrast, the maximum response at 4 kHz, a region with 30–40 dB of hearing loss, was similar to that before the exposure as schematized in Figure 6.3c (Salvi et al., 1990). These results suggest that the amplitude enhancement at frequencies below the maximum hearing loss (< 4 kHz) could be due to the loss of lateral inhibition emanating from higher frequencies. This hypothesis has gained support from single-unit experiments.

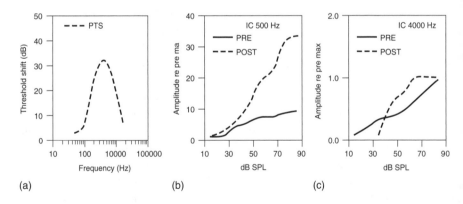

(a)                                  (b)                                  (c)

**Figure 6.3** Schematics illustrating the changes in the local field potentials recorded from chinchilla inferior colliculus (IC) before and after a 5-day exposure to a 2-kHz, 105 dB SPL tone. (a) Exposure results in a threshold shift at the mid-frequencies. (b) Amplitude-level functions recorded at 500 Hz before (dashed line) and after (solid line) the exposure. Note large increase in response amplitude after the exposure. (c) Amplitude-level functions recorded at 4000 Hz before (dashed line) and after (solid line) the exposure. Post-exposure function is shifted to the right of pre-exposure function due to the elevation of threshold; however, the post-exposure function increases rapidly with level so that the maximum post-exposure amplitude is approximately equal to the pre-exposure maximum. PTS, permanent threshold shift. (Adapted from Salvi et al., 1992.)

# Acoustic trauma, lateral inhibition and single-unit activity

Several single-unit studies have examined the effects of acoustic trauma on the excitatory and inhibitory response areas in the central auditory pathway. Many neurons in the central auditory pathway have inhibitory response areas located above, within and below the neuron's excitatory response area (Figure 6.4a). It is possible to attenuate the inhibitory response area selectively by presenting a traumatizing tone above the characteristic frequency (CF), outside the excitatory response area. The general strategy of these experiments is to measure the normal inhibitory and excitatory response areas before and after presenting a high intensity tone (typically 110–115 dB SPL, 15–20 minutes) above CF (arrow in Figure 6.4a). With this approach, the traumatizing tone causes maximum activation in the inhibitory area above the CF, but has no effect on the excitatory response area. If the traumatizing tone damages the inhibitory inputs impinging on the neuron,

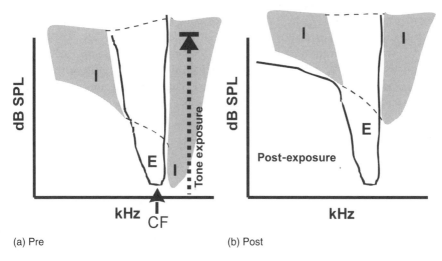

(a) Pre                                        (b) Post

**Figure 6.4** Schematic illustrating the changes seen in the excitatory and inhibitory response areas of sharply tuned neurons in the inferior colliculus (IC) before (a) and after (b) acute acoustic overstimulation. Solid line and open area show excitatory response area (E). Shaded areas and dashed lines show inhibitory response area (I). Inhibitory area bounded by dashed line 'covered over' by excitatory region. Note that inhibitory region (shaded area plus dashed line) extend though the excitatory response area (a): the IC neuron has excitatory response area with narrow tip near the characteristic frequency (CF), but lacks a low-frequency tail. Inhibitory response areas present above and below the excitatory response area. A traumatizing tone is presented at a frequency within the inhibitory response area above the CF (b). After the traumatizing exposure, the threshold for the inhibitory areas above and below the CF increase, unmasking the full extent of the excitatory response area. The tip of excitatory response area near the CF remains unchanged, but the excitatory response area below the CF develops a high-threshold, broadly tuned tail. (Adapted from Salvi et al., 2000b.)

then the excitatory response should increase due to the loss of inhibition. Figure 6.4b is a schematic that illustrates the basic functional changes that occur in many sharply tuned IC neurons. As expected, the traumatizing tone causes the threshold of the inhibitory area above CF to increase while the threshold at CF remains unchanged. However, unexpected changes occur in the tail of the tuning curve. First, the threshold for activating the inhibitory region below the CF increased even though the traumatizing tone was not presented in this frequency region. Second, the loss of inhibition below the CF leads to an expansion of the excitatory response area in the tail of the excitatory tuning curve and a lowering of the threshold. Thus, the tail of the excitatory tuning curve is 'unmasked' by the reduction in inhibition.

These results suggest a model (Figure 6.5a) in which the inhibitory region above the CF normally extends through the excitatory tuning curve into its low-frequency tail – an inhibitory tuning curve similar to the excitatory tuning curve, but shifted to higher frequencies. In the tail region, inhibition has a lower threshold and is normally stronger than excitation. Therefore, the excitatory inputs in this frequency region are suppressed, thereby limiting the spread of excitation towards the low frequencies. However, near the CF, the excitatory threshold is lower and more potent than the inhibitory inputs. Therefore, at low intensities, the response at the CF will be dominated by excitation whereas, at high intensities, the excitatory response will be opposed by inhibition. Thus, the neuron's firing rate at the CF will initially increase above it spontaneous discharge rate, and then roll over at high intensities as the inhibitory inputs 'kick in' (Figure 6.5c). When a traumatizing tone is presented above the CF, the threshold for inhibition increases, exposing a large portion of the tail of the excitatory tuning curve (Figure 6.5b). The increase in the threshold for inhibition also causes the firing rate to increase at suprathreshold intensities (Figure 6.5c). In addition, the loss of inhibition sometimes results in an increase in the spontaneous discharge rate as indicated in the lower left of Figure 6.5c. The increase in spontaneous activities implies that there is baseline level of inhibition present in quiet.

Approximately 45% of IC neurons had extremely narrow excitatory tuning curves similar to those shown in Figure 6.4a (so-called level-tolerant or upper threshold tuning curves). After the traumatizing exposure, most of these (about 85%) showed a striking decrease in threshold and expansion of the tail of the tuning curve, but little change in the tip of the excitatory tuning curve (Wang, Salvi and Powers, 1996). By contrast, the traumatizing tone had little effect on IC neurons with a conventional tuning curve with a low-threshold tip and high-threshold, broadly tuned tail. These results suggest that the loss of inhibition could contribute to the enhancement of the evoked response amplitude in the IC.

Neurons in the contralateral IC receive many inputs from the ipsilateral dorsal cochlear nucleus (DCN). When the same noise-exposure protocol was applied in the ipsilateral DCN, approximately 44% of the neurons

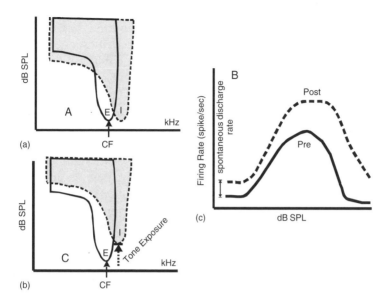

**Figure 6.5** (a, b) Model illustrating the overlap of the true excitatory and inhibitory response areas and the characteristic frequency (CF) discharge rate-level functions measured before and after acoustic overstimulation. (a) Open areas show boundary of excitatory response area; shaded area shows boundary of inhibitory response area. Note that both the excitatory and inhibitory response areas have a narrowly tuned tip and a high-threshold, broadly tuned tail. The tip of the inhibitory response area is displaced towards high frequencies so that the tail of the inhibitory response area overlaps the tip and tail of the excitatory response area. (b) A traumatizing tone (dashed vertical line) in the inhibitory response area above the CF causes an increase in the inhibitory response area that exposes the tail of the excitatory response area. (c) CF discharge rate-level functions are measured before and after the presentation of a traumatizing tone above the CF. Pre-exposure discharge rate initially increases above the spontaneous rate as intensity increases. At low intensities, the response is mainly from the low-threshold tip of the excitatory tuning curve. At moderate intensities, the discharge rate reaches a plateau as the inhibitory response begins to suppress the excitatory response. At high intensities, the discharge rate decreases because the inhibitory inputs are becoming stronger. After the traumatizing exposure, the inhibitory response is weaker, resulting in an increase in the spontaneous discharge rate (lower left) and an increase in the suprathreshold discharge rate. (Adapted from Salvi et al., 2000b.)

showed an expansion of the low-frequency tail and decrease in threshold similar to that shown in Figure 6.4 (Salvi and Wang, 1997). These effects were mainly confined to DCN neurons with narrow excitatory response areas and prominent inhibitory sidebands above and below CF – neurons that would be classified as type III neurons (Young, 1984). Thus, some of effects seen in the IC may be mediated in part by changes occurring in the DCN.

# Biochemical mechanisms

The EVP enhancement (Gerken, Simhadri-Sumithra and Bhat, 1986; Popelar et al., 1994) and increased single-unit activity seen in the central auditory pathway after acoustic overstimulation could be due to the loss of inhibition (disinhibition) (Willott and Lu, 1982; Rajan et al., 1992; Boettcher and Salvi, 1993; Calford, Rajan and Irvine, 1993; Irvine and Rajan, 1995; Wang, Salvi and Powers, 1996; Salvi and Wang, 1997). Neuropharmacological studies have shown that $\gamma$-aminobutyric acid (GABA) is a potent inhibitory neurotransmitter in the central auditory pathway. Blocking GABA-mediated inhibition causes a significant increase in discharge rate around CF in the cochlear nucleus, IC and AC (Yang, Pollak and Resler, 1992; Palombi and Caspary, 1992, 1996; Wang, Caspary and Salvi, 2000). In addition, type A GABA antagonists cause a broadening of the tails of sharply tuned IC neurons (Yang, Pollak and Resler, 1992) and substantial widening of tuning curves in the AC (Wang, Caspary and Salvi, 2000). Thus, the effects of blocking GABA-mediated inhibition closely resemble those seen in the central auditory pathway following acoustic overstimulation (Salvi and Wang, 1997; Wang, Salvi and Powers, 1996). If the enhancement of neuronal activity following acoustic overstimulation is due to the downregulation of GABA-mediated inhibition, then one might expect to find evidence for altered GABA release or binding in the central auditory system. In fact, acoustic overstimulation has been shown to decrease the sensitivity of IC neurons to the type A GABA antagonist, bicuculline (Szczepaniak and Moller, 1995b, 1996a), suggesting a decreased function of GABA-mediated inhibition in damaged ears. Consistent with these findings is the reduction in the number of IC neurons that could be inhibited by contralateral cochlear electrical stimulation after bilateral deafness (Bledsoe et al., 1995).

---

**Proposed mechanisms of CANS changes following experimental acoustic overstimulation**

- Downregulation of GABA-mediated inhibition
- Decreased sensitivity of IC neurons to Type A GABA antagonist, bicuculline
- Decrease in GAD synthesis (2-30 days) post acoustic exposure

---

For further evaluation of the role of GABA-mediated inhibition following acoustic overstimulation, GABA levels were assessed in the IC by measuring the level of glutamic acid decarboxylase (GAD), the rate-limiting enzyme involved in the synthesis of GABA (Martin and Rimvall, 1993; Rimvall, Sheikh and Martin, 1993; Rimvall and Martin, 1994). GAD levels in the cytosol and membrane fractions of IC homogenates of rats were

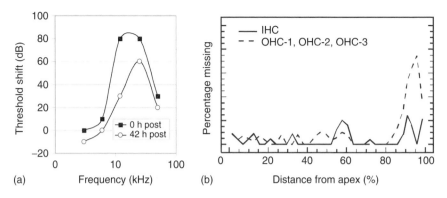

**Figure 6.6** (a) Threshold shift of inferior colliculus (IC)-evoked response from a rat exposed to a 12-kHz, 106 dB SPL tone for 10 hours. Threshold shift at 0 hours post-exposure was approximately 80 dB between 12 and 25 kHz decreasing to around 60 dB at 25 kHz at 42 hours post-exposure. (b) Cytocochleogram showing the pattern of outer hair cell (OHC) and inner hair cell (IHC) loss from rat exposed to the traumatizing tone. Note hair cell lesion near the high-frequency basal end of the cochlea. (Adapted from Milbrandt et al., 2000.)

assessed after high-intensity noise exposure (12 kHz, 10-hour exposure, 106 dB SPL) (Milbrandt et al., 2000). The exposure caused a threshold shift in the IC-evoked response of approximately 80 dB between 12 and 25 kHz 0 hours post-exposure (Figure 6.6a). At 42 hours post-exposure, the threshold shift had decreased to 60 dB at 25 kHz. The hair cell loss resulting from the exposure was greatest in the high-frequency region of the cochlea (90% of distance from apex) where the outer hair cell (OHC) loss was approximately 75% and the inner hair cell (IHC) loss was around 25%. Figure 6.7a shows the GAD65 levels in the IC expressed as a percentage of the levels seen in normal control animals. Cytosolic GAD levels were reduced to approximately 75% of control levels between 0 and 42 hours post-exposure and recovered to approximately 90% by 30 days post-exposure. Membrane-bound GAD levels were reduced to 55% of control levels ($p < 0.05$) immediately after the exposure and recovered to approximately 90% of control levels at 30 days post-exposure. These results suggest that severe acoustic trauma causes a decrease in GAD65 levels in the IC, particularly in the membrane bound levels of GAD65.

Another study, involving an exposure (10 kHz, 100 dB SPL, 9 hours) that caused significantly less threshold shift (30 dB) than the preceding one (80 dB), resulted in a complex pattern of GAD protein expression and neuronal immunolabelling in the IC (Abbott et al., 1999). At 0 hours post-exposure, protein levels of the 67-kDa isoform of GAD increased significantly (118%) in the IC. In addition, the optical density of GAD-immunolabelled cells also increased (35%) significantly. However, at 2 days post-exposure, protein levels of both the 67-kDa and 65-kDa isoforms of GAD had decreased below control levels and at 30 days post-exposure, the 67-kDa and 65-kDa isoforms were significantly below normal (21% and 39% respectively).

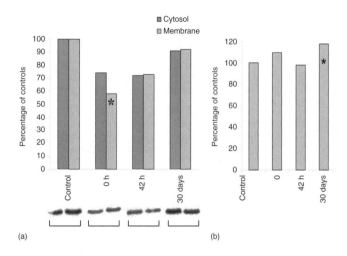

(a)                                                              (b)

**Figure 6.7** (a) Graph showing relative levels of membrane and cytosolic glutamic acid decarboxylase (GAD) in the inferior colliculus (IC) of rats measured 0 hours, 42 hours and 30 days post-exposure (12 kHz, 10 hours, 106 dB SPL). GAD levels were compared with those in unexposed controls. Western blots from controls and noise-exposed animals are shown beneath graph. (b) Percentage change in [$^3$H]muscimol binding in the IC of rats at 0 hours, 42 hours and 30 days post-exposure (12 kHz, 10 hours, 106 dB SPL). Measures normalized to those in unexposed controls. (*, $p < 0.05$) (Adapted from Milbrandt et al., 2000.)

Collectively, the preceding studies suggest that noise-induced cochlear damage leads to a decrease in GAD synthesis in the IC from 2 to 30 days post-exposure (Abbott et al., 1999; Milbrandt et al., 2000).

The reduction in GAD synthesis presumably leads to less GABA release from presynaptic neurons. An important question that arises from these observations is how do the post-synaptic neurons compensate for these changes? To address this question, [$^3$H]muscimol receptor autoradiography was used to localize and quantify GABA-A receptor-binding sites in the IC after acoustic stimulation (Abbott et al., 1999). Thirty days after acoustic overstimulation, there was significant increase (+20%) in GABA-A receptor-binding sites in the IC. These results suggest that there is an upregulation of GABA-A receptors to compensate for the reduction in GABA release.

## Conclusion and future direction

When the cochlea is damaged by acoustic overstimulation, the central auditory system compensates for the lack of activity. The cortical tonotopic map undergoes significant rearrangement so that inactivated frequency regions begin to respond to higher or lower frequencies where hearing is relatively intact. The mechanisms underlying these changes are not fully understood but could involve synaptic reorganization or reactivation of pre-existing, but previously silent, neural circuits (Calford and Tweedale, 1988; Calford and Tweedale, 1990; Darian-Smith and Gilbert, 1994; Benson et al., 1997; Bilak et al., 1997; Illing et al., 1999). The tonotopic reorganization seen in auditory cortex following cochlear pathology is reminiscent of the plastic changes that occur in learning paradigms (Weinberger, 1993; Cruikshank and Weinberger, 1996; Weinberger and Bakin, 1998). Thus, the dynamic changes in the tonotopic maps may be a normal response of the central auditory system to changes in the significant features of the external sound environment. Damaged regions of the cochlea that transmit little or no information to the central auditory brain are eliminated in favour of frequencies that provide information for the organism's survival.

Acoustic trauma can also cause a striking increase in the gain of the central auditory system that compensates, or in some cases overcompensates, for the reduced input from the cochlea. Changes similar to this have also been seen in the central auditory system after cochlear damage from ototoxic drugs (Popelar et al., 1994; Qiu et al., 2000). One factor that appears to contribute to this hyperactivity is the loss of GABA-mediated inhibition (see Figure 6.6) (Szczepaniak and Moller, 1995a.; Abbott et al., 1999; Salvi et al., 2000; Milbrandt et al., 2000). Disinhibition increases the gain of the system, making it more responsive to weak inputs from the periphery, but probably compromising other important coding circuits. Although GABA-mediated inhibition appears to be an important factor, other excitatory and inhibitory neurotransmitter systems are likely to be involved (Potashner, Suneja and Benson, 1997; Suneja, Benson and Potashner, 1998a; Suneja, Potashner and Benson, 1998b). The time course of these changes appears to vary significantly over time and place within the central auditory system. Defining the cellular basis, location and temporal pattern of changes is a major challenge for auditory neuroscience.

## Tinnitus and hyperacusis

Tinnitus and hyperacusis are two of the most debilitating consequences of sensorineural hearing loss induced by acoustic trauma and other oto-traumatic agents. These symptoms have long been attributed to aberrant signals from the cochlea. Tinnitus has often been attributed to an irritative lesion in the cochlea that results in abnormally high rates of spontaneous activity in auditory nerve fibres while hyperacusis was attributed to the rapid growth in the neural output of the cochlea. In general, data from the auditory nerve of damaged ears have found little or no evidence to corroborate these models (Kiang, Moxon and Levine, 1970; Salvi, Henderson and Hamernik, 1983). For example, patients who have had the eighth cranial nerve transected for the removal of an acoustic neuroma often experience tinnitus despite the fact that there is no neural activity from the auditory nerve (House and Brackmann, 1981). The paucity of data supporting peripheral models of tinnitus and hyperacusis has led to the notion that tinnitus and hyperacusis may originate in the central auditory system (see Chapter 12).

The hyperactive responses seen in the central auditory system following cochlear damage makes a strong argument for a central mechanism for hyperacusis and loudness recruitment.

Indeed, recent human brain-imaging studies have found evidence of sound-induced hyperactivity in subjects with high-frequency hearing loss (Lockwood et al., 1998). Moreover, some neurons in the central auditory system increase their rate of spontaneous activity after acoustic overstimulation that causes temporary hearing loss (Boettcher and Salvi, 1993; Wang et al., 1997a) or permanent cochlear damage (Kaltenbach et al., 1998). Acoustic overstimulation causes direct damage to the sensory and supporting cells in the inner ear, but it is becoming increasingly clear that these peripheral changes lead to widespread physiological, anatomical and biochemical consequences in the central auditory system. Clearly, further work is needed to define when, where and how these changes occur.

# References

Abbott SD, Hughes LF, Bauer CA, Salvi R, Caspary DM (1999) Detection of glutamate decarboxylase isoforms in rat inferior colliculus following acoustic exposure. Neuroscience 93: 1375–81.

Benson CG, Gross JS, Suneja SK, Potashner SJ (1997) Synaptophysin immunoreactivity in the cochlear nucleus after unilateral cochlear or ossicular removal. Synapse 25: 243–57.

Bilak M, Kim J, Potashner SJ, Bohne BA, Morest DK (1997) New growth of axons in the cochlear nucleus of adult chinchillas after acoustic trauma. Experimental Neurology 147: 256–68.

Bledsoe SC, Jr, Nagase S, Miller JM, Altschuler RA 1995 Deafness-induced plasticity in the mature central auditory system. Neuroreport 7, 225–9.

Boettcher FA, Salvi RJ (1993) Functional changes in the ventral cochlear nucleus following acute acoustic overstimulation. Journal of the Acoustical Society of America 94: 2123–34.

Calford MB, Tweedale R (1988) Immediate and chronic changes in responses of somatosensory cortex in adult flying-fox after digit amputation. Nature 332: 446–8.

Calford MB, Tweedale R (1990) Interhemispheric transfer of plasticity in the cerebral cortex. Science 249: 805–7.

Calford MB, Rajan R, Irvine DR (1993) Rapid changes in the frequency tuning of neurons in cat auditory cortex resulting from pure-tone-induced temporary threshold shift. Neuroscience 55: 953–64.

Caspary DM, Salvi RJ, Helfert RH, Brozoski TJ, Bauer CA (2005) Neuropharmacology of noise induced hearing loss in brainstem auditory structures. In D Henderson, D Prasher, RJ Salvi, R Kopke (eds) Proceedings of the Sixth International Symposium on Noise Induced Hearing Loss (in press).

Cruikshank SJ, Weinberger NM (1996) Receptive-field plasticity in the adult auditory cortex induced by Hebbian covariance. Journal of Neuroscience 16: 861–75.

Darian-Smith C, Gilbert CD (1994) Axonal sprouting accompanies functional reorganization in adult cat striate cortex. Nature 368: 737–40.

Eldredge DH, Mills JH, Bohne BA (1973) Anatomical, behavioral, and electro-physiological observations on chinchillas after long exposures to noise. Advances in Oto-Rhino-Laryngology 20: 64–81.

Eysel UT, Gonalez-Aguilar F, Mayer U (1980) A functional sign of reorganization in the visual system of adult cats: lateral geniculate neurons with displaced receptive fields after lesions of the nasal retina. Brain Research 191: 285–300.

Eysel UT, Gonzalez-Aguilar F, Mayer U (1981) Time-dependent decrease in the extent of visual deafferentation in the lateral geniculate nucleus of adult cats with small retinal lesions. Experimental Brain Research 41: 256–63.

Gerken G, Simhadri-Sumithra R, Bhat HHV (1986) Increase in central auditory responsiveness during continuous tone stimulation or following hearing loss. In RJ Salvi, RP Hamernik, D Henderson, V Colletti (eds) Basic and Applied Aspects of Noise Induced Hearing Loss. New York: Plenum Press, pp. 195–212.

Hamernik RP, Turrentine G, Roberto M, Salvi RJ, Henderson D (1984) Anatomical correlates of impulse noise induced mechanical damage to the cochlear. Hearing Research 13: 229–47.

Harrison RV, Nagasawa A, Smith DW, Stanton S, Mount RJ (1991) Reorganization of auditory cortex after neonatal high frequency cochlear hearing loss. Hearing Research 54: 11–19.

House JW, Brackmann DE (1981) Tinnitus: surgical treatment. Ciba Foundation Symposium 85: 204–16.

Illing RB, Horvath M, Laszig R (1997) Plasticity of the auditory brainstem: effects of cochlear ablation on GAP-43 immunoreactivity in the rat. Journal of Comparative Neurology 382: 116–38.

Illing R, Cao QL, Forster CR, Laszig R (1999) Auditory brainstem: development and plasticity of GAP-43 mRNA expression in the rat. Journal of Comparative Neurology 412: 353–72.

Irvine DRF, Rajan R (1995) Plasticity in the mature auditory system. In GA Manley, GM Klump, C Koppl, H Fastl, H Oeckinghaus (eds) Advances in Hearing Research. Singapore: World Scientific, pp. 3–23.

Kaas JH, Krubitzer LA, China YM, Langston AL, Polley EH, Blair N (1990) Reorganization of retinotopic maps in adult mammals after lesions of the retina. Science 248: 229–31.

Kaltenbach JA, Czaja JM, Kaplan CR (1992) Changes in the tonotopic map of the dorsal cochlear nucleus following induction of cochlear lesions. Hearing Research 59: 213–23.

Kaltenbach JA, Godfrey DA, Neumann JB, McCaslin DL, Afman CE, Zhang J (1998) Changes in spontaneous neural activity in the dorsal cochlear nucleus following exposure to intense sound: relation to threshold shift. Hearing Research 124: 78–84.

Kiang NY, Moxon EC, Levine RA (1970) Auditory-nerve activity in cats with normal and abnormal cochleas. In Sensorineural Hearing Loss. Ciba Foundation Symposium, pp. 241–73.

Lockwood AH, Salvi RJ, Coad ML, Towsley M, Wack DS, Murphy BW (1998) The functional neuroanatomy of tinnitus: evidence for limbic system links and neural plasticity. Neurology 50: 114–20.

Lonsbury-Martin BL, Martin GK (1981) Temporary hearing loss from exposure to moderately intense tones in rhesus monkeys. American Journal of Otolaryngology 2: 321–35.

Martin DL, Rimvall K (1993) Regulation of gamma-aminobutyric acid synthesis in the brain. Journal of Neurochemistry 60: 395–407.

Merzenich MM, Kaas JH (1982) Organization of mammalian somatosensory cortex following peripheral nerve injury. Trends in Neuroscience 5: 4428–36.

Milbrandt JC, Holder TM, Wilson MC, Salvi RJ, Caspary DM (2000) GAD levels and muscimol binding in rat inferior colliculus following acoustic trauma. Hearing Research 147: 251–60.

Morest DK, Kim J, Bohne BA (1997) Neuronal and transneuronal degeneration of auditory axons in the brainstem after cochlear lesions in the chinchilla: cochleotopic and non-cochleotopic patterns. Hearing Research 103: 151–68.

Palombi PS, Caspary DM (1992) GABAA receptor antagonist bicuculline alters response properties of posteroventral cochlear nucleus neurons. Journal of Neurophysiology 67: 738–46.

Palombi PS, Caspary DM (1996) GABA inputs control discharge rate primarily within frequency receptive fields of inferior colliculus neurons. Journal of Neurophysiology 75: 2211–19.

Popelar J, Syka J, Berndt H (1987) Effect of noise on auditory evoked responses in awake guinea pigs. Hearing Research 26: 239–47.

Popelar J, Erre JP, Aran JM, Cazals Y (1994) Plastic changes in ipsi-contralateral differences of auditory cortex and inferior colliculus evoked potentials after injury to one ear in the adult guinea pig. Hearing Research 72: 125–34.

Potashner SJ, Suneja SK, Benson CG (1997) Regulation of D-aspartate release and uptake in adult brain stem auditory nuclei after unilateral middle ear ossicle removal and cochlear ablation. Experimental Neurology 148: 222–35.

Qiu C, Salvi R, Ding D, Burkard R (2000) Inner hair cell loss leads to enhanced response amplitudes in auditory cortex of unanesthetized chinchillas: evidence for increased system gain. Hearing Research 139: 153–71.

Rajan R, Irvine DRF, Calford MB, Wise LZ (1992) Effects of frequency-specific losses on cochlear neural sensitivities in the processing and representation of frequency in primary auditory cortex. In A Dancer, D Henderson, RJ Salvi, RP Hamernik (eds) Noise Induced Hearing Loss. St Louis, MO: Mosby Year Book, pp. 119–29.

Rimvall K, Martin DL (1994) The level of GAD67 protein is highly sensitive to small increases in intraneuronal gamma-aminobutyric acid levels. Journal of Neurochemistry 62: 1375–81.

Rimvall K, Sheikh SN, Martin DL (1993) Effects of increased gamma-aminobutyric acid levels on GAD67 protein and mRNA levels in rat cerebral cortex. Journal of Neurochemistry 60: 714–20.

Robertson D, Irvine DR (1989) Plasticity of frequency organization in auditory cortex of guinea pigs with partial unilateral deafness. Journal of Comparative Neurology 282: 456–71.

Salvi RJ, Wang J (1997) Evidence for rapid reorganization in inferior colliculus and cochlear nucleus. In J Syka (ed.) Acoustical Signal Processing in the Central Auditory System. New York: Plenum Publishing Corp., pp. 477–88.

Salvi R, Henderson D, Hamernik RP (1979) Single auditory nerve fiber and action potential latencies in normal and noise-treated chinchilla. Hearing Research 1: 237–51.

Salvi RJ, Perry J, Hamernik RP, Henderson D (eds) (1982) Relationship between Cochlear Pathologies and Auditory Nerve and Behavioral Responses following Acoustic Trauma. New York: Raven Press.

Salvi RJ, Henderson D, Hamernik RP (1983) Physiological basis of sensorineural hearing loss. In J Tobias, E Schubert (eds) Hearing Research and Theory. 2 edn. New York: Academic Press, pp. 173–231.

Salvi RJ, Saunders SS, Gratton MA, Arehole S, Powers N (1990) Enhanced evoked response amplitudes in the inferior colliculus of the chinchilla following acoustic trauma. Hearing Research 50: 245–58.

Salvi RJ, Henderson D, Boettcher FA, Powers N (1992) Functional changes in central auditory pathways resulting from cochlear diseases. In J Katz, N Stecker, D Henderson (eds) Central Auditory Processing: A transdisciplinary view. St Louis, MO: Mosby Year Book, pp 47–60.

Salvi RJ, Wang J, Powers NL (1996) Plasticity and reorganization in the auditory brainstem: implications for tinnitus. In G Reich, J Vernon (eds) Proceedings of the Fifth International Tinnitus Seminar. Portland: American Tinnitus Association, pp. 457–66.

Salvi RJ, Sun W, Wang J, Guo Y-Q, Ding D-L, Burkard R (2000a) Diminished GABA-A mediated inhibition in auditory cortex following carboplatin-induced inner hair cell loss. Abstract of Association for Research in Otolaryngology 23: 522.

Salvi R, Wang J, Ding D (2000b) Auditory plasticity and hyperactivity following cochlear damage. Hearing Research 147: 261–74.

Suneja SK, Benson CG, Potashner SJ (1998a) Glycine receptors in adult guinea pig brain stem auditory nuclei: regulation after unilateral cochlear ablation. Experimental Neurology 154: 473–88.

Suneja SK, Potashner SJ, Benson CG (1998b) Plastic changes in glycine and GABA release and uptake in adult brain stem auditory nuclei after unilateral middle ear ossicle removal and cochlear ablation. Experimental Neurology 151: 273–88.

Syka J, Rybalko N, Popelar J (1994) Enhancement of the auditory cortex evoked responses in awake guinea pigs after noise exposure. Hearing Research 78: 158–68.

Szczepaniak WS, Moller AR (1995a) Effects of L-baclofen and D-baclofen on the auditory system: a study of click-evoked potentials from the inferior colliculus in the rat. Annals of Otology, Rhinology and Laryngology 104: 399–404.

Szczepaniak WS, Moller AR (1995b) Evidence of decreased GABAergic influence on temporal integration in the inferior colliculus following acute noise exposure: a study of evoked potentials in the rat. Neuroscience Letters 196: 77–80.

Szczepaniak WS, Moller AR (1996a) Effects of (–)-baclofen, clonazepam, and diazepam on tone exposure- induced hyperexcitability of the inferior colliculus in the rat: possible therapeutic implications for pharmacological management of tinnitus and hyperacusis. Hearing Research 97: 46–53.

Szczepaniak WS, Moller AR (1996b) Evidence of neuronal plasticity within the inferior colliculus after noise exposure: a study of evoked potentials in the rat. Electroencephalography of Clinical Neurophysiology 100: 158–64.

Wang J, Salvi RJ, Powers N (1996) Plasticity of response properties of inferior colliculus neurons following acute cochlear damage. Journal of Neurophysiology 75: 171–83.

Wang J, Ding DL, Salvi RJ, Powers N (1997a) Rapid functional plasticity of the neurons in the inferior colliculus and dorsal cochlear nucleus after brief exposure to intense tone. Chinese Journal of Otorhinolaryngology 32: 218–21.

Wang J, Powers NL, Hofstetter P, Trautwein P, Ding D, Salvi R (1997b) Effects of selective inner hair cell loss on auditory nerve fiber threshold, tuning and spontaneous and driven discharge rate. Hearing Research 107: 67–82.

Wang J, Caspary D, Salvi RJ (2000) GABA-A antagonist causes dramatic expansion of tuning in primary auditory cortex. NeuroReport 11: 1137–40.

Weinberger NM (1993) Learning-induced changes of auditory receptive fields. Current Opinion in Neurobiology 3: 570–7.

Weinberger NM, Bakin JS (1998) Learning-induced physiological memory in adult primary auditory cortex: receptive fields plasticity, model, and mechanisms. Audiology and Neuro-Otology 3: 145–67.

Willott JF, Lu SM (1982) Noise-induced hearing loss can alter neural coding and increase excitability in the central nervous system. Science 216: 1331–2.

Willott JF, Aitkin LM, McFadden SL (1993) Plasticity of auditory cortex associated with sensorineural hearing loss in adult C57BL/6J mice. Journal of Comparative Neurology 329: 402–11.

Yang L, Pollak GD, Resler C (1992) GABAergic circuits sharpen tuning curves and modify response properties in the mustache bat inferior colliculus. Journal of Neurophysiology 68: 1760–74.

Young E (1984) Response characteristics of neurons of the cochlear nucleus. In C Berlin (ed.) Hearing Science. San Diego, CA: College-Hill, pp. 423–60.

# CHAPTER 7

# Factors determining an individual's susceptibility to noise damage

*Noise and Its Effects:* Edited by Linda Luxon and Deepak Prasher © 2007
John Wiley & Sons Ltd.

DEEPAK PRASHER

## Introduction

Excessive exposure to noise damages the sensitive cochlear structures through direct mechanical damage or through metabolic overload due to overstimulation. Direct shearing forces damage the outer hair cells of the organ of Corti in the cochlea and the delicate displacement-detecting stereocilia that are the weakest link in the transduction of sound information to the cochlea. Outer hair cells provide biomechanical feedback to enhance cochlear sensitivity and frequency selectivity, whereas the inner hair cells relay signals to the brain via the eighth cranial nerve.

With overstimulation, pathological changes can be observed in the nucleus and cytoplasmic structures. Furthermore, membrane alterations lead to changes in ionic composition and herniation of cell contents. Vascular changes in the stria vascularis and the spiral ligament have also been reported. No direct relationship between pathophysiological changes and function has yet been defined. Thresholds may be normal despite substantial loss of outer and inner hair cells and cannot be predicted accurately on the basis of the extent of hair cell loss; nor can pathological changes be predicted from threshold. However, noise characteristically causes a notch in auditory sensitivity in the region of 2–8 kHz, with reduction in the dynamic range of hearing and impairment of the ability to enhance selectively the detection of a specific frequency of signal. There may also be pitch distortion, impairment of speech perception and tinnitus. Molecular alterations may precede detectable structural and physiological changes, so knowledge of molecular events in the cochlea provides not only a basis for the understanding of the pathogenesis of noise-induced hearing loss (NIHL) but also a means of identifying vulnerable individuals early.

A number of endogenous factors may contribute in the different stages of sound transduction and processing which leads to the large variation observed across individuals when overexposed to noise.

The large variation in susceptibility to noise damage means that it is extremely difficult to define a relationship between the extent of exposure and auditory effects. Even when precise measurement of noise exposures has been possible, as in animal experiments, the extent of the effect observed in terms of both function and pathology has shown considerable variation across individual animals.

## Extent of variability of hearing loss across individuals

Shapiro (1959) was the first to show that extreme differences in hearing loss can be seen with similar exposures over long time. One of his two drop-forge workers with 28 years' exposure had essentially normal hearing whilst the other was almost totally deaf. Taylor et al. (1965) reported a range from 0 to 60 dB hearing loss observed at 4 kHz after 40 years of exposure to industrial noise at 115 dB. The UK Health and Safety Executive report that, if 100 workers are exposed to 100 dB (A) for 40 years, 32 of the 100 will have an average hearing loss greater than 50 dB. Henderson and Hamernik (1995) were able to confirm the variability in threshold change with exact exposure at 161 dB impulse noise in five chinchillas producing a range of 40–70 dB hearing loss.

Same noise exposure in different individuals can result in a range of effects on hearing threshold from no loss to near total loss.

## Relationship between pathology and function

The large variation in the hearing thresholds of people exposed to the same noise over the same time may partly stem from the fact that the relationship between the loss of hearing function and auditory pathology remains obscure. The redundancy in the auditory system means that sometimes significant pathological changes may exhibit only slight change in hearing thresholds and conversely significant functional loss may appear to have only slight morphological change.

Normal thresholds have been reported with considerable outer hair cell and inner hair cell loss. Accurate threshold prediction on the basis of hair cell loss has not been possible, nor has the prediction of underlying pathology for a given threshold.

It is possible to have a loss of 30–40 dB in hearing threshold purely on the basis of loss of active processing function of the outer hair cells.

The wide variation in pathology and its relationship with function may be partly responsible for the variability in hearing observed across individuals after noise exposure.

There is no clearly defined relationship between hearing function and pathology of the auditory system.

# Establishing risk factors and protective mechanisms

It is important to establish the factors that may be responsible for the variation in susceptibility to noise damage as it may lead to means of protection for particularly vulnerable individuals. A number of questions may be posed that may affect the individual's risk of noise damage:

- Does efficient transmission of sound to the inner ear increase risk?
- Does an inefficient efferent control system increase risk?
- Does reduced microcirculation and oxygenation of the cochlea increase risk?
- Does genetic predisposition increase risk?
- Does pre-exposure conditioning alter risk?
- Do melanin and magnesium affect risk?
- Does ageing alter risk?

Of course for each element that poses a risk, if a means of averting the risk can be found, or the means of action can be established, it may be turned to a protective mechanism, such as by reducing sound transmission, increasing cochlear blood flow, increasing levels of magnesium or using gene therapy.

This chapter will assess the evidence for each of the questions posed.

# Risk factor/protective mechanism

## Transmission of sound to the inner ear

*Response of auditory system to noise: external ear canal*

It is clear that increasing the intensity level of noise increases the damage in any individual. The more acoustic energy that is delivered to the cochlea, the greater is the detrimental effect. Thus the variability in the efficiency of sound transmission from the environment to the tympanic membrane must play a crucial role in determining the extent of auditory damage experienced by individuals.

Sounds from the environment are directed to the ear canal by the pinna, which helps in sound localization and amplification of sound in the human speech range. There can be a 3-dB sound pressure gain within the 3 to 6 kHz frequency range. The concha acts as a cavity resonator with around 10-dB sound pressure gain within the 4- to 5-kHz range. The external ear canal with, on average, a length of 25 mm, a diameter of 7 mm and a volume of 1 ml can provide a sound pressure gain of 12 dB at the tympanic membrane with a peak between 3400 and 3900 Hz compared with that at the ear canal opening.

The resonant frequency depends on the length of the canal and the 'amplification' depends on the angle of incidence, canal volume and length. In an average ear canal the resonant frequency is around 3400 Hz where the gain can be as much as 20 dB. There is a decrease in the resonance peak with decreased canal opening size. Chandler (1964) showed that a decrease in canal opening from 3 to 2 mm may produce an increase in hearing loss from 14 dB at 4 kHz to 21 dB. Changing ear canal length by 2 cm to Kemar's ear canal from 2 to 4 cm results in downward shift of resonance peak to around 2400 Hz. Short ear canal lengths shift the resonant frequency above the speech frequency range, for example 1.7 cm, resulting in a peak at 5 kHz.

Gerhardt et al. (1987) showed that the higher the resonant frequency the higher will be the frequency of maximum temporary threshold shift (TTS) (Rodriguez and Gerhardt, 1991) or permanent threshold shift (PTS) (Pierson et al., 1994). The ear canal characteristics therefore determine the acoustic energy transferred to the middle ear and into the cochlea. With the resonance at around 3 kHz in an average ear canal, the characteristic loss of hearing as a result of noise exposure is therefore observed at half an octave shift of the fundamental resonance resulting in the characteristic 4-kHz notch.

The variability in the efficiency with which the ear canal transfers sound to the cochlea in individuals may be partly responsible for the variation observed in the hearing loss due to noise exposure. The geometry of the ear canal is therefore partly responsible for the variation in the level and frequency of the hearing loss. Ear wax, for example, can, by reducing transmission of sound, act as a protector.

Hellstrom (1995) has shown a significant relationship between the dimensions of the ear canal and hearing levels. Large, rather than small, ear canal volumes resulted in a shift of sound transfer functions (STFs) towards lower frequencies. Sound transfer function spectra and magnitudes had a significant effect on hearing levels. He reported that subjects with low-frequency-dominated STFs have higher hearing thresholds than subjects with lower magnitude STFs. A difference in thresholds of 6–8 dB can exist between individuals with high and low sound transfer functions.

Ear canal characteristics determine acoustic energy transferred to the middle ear and into the cochlea.

## Acoustic reflex

*Response of auditory system to noise: middle ear*

The sound entering through the ear canal sets the tympanic membrane in motion transferring the pressure variations via the mechanical system of the middle ear to the cochlea fluids. As the sound medium changes from air to fluid the impedance mismatch can result in a significant loss of sound energy due to the substantial mismatch. However, the middle-ear mechanism, with the surface area ratio change of the ossicular chain and tympanic membrane to oval window is able to effect a significant increase in pressure at the oval window. This mechanical advantage results in an impedance change matching the impedance of the cochlea to that of the ear canal. This provides for an efficient transfer of energy from the tympanic membrane to the cochlear fluids.

It is not clear how variations in the middle-ear system may contribute to the variability in the noise exposure effects but Henderson and Hamernik (1995) have shown that at 220 Hz and 660 Hz the human impedance is two to three times greater than that of the chinchilla and that the chinchillas are 10–15 dB more susceptible to NIHL. The middle-ear system also behaves like a low-pass filter with a cutoff of 1200 Hz, which means that its performance at higher frequencies may be compromised.

The acoustic reflex also provides a means of protection from intense sound exposure. The stapedius muscle attached to the head of the stapes is controlled by the facial nerve (VII) and the tensor tympani muscle, attached to the malleus, is controlled by the trigeminal nerve (V). Loud sounds activate both muscles, which lead to tensor tympani stiffening the tympanic membrane and the stapedius reducing the motion at the oval window, thereby reducing the overall sound transmission through the system and protecting the cochlea from damage. The stiffening of the middle-ear system results in attenuation of sounds below 2000 Hz. The reflex system is activated by sounds just below 80 dB above the threshold of normal hearing. The reduction in sound transmission from acoustic reflex activation can be up to 20 dB in the 125- to 500-Hz frequency range but decreases with increasing frequency up to 2 kHz. Several studies (Brask 1979; Nilsson and Borg 1983; Lonsbury-Martin et al., 1987; Henderson et al., 1993; Quaranta et al., 2003) have shown that workers with efficient reflexes develop less PTS and those with Bell's palsy with no reflex action have increased TTS as a result of noise exposure.

Zakrisson et al. (1975) showed that individuals with Bell's palsy have a greater TTS at low audiometric frequencies than controls. Any ossicular chain defect should theoretically reduce TTS and PTS. Anderson and Barr (1986) showed that the amount of protection depends on the nature of the loss. Interruption of the ossicular chain has a greater effect than fixation.

It is clear that an efficient external and middle-ear system will deliver a greater acoustic stimulation level to the cochlea and thus it will experience a greater loss than the ear that impedes the delivery of the sound stimulus. The structural characteristics and the efficiency of the acoustic reflex mechanism must play a crucial role in determining the variation in the auditory effects observed across people.

Structural characteristics and the efficiency of the acoustic reflex mechanism play a crucial role in determining the extent of the noise effect observed.

### Response of auditory system to noise: cochlea

Once the sound reaches the cochlea, the structural and functional properties of the cochlear mechanisms including the metabolic, vascular, afferent and efferent systems as well as the stiffness of the membranes must play a part in the variability.

Movements of the oval window induce disturbances in the cochlear fluid resulting in a travelling wave in the basilar membrane. Although the frequency of the sound determines the extent of travel with the low frequencies reaching the apex and high frequencies only affecting the basal end, all sounds excite the basal end, which may partially explain the deterioration of hearing from the high frequency end of the range.

The inner hair cells (IHCs) and outer hair cells (OHCs) are responsible for turning the travelling wave mechanical energy into the receptor potentials, which in turn activate the auditory nerve. Noise exposure leads to greater damage or loss of OHCs than IHCs. The OHCs are subject to direct shearing forces at the stereocilia, and are largely unsupported and closer to the maximum travelling wave of the basilar membrane to displacement according to Henderson and Hamernik (1995).

### Cochlear blood supply

Noise exposure can reduce cochlear blood flow, which in turn may lead to hearing loss. Thorne and Nuttall (1987) showed that loud sounds resulted in reduced blood flow in the cochlea. It has been known for some time that acute acoustic trauma results in peripheral vasoconstriction. Spiral modiolar artery provides the main blood supply to the cochlea and its regulation to control cochlear blood flow is crucial for auditory function as the cochlea is sensitive to hypoxia. Nuttall (1999) considers that sound-induced cochlear ischaemia/hypoxia is a mechanism of hearing loss.

Quirk and Seidman (1995) stated that, although the influence of noise on cochlear microcirculation was controversial, investigations had identified a number of microvascular alterations during noise exposure including changes in cochlear lateral wall vessels, red blood cell velocity and capillary vasoconstriction within the cochlea. They suggested that these alterations were sufficient to induce localized periods of stasis, alterations in vascular permeability and local ischaemia, which may result in reduced auditory sensitivity. Evidence (Seidman et al., 1999) suggests that these microcirculatory events are mediated in part by several circulating factors, including the potent vasoactive peptide angiotensin. Goldwin et al. (1998) pretreated guinea pigs with the angiotensin receptor antagonist, sarthran, during noise exposure and showed that sarthran prevents noise-induced microcirculatory ischaemia and preserves auditory sensitivity at the low frequencies tested. Their findings further support the relationship of cochlear blood flow to auditory sensitivity. Latoni et al. (1996) showed that treatment with pentoxifylline maintains cochlear microcirculation, as assessed by continuous red blood cell movement through capillaries, and prevents vasoconstriction or increased permeability often observed in the cochlear microvasculature during noise and reduces noise-induced TTS. Haupt and Schiebe (2002) have demonstrated in the guinea pig that preventive dietary magnesium supplementation can protect the cochlea against noise-induced impairment of blood flow and oxygenation, which may be partly responsible for NIHL.

Alteration of cochlear blood flow may be involved in the aetiology of sudden and fluctuating hearing loss and tinnitus (Herzog et al., 2002). There are vascular changes in the stria vascularis and the spiral ligament as a result of noise exposure, which implies that those with generalized blood circulation problems may be at increased risk of NIHL. Some ciliary changes are reversible and may partly explain the variability of recovery from TTS.

Noise exposure induces the formation in the cochlea of 8-isoprostaglandin F2$\alpha$ (8-iso-PGF2$\alpha$), a marker for reactive oxygen species (Ohinata et al., 2000) and a potent vasoconstrictor, raising the possibility that 8-iso-PGF2$\alpha$ may be responsible for noise-induced reductions in cochlear blood flow (CBF).

Miller et al. (2003) tested this hypothesis; CBF was assessed in the guinea pig in response to 'local' (via the antero-inferior cerebellar artery) and systemic intravenous delivery of 8-iso-PGF2$\alpha$ using laser Doppler flowmetry. Local 8-iso-PGF2$\alpha$ induced a clear reduction in CBF. With systemic infusion, vascular conductance (VC), the ratio of CBF to systemic blood pressure, decreased in a dose-dependent manner up to 30%, consistent with an 8-iso-PGF2$\alpha$-induced constriction of the cochlear vasculature. Infusion of SQ29548, a specific antagonist of 8-iso-PGF2$\alpha$, appropriately blocked an 8-iso-PGF2$\alpha$-induced CBF response. Similarly, noise-induced changes in CBF and VC were prevented by infusion of SQ29548 during noise exposure or by antioxidant treatment (glutathione monoethyl ester) prior to exposure. They suggested that isoprostane-mediated vasoconstriction may be valuable in the protection against NIHL.

It is becoming increasingly clear that the blood supply to the cochlea is vitally important in terms of oxygenation and hence the function of the cochlea and maintenance of the auditory sensitivity. Another condition that affects the blood supply is atherosclerosis, which would have an impact on the susceptibility of the cochlea to damage.

Noise can induce a reduction in cochlear blood flow.

## Smoking

The effect of smoking is most often observed in high-frequency loss and may be mediated via the alterations that it may cause in the vascular system.

Smoking has been shown as an independent risk factor for hearing loss among workers by some researchers (Virokannas and Anttonen 1995; Fuortes et al., 1995; Starck et al., 1999; Nakanishi et al., 2000) whilst others (Friedman et al., 1969; Drettner et al., 1975; Barone et al., 1987; Brant et al., 1996; Karlsmose et al., 1999) have reported no such associations. Cocchiarella et al. (1995) observed that ever-smokers had a hearing loss that was worse by 6.8 dB than never-smokers. A number of reports indicate an association between smoking and high-frequency hearing loss but not with low-frequency loss. It has also been shown (Browning et al., 1986) that high-frequency loss may be associated with high shear blood viscosity, which may also occur with smoking. The differential effect on high frequency may explain why some studies using average hearing thresholds across all frequencies may not have shown an association. More recently, Mizoue et al. (2003), after examining the association between exposure to noise and hearing loss among 4624 steel workers in Japan, reported that smoking was associated with an increased odds of having high-frequency hearing loss in a dose–response manner with a prevalence rate ratio (PRR) of 2.56 among workers exposed to noise whilst the PRR for smokers not exposed to noise was 1.57 and for non-smokers exposed to noise it was 1.77. The combined effect of smoking and exposure to occupational noise was comparable to the sum of the independent effects of each factor at 4 kHz but not at 1 kHz where no significant effect was observed.

The mechanism by which smoking may damage hair cells is hypothesized to be through reduced blood flow or by increasing carboxyhaemoglobin (Hawkins, 1971; Fechter et al., 1987). Nicotinic-type receptors have also been found in hair cells, which may contribute direct ototoxic effects on hair cell function (Blanchet et al., 1996).

There appears to be growing evidence (Toppila et al., 2000; Hong and Kim 2001) that smoking is a contributory factor for high-frequency hearing loss and combined with noise exposure increases the risk for hearing loss.

## Ageing

It is not clear whether the ageing ear is more vulnerable than a younger one. Hetu et al. (1977) showed that TTS was not significantly different in 12-year-olds compared with adults. There is no clear evidence that the aged ear is tougher than the young one or vice versa but there is evidence that ageing effects combined with those due to noise exposure can leave the individual with greater disability than if either existed on its own. Furthermore, the audiometric threshold change with age affects the high-frequency region and combines with the noise effects in that region to reach a plateau after a certain age or noise exposure.

Campo et al. (2003) examined noise-induced hearing and hair cell loss in young (3 months) and aged (24–26 months) Long-Evans rats. The animals were exposed 6 h/days, 5 days/week for 4 weeks to broadband noise centred at 8 kHz (92 or 97 dB SPL). Aged controls showed OHC loss at the basal and apical regions of the organ of Corti, and an increase in pigmentation concomitant with a decrease in vascularization of the stria vascularis, along with elevated thresholds relative to young controls. The 92-dB noise caused similar threshold shifts in both age groups, whereas the 97-dB noise caused more threshold shifts in the aged group compared with the young.

However, Boettcher (2002), investigating the susceptibility to acoustic trauma in young and aged gerbils, suggested that no differences exist in susceptibility as a function of age. Similarly, Frenkel et al. (2003) found that the noise exposures caused elevations in auditory brain-stem response threshold and reductions in distortion product otoacoustic emission (DPOAE) amplitude and transient evoked otoacoustic emission (TEOAE) energy content that were similar in both the old and young rats.

## Temporary threshold shift

### Response of auditory system to noise: nerve VIII

Pujol, Puel and co-workers have shown that, in guinea pigs, noise overstimulation produces a TTS, partly through excitotoxic damage to primary auditory dendrites due to excessive release of glutamate, an excitatory amino acid used as a neurotransmitter by the IHCs. Application of kynurenate, a glutamate antagonist, during intense sound exposure prevents dendritic damage and limits the TTS. Part of the recovery from the TTS is attributed to the synaptic repair and reconnection of IHCs by new dendritic processes. The permanent loss is due to loss or damage of OHCs, which were unaffected by the treatment.

Although TTS has, for some time, been suggested as means of identifying vulnerable individuals, very few studies have shown a positive correlation between TTS and PTS. Lawton and Robinson (1986) examined a number of indices in tough ears (those having minimal change in thresholds after many years of noise exposure) and compared them with normal unexposed ears, but found none to be of value in predicting susceptibility. It may, however, be presumed that repeated TTS with regular exposures may lead to increasing TTS with an ever-reducing recovery, which then manifests itself as PTS. Hetu and Parrot (1978) reported that empirical rules predicting exponential growth and recovery of TTS during and following a work day apply in men who have a significant PTS from repeated exposures to the same work-day noise for a number of previous years. However, it has also been reported (Hamernik et al., 2003) that repeated exposures can result in reduced TTS after initial 'toughening' of the auditory system. This reduction of threshold shift, despite the continuing daily exposure regimen, has been called a cochlear toughening effect and the exposures referred to as toughening exposures. It appears that behavioural and physiological recovery from noise exposure follows an increasing resistance to the effects of repeated exposure. Clark (1991) in reviewing the literature indicated that, with continuous exposures to moderate-level noise, thresholds reach asymptotic levels within 18–24 hours; however, PTSs depend upon the level, frequency and duration of exposure. He reported further that periodic rest periods inserted in an exposure schedule are protective and result in less hearing loss and cochlear damage than equal energy continuous exposures and, under some schedules of periodic exposure, threshold shifts increase over the first few days of exposure, then recover as much as 30 dB as the exposure continues.

A number of factors may be identified that may affect the variability observed in the TTS after noise exposure. The extent of stereocilia rigidity may be a significant factor as well as the extent of loss of receptor currents due to disruption of transduction channels. The extent to which the increased noise levels lead to high metabolic activity resulting in excitotoxic damage such as swelling and loss of dendritic terminals at IHCs and high densities of synaptic vesicles at the efferent endings of OHCs may also contribute to the level of TTS observed. Glutamate excitotoxicity has also been implicated in the pathological processes. The degree of disruption of the active biomechanical feedback mechanism may also play a part in determining the initial threshold shift.

Ruel et al. (2001) have shown that tonic inhibition at the first synapse through the lateral olivocochlear efferent system acts as a gain control of the auditory nerve response. Furthermore, they state that dysfunction of this system may lead to the development of glutamate-induced excitotoxicity and consequently increased cochlear vulnerability to sound.

It appears that the extent of initial TTS following noise exposure is unable to predict the final PTS as a number of variables affect the final threshold including the 'toughening' phenomenon, extent of the natural recovery mechanisms in place, nature of the exposure in terms of the time course and spectral composition. Thus the initial threshold change does not appear to be a valuable indicator of long-term effects. It appears that the vulnerability to continued noise exposure is dynamic and dependent on features of the exposure and recovery/protective mechanisms available. TTS itself may be a means of protection of the auditory system as it results in a reduction in the influence of further exposure.

# Genes

Susceptibility to NIHL is poorly understood at the genetic level. There is evidence that genetic and environmental factors contribute to hearing loss. The genetic effects implicate the *Ahl* gene as contributing to susceptibility for NIHL. According to Davis et al. (2001) all the evidence supports the role of the *Ahl* gene in both age-related hearing loss and NIHL among certain strains of mice. The mice that show pronounced age-related hearing loss are also especially vulnerable to noise, which supports the notion that genes associated with age-related hearing loss often act by rendering the cochlea susceptible to insults (Ohlemiller et al., 2000).

As Fridberger et al. (1998) had observed that OHC cytoplasmic calcium concentration rises following acoustic overstimulation, this led Kozel et al. (2002) to examine mice with deficiency in plasma membrane calcium ATPase isoform 2 which is expressed on OHC stereocilia, to determine whether this increased susceptibility to NIHL. They confirmed this to be the case.

Cells produce heat-shock proteins (hsps) in response to any form of stress, including acoustic overstimulation. According to Altschuler and co-workers (2002), these proteins facilitate cellular repair by binding to damaged proteins and preventing further damage; after noise exposure, hsp70i, hsp72, hsp27, and hsp90 are expressed in the OHCs and the stria vascularis, and the greater the expression of hsp72, the greater the protection. Neurotrophic factors can also protect against noise-induced damage, perhaps by acting on oxidative stress-driven increases in intracellular calcium through induced expression of calcium-binding proteins or antioxidant enzymes. Glia-derived neurotrophic factors (GDNFs) have been applied directly to the inner ear, by microcannulation of the scala tympani, with expression of GDNF mRNA in IHC of mature rats and expression of GDNF-α in the spiral ganglion cells. Brain-derived neurotrophic factors and neurotrophin 3 (NT3) provide dose-dependent protection against NIHL. Studies of how growth factors might be used in gene therapy to protect against NIHL are in progress. Inoculation of an adenoviral vector encoding the human GDNF gene into the perilymph before trauma has reduced damage to OHCs.

Initial temporary threshold shift following noise exposure is unable to predict the final permanent loss.

## Oxidative stress

Oxygen free radicals are produced in hair cells after metabolic overload from intense sound exposure, so they have been implicated in the development of NIHL, probably when they are converted to the highly destructive hydroxyl radicals in the stria vascularis. These radicals induce membrane lipid peroxidation, which alters ion homoeostasis and energy metabolism and destroys plasma membranes. These processes can lead to a cascade of events culminating in apoptosis.

Ohlemiller et al. (1999) have shown that targeted deletion of the cytosolic Cu/Zn superoxide dismutase gene (*Sod1*) increases vulnerability to NIHL. Antioxidant enzymes such as superoxide dismutase (SOD) play a vital role in reducing reactive oxygen species. Yamasoba et al. (1998) have shown that inhibition by the antioxidant glutathione increases susceptibility to NIHL and replenishing glutathione by enhancing availability of cysteine reduces noise-induced cochlear damage.

The proposed strategies for protection include the enhancement of the natural mechanisms – by, for example, antioxidative processes to inhibit free-radical generation or to accelerate removal of superoxide, iron or derived free radicals. Agents that upregulate the antioxidant enzyme activity reduce the damage expected from acoustic trauma, whereas a reduction in glutathione concentrations increases NIHL. Transgenic mice overexpressing SOD show a significantly reduced TTS after noise exposure. Intraperitoneal injections of antioxidants such as allopurinol, lazaroids, α-D-tocopherol and mannitol have helped in reducing the threshold shift after noise exposure.

This means that endogeneous levels of antioxidant enzymes are important determinants of susceptibility to NIHL.

Metabolic overload due to noise exposure resulting in the production of oxygen free radicals leading to a cascade of events to cell death may be one possible mechanism.

# Efferent control of cochlear mechanics

It is becoming clear that the cochlear biomechanical amplification occurs via the motile OHCs under efferent control. This mechanism provides the gain control of the active, non-linear cochlear-processing system. The efferent medial olivocochlear system originating at the medial superior olivary complex acts through synapses with OHCs whilst the lateral olivocochlear system from the lateral superior olive acts through synapses with afferent dendrites of auditory neurons below the IHCs. It has been estimated that the mechanical sensitivity may be increased by 55–60 dB when the OHCs are operating normally (Patuzzi and Thompson, 1991) and reduced as the ability of the OHCs to generate their receptor currents is impaired. Loss of receptor currents may be due to a number of causes including saturation of current generation processes at the apex of OHCs by large movements of hair bundles, such as may be experienced with loud sounds.

This may be one of the earliest indications of change in the auditory system as a result of overstimulation. In this regard, otoacoustic emissions, which reflect OHC function, have been found to be very useful and particularly sensitive to acoustic trauma, drugs, hypoxia and so forth.

A number of studies (Desai et al., 1999; Plinkert et al., 1999; Prasher and Sulkowski, 1999; Hall and Lutman 1999; Attias et al., 2001) indicate that otoacoustic emissions provide an indication of OHC damage from overstimulation by noise prior to any change in the pure-tone audiometric threshold. There is also some evidence that the medial efferent system evaluation using contralateral sound-activated suppression of transient emissions indicates dysfunction after noise exposure. Increased variability of spontaneous emissions has also been shown to be associated with the presence of tinnitus in various aetiologies. Contralateral sound-activated efferent suppression of otoacoustic emissions can be used to examine the integrity of the auditory efferent system. It has been shown that prior to changes in otoacoustic emissions as a result of noise exposure, the efferent suppression of emissions is affected. The possible deactivation of active processes of OHCs may partially explain the variability of noise damage. The relative risk for an individual may depend on the strength of efferent control and reflex protective mechanisms.

Henderson et al. (2001) have shown that stimulation of the cochlear efferent system, either with electrical shocks to the floor of the fourth ventricle or sound at the contralateral ear, reduces the TTS from a moderate-level short-duration exposure. Those chinchillas with ablation of the efferent system developed more hearing loss and greater loss of hair cells than controls.

Yamasoba and Dolan (1997) investigated whether elimination of the medial efferent system influences PTS following noise exposure, in which strychnine was chronically delivered into the cochlea via an osmotic pump. Their study showed that chronic strychnine administration into the cochlea inactivates the medial efferents without changing hearing threshold and that the medial efferents help to protect against PTS following noise exposure.

Attanasio et al. (1999) demonstrated that sectioning of the olivocochlear bundle (OCB) in guinea pigs causes persistent hearing loss during noise exposure, in contrast to the unoperated ear. According to Zheng et al. (1997a) sectioning the olivocochlear fibres decreased cochlear microphonics whilst DPOAEs were unchanged but, following noise exposure, the ears that were de-efferented showed significantly more depression of DPOAEs and greater decrement of CM amplitude. De-efferentation resulted in an increase in susceptibility to noise-induced hearing damage across all frequencies. Furthermore, de-efferented ears showed substantially more TTS, greater PTS and larger cochlear lesions of OHCs (Zheng et al., 1997b).

The crossed and uncrossed medial olivocochlear systems terminate on cochlear outer hair cells and mediate their effects via the nicotinic cholinergic receptors.

Maison et al. (2002) have demonstrated that the efferent protection is mediated via the cholinergic system α-9-nicotinic acetylcholine receptor (nAChR) complex in the OHCs. Luebke and Foster (2002) suggest that the variation in inter-animal susceptibility to noise damage is associated with AChR subunit expression level as this was correlated with the animals' average efferent strength.

There is growing evidence that the active processing mediated via the efferent control of the OHCs may be the first casualty of overstimulation of the cochlea leading to problems of frequency selectivity. The strength or vulnerability of the efferent control mechanism in individuals may provide the first indication of vulnerability of the individual to excessive stimulation-induced auditory system damage. The contralateral sound-activated suppression of the otoacoustic emissions provides a means of evaluating the efferent pathway function. Reduced or absent efferent suppression of otoacoustic emissions may be an indication of a compromised functional pathway. Furthermore, evidence suggests that the efferent system may contribute to the protection mechanism of the cochlea possibly by altering the cochlear gain. Alterations in the efferent system of control of the cochlear mechanics may also explain the possible mechanism for the generation of noise-induced tinnitus.

Thus, measures of the efferent system may be a very effective means of early detection of the effects of noise on the auditory system and a possible means of identifying vulnerable individuals. Clearly these changes manifest themselves much earlier than the audiometric threshold alterations observed using standard audiometric techniques and therefore provide a means of early investigation of susceptibility.

Maison and Liberman (2000) demonstrated, in an animal model, that the measures of the strength of the sound-evoked neuronal feedback pathway to the cochlea, the olivocochlear efferents, were inversely correlated with the degree of hearing loss after subsequent noise exposure. They suggest that this reflex strength would be useful in screening individuals most at risk in noisy environments.

Veuillet et al. (2001) investigated the relationship between recovery of cochlear function after acoustic trauma and variables that may serve as predictors of vulnerability to NIHL. No significant change in transient emissions or efferent suppression was observed whereas the incidence of spontaneous emissions was found to increase in the affected ear. There was no correlation between NIHL and efferent suppression on the day of trauma but significant correlations were obtained between audiometric threshold improvements by day 3 and extent of suppression, with better recovery in those with the greater suppression.

In our study (Desai et al., 1999) of subjects exposed to noise but having a hearing threshold better than 30 dB, it was observed that they had reduced transient emissions compared with controls and 54% had absent transient emissions and 60% of those with emissions present had absence of efferent suppression. This was in contrast to those with similar thresholds but suffering from Ménière's disease, in whom only 8% had absence of emissions and none had absence of suppression. It appears that the earliest indication of auditory damage from noise exposure prior to any audiometric change is the absence of emission suppression followed by absence of transient emissions. These techniques provide an early indication of noise effects in susceptible individuals.

Noise exposure may affect the auditory efferent control mechanisms early in the chain of effects.

# Magnesium

Noise overstimulation increases energy consumption, which is heavily dependent on magnesium and calcium metabolism. Decreases in extracellular magnesium affect the intracellular ion content of the hair cells, especially the calcium concentrations. The potential for hearing loss is increased if magnesium concentrations are low or reduced by noise exposure. Oral supplements of magnesium have been shown in army recruits to reduce significantly the temporary and permanent hearing loss caused by noise.

A number of studies (Joachims et al., 1993; Attias et al., 1994) have shown the beneficial effects of magnesium in protecting against NIHL. Noise-induced hearing loss increased with decreasing serum magnesium (Gunther et al., 1989) but no associations were observed between hearing levels and naturally occurring body magnesium. Walden et al. (2000) showed that a small change in magnesium intake leads to significant changes in inner-ear susceptibility to NIHL in guinea pigs exposed to impulsive noise.

Schiebe et al. (2001) examined the therapeutic effect of magnesium on noise trauma in guinea pigs. They showed that PTS and perilymph magnesium levels showed a close negative correlation suggesting that intracochlear magnesium is important in the protective effect. The therapeutic effect decreased with the time elapsed between the end of exposure and beginning of treatment.

A recent study (Konig et al., 2003) demonstrated that magnesium is protective in hypoxia-induced hair cell loss using an in vitro model of the newborn rat cochlea.

## Sound conditioning

Another interesting approach to protection has come from the observations of Canlon (1997), who showed that low-level exposure to an acoustic stimulus before noise trauma can alter the susceptibility to and reduce the PTS. This approach is termed 'sound conditioning'. Another approach – intermittent pre-exposure to high sound levels that produce a TTS – is termed 'toughening'. Although precisely how conditioning or toughening protects against TTS is unknown, sound conditioning boosts endogenous antioxidant systems, which can protect against noise trauma. It has been shown by a number of studies that conditioning the ear with low-level sound stimulation or toughening with a louder sound prior to a noise exposure results in reduced damage. It has been suggested that conditioning effects may involve efferent olivocochlear pathways or stress-induced gene expression. Wang and Liberman (2002) have shown that mild physical restraint of mice significantly reduced PTS from subsequent acoustic overexposure as long as the treatment–trauma was short (2 hours). The period of protection coincided with the period of elevated corticosterone levels. This study suggests that stress pathways and glucocortcoid levels may be important in cochlear protection. Niu and Canlon (2002) have demonstrated that tyrosine hydroxylase in the lateral efferents are upregulated during sound conditioning and suggest a role for the lateral efferent system in protecting against acoustic trauma by sound conditioning.

## Melanin

It has been shown (Kleinstein et al., 1984; Barrenas and Lindgren, 1991) that a significant difference exists between the susceptibility to noise in people with brown eyes and that in those with blue eyes. Those with brown eyes develop less TTS than those with blue eyes. This is explained on the basis of inner-ear melanin. Race differences have also been reported (Royster et al., 1980; Jerger et al., 1986) which show that black people are less susceptible to noise than their white counterparts, again implicating melanin as a protector. It has been suggested that eumelanin and pheomelanin may have differing effects within the stria vascularis. It is interpreted as a toxic interaction in the strial melanocytes between pheomelanin and noise. Melanin can both generate and neutralize reactive oxygen species depending on the type.

## Tinnitus

Tinnitus may be an early indicator of the effect of excessive noise stimulation.

Overstimulation of the cochlea may lead to increased instability of spontaneous and neural activity resulting in the perception of tinnitus. A recent investigation of spontaneous emissions found significantly more variable spontaneous emissions in subjects with tinnitus than without (Prasher et al., 2001). Continued stimulation at a high sound level may result in the efferent-mediated gain control suppressing the auditory input as much as possible. Excessive stimulation results in the disruption of the feedback control of active processing which may play a role in the generation of tinnitus after noise exposure. The resetting of control mechanisms after noise exposure may result in the tinnitus subsiding after a few hours or sometimes days. It is not clear whether those individuals who suffer from post-noise exposure tinnitus are more vulnerable to noise damage. Conversely those with similar noise exposure but absence of tinnitus post-exposure have more robust auditory systems. Furthermore, whether repeated exposures contribute to continuous presence of tinnitus has not been established.

# Conclusions

Noise initially impairs active processing of OHCs under efferent control. Noise subsequently leads to reduced otoacoustic emissions as a consequence of OHC dysfunction. Further noise damages OHCs leading to raised auditory thresholds.

A number of factors have been identified that may contribute to the variability observed in an individual's susceptibility to noise damage. It is clear that some factors may also trigger protective mechanisms against damage. It may be possible to use some of the risk factor assessments and the level of protection afforded by some measures to determine the extent of vulnerability of an individual. For example, an assessment of the relative strength of the acoustic reflex, or the efferent suppression or otoacoustic emission amplitude, may provide an indication of relative functional response to noise of the auditory system. Furthermore, the levels of melanin or magnesium, or the relative protection from sound conditioning may also provide an indication of the tolerance to noise available to an individual. Other indicators of noise effects on the auditory system may be the presence of and recovery from noise-induced tinnitus.

# References

Altschuler RA, Fairfield D, Cho Y, Leonova E, Benjamin IJ, Miller JM et al. (2002) Stress pathways in the rat cochlea and potential for protection from acquired deafness. Audiol Neuro-otol 7: 152–6.

Anderson H, Barr B (1986) Conductive recruitment. Acta Otolaryngol 62: 171–84.

Attanasio G, Barbara M, Buongiorno G, Cordier A, Mafera B, Piccoli F et al. (1999) Protective effect of the cochlear efferent system during noise exposure. Ann NY Acad Sci 28: 361–7.

Attias J, Weisz G, Almog S, Shahar A, Wiener M, Joachims Z et al. (1994) Oral magnesium intake reduces permanent hearing loss induced by noise exposure. Am J Otolaryngol 15: 26–32.

Attias J, Horovitz G, El-Hatib N, Nageris B (2001) Detection and clinical diagnosis of noise-induced hearing loss by otoacoustic emissions. Noise Health 3(12): 19–31.

Barone JA, Peters JM, Garabrant DH, Bernstein L, Krebsbach R (1987) Smoking as a risk factor in noise-induced hearing loss. J Occup Med 29: 741–5.

Barrenas ML, Lindgren F (1991) The influence of eye colour on susceptibility to TTS in humans. Br J Audiol 25: 303–7.

Blanchet C, Erostegui C, Sugasawa M, Dulon D (1996) Acetylcholine-induced potassium current of guinea pig outer hair cells: its dependence on a calcium influx through nicotinic-like receptors. J Neurosci 16: 2574–84.

Boettcher FA (2002) Susceptibility to acoustic trauma in young and aged gerbils. J Acoust Soc Am 112: 2948–55.

Brant LJ, Gordon-Salant S, Pearson JD, Klein LL, Morrell CH, Metter EJ et al. (1996) Risk factors related to age-associated hearing loss in the speech frequencies. J Am Acad Audiol 7: 152–60.

Brask T (1979) The noise protection effect of the stapedius reflex. Acta Otolaryngol Suppl 360: 116–17.

Browning GG, Gatehouse S, Lowe GD (1986) Blood viscosity as a factor in sensorineural hearing impairment. Lancet i: 121–3.

Campo P, Pouyatos B, Lataye R, Morel G (2003) Is the aged rat ear more susceptible to noise or styrene damage than the young ear? Noise Health 5(19): 1–18.

Canlon B (1997) Protection against noise trauma by sound conditioning. Ear Nose Throat J 76: 248–50.

Chandler JR (1964) Partial occlusion of the external auditory meatus; its effect upon air and bone conduction hearing acuity. Laryngoscope 74: 22–54.

Clark WW (1991) Recent studies of temporary threshold shift (TTS) and permanent threshold shift (PTS) in animals. J Acoust Soc Am 90: 155–63.

Cocchiarella LA, Sharp DS, Persky VW (1995) Hearing threshold shifts, white-cell count and smoking status in working men. Occup Med 45: 179–85.

Davis RR, Newlander JK, Ling X, Cortopassi GA, Krieg EF, Erway LC (2001) Genetic basis for susceptibility to noise-induced hearing loss in mice. Hear Res 155(1–2): 82–90.

Desai A, Reed D, Cheyne A, Richards S, Prasher D (1999) Absence of otoacoustic emissions in subjects with normal audiometric thresholds implies exposure to noise. Noise Health 1(2): 58–65.

Drettner B, Hedstrand H, Klockhoff I, Svedberg A (1975) Cardiovascular risk factors and hearing loss. A study of 1000 fifty-year-old men. Acta Otolaryngol 79: 366–71.

Fechter LD, Thorne PR, Nuttall AL (1987) Effects of carbon monoxide on cochlear electrophysiology and blood flow. Hear Res 27: 37–45.

Frenkel R, Freeman S, Sohmer H (2003) Susceptibility of young adult and old rats to noise-induced hearing loss. Audiolo Neuro-otol 8: 129–39.

Friedman GD, Siegelanb AB, Seltzer CC (1969) Cigarette smoking and exposure occupational hazards. Am J Epidemiol 98: 175–183

Fridberger A, Flock A, Ulfendahl M, Flock B (1998) Acoustic overstimulation increases outer hair cell $Ca^{2+}$ concentrations and causes dynamic contractions of the hearing organ. Proc Natl Acad Sci USA 95: 7127–32.

Fuortes LJ, Tang S, Pomrehn P, Anderson C (1995) Prospective evaluation of associations between hearing sensitivity and selected cardiovascular risk factors. Am J Ind Med 28: 275–80.

Gerhardt KJ, Rodriguez, GP, Hepler EL, Moul ML (1987) Ear canal volume and variability in the patterns of temporary threshold shifts. Ear Hear 8: 316–21.

Goldwin B, Khan MJ, Shivapuja B, Seidman MD, Quirk WS (1998) Sarthran preserves cochlear microcirculation and reduces temporary threshold shifts after noise exposure. Otolaryngol Head Neck Surg 118: 576–83.

Gunther T, Ising H, Joachims Z (1989) Biochemical mechanisms affecting susceptibility to noise-induced hearing loss. Am J Otol 10: 36–41.

Hall AJ, Lutman ME (1999) Methods for early identification of noise-induced hearing loss. Audiology 38: 277–80.

Hamernik RP, Qiu W, Davis B (2003) Cochlear toughening, protection, and potentiation of noise-induced trauma by non-Gaussian noise. J Acoust Soc Am 113: 969–76.

Haupt H, Scheibe F (2002) Preventive magnesium supplement protects the inner ear against noise-induced impairment of blood flow and oxygenation in the guinea pig. Magnes Res 15(1–2): 17–25.

Hawkins JE Jr (1971) The role of vasoconstriction in noise-induced hearing loss. Ann Otol Rhinol Laryngol 80: 903–13.

Hellstrom PA (1995) The relationship between sound transfer functions and hearing levels. Hear Res 88(1–2): 54–60.

Henderson D, Hamernik RP (1995) Biologic bases of noise-induced hearing loss. Occup Med 10: 513–34.

Henderson D, Subramaniam M, Boetttcher FA (1993) Individual susceptibility to noise-induced hearing loss: an old topic revisited. Ear Hear 14: 152–68.

Henderson D, Zheng X, McFadden SL (2001) Cochlear efferent system: A factor in susceptibility to noise. In D Henderson, D Prasher, R Kopke, R Salvi, R Hamernik (eds) Noise Induced Hearing Loss: Basic mechanisms, prevention and control. London: nRn Publications.

Herzog M, Scherer EQ, Albrecht B, Rorabaugh B, Scofield MA, Wangemann P (2002) CGRP receptors in the gerbil spiral modiolar artery mediate a sustained vasodilation via a transient cAMP-mediated $Ca^{2+}$-decrease. J Membr Biol 189: 225–36.

Hetu R, Parrot J (1978) A field evaluation of noise-induced temporary threshold shift. Am Ind Hyg Assoc J 39: 301–11.

Hetu R, Dumont L, Legare D (1977) TTS at 4 kHz among school age children following continuous exposure to broad band noise. J Acoust Soc Am 62(suppl 1): S96.

Hong OS, Kim MJ (2001) Factors associated with hearing loss among workers of the airline industry in Korea. ORL Head Neck Nurs 19(1): 7–13.

Jerger J, Jerger S, Pepe P, Miller R (1986) Race difference in susceptibility to noise-induced hearing loss. Am J Otol 7: 425–9.

Joachims Z, Netzer A, Ising H, Rebentisch E, Attias J, Weisz G et al. (1993) Oral magnesium supplementation as prophylaxis for noise-induced hearing loss: results of a double blind field study. Schriftenr Ver Wasser Boden Lufthyg 88: 503–16.

Karlsmose B, Lauritzen T, Parving A (1999) Prevalence of hearing impairment and subjective hearing problems in a rural Danish population aged 31–50 years. Br J Audiol 33: 395–402.

Kleinstein RN, Seitz MR, Barton TE, Smith CR (1984) Iris color and hearing loss. Am J Optom Physiol Opt 61: 145–9.

Konig O, Winter E, Fuchs J, Haupt H, Mazurek B, Weber N et al. (2003) Protective effect of magnesium and MK 801 on hypoxia-induced hair cell loss in newborn rat cochlea. Magnes Res 16(2): 98–105.

Kozel PJ, Davis RR, Krieg EF, Shull G, Erway LC (2002) Deficiency in plasma membrane calcium ATPase isoform 2 increases susceptibility to noise-induced hearing loss in mice. Hear Res 164: 231–9.

Latoni J, Shivapuja B, Seidman MD, Quirk WS (1996) Pentoxifylline maintains cochlear microcirculation and attenuates temporary threshold shifts following acoustic overstimulation. Acta Otolaryngol 116: 388–94.

Lawton BW, Robinson DW (1986) An investigation of tests of susceptibility to noise-induced hearing loss. Institute of Sound and Vibration Research, University of Southampton, technical report 138. Southampton, UK.

Lonsbury-Martin BL, Martin GK, Bohne BA (1987) Repeated TTS exposures in monkeys: alterations in hearing, cochlear structure, and single-unit thresholds. J Acoust Soc Am 81: 1507–18.

Luebke AE, Foster PK (2002) Variation in inter-animal susceptibility to noise damage is associated with alpha 9 acetylcholine receptor subunit expression level. J Neurosci 22: 4241–7.

Maison SF, Liberman MC (2000) Predicting vulnerability to acoustic injury with a noninvasive assay of olivocochlear reflex strength. J Neurosci 20: 4701–7.

Maison SF, Luebke AE, Liberman MC, Zuo J (2002) Efferent protection from acoustic injury is mediated via alpha9 nicotinic acetylcholine receptors on outer hair cells. J Neurosci 22: 10838–46.

McFadden SL, Campo P, Ding D, Quaranta N (1998) Effects of noise on inferior colliculus evoked potentials and cochlear anatomy in young and aged chinchillas. Hearing Research 117(1-2): 81–96.

McFadden SL, Ohlemillier KK, Ding D, Shero M, Salvi RJ (2001) The influence of superoxide dismutase and glutathione peroxidase deficiencies on noise-induced hearing loss in mice. Noise and Health 3(11): 49–64.

Miller JM, Brown JN, Schacht J (2003) 8-Iso-prostaglandin F(2alpha), a product of noise exposure, reduces inner ear blood flow. Audiol Neuro-otol 8: 207–21.

Mizoue T, Miyamoto T, Shimizu T (2003) Combined effect of smoking and occupational exposure to noise on hearing loss in steel factory workers. Occup Environ Med 60: 56–9.

Mom T, Bonfils P, Gilain L, Avan P (1999) Vulnerability of the gerbil cochlea to sound exposure during reversible ischemia. Hear Res 136(1–2): 65–74.

Nakanishi N, Okamoto M, Nakamura K, Suzuki K, Tatara K (2000) Cigarette smoking and risk for hearing impairment: a longitudinal study in Japanese male office workers. J Occup Environ Med 42: 1045–9.

Nilsson R, Borg E (1983) Noise-induced hearing loss in shipyard workers with unilateral conductive hearing loss. Scand Audiol 12: 135–40.

Niu X, Canlon B (2002) Protective mechanisms of sound conditioning. Advances Otorhinolaryngol 59: 96–105.

Nuttall AL (1999) Sound-induced cochlear ischemia/hypoxia as a mechanism of hearing loss. Noise Health 2(5): 17–32.

Ohinata Y, Miller JM, Altschuler RA, Schacht J (2000) Intensive noise induces formation of vasoactive lipid peroxidation products in the cochlea. Brain Res 878: 163–73.

Ohlemiller KK, McFadden SL, Ding DL, Flood DG, Reaume AG, Hoffman EK et al. (1999) Targeted deletion of the cytosolic Cu/Zn-superoxide dismutase gene (Sod1) increases susceptibility to noise-induced hearing loss. Audiol Neuro-otol 4: 237–46.

Ohlemiller KK, Wright JS, Heidbreder AF (2000) Vulnerability to noise-induced hearing loss in 'middle-aged' and young adult mice: a dose-response approach in CBA, C57BL, and BALB inbred strains. Hear Res 149: 239–47.

Patuzzi RB, Thompson ML (1991) Cochlear efferent neurones and protection against acoustic trauma: protection of outer hair cell receptor current and interanimal variability. Hear Res 54(1): 45–58.

Pierson LL, Gerhardt KJ, Rodriguez GP, Yanke RB (1994) Relationship between outer ear resonance and permanent noise-induced hearing loss. Am J Otolaryngol 15: 37–40.

Plinkert PK, Hemmert W, Wagner W, Just K, Zenner HP (1999) Monitoring noise susceptibility: sensitivity of otoacoustic emissions and subjective audiometry. Br J Audiol 33: 367–82.

Prasher D, Sulkowski W (1999) The role of otoacoustic emissions in screening and evaluation of noise damage. Int J Occup Med Environ Health 12: 183–92.

Prasher D, Ceranic B, Sulkowski W, Guzek W (2001) Objective evidence for tinnitus from spontaneous emission variability. In D Henderson, D Prasher, R Kopke, R Salvi, R Hamernik (eds) Noise Induced Hearing Loss: Basic mechanisms. prevention and control. London: nRn Publications, pp. 471–83.

Quaranta A, Scaringi A, Fernandez-Vega S, Quaranta N (2003) Effect of ipsilateral and contralateral low-frequency narrow-band noise on temporary threshold shift in humans. Acta Otolaryngol 123: 164–7.

Quirk WS, Seidman MD (1995) Cochlear vascular changes in response to loud noise. Am J Otol 16: 322–5.

Rodriguez GP, Gerhardt KJ (1991) Influence of outer ear resonant frequency on patterns of temporary threshold shift. Ear Hear 12: 110–14.

Royster LH, Royster JD, Thomas WG (1980) Representative hearing levels by race and sex in North Carolina Industry. J Acoust Soc Am 68: 551–66.

Ruel J, Gervais d'Aldin C, Nouvian R, Pujol R, Puel JL (2001) Tonic dopamine inhibition from the lateral olivo-cochlear efferents protects the auditory nerve dendrites from glutamate-induced excitotoxicity. In D Henderson, D Prasher, R Kopke, R Salvi, R Hamernik (eds) Noise Induced Hearing Loss: Basic mechanisms, prevention and control. London: nRn Publications, pp. 141–53.

Schiebe F, Haupt H, Mazurek B, Konig O (2001) Therapeutic effect of magnesium on noise-induced hearing loss. Noise Health 3(11): 79–84.

Seidman MD, Quirk WS, Shirwany NA (1999) Mechanisms of alterations in the microcirculation of the cochlea. Ann NY Acad Sci 884: 226–32.

Shapiro SL (1959) Deafness following short-term exposure to industrial noise. Ann Otol 68: 1170–81.

Starck J, Toppila E, Pyykko I (1999) Smoking as a risk factor in sensory neural hearing loss among workers exposed to occupational noise. Acta Otolaryngol 119: 302–5.

Taylor W, Pearson J, Main A, Burns W (1965) Study of noise and hearing. J Acoust Soc Am 38: 113–120.

Thorne PR, Nuttall AL (1987) Laser Doppler measurements of cochlear blood flow during loud sound exposure in the guinea pig. Hear Res 27(1): 1–10.

Thorne PR, Nuttall AL (1995) Dose-response relationship between smoking and impairment of hearing acuity in workers exposed to noise. Scand Audiol 24: 211–6.

Toppila E, Pyykko II, Starck J, Kaksonen R, Ishizaki H (2000) Individual risk factors in the development of noise-induced hearing loss. Noise Health 2(8): 59–70.

Veuillet E, Martin V, Suc B, Vesson JF, Morgon A, Collet L (2001) Otoacoustic emissions and medial olivocochlear suppression during auditory recovery from acoustic trauma in humans. Acta Otolarynngol 121: 278–83.

Virokannas H, Anttonen H (1995) Dose-response relationship between smoking and impairment of hearing acuity in workers exposed to noise. Scand Audiol 24(4): 211–16.

Walden BE, Henselman LW, Morris ER (2000) The role of magnesium in the susceptibility of soldiers to noise-induced hearing loss. J Acoust Soc Am 108: 453–6.

Wang Y, Liberman MC (2002) Restrain stress and protection from acoustic injury in mice. Hear Res 165(1–2): 96–102.

Wangemann P (2002) Cochlear blood flow regulation. Adv Otorhinolaryngol 59: 51–7.

Yamasoba T, Dolan DF (1997) Chronic strychnine administration into the cochlea potentiates permanent threshold shift following noise exposure Hear Res 112(1–2): 13–20.

Yamasoba T, Nuttall AL, Harris C, Raphael Y, Miller JM (1998) Role of glutathione in protection against noise-induced hearing loss. Brain Res 784(1–2): 82–90.

Zakrisson JE, Borg E, Diamant H et al. (1975) Auditory fatigue in patients with stapedius muscle paralysis. Acta Otolaryngol 79: 228–32.

Zakrisson JE, Borg E, Diamant H, Mlller AR (1987) Laser Doppler measurements of cochlear blood flow during loud sound exposure in the guinea pig. Hear Res 27(1): 1–10.

Zheng XY, Henderson D, Hu BH, Ding DL, McFadden SL (1997a) The influence of the cochlear efferent system on chronic acoustic trauma. Hear Res 107(1–2): 147–59.

Zheng XY, Henderson D, McFadden SL, Hu BH (1997b) The role of the cochlear efferent system in acquired resistance to noise-induced hearing loss. Hear Res 104(1–2): 191–203.

# CHAPTER 8

# Measurement of hearing thresholds

*Noise and Its Effects:* Edited by Linda Luxon and Deepak Prasher © 2007
John Wiley & Sons Ltd.

STIG ARLINGER

## Background

Hearing thresholds have long constituted a very basic characteristic of the auditory organ, describing its sensitivity in detecting very soft sounds. As the primary purpose of hearing, like other sensory functions, is to inform the human being of changes in the environment, it responds better to transient stimuli than to steady-state situations. Therefore, test methods normally used in the determination of hearing thresholds present test sounds of limited duration.

The threshold of hearing is defined as the 'level of a sound at which, under specified conditions, a person gives 50% of correct detection responses on repeated trials' (ISO 389-1). 'Specified conditions' refer to the type of sound and ways of presenting the test sound. The normal test sound is pure-tone pulses at standardized frequencies in the range 125–8000 Hz and the normal presentation mode is monaurally by means of a standardized type of earphone. The standardized test procedure for the determination of hearing threshold levels for pure tones is called pure-tone audiometry and the graphical presentation of the test results is the pure-tone audiogram.

---

**Pure-tone audiometry**

- is the standard method to determine hearing thresholds for pure tones;
- covers the frequency range from 125 to 8000 Hz in discrete steps;
- testing is performed monaurally, i.e. one ear at a time by means of earphones;
- is used on listeners from about school age and up.

---

Focus for this chapter is on pure-tone audiometry performed on subjects who are able and willing to cooperate in the psychophysical procedure. In terms of age, this usually implies listeners from approximately school age and up. It is also assumed that the listener understands the instructions given and has no obvious reason to influence the outcome by simulation or aggravation. However, some of these exceptions are discussed later in this chapter.

Hearing thresholds are relatively sensitive indicators of the functional state of the peripheral part of the auditory sense organ. The most common type of damage occurs among the hair cells in the cochlea, and noise-induced hearing loss is due to hair cell damage. Although pure-tone audiometry has several limitations in reflecting the location and extent of loss of hair cell function, it is still the method with the best overall sensitivity to quantify noise-induced hearing loss (NIHL).

# Equipment

The equipment to be used, a pure-tone audiometer, has a functional design in terms of a set of basic building blocks as illustrated in Figure 8.1. Technical specifications for the instrument are given in the international standard IEC 60645-1, in which four different types are identified relating

**The international standard IEC 60645—1 specifies technical requirements of the equipment**

- test frequencies;
- calibration of signal levels;
- rise and fall times of tone pulses.

to the complexity of functions and working range of various variables offered. Sinusoidal signals of standardized frequencies at octave steps from 125 Hz to 8000 Hz and the intermediate frequencies 1500, 3000 and 6000 Hz are generated in the oscillator. Tone pulses are formed by the pulse former, which controls rise time, duration and fall time. Too short rise and fall times will result in spectral smear, audible as clicks at the beginning and end of the tone pulse. Too long rise and fall times, on the other hand, will result in weaker activation of the sensory organ. A suitable compromise is rise and fall times in the range 20–50 ms. Making the tone pulse duration too short may give rise to increased threshold levels because of auditory temporal integration. Detection of barely audible tone pulses primarily relies on the detection of the changes that occur at the onset and offset of the pulse, so it is essential that these are not too far apart. Thus, a suitable compromise for the tone pulse duration is in the range 1–2 s.

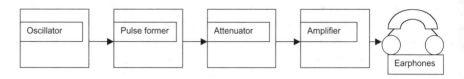

**Figure 8.1** The basic design of a pure-tone audiometer.

The attenuator is a volume control that allows the change of signal level in calibrated steps along a decibel scale. For the normal manual procedures as well as computer-controlled versions of it, the optimum step size is 5 dB. Larger step size reduces the accuracy of the measurement whereas smaller step size does not increase it because of the limited resolution of the human auditory system close to threshold (Jerlvall and Arlinger, 1986; Marshall et al., 1996). The attenuator scale is calibrated in decibels hearing level (dB HL). This scale has its zero at a sound level that, for each tone frequency, corresponds approximately to the average normal threshold of hearing for young otologically normal subjects (ISO 8253-1).

After suitable amplification, the signal is finally delivered to one of the earphones. The most commonly used earphone type is the supra-aural Telephonics TDH-39. Other types of supra-aural earphone used for audiometry are Beyer DT48 and Telephonics TDH-49 and 50. Larger circum-aural earphones, Sennheiser HDA-200, housed in relatively effective noise-excluding muffs, have also appeared on the market. Insert earphones of type EAR-Tone 3-A or ER-5A, coupled to the ear canal by means of foam inserts, offer another alternative with superior attenuation of ambient noise compared with supra-aural earphones. They also prevent problems due to a collapsing ear canal caused by a supra-aural earphone pressing on a too soft tragus of the external ear. In addition the risk of cross-hearing to the other ear is considerably lower than for other earphone types, reducing the need for contralateral masking (see below).

The supra-aural earphone Telephonics TDH-39 has been manufactured over a large number of years and unfortunately been subject to some minor changes that affect its acoustic performance. This has been shown to generate uncertainty mainly at 6 kHz, close to the resonance frequency of the earphone, where samples from different batches may have significantly different sensitivity (Canning, 1991; Dowson et al., 1991).

---

**Audiometers may be calibrated for earphones of different types**

- supra-aural (Telephonics TDH 39, 49, or 50; Beyer DT48);
- circum-aural (Sennheiser HDA 200);
- insert (E-A-R-tone ER-3A or ER-5A).

Clinical audiometers offer functions in addition to this basic pure-tone stimulus channel. One is the choice of a bone vibrator as alternative output transducer, whereby mechanical vibrations coupled to the skull bone at the mastoid process behind the external ear are used to stimulate the cochlea through bone conduction. In a first approximation, the sensitivity to detect these mechanical vibrations depends on the sensorineural (inner ear and auditory nerve) function alone with negligible influence from the outer and middle ears. Thus, a comparison of results obtained by air and by bone conduction provides evidence for the localization of a lesion either in the conduction mechanism of the outer and middle ear or in the sensorineural function of the cochlea or the cochlear nerve.

In order to allow reliable measurements of hearing thresholds for bone conduction in general as well as for air conduction in the poorer ear when there is a side difference of 40 dB or more in air conduction hearing thresholds, masking of the contralateral non-test ear is necessary (the 40-dB value holds for supra-aural earphones; for insert earphones the corresponding value is 60 dB). This is performed by presenting narrow-band filtered random noise to that ear, with a centre frequency equal to the test tone frequency being used. Thus, a clinical pure-tone audiometer needs a second channel in which random noise is generated, band-pass filtered, attenuated and amplified in order to be presented as a continuous sound through one of the earphones available. The calibration of the attenuator when used for adjusting the masking noise level is in decibel effective masking level. The effective masking level of a masker is defined as the hearing level of a pure tone of a frequency equal to the masker band centre frequency to which the threshold of hearing is raised by the presence of the masking noise. A detailed review of the concept of masking can be found in Goldstein and Newman (1994).

# Calibration of audiometric equipment

Two concepts need to be defined with regard to the procedures needed to make sure that the equipment performs as required. *Verification* is a concept that represents the measurements needed in order to be able to verify that the equipment intended for a certain type of audiometry fulfils all requirements for such equipment. Such requirements are specified in the IEC 60645, ISO 389 and to some extent ISO 8253 series of international standards. *Calibration* refers to the process where the equipment is adjusted in order to fulfil all these requirements, for example the sound pressure levels of the pure tones of an audiometer are adjusted to the specifications given in ISO 389-1 within tolerances given in IEC 60645-1.

Equipment checks require basic verification and calibration (daily subjective and periodic objective) assessments.

For the verification of test signals delivered by means of earphones, the earphone must be coupled to a device that provides a realistic acoustic load to the earphone, and offers an acoustic environment that is representative of the situation when the earphone is placed on a human ear. Such a device is called an acoustic coupler or ear simulator. In addition to providing the proper acoustic load, it contains a measurement microphone by which various characteristics of the acoustic signal can be measured. Depending on the type of earphone being used, different types of standardized couplers or ear simulators have to be used.

**Verification and calibration:**

- Verification is the process where an audiometer is tested with regard to all essential characteristics that are specified in the international standards IEC 60645-1 and ISO 389.
- Calibration is the process where the equipment is adjusted to fulfil all electroacoustical requirements.
- A subjective check of audiometer functions should be performed by the user regularly, ideally on a daily basis.
- An objective check, based on electroacoustic verification, should be made at least once a year.

The two most common types of supra-aural earphone are the Telephonics TDH-39 with MX41/AR or Model 51 cushion and Beyer DT48. For these transducers the acoustic coupler specified in IEC 60318-3 (often called a 6 cm$^3$ coupler) shall be used for the verification. Pure tones shall be calibrated to the reference levels specified in ISO 389-1. Reference levels for narrow-band-masking noise are specified in ISO 389-4.

Other types of supra-aural earphones fulfilling requirements specified in ISO 389-1 regarding physical design shall be tested on an artificial ear as specified in IEC 60318-1. This requirement thus also refers to earphones of type Telephonics TDH-49 and TDH-50.

For verification of test signals presented by means of circum-aural earphones, only an interim coupler is specified in the standard IEC 60318-2, based on the ear simulator described in IEC 60318-1 equipped with a flat plate adapter. Internationally standardized reference sound levels for pure tones are at present available only for the extended high-frequency range (ISO 389-5). However, single laboratory data exist also for pure tones in the conventional frequency range for the earphone Sennheiser HDA 200 (Richter, 1992; Han and Poulsen, 1997).

For verification of test signals produced by insert earphones, the earphone should be connected to either a coupler as specified in IEC 60126 (often called a 2 cm$^3$ coupler) or to an occluded-ear simulator according to IEC 60711. Reference levels for pure tones are specified in ISO 389-2. The data apply to insert earphones of type Etymotic Research ER-3A or HER-5A, coupled to the ear by foam eartips.

The functional state of audiometric equipment should be checked in different, complementary ways with different time intervals. The following suggestions are in accordance with the ISO 8253 standards.

### Subjective check

Routine checks based on listening and subjective assessment should be made each day before the equipment is to be used. An experienced person with known hearing thresholds within normal range should listen to all test signals with regard to approximately correct sound levels, absence of distortion and absence of any unwanted sound for all transducers available. The condition of all earphones' cables should be checked by pulling and twisting with a continuous test signal on at a clearly audible sound level. Headbands of earphones and bone vibrator need to be checked with regard to elastic force and mobility in swivel joints.

### Periodic objective check

Periodic objective checks should be performed at intervals not exceeding one year. This procedure involves verification and calibration if needed of a number of basic characteristics of the signals. For all test and masking signals available sound pressure levels or vibratory force levels should be determined using relevant equipment and methods at suitable attenuator settings. The measurements should also cover the attenuator steps over a significant part of its/their range (especially below 60 dB HL). For pure tones, the tone frequencies should also be measured. For all types of equipment harmonic distortion should be determined. For equipment used to present speech signals, the frequency response should be verified.

### Basic verification and calibration

A basic verification and calibration concerns virtually all characteristics of the equipment that are specified in relevant parts of the IEC 60645 and ISO 8253 series of standards. It need not be used on a routine basis if the subjective checks and periodic objective checks are regularly performed. A basic test will be required only when a serious equipment failure occurs or when for some reason it is suspected that the equipment is no longer performing fully to its specifications. A recommendation is to have a basic verification performed at intervals not exceeding 5 years.

# Test environment

The test environment for audiometry is a potential source of error.

The test environment for audiometry is a potential source of error. The ambient noise levels need to be sufficiently low in order to guarantee non-interference with the test tones even at very low test tone levels. The better the noise attenuation characteristics of the earphones used, the higher the permissible ambient sound levels. The international standard for pure-tone audiometry, ISO 8253-1, contains specifications on maximum ambient sound levels that allow the measurement of hearing threshold levels down to 0 dB HL with a maximum error of 2 dB (Table 8.1). They are based on the use of Telephonics supra-aural earphones TDH-39 with MX41/AR or Model 51 cushions, but are also valid for Telephonics TDH-49 and 50. For other earphone types correction has to be made with regard to the difference in noise attenuation properties between the earphone patterns.

**Table 8.1** Maximum permissible ambient sound pressure levels in one-third octave bands for air-conduction audiometry when typical current supra-aural earphones are used, allowing measurement of hearing threshold levels down to 0 dB HL with a maximum error of 2 dB. Data are specified for test tone frequency ranges 125-8000 and 250-8000 HZ.

| Mid-frequency of one-third octave band (Hz) | Maximum permissible ambient sound pressure levels $L_{max}$ (reference: 20 mPa) (dB) | |
|---|---|---|
| | *125–8 000 Hz* | *250–8 000 Hz* |
| 31.5 | 56 | 66 |
| 40 | 52 | 62 |
| 50 | 47 | 57 |
| 63 | 42 | 52 |
| 80 | 38 | 48 |
| 100 | 33 | 43 |
| 125 | 28 | 39 |
| 160 | 23 | 30 |
| 200 | 20 | 20 |
| 250 | 19 | 19 |
| 315 | 18 | 18 |
| 400 | 18 | 18 |
| 500 | 18 | 18 |
| 630 | 18 | 18 |
| 800 | 20 | 20 |
| 1000 | 23 | 23 |
| 1250 | 25 | 25 |
| 1600 | 27 | 27 |
| 2000 | 30 | 30 |
| 2500 | 32 | 32 |
| 3150 | 34 | 34 |
| 4000 | 36 | 36 |
| 5000 | 35 | 35 |
| 6300 | 34 | 34 |
| 8000 | 33 | 33 |

In addition to the acoustic environment it is also important to eliminate other possible distractions to the person being tested. He or she should be comfortably seated in a room with sufficient noise-free ventilation to provide thermal comfort. Preferably the test subject should be placed in a room separate from where the tester and the equipment are housed in order to allow for as low ambient sound levels as possible and eliminate any visual cues as to when stimuli are being presented.

# Procedure for audiometric testing

The procedure for the measurement of hearing thresholds is specified in the international standard ISO 8253-1. Before commencing the test and applying the tranducers, the test subject should be instructed in appropriate language about:

- the response task;
- the importance of responding whenever the tone is heard in either ear, no matter how faint it may be;
- the need to respond as soon as the tone is heard and stop responding immediately once the tone is no longer heard;
- the general pitch sequence of the sound;
- which ear will be tested first.

After instructing the test subject, spectacles and head ornaments and hearing aids should be removed before placement of the transducers. Hair should be moved from between the head and the transducers. The sound opening of an earphone should face the ear canal entrance. The manual procedure for determination of hearing threshold levels should be as follows, according to either the ascending or the bracketing method. The order of presentation of test tones should be from 1000 Hz upwards, followed by the lower frequency range in descending order. A repeat test should be carried out at 1000 Hz on the ear tested first. Test tones should be presented with a duration in the range 1–2 s. When a response occurs, the interval between test tones should be varied but should not be shorter than the duration of the test tone. Automatically pulsed tones are sometimes used as an alternative stimulus. However, correlative data are not currently available. The use of such a stimulus should be noted on the audiogram.

The test subject should be familiarized with the task prior to threshold determination by presenting a signal at 1000 Hz of sufficient intensity to evoke a definite response. Usually 40 dB is sufficient. If not, increase the level in steps of 20 dB until a response is obtained. Then reduce the level in steps of 20 dB until no response occurs. Increase the level in steps of 10 dB until a response occurs. Repeat this and then proceed to the actual testing as follows.

*Step 1*

Present the first test tone at a level that is 10 dB below the lowest level of the test subject's response during the familiarization. After each failure to respond to a test tone, increase level of the test tone in steps of 5 dB until a response occurs.

*Step 2: ascending method*

After the response, decrease the level in steps of 10 dB until no response occurs and then begin another ascent. Continue until three responses occur at the same level out of a maximum of five ascents. If less than three responses out of five ascents have been obtained at the same level, present a test tone at a level 10 dB higher than the level of the last response. Then repeat the test procedure.

A shortened version of the ascending method has been shown to yield nearly equivalent results and may be appropriate in some cases. In this version, continue testing until at least two responses have occurred at the same level out of three ascents.

*Step 2: bracketing method*

After the response, increase the level of the test tone by 5 dB and begin a descent in which the level of the tone is decreased in steps of 5 dB until no response occurs. Then decrease the level of the test tone another 5 dB and begin the next ascent at this level. This should be continued until three ascents and three descents have been completed. Shortened versions of the bracketing method may be appropriate in some cases. This consists of omitting the further descent of 5 dB after no response occurred or requiring only two ascents and two descents in series, provided that the four minimal response levels differ by no more than 5 dB.

*Step 3*

Proceed to the next test frequency at an estimated clearly audible level, as indicated by the previous responses, and repeat step 2. For any frequency, the familiarization or an abbreviated form of it may be repeated. Finish all test frequencies on one ear.

*Step 4*

Finally repeat the measurement at 1000 Hz. If the results of the repeat measurement for that ear agree to 5 dB or less with the first measurement for the same ear, proceed to the other ear. If not, retest at further frequencies in the same order until agreement to 5 dB or less has been obtained. Proceed until both ears have been tested.

## Testing with masking

To avoid the test tone being heard in the ear not under test, it may be necessary to apply masking noise to that ear.

This situation occurs when:

- Testing the poorer ear of a listener whose better ear bone conduction threshold is 40 dB or more better than the test signal levels used on the test ear and when conventional supra-aural earphones are used.
- When foam-type insert earphones are used, contralateral masking is typically needed when the bone-conduction threshold of the non-test ear is 60 dB or more better than the test signal level used in the test ear.
- If bone-conduction thresholds of the non-test ear are unknown, worst case assumptions would be to consider them normal. The following procedure is recommended to determine the hearing threshold level with masking:

*Step 1*

Present a test tone to the ear being tested at a level equal to the hearing threshold level without masking. Present masking noise to the ear not under test with an effective masking level equal to the hearing threshold level of the ear not under test. Increase the level until the test tone becomes inaudible or until the masker level exceeds the test tone level.

*Step 2*

If the test tone is still audible when the noise level equals the test tone level, assume this to be the masked hearing threshold level. If the tone is masked, increase its level until it becomes audible again.

*Step 3*

Increase the noise level by 5 dB. If the test tone is inaudible, increase the test tone level until the tone becomes audible again. Repeat this procedure until the test tone remains audible although the level of the masking noise has been increased by more than 10 dB. This masking level, i.e. the level above which no further increase in the tone level was required for its audibility, is the correct masking level and this procedure should have produced the correct hearing threshold level for that test frequency.

## Determination of hearing threshold level for the ascending method

For each frequency and ear the hearing threshold level is defined as the lowest level at which responses occur in more than half of the ascents. If, however, the lowest response levels span more than 10 dB at a given frequency, the test should be considered of doubtful reliability and should be repeated.

## Determination of hearing threshold level for the bracketing method

For each frequency and ear, determine the average of the lowest levels at which responses occur in the ascents as well as in the descents. The hearing threshold level is defined as the mean value of these two averages, rounded to the nearest whole number in decibels. If the lowest response levels in the ascents deviate by more than 10 dB among themselves and/or if the lowest response levels in the descents deviate by more than 10 dB among themselves the test should be considered of doubtful reliability and should be repeated.

### Screening audiometry

In screening audiometry the test tones at the screening level are either audible or inaudible to the subject. The test results show whether the hearing threshold levels are better or equal to or worse than the screening level used. Screening audiometry may be combined with hearing threshold measurements at those frequencies where the test subject fails the screening test.

First present a tone at 1000 Hz and a hearing level of 40 dB to the subject's right ear to check that the instructions have been understood. Adjust the signal level to the required screening level and present two tones with an interval of 3–5 s. If both are perceived, the subject has passed the screening test at this frequency. If only one tone was heard, present a third tone. If this third tone is heard, the subject has passed the screening test at this frequency. If it is not heard or if neither of the first two tones was heard, the test subject has failed the screening test at 1000 Hz at the screening level chosen. Continue with other test frequencies as required and then proceed to the left ear.

### Self-recording (Békésy) audiometry

Self-recording or Békésy audiometry refers to a method of adjustment in which the listener adjusts the sound level of a pulsed test tone between the limits of just audible and just inaudible tone. The range between these limits is normally 5–10 dB, and the hearing threshold level is calculated as the

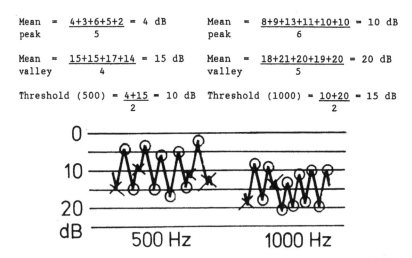

$$\text{Mean peak} = \frac{4+3+6+5+2}{5} = 4\ dB \qquad \text{Mean peak} = \frac{8+9+13+11+10+10}{6} = 10\ dB$$

$$\text{Mean valley} = \frac{15+15+17+14}{4} = 15\ dB \qquad \text{Mean valley} = \frac{18+21+20+19+20}{5} = 20\ dB$$

$$\text{Threshold (500)} = \frac{4+15}{2} = 10\ dB \qquad \text{Threshold (1000)} = \frac{10+20}{2} = 15\ dB$$

**Figure 8.2** Recording of stimulus level variations between just audible and just inaudible tone signal in Békésy audiometry and examples of calculation of hearing threshold level.

mean level between the average of six upper and six lower turning points. The audiometer used for this procedure differs with respect to step size for the variation of test tone level by using small steps, usually less than 1 dB. The nominal rate of change is 2.5 dB/s. The testing may be performed at discrete fixed frequencies or by means of a continuous frequency sweep. Normally, the Békésy-audiometer generates a graphic recording of the stimulus level variations that the listener produces (see Figure 8.2).

# Graphical symbols

When the measured hearing threshold levels are recorded graphically, standardized symbols are to be used in the pure-tone audiogram. Circles represent right ear air-conduction thresholds and crosses left ear data for thresholds determined without contralateral masking.

**Contralateral masking, i.e. presentation of narrow-band noise to the non-test ear is required**

- always for bone conduction measurements;
- in air conduction measurements using supra-aural earphones when testing an ear with hearing threshold levels that are 40 dB or more poorer than those of the better ear;
- in air conduction measurements using insert earphones when testing an ear with hearing threshold levels that are 60 dB or more poorer than those of the better ear.

# Reliability

All measurement methods are subject to influence by various sources of error. Test–retest reliability of a measurement method is an important characteristic that is often used to quantify the effects of the sources of error. Unless test reliability is known, there is no reliable way to assess a difference in measurement results obtained at two different occasions on the same subject and decide whether the difference recorded represents a significant difference or is likely to be due to the various sources of error.

**Pure tone threshold variables**

- Equipment variables.
- Environment variables.
- Technique variables.
- Subject variables.

A large number of potential sources of error exist in pure-tone audiometry. The probability of detecting a barely audible signal in a background of physiological noise depends on random fluctuations. Psychological factors, mainly related to the listener's limited ability to keep his or her concentration on the task constantly high, probably represent the main source of uncertainty. Forced-choice methods have been shown to reduce test–retest variability compared with the conventional clinical method (Marshall et al., 1996) but are more difficult to apply in general clinical practice. Variations in the test method may also affect the outcome: how the stimulus level is varied, temporal pattern of stimulus presentation, threshold criterion, the use of masking are examples of parameters of importance. Physical factors involve, among other aspects, placement of transducers – at repeated testing there will invariably be differences in this respect. Variations in physical dimensions of the enclosed air volume (Hudde et al., 1999), placement relative to the ear canal (Erlandsson et al., 1980), and leakage between earphone and ear (Voss et al., 2000) may significantly affect the sound pressure at the eardrum and thus the hearing threshold level recorded.

**Test reliability is affected by**

- physiological factors — barely audible signal in random physiological noise;
- psychological factors, mainly the listener's concentration;
- methodological factors: presentation of stimuli and interpretation of responses;
- physical factors: calibration of equipment, placement of transducers, ambient sound levels in test room.

The main purpose of using standardized test methods is to minimize the effects of variations in test procedure on the measurement results. Thus, if the equipment used fulfils the specifications according to IEC 60645-1, and the acoustic test environment and the test procedure follows the specifications in ISO 8253-1, variations in test results related to the hearing centre and person who performs the test should be reduced to a minimum.

One way of determining test–retest reliability is to perform tests at two different occasions on a large group of test subjects and assess the difference in outcome between the two measurements. The choice of test subjects, the procedures used at testing and the interval between the test sessions should as far as possible represent the normal clinical use of the test method. The mean difference is usually close to zero unless there is a significant learning effect. The standard deviation of the test–retest difference is the most common measure of test reliability. If, in a practical situation, the measurement of a hearing threshold level on a test subject shows a result that is worse than the result obtained at a previous test occasion by more than two standard deviations, then, by a probability of more than 97%, the recorded change in hearing threshold level represents a true change.

In a study of test–retest reliability in manually performed pure-tone audiometry we tested 25 young normal hearing subjects and 60 hearing-impaired subjects selected at random from the clinical patients. Figure 8.3 illustrates the standard deviations for the test–retest differences in hearing threshold levels obtained for these two groups. The values vary between approximately 4 dB and 6 dB for the normal hearing group and between 5 dB and 7 dB for the hearing-impaired group.

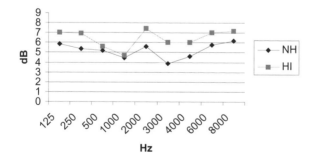

**Figure 8.3** Standard deviation (dB) for test-retest differences in air conduction pure-tone audiometry determined on groups of normal-hearing (NH) and hearing-impaired (HI) subjects.

Sometimes averages are formed of hearing threshold levels at neighbouring frequencies. When assessing NIHL a meaningful approach may be to form an average of the thresholds at 4 and 6 kHz or 3, 4 and 6 kHz. The standard deviation for test–retest difference for such averages will be smaller than for thresholds at single frequencies because random errors to some extent balance out. However, there is also some correlation between the variations at neighbouring frequencies, which makes the reduction of the test–retest difference variance less than theoretically possible. Figure 8.4 illustrates the reduction of the average standard deviation when averages are formed as a function of the number of test frequencies making up the average. The data are based on test results obtained on the group of normal hearing subjects.

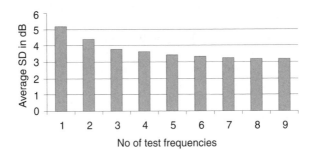

**Figure 8.4** Average standard deviations for test–retest differences when hearing threshold levels are averaged over several test frequencies. Data based on normal hearing test subjects.

## Measurements in special populations

Measuring hearing thresholds in children below school age often requires modifications of the method described here, in particular with regard to response mode. For children below the age of 2 or 3 years entirely different methods are used, based on the child's spontaneous reactions to sound stimuli.

Pure-tone audiometry in medicolegal cases requires some special caution. The outcome of the test may affect the test subject in some essential way, for example in terms of insurance compensation, and this fact may tempt him or her to aggravate or simulate. Type and degree of audiometric loss may cause suspicion, and so may poor reproducibility at repeated tests, or a significant discrepancy between the results of pure-tone audiometry and speech audiometry. If the average pure-tone hearing threshold level at 500, 1000 and 2000 Hz differs by more than 10 dB from the speech recognition threshold level (usually exceeding it) this indicates unreliable pure-tone hearing thresholds. There is no easy alternative way to determine hearing threshold levels in a subject who is unwilling to cooperate reliably in pure-tone audiometry. Electrophysiological test methods can usually verify suspected malingering but the hearing threshold estimates that may be made by such methods are usually less precise than what is obtained in pure-tone audiometry with a cooperative listener.

# Conclusions

The measurement of hearing threshold levels will remain a basic and important test method in audiology in general and not least when assessing NIHL. Although the method by which thresholds are determined as such is relatively straightforward, the adherence to a standardized method is essential. A number of sources of error exist that may influence the outcome, and it is essential to minimize the effect of these. However, there will always be an uncertainty in the test result, the magnitude of which is necessary to know in order to be able to assess the results.

# References

Arlinger S (1998) How to combine data harvested using different audiometric techniques. Advances in Noise Research, Vol.II. Protection against noise. London: Whurr Publishers pp. 119–21.

Canning DM (1991) An initial investigation into the equivalence of the metal and plastic-cased TDH39 earphones. British Journal of Audiology 25: 429–31.

Dowson SP, McNeill HA, Torr GR (1991) The performance and calibration of TDH39 earphones fitted with Model 51 and MX41/AR cushions. British Journal of Audiology 25: 419–22.

Erlandsson B, Håkansson H, Ivarsson A, Nilsson P (1980) The reliability of Békésy sweep audiometry recording and effects of the earphone position. Acta Otolaryngologica, Supplementum 366: 99–112.

Goldstein BA, Newman CW (1994) Clinical masking: a decision-making process. In J Katz (ed.) Handbook of Clinical Audiology, 4th edn. Baltimore: Williams & Wilkins, pp. 109–31.

Han LA, Poulsen T (1997) Equivalent threshold sound pressure levels for Sennheiser HDA 200 earphone and Etymotic Research ER-2 insert earphone in the frequency range 125 Hz to 16 kHz. Scandinavian Audiology 27: 105–12.

Hudde H, Engel A, Lodwig A (1999) Methods for estimating the sound pressure at the eardrum. Journal of the Acoustical Society of America 106: 1977–92.

IEC 60126. IEC reference coupler for the measurement of hearing aids using earphones coupled to the ear by means of ear inserts (to be re-issued as IEC 60318-5). Geneva: International Electrotechnical Commission.

IEC 60318-1. Electroacoustics – Simulators of human head and ear – Part 1: Ear simulator for the calibration of supra-aural earphones. Geneva: International Electrotechnical Commission.

IEC 60318-3. Electroacoustics – Simulators of human head and ear – Part 3: Acoustic coupler for the calibration of supra-aural earphones used in audiometry. Geneva: International Electrotechnical Commission.

IEC 60645-1. Audiometers – Part 1: Pure tone audiometers. Geneva: International Electrotechnical Commission.

IEC 60711. Occluded-ear simulator for the measurement of earphones coupled to the ear by means of ear inserts (to be re-issued as IEC 60318-4). Geneva: International Electrotechnical Commission, Geneva.

ISO 389-1. Acoustics – Reference zero for the calibration of audiometric equipment – Part 1: Reference equivalent threshold sound pressure levels for pure tones and supra-aural earphones. Geneva: International Organization for Standardization.

ISO 389-2. Acoustics – Reference zero for the calibration of audiometric equipment – Part 2: Reference equivalent threshold sound pressure levels for pure tones and insert earphones. Geneva: International Organization for Standardization.

ISO 8253-1. Acoustics – Audiometric test methods – Part 1: Basic pure tone air and bone conduction threshold audiometry. Geneva: International Organization for Standardization.

Jerlvall L, Arlinger S (1986) A comparison of 2 and 5 dB step size in pure tone audiometry. Scandinavian Audiology 15: 51–6.

Jerlvall L, Dryselius H, Arlinger S (1983) Comparison of manual and computer-controlled audiometry using identical procedures. Scandinavian Audiology 12: 209–13.

Marshall L, Hanna TE, Wilson RH (1996) Effect of step size on clinical and adaptive 2IFC procedures in quiet and in a noisy background. Journal of Speech and Hearing Research 39: 687–96.

Richter U (1992) Kenndaten von Schallwandlern der Audiometrie. PTB-Bericht PTB-MA-27, Physikalisch Technische Bundesanstalt, Braunschweig.

Voss SE, Rosowski JJ, Shera CA, Peake WT (2000) Acoustic mechanisms that determine the ear-canal sound pressures generated by earphones. Journal of the Acoustical Society of America 107: 1548–65.

# CHAPTER 9

# Noise-induced hearing loss and tinnitus in children – a matter of diagnostic criteria?

*Noise and Its Effects:* Edited by Linda Luxon and Deepak Prasher © 2007 John Wiley & Sons Ltd.

KM HOLGERS, Å BRATTHALL, ML BARRENÄS

## Introduction

Occupational noise has been generally recognized as a public health problem among adults. Non-occupational activities, however, such as rock concerts, discotheques and personal cassette players (PCPs), which may cause hazardous environmental noise for both children and adults, have not been regarded as a health risk to the same extent. There are many reports on the impact of leisure noise on hearing, but the scientific evidence of a relationship between leisure-time noise and sensorineural high-frequency hearing loss (SHFHL) in young people is inconclusive. Nevertheless, there are reasons to believe that leisure noise may be an important health risk in children.

Besides temporary and permanent noise-induced sensorineural hearing loss, noise exposure may also have non-auditory health effects. Noise-induced blood pressure increase and cortisol elevation are consistently seen in children exposed to noise from the environment, such as road noise and aircraft noise (Karlsdorf and Klappach, 1968; Karagodina et al., 1969; Cohen et al., 1980, 1981). It has also been reported that children in high noise areas have worse results in reading tests, auditory discrimination and long-term memory recall, than children in low noise areas (Hygge et al., 2002). For further reading see Chapter 25 in this book.

The objective of this chapter is to describe the auditory effects of noise exposure in children. The goal is not to present all reports that are available in this area but to describe the main findings by discussing:

* common conclusions about noise effects on tinnitus and hearing in children;
* pitfalls in the present literature.

# Noise-induced hearing loss in children

There is no consensus about how to diagnose noise-induced hearing loss (NIHL). Usually, NIHL or noise-induced permanent threshold shift (NIPTS) is defined as the amount of hearing threshold shift that remains after subtracting an amount for 'normal' age-induced hearing loss from the hearing level of a noise-exposed person or population.

**In children, the definition of NIHL is compounded by two factors:**

* knowledge about damaging noise exposure dosages in children is lacking;
* normative hearing threshold levels for children are not available.

The normal hearing thresholds according to age as estimated by the ISO 389 standard include adults 18 years and above. As the hearing thresholds in children without hearing pathology and known hazardous noise exposure appear to be around zero (Roberts, 1972; Lutman and Davies, 1994; Haapaniemi, 1996), children need their own hearing standard to diagnose NIHL.

# NIPTS/NIHL audiometric classification

To diagnose a hearing loss as noise induced, there has to be both a damaging noise exposure and a threshold shift in the audiogram. The best evidence for NIHL is if the change in hearing level thresholds is documented by a baseline audiogram and a follow-up audiogram covering the time period of documented noise exposure. In the absence of specific evaluation in children, the criteria used for the diagnosis of NIHL in children rely on data in adults. According to National Institute for Occupational Safety and Health (NIOSH, 1996), a threshold shift relative to baseline is present if there is a shift of 15 dB or more at 0.5, 1, 2, 3, 4 or 6 kHz in either ear, and the same shift at the same test frequency in the same ear on an immediate retest. NIOSH also recommends a confirmation test after 30 days preceded by a quiet period of at least 14 hours. The latter recommendation is to avoid temporary threshold shift being present at the time of audiometry. However, most of the studies in the literature do not include baseline audiometry.

A notch at 3, 4 or 6 dB HL in the audiogram is not sufficient to diagnose NIPTS because of a large number of other medical conditions causing notches in the audiogram (Sataloff, 1980). Nevertheless, different definitions of the audiometric profile are used to diagnose NIHL:

* A common classification of NIHL is a notch at 4 kHz (Passchier-Vermeer, 1974; McBride and Williams, 2001a,b).
* Niskar et al. (2001) used the following criteria: the threshold values for

0.5 kHz and 1 kHz should be ≤ 15 dB HL better than the poorest threshold value at 3, 4 and 6 kHz. The threshold value at 8 kHz has to be at least 10  dB HL better than the poorest value for 3, 4 or 6 kHz.

- Schmidt et al. (1994) described NIHL as a hearing loss in one or both ears 20 dB for frequencies 3, 4 or 6 kHz with the loss at the two nearest frequencies on both sides of the dip amounting to at least 5 dB less. The authors described their definition as their 'intuitive interpretation of audiograms'. By including subjects with SHFHL of aetiologies other than noise in the study, the prevalence of NIHL will be overestimated.

# Safety limits at work

With regard to diagnosis, the safety limits for noise exposure in children must be extrapolated from the work in adults. The Swedish Occupational Safety and Health Administration has regulations and recommendations for calculated NIHL risk. The regulations are based on the exposure of 85 dB $L_{Aeq, 8h}$, continuous noise, with maximum levels of 115 dB (A) and 140 dB (C) peak (See Chapter 2). Data from workers exposed to noise during many years without wearing hearing protectors, such as workers at jute weaving factories, have been considered (Taylor et al., 1965). It was also shown that if individuals were exposed to a 4-kHz noise above 74 dB, a temporary threshold shift (TTS) was detected (Mills, 1979). Therefore, it was concluded that the risk of inner-ear damage was very small if the noise exposure was below this level. The relationship between TTS and permanent threshold shift (PTS) is still unclear but it is considered that the PTS will not be more than the TTS. Nevertheless, the 85 dB $L_{Aeq}$ level could be disputed because it is set at a statistical level of 9% probability, which means that 9% of an exposed population is at risk of developing NIHL. If the statistical level is set to 80 dB, this risk could be reduced to 4%.

# Music and safety limits

Music often includes impulse noise and much circumstantial evidence exists to support the view that impulse noise is more harmful than continuous noise. In Sweden, the safety limits for music exposure have been considered to be acceptable on a 90 dB $L_{Aeq, 8h}$. This is 5 dB higher than for occupational noise exposure. The assumption that music is less hazardous than occupational noise is generally based on studies of hearing in professional musicians and one experimental study on 10 volunteers (Axelsson and Lindgren, 1981a,b; Lindgren and Axelsson,1983).

Reviewing 139 professional pop musicians with an average exposure of 9 years, a recent study concluded that the incidence of hearing loss was surprisingly low and suggested that music exposure, compared with non-music exposure, could have a lower risk of NIHL (Kahari et al., 2003).

However, other explanations could be a selection bias of persons with less susceptibility for hearing loss, as these persons have continued to work with music. The finding could also be explained by reluctance to participate in interventions that include hearing tests, which is a well-known behaviour for persons with noise-induced hearing. In an experimental study, TTS were investigated in 10 volunteers who were exposed to musical and non-musical noise stimuli. The TTSs showed almost equal sensitivity to the two stimuli in four subjects, but in the other six subjects a difference in sensitivity was found to the non-musical noise stimuli (Lindgren and Axelsson, 1983). However, 20-year-old music students in Göteborg reported a seven times higher occurrence of subjective hearing loss, compared with the normal population, 20% and 2.7%, respectively (Nebeska et al., 2000; Statistiska Centralbyrån (SCB), Sweden, 2001).

In a thorough review of the literature, a firm association between live rock-and-roll music and hearing loss was found in rock musicians but for classical musicians the reports were conflicting (Palin, 1994). This supports a recent follow-up study in which 74% of professional rock and jazz musicians had hearing loss, while in classical professional musicians, no severe hearing loss could be directly attributed to exposure to musical noise (Kahari, 2002).

There is no strong evidence in the literature to support the view that music exposure is less harmful than other noise exposure. Until more knowledge has been gained, safety limits similar to other noise legislation should be used for music exposure.

## Pitfalls in reports of NIHL in children

Table 9.1 presents a review of NIHL in children, including confounding factors such as familial hearing loss, noise exposure and recurrent otitis media. Longitudinal and cross-sectional studies controlling for the most important confounding factors are rare. Most reports lack both controls and basic background data about heredity and noise exposure.

The occurrence of NIHL in children varies greatly between studies. This is probably due to the limitations in knowledge of noise exposure and adjustments for important confounders. Usually, exposure data are collected by a questionnaire, although in some studies objective measurements with dosimetry are used. However, dosimetry only gives information on the noise exposure for a specific time, and questionnaires are notoriously unreliable in providing retrospective detail about the extent of noise exposure.

**Sources of inaccuracy in assessing NIHL in children**
- Objective noise measurements are rare.
- Retrospective evaluation of noise exposure has used questionnaires.
- Few studies have evaluated noise exposure in children with and without hearing loss.
- There have been few controlled studies.

**Table 9.1** Review of NIHL in children

**Longitudinal studies**

| Author | Study sample | Audiometry screening level | Hearing loss | Noise exposure and comments |
|---|---|---|---|---|
| Richardson and Peckham (1977) | 11 000 children tested at age 7, 11 and 16 | 20 dB for 0.25, 0.5, 1, 2, 4 and 8 kHz. Better ear | HL at 2 kHz: 2%, HL at 4 kHz: 3%, HL at 8 kHz: 5% (16 year olds) | Data about exposure to noise was not collected. Children of fathers in manual occupations had higher thresholds on all frequencies than those of non-manual workers. Hearing loss in the family was not investigated |
| Carter et al. (1984) | 69 boys and 72 girls 10–12-year-olds at first test | HT tested 1972–74, and 1980 at 0.5, 1, 2, 3, 4, 6 and 8 kHz | All participants had normal hearing | No evidence for noise-induced hearing deterioration was found during a 6–8 year period. Hearing loss in the family was not investigated |
| Klockhoff et al. (1986) | 38 294 conscripts, aged 18–19 | 20 dB at 0.5, 1, 2, 3, 4 and 6 kHz | HL: 29% Deterioration (at least 5 dB in the PTA at 3, 4 and 6 kHz) during training was found in 5% | Hearing deterioration during military training was related to hearing status on reporting. High-frequency deterioration most common. No significant correlation between hearing deterioration in relation to type of military unit. Hearing loss in the family was not investigated |
| Lindeman et al. (1987) | 163 male adolescents, aged 17–23 | HT tested 1977, 1980 and 1983 at 0.5, 1, 2, 3, 4, 6 and 8 kHz | All subjects had normal hearing at first test | No hearing impairment developed in boys with normal hearing aged 17 and up to the age of 23. Hearing loss in the family was not investigated |

**Table 9.1** Review of NIHL in children (contd)

Cross-sectional studies controlled for heredity and noise exposure

| Author | Study sample | Audiometry screening level | Hearing loss | Hearing loss in the family | Noise exposure and comments |
|---|---|---|---|---|---|
| Axelsson et al. (1994) | 500 conscripts, aged 18–19 years | 20 dB at 0.25, 0.5, 1, 2, 3, 4, 6 and 8 kHz | SNHL: 14%<br>SNHL: 15%<br>HF dips: 8% | A conscript was three times more likely to have HL if there was HL in his family | No significant correlation to noise exposure. Plausible causes described were previous otitis media, hereditary factors, skull trauma and noise |
| Axelsson et al. (1981) | 538 boys aged 17–20 years | 20 dB for 0.25, 0.5, 1, 2, 3, 4, 6 and 8 kHz | Not applicable | HL in the family was significantly correlated to HFHL | No significant correlation between noisy leisure time activities and HL was found. Authors 'believe that the HFHL speaks in favour of noise exposure rather than a genetic deficiency' |
| Klockhoff and Lyttkens (1982) | 30 unexposed children with a 4 kHz dip and 42 unexposed controls with normal hearing (mean: 14 years) | Békésy audiometry | No epidemiological study | A positive family history was found in 76% of the cases, and 17% among controls (OR=4.5) | Subjects had no history of noise exposure, complications during pregnancy and delivery, head trauma, use of ototoxic drugs or relevant diseases |

**Table 9.1** Review of NIHL in children (continued)

**Cross-sectional studies controlled for noise, but not heredity**

| Author | Study sample | Audiometry screening level | Hearing loss | Noise exposure and Comments |
|---|---|---|---|---|
| Lipscomb (1972) | 2769 university freshmen tested in 1968 + 1410 freshmen in 1969, age 16–21 years | 15dB for 2, 3, 4 and 6 kHz | HFHL: Boys: 40%; 73% Girls: 24%; 52% | Significant correlation between HFHL and gunfire in 1969 students. Authors conclude that something is causing this rise in the prevalence of impairment. The rise in recreational noise levels must be considered a contributing factor |
| Axelsson and Lindgren (1987) | 701 schoolchildren exposed to fire-crackers. 482 unexposed controls age 10–15 years | Pre- and post-exposure tests: HT tested at 1, 2, 3, 4, 6 and 8 kHz before and after Easter in 1985 | HL among exposed children: 4%. HL among unexposed children: 4% | Equal risk between exposed and unexposed firecracker groups to develop a hearing deterioration. Hearing thresholds in the exposed groups were better after than before exposure |
| Wong et al. (1990) | 78 users and 25 non-users of PCPs, aged 15–24 years | HT tested at 0.5,1,2,4 and 8 KHz. | No difference between users and non-users. | No difference between the exposed and unexposed group |
| Schmidt et al. (1994) | 50 male+29 female conservatory students (21–40 years) v. 20 male+29 female medical students (21–48 years) | HT tested at 0.25, 0.5, 1, 2, 3, 4, 6 and 8 kHz + high frequency audiometry | HFHL: Musicians: 16% Medical students: 14% | No difference between the exposed and unexposed group |
| Meyer-Bisch (1996) | N1 = 54, PCP < 7 h/week; N2: 195, 2–7 h/week; N3: 87, 2 rock concerts/month; N4: matched controls | Audio-Scan 0.5–16 kHz | Exposed groups had worse hearing thresholds than controls | A dose–response relationship was reported between hearing and exposure |

**Table 9.1** Review of NIHL in children (continued)

**Cross-sectional studies controlled for noise, but not heredity (continued)**

| Author | Study sample | Audiometry screening level | Hearing loss | Noise exposure and comments |
|---|---|---|---|---|
| Job et al. (2000) | 1208 conscripts, aged 18–24 years | HT tested at 0.5 1, 2, 3, 4, 6 and 8 kHz | MFHL: 9% HFHL: 15% | Among noise-exposed men, those having had recurrent otitis media during childhood showed an increased risk of hearing loss. Among men with no previous otitis problems, no difference was found between noise-exposed and non-exposed subjects |

**Cross-sectional studies controlled for heredity but not noise**

| Author | Study sample | Hearing loss | Noise exposure and comments |
|---|---|---|---|
| | **Children born in the UK** | | |
| Fortnum et al. (2001) | 1985–93 with a hearing loss > 40 dB HL | 1.3 : 1000 | |
| Fortnum and Davis (1997) | 1980–95 with a hearing loss > 40 dB HL | 1.7 : 1000 | A 14-fold increase in prevalence if a positive family history |
| Das (1996) | 1981–90 with a hearing loss > 30 dB HL | 1.1 : 1000 ♂:♀=1,4 | Heredity was found in about 23% of cases |
| Sutton and Rowe (1997) | 1984–88 with a hearing loss > 30 dB HL | 0.9 : 1000 ♂:♀=1,2 | Heredity was found in about 25% |
| | **Preschool children born in Sweden** | | |
| Thiringer et el. (1984) | 1970–74 with a hearing loss > 20 dB HL | 3.8 : 1000 ♂:♀=1,7 | Heredity was found in 39% |
| Darin et al. (1997) | 1980–84 with a hearing loss > 20 dB HL | 2.0 : 1000 ♂:♀=1 | Heredity was found in 33% |
| Sehlin et al. (1990) | 1964–83 with a hearing loss > 30 dB HL | 2.6 : 1000 | Heredity was found in 33% |

**Table 9.1** Review of NIHL in children (continued)

**Uncontrolled cross-sectional studies: no hearing loss in the family or noise exposure were investigated**

| Author | Study sample | Audiometry screening level | Hearing loss | Noise exposure and Comments |
|---|---|---|---|---|
| Weber et al. (1967) | 1000 children with hearing loss; 3–16 years | 10 dB for 0,5, 1, 2 kHz; 20 dB for 4 kHz | 4-kHz dip: boys: 25%; girls: 5% of children with hearing impairment | 4-kHz dip occurred more frequently in children living in noisy counties, and more often in boys than girls. NIHL assumed but not proved, as noise exposure data was not collected for each individual |
| Barr et al. (1973) | 1. 500 000 school children: 7, 10, 13, 17 years; 2. 2135 children; 4 years; 3. 9766 conscripts; 18 years | 20dB for 0.25, 0.5, 1, 2, 4 and 8 kHz | 1. SNHL: 2.7% boys; 1.5% girls. HFHL: 1.3% boys; 0.5% girls. 2. HFHL: 0.2% boys; 0.1% girls. 3. HFHL: 4% | Differences in prevalence of HFHL between boys and girls were observed from the age of 4. Genetic causes suggested |
| Rytzner and Rytzner (1981) | 14391 children; 7,10 and 13 years | 20 dB for 0.25, 0.5, 1, 2, 4 and 8 kHz | 4-kHz dip: Boys: 2%, 3%, 5% Girls: 1%, 1%, 2% | Noise exposure data were only collected among individuals with hearing loss. Even though no comparison to noise exposure among the normal hearing children was conducted, noise was assumed to have caused the dips |
| Axelsson et al. (1987) Costa et al. (1988) | 2543 children, followed at age 7, 10 and 13 | 20 dB for 0.25, 0.5, 1, 2, 4, 6 and 8 kHz | Boys: 14%; 16%;16% Girls: 12%; 12%; 9% | The increased prevalence of hearing loss in boys with age is assumed to be noise induced and/or inherited. Hearing loss in the family was not investigated. Noise exposure was not investigated |
| Niskar et al. (2001) | 5249 US children, aged 6–19 years | Thresholds for 0.5, 1, 2, 3, 4, 6 and 8 kHz | HFHL: Boys: 15% Girls: 10% | NIHL was suggested, but criticized (Green, 2002) due to the lack of exposure data |

HFHL, high-frequency hearing loss; HT, hearing threshold; NIHL, noise-induced hearing loss; OR, odds ratio; PCP, Personal Cassette Player; SNHL, sensorineural hearing loss; HL, hearing loss, MFHL, mid-frequency hearing loss.

There are also differences between studies in the definition of NIHL or NIPTS as described above. Unfortunately, such definitions may even include unexposed people. Other sources of bias include data in which noise exposure is only evaluated in subjects with hearing loss but not in subjects with normal hearing, and studies reporting only a noise-exposed group, without a proper unexposed control group for comparison.

Longitudinal studies are reliable, but rare. No study supports the view that high-frequency dips in children are noise induced. On the contrary, heredity seems the more likely cause, even though hearing loss among family members was not investigated (Table 9.1).

In the literature there are more cross-sectional studies than longitudinal. All the cross-sectional studies controlled for both heredity and noise exposure show a positive correlation to heredity but could not verify a relationship to noise exposure (Table 9.1). Nevertheless, the authors suggest that 'the high-frequency hearing loss speaks in favour of noise exposure rather than a genetic deficiency' (Axelsson et al., 1981).

Among cross-sectional studies controlled for noise but not heredity, most studies report that the occurrence of high-frequency hearing loss (HFHL) did not differ between noise-exposed and unexposed groups. Lipscomb (1972) reported a dramatic increase from 1968 to 1969, which he regarded as due mainly to recreational noise. The possibility of experimental errors was not elucidated.

In 1996, Meyer-Bisch reported a significant increase in hearing thresholds in young people using Personal CD Player (PCP) for more than 7 hours per week compared with those using PCP 2–7 hours per week and compared with their matched controls. The same was true for subjects who went to rock concerts at least twice a month compared with their matched controls. These results contradict Wong et al. (1990), who reported no difference between PCP users and non-users. Job et al. (2000) found an increased risk only in persons who had suffered from recurrent otitis media during childhood.

As these uncontrolled cross-sectional studies provide no background data but only hearing thresholds, the conclusions concerning the aetiology of sensorineural hearing loss (SNHL) in children are open to bias based on the beliefs of the authors. For example, despite the lack of exposure data, the prevalence of noise-induced hearing threshold shift among American children aged 6–19 years was estimated to be as high as 12.5% (Niskar et al., 2001). This prevalence has been discussed by Green (2002) who pointed out experimental error and the lack of baseline audiograms.

The two main arguments for the assumption of leisure noise as a risk factor in teenagers are:

- the audiometric configuration resembles that of NIHL (the 4-kHz notch);
- the sex distribution, accepting that boys are exposed to noisy activities more often than girls.

However, even at the age of 4 years a gender difference of 4-kHz notches is present (Barr et al., 1973). This finding can hardly be explained by differences in noise exposure, as such small children are rarely exposed to noise at all. Even though most studies show that HFHL occurs more frequently in boys than girls, and that the proportion of boys with a HFHL increases with age, there are differences other than noise exposure between the genders. Not only are men believed to be more susceptible to noise than women (Royster et al., 1980), but also to age-induced SNHL at all ages and to recurrent otitis media (Stenström and Ingvarsson, 1994). Interestingly, Job et al. (2000) reported recurrent otitis media as a risk factor for hearing loss among noise-exposed men, whereas no difference in hearing was found between noise-exposed and unexposed men with no history of recurrent otitis media during childhood. One interpretation of these results is that intrinsic factors are just as important as the external exposure. In our opinion, individuals with an inherited predisposition to SNHL are probably more susceptible to noise than those with no such genetic predisposition.

# The prevalence of noise-induced tinnitus in children

Data on tinnitus and, in particular, the effects of tinnitus in childhood are limited. There are no reports available where statistical analyses have been performed, identifying predictors of the severity of tinnitus. For children with normal hearing the prevalence has been reported to vary between 6% and 36% (Nodar, 1972; Graham, 1981; Graham and Butler, 1984; Nodar and Lezak, 1984; Mills et al., 1986; Stouffer et al., 1991; Baguley and McFerran, 1999). The variation of the prevalence between different studies is greater in children than in adults, which might reflect the difficulties faced when interviewing children. Therefore, in order to increase the reliability, other authors included only children ($n = 120$) who at the beginning of the interview had given reliable answers to practical questions not concerning tinnitus (Stouffer et al., 1991). When using this method, 6 or 13% of the children with normal hearing reported having experienced tinnitus, depending on the criterion for response consistency. This method has its advantages, because the answers from the participating children are more likely to be accurate. However, one disadvantage with the selection of children by this method is that the personality of the child may affect the outcome (Newman et al., 1997).

**Tinnitus in children**

- Prevalence 6–36%
- Prevalence higher in hearing-impaired than in normally hearing individuals
- More often perceived in mild-to-moderate hearing loss than severe hearing loss
- Girls perceive tinnitus more than boys

The prevalence of tinnitus is higher in children having a hearing loss than in normal hearing subjects and has been reported as high as 76% (Nodar, 1972; Graham, 1981; Nodar and Lezak, 1984; Mills et al., 1986; Baguley and McFerran, 1999). Unexpectedly, Graham and Butler (1984) reported that tinnitus is more often perceived in children with mild-to-moderate hearing loss (66%) than among children with severe hearing loss (29%). A higher prevalence of tinnitus correlated to better hearing is contradictory to the findings in adults (Axelsson and Ringdahl, 1989).

In a study based on individual structural interviews and hearing tests of 961 children, 12% of the 7-year-old children had experience of tinnitus, including noise-induced tinnitus (NIT) (2.5%). Screening audiometry at 20 dB HL was performed and, if the child failed at this level, thresholds were performed. There were no differences in hearing between boys and girls and the auditory parameters did not correlate to the prevalence of tinnitus.

Data about the severity of tinnitus in childhood are limited. Since knowledge of tinnitus suffered by children is lacking, we have to rely on reports of adults. In a report on 93 schoolchildren 5–16 years of age, 27 (29%) reported that they had 'noise' in their ears and 9 children (9/93 = 10%) were troubled by their tinnitus (Mills et al., 1986). Other researchers have estimated, that only 3% of the children spontaneously complain about tinnitus (Nodar, 1972). In a small school in Sweden, lectures were given on hearing and tinnitus. All students in school, aged between 9 and 16 years, participated in the lecture and filled in a questionnaire ($n = 274$: 139 girls, 135 boys). Noise-induced tinnitus was experienced by 53% of the children and this great increase may be due to change of behaviour and attitudes to noise exposure. The mean age for the group with experience of NIT was higher than the group without NIT, 12 and 11 years respectively. Compared with boys, girls seem to have more experiences of NIT. However, when investigating the literature, it is reported that more boys than girls have noise-induced hearing loss.

Forty-six per cent of the children also experienced spontaneous tinnitus (ST) without preceding noise. When girls and boys were analysed together, 14% of the children experienced tinnitus every day and 2.2% always had tinnitus, but the girls perceived tinnitus more often than the boys. Almost 23% of the children, and girls in particular, reported that they were annoyed by tinnitus (Holgers, 2003). Preliminary results from another study (Holgers and Pettersson, 2005), including almost 700 children aged 13–16 years, showed that the more the student went to discotheques or music clubs, the more often they perceived TTSs and NIT. An interesting finding was that these symptoms were found more frequently with increasing anxiety levels as well as heredity for hearing loss and older age.

Some of these findings in children differ from findings in adults. In adults, the prevalence of tinnitus is higher in men than in women, but in children there is no difference or a reversed difference between genders. In adults, one could speculate that the severity of tinnitus is higher in men than women, judging from the number of men who seek help for tinnitus at an audiology clinic, compared with women. However, it is not that simple as, despite the finding that more girls are annoyed by tinnitus and perceive tinnitus more often, more boys seek help for tinnitus.

Predictors for the severity of tinnitus have been described in adults by many authors. Unfortunately, most studies on tinnitus in children include only a small number of individuals and, consequently, statistical analyses revealing predictive factors for development of severe tinnitus in children have not been made. However, there are some reports pointing to the importance of psychological factors in determining the level of suffering from tinnitus (Rosanowski et al., 1997; Kentish et al., 2000). As a conclusion, one can say that the relationship between audiometry and tinnitus severity seems to be weaker than the correlation between tinnitus severity and psychological factors, for example depression, concentration problems and irritability (Collet et al., 1990; Halford et al., 1991; Erlandsson et al., 1992; Newman et al., 1994; Holgers et al., 2000). For further reading, see a recent review by Holgers et al. (2000).

It is possible that the reason for the over-representation of men and boys seeking help for tinnitus has to do with old attitudes. It is very likely that girls have other ways to handle their symptoms and have not the same need for seeking professional help as boys. It can be suggested that it is more socially acceptable for men to seek help for somatic symptoms, such as tinnitus, than for psychological or psychiatric symptoms. This attitude may also be reflected in the reported prevalence of depressive and anxiety disorders, where women outnumber men.

# Conclusion

The epidemiology of NIHL and tinnitus in children is much less well defined than in adults. The experience of NIT was 20 times higher in the group of 9 to 16-year-old children compared with younger children. This increase may be due to change of behaviour and attitudes to noise exposure. Some evidence indicates that children are more susceptible to noise than adults. Still, the scientific evidence of a relationship between leisure-time noise and HFHL in young people is inconclusive because of the limitations in exposure characteristics, adjustments for important confounders and the occurrence of publication bias – misinterpretation of results (see Table 9.1). Dose–response relationships have been found in some retrospective studies, but results were not adjusted for heredity. Longitudinal studies and controlled cross-sectional studies are rare and do not verify any causality of noise exposure to HFHL in young people. Nevertheless, some authors have considered noise as a more likely cause of HFHL than heredity, despite having shown significant relationship to heredity but not to noise. Uncontrolled cross-sectional studies do not allow any interpretation due to low reliability. Future studies are necessary to sort out the impact of genetic factors from those due to the noise exposure itself. So far, our interpretation of the present literature is that the importance of the genetic factors is underestimated and that of noise exposure probably overestimated. We recommend that all future epidemiological studies on this topic should be controlled for both heredity and noise exposure.

# References

Axelsson A, Lindgren F (1987). Firecrackers - a risk of hearing injuries. Lakärtidningen 15; 84(16): 1341–6.

Axelsson A, Lindgren F (1981a) Hearing in classical musicians. Acta Otolaryngologigica 377:3–74.

Axelsson A, Lindgren F (1981b) Pop music and hearing. Ear and Hearing 2:64–9.

Axelsson A, Ringdahl A (1989) Tinnitus – a study of its prevalence and characteristics. British Journal of Audiology 23:53–62.

Axelsson A, Jerson T, Lindberg U, Lindgren F (1981) Early noise-induced hearing loss in teenage boys. J Scandinavian Audiology 10:91–6.

Axelsson A, Aniansson G, Costa O (1987) Hearing loss in school children. A longitudinal study of sensorineural hearing impairment. Journal of Scandinavian Audiology 16:137–43.

Axelsson A, Rosenhall U, Zachau G (1994) Hearing in 18-year-old Swedish males. Journal of Scandinavian Audiology 23:129–34.

Baguley DM, McFerran DJ (1999) "Tinnitus in childhood." International Journal of Pediatric Otorhinolaryngology 5;49(2):99–105.

Barr B, Anderson H, Wedenberg E (1973) Epidemiology of hearing loss in childhood. Auidiology 12(5):426–37.

CDC/NIOSH (1998) Criteria for a Recommended Standard: Occupational Noise Exposure revised Criteria 1998. Cincinnati, OH: US Department of health and Human Services.

Carter NLM, Khan A, Waugh RL (1984) A longitudinal study of recreational noise and young people's hearing. Australian Journal of Audiology 6:45–53.

Cohen S, Evans GW, Krantz DS, Stokols D (1980) Psychological, motivational and cognitive effects of aircraft noise on children. American Psychologist 35:231–43.

Cohen S, Evans GW, Krantz DS, Stokols D, Kelly S (1981) Aircraft noise and children: longitudinal and cross-sectional effectiveness of noise abatement. Journal of Personality and Social Psychology 40: 331–45.

Collet L, Moussu MF, Disant F, Ahami T, Morgan A (1990) Minnesota multiphasic personality inventory in tinnitus disorders. Audiology 28:101–6.

Costa OA, Axelsson A, Aniansson G (1988) Hearing loss at age 7, 10 and 13-an audiometric follow-up study. Scand Audiol Suppl 30:25–32.

Darin N, Hanner P, Thiringer K (1997) Changes in prevalence, aetiology, age at detection, and associated disabilities in preschool children with hearing impairment born in Goteborg. Journal of Developmental & Behavioral Pediatrics 39:797–802.

Das VK (1996) Aetiology of bilateral sensorineural hearing impairment in children: a 10 year study. Archives of Diseases in Childhood 74:8–12.

Erlandsson S, Hallberg L, Axelsson A (1992) Psychological and audiological correlates of perceived tinnitus severity. Audiology 31:168–79.

Fortnum H, Davis A (1997) Epidemiology of permanent childhood hearing impairment in Trent Region, 1985–1993. British J Audiology 31:409–46.

Fortnum HM, Summerfield AQ, Marshall DH, Davis AC, Bamford JM (2001) Prevalence of permanent childhood hearing impairment in the United Kingdom and implications for universal neonatal hearing screening: questionnaire based ascertainment study. British Medical Journal 323:536–40.

Franks JR, Stephanson MR, Merry CJ (1996) Preventing occupational hearing loss - a pratical guide, U.S. National Institute for Occupational safety on Health. Department of Health and Human Services, Public Health Service Centers for Diseases Control and Prevention, National Institute for Occupation Safety and Health DHHS (NIOSH) Publication 96–110.

Graham J (1981) Paediatric tinnitus. Journal of Laryngology and Otology 4:117–20.

Graham J, Butler J (1984) Tinnitus in children. Journal of Laryngology and Otology 9:236–41.

Green J (2002) Noise induced hearing loss. Pediatrics 109:987–8.

Goebel G, Hiller W (1998) Tinnitus-Fragebogen (TF) Ein instrument zur Erfassung von Belastung und Scheregrad bei Tinnitus (Mannual). Göttingen: Hogrefe Verlag.

Haapaniemi J (1995) The 6 kHz acoustic dip in school-aged children in Finland. European Archives of Otorhinolaryngology 252:391–4.

Haapaniemi JJ (1996) The hearing threshold levels of children at school age. Ear and Hearing 17:469–77.

Halford JBS, Stewart D, Andersson M (1991). Tinnitus severity measured by a subjective scale, audiometry and clinical judgement Journal of Laryngology and Otology 105: 89–93

Holgers KM (2002) Noise induced tinnitus in young people. Noise and Health 5:65–6.

Holgers KM (2003) "Tinnitus in 7 years-old children." European Journal of Pediatrics 162:276–8.

Holgers KM, Pettersson B (2005) Tinnitus and noise exposure among school children in Sweden. Noise and Health 7(27):27–37.

Holgers KM, Erlandsson SI, Barrenäs ML (2000) Predictive factors for the severity of tinnitus. Audiology 39:284–291.

Hygge S, Evans GW, Bullinger M (2002) A prospective study of some effects of aircraft noise on cognitive performance in schoolchildren. Psychological Sciences 13:469–74.

Job A, Raynal M, Tricoire A, Signoret J, Rondet P (2000) Hearing status of French youth aged from 18 to 24 years in 1997: a cross-sectional epidemiological study in the selection centres of the army in Vincennes and Lyon. Revue De Epidemiologie et de Sante Publique 48:227–37.

Kahari K (2002) The Influence of Music on Hearing. Doctorial Thesis, Dept of Otolaryngology, Faculty of Medicine, Goteborg University.

Kahari K, Zachau G, Eklof M, Sandsjo L, Moller C (2003) Assessment of hearing and hearing disorders in rock/jazz musicians. International Journal of Audiology 42(5): 279–88.

Karagodina IL, Soldatkin SA, Vinokur IL, Kilmunkhin A (1969) Effects of aircraft noise on the population near airports. Hygiene Sanitation 34:182–7.

Karlsdorf G, Klappach H (1968) Einflüsse des Verkehrslärms auf Gesundheit und Leistung bei Oberschülern einer GroBstadt. Zeitschrift für die gesamte. Hygiene 14: 52–4.

Kentish RC, Crocker SR, McKenna L (2000) Children's experience of tinnitus: a preliminary survey of children presenting to a psychology department. British Journal of Audiology 34(6):335–40

Klockhoff I, Lyttkens L (1982) Hearing defects of noise trauma type with lack of noise exposure. J Scandinavian Audiology 11:257–60.

Klockhoff I, Lyttkens L, Svedberg A (1986) Hearing damage in military service. A study on 38,294 conscripts. Scandinavian Audiology 15:217–22.

Lindeman HE, van der Klaauw MM, Platenburg-Gits FA (1987) Hearing acuity in male adolescents (young adults) at the age of 17 to 23 years. Audiology 26:65–78.

Lindgren F, Axelsson A (1983) Temporary threshold shift after exposure to noise and music of equal energy. Ear and Hearing 4:197–201.

Lipscomb DM (1972) The increase in prevalence of high frequency hearing impairment among college students. Audiology 11:231–7.

Lutman ME, Davies AE (1994) The distribution of hearing threshold levels in general population aged 18–30 years. Audiology 33:327–50.

McBride D, Williams S (2001a) Characteristics of the audiometric notch as a clinical sign of noise exposure. Scandinavian Audiology 30:106–11.

McBride DI, Williams S (2001b) Audiometric notch as a sign of noise induced hearing loss. Journal of Occupational and Environmental Medicine 58:46–51.

Meyer-Bisch C (1996) Epidemiological evaluation of hearing damage related to strongly amplified music (personal cassette players, discotheques, rock concerts) –high-definition audiometric survey on 1364 subjects. Audiology 35:121–42.

Mills JM, Gilbert RM, () Temporary threshold shifts in humans exposed to octave bands of noise for 16 to 24 hours. J Acoust Soc Am 65(5):1238–48.

Mills RP, Albert DM, Brain CE (1986) Tinnitus in childhood. Journal of Clinical Otolaryngology 11:431–4.

Nebeska M, Stig-Magnus T, Wenneburg B, Holgers K (2000) Har musikstuderande högre nsk för tinitus och bettstörniga! The Annual Swedish Medical Society Congress. Göteburg, 29 November–1 December 2000.

Nebeska M, Stig-Magnus T, Wenneberg B, Holgers K (2002) Tinnitus, hyperacusis and tempromandibular disorders in young musicians, 7th Int Tinnitus Seminar, Freemantle, Australia 5–9 March.

Newman CW, Wharton JA, Shivapuja BG, Jacobson GP (1994) Relationships among psychoacoustic judgements, speech understanding ability and self-perceived handicap in tinnitus subject. Audiology 33:47–60

Newman CW, Wharton JA, Jacobson GP (1997) Self-focused and somatic attention in patients with tinnitus, Journal of the American Academy of Audiology 8:143–9

Niskar AS, Kieszak SM, Holmes AE, Esteban E, Rubin C, Brody DJ ( 2001) Estimated prevalence of noise-induced hearing threshold shifts among children 6 to 19 years of age: the Third National Health and Nutrition Examination Survey, 1988–1994, United States. Pediatrics 108:40–3.

Nodar, RH (1972) Tinnitus aurium in school age children: a survey. Journal of Audiological Research 12:133–5

Nodar RH, Lezak MHW (1984) Pediatric tinnitus:a thesis revised. Journal of Laryngology and Otology 98:234–5

Palin SL (1994) Does classical music damage the hearing of musicians? A review of the literature. Occupational Medicine 44:130–6.

Passchier-Vermeer W (1974) Hearing loss due to continuous exposure to steady-state broad-band noise. Journal of the Acoustical Society of America 56:1585–93.

Richardson KHD, Peckham CS (1977). Audiometric thresholds of a national sample of British 16-year-olds: longitudinal study. Journal of Developmental & Behavioral Pediatrics 19:797–802.

Roberts J (1972a) Hearing levels of children by demographic and socioeconomic characteristics. National Health Survey. Vital and Health Statistics. Series II. Number III. DHEW Publication No. (HSM) 72–1025 (PDF download from www.cdc.gov)

Roberts J (1972b) Symposium: conservation of hearing in children. Hearing sensitivity and related medical findings among children in the United States. Transactions of the American Academy of Ophthalmology and Otolaryngology 76:355–9.

Rosanowski F, Hoppe U, Proschel U, Eysholdt U (1997) (Chronic tinnitus in children and adolescents) Deutsche Gessellschaft fur Hals-Nasen-Ohren-Heillande,kopf-und Hals Chirurgie vol. 45, pp. 927–32

Royster LH, Royster JD, Thomas WG (1980) Representative hearing levels by race and sex in North Carolina industry. 1: J Acoust Soc Am. Aug; 68(2):551–66.

Royster Jd (2002) Audiometric monitoring phase of HCP. In EH Berger, LH Royster, DP Driscoll, J Doswell Royster, M Layne (eds) The Noise Manual, 5th edition. Fairfax, VA: American Industrial Hygiene Association, pp 455–516.

Rytzner B, Rytzner C (1981) Schoolchildren and noise. The 4 kHz diptone screening in 14391 schoolchildren. Scandinavian Audiology 10:213–6.

Sataloff RT (1980) The 4000 -Hz Audiometric dip. Entechnology 59: 251–7

Schmidt JM, Verschuure J, Brocaar MP (1994) Hearing loss in students at a conservatory. Audiology 33(4):185–94.

Sehlin P, Holmgren G, Zakrisson J (1990) Incidence, prevalence and etiology of hearing impairment in children in the county of Vasterbotten, Sweden. Scandinavian Audiology 19:193–200.

Statistiska Centralbyrån (2001) Swedish Central Government Authority for Official Statistics. Statistical Database–living conditions; poor health and care (ULF) hearing loss, 20 years old. www.scb.se

Stenstrom C, Ingvarsson L (1994) General illness and need of medical care in otitis prore children. Int J Pediatr Otorhinolaryngol 29(1):23–32.

Stenstrom C, Ingvarsson L (1995) Late effects on ear disease in otitis-prone children: a long-term follow-up study. Acta Otolaryngologica 115:658–63.

Stenstrom C, Ingvarsson L (1997) Otitis-prone children and controls: a study of possible predisposing factors. 2. Physical findings, frequency of illness, allergy, day care and parental smoking. Acta Otolaryngologica 117: 696–703.

Stouffer JL, Tyler RS, Booth JC, Buckrell B (1991) "Tinnitus in Normal-Hearing and Hearing-Impaired Children." presented at Fourth International Tinnitus Seminar, Bordeaux.

Sutton GJ, Rowe SJ (1997) Risk factors for childhood sensorineural hearing loss in the Oxford region. British Journal of Audiology 31:39–54.

Taylor, W, Pearson JC, Mair A, Burns W (1965) Study of noise and hearing loss in jute weavers. Journal of the Acoustical Society of America 38:13–20.

Thiringer K, Kankkunen A, Liden G, Niklasson A (1984) Perinatal risk factors in the aetiology of hearing loss in preschool children. Journal of Developmental & Behavioral Pediatrics 26:799–807.

Weber HJ, McGovern FJ, Zink D (1967) An evaluation of 1000 children with hearing loss. Journal of Speech and Hearing Disorders 32:343–54.

Wong TW, Van Hasselt CA, Tang LS, Yiu PC (1990) The use of personal cassette players among youths and its effects on hearing. Public Health 104(5):327–30.

# CHAPTER 10

# Clinical diagnosis of noise-induced hearing loss

*Noise and Its Effects:* Edited by Linda Luxon and Deepak Prasher © 2007
John Wiley & Sons Ltd.

IAN COLVIN, LINDA LUXON

## Introduction

Noise-induced hearing loss (NIHL) is a common problem. In 1997, a consultation was undertaken by the World Health Organization (WHO) in order to gain a worldwide perspective on the problem and consider mechanisms of prevention (WHO, 1997).

**Key points from WHO consultation (1997)**

- Exposure to noise represents the principal avoidable cause of permanent hearing impairment worldwide.
- In many regions, noise is the occupational hazard that accounts for most compensation awards.
- The global prevalence of people with a hearing impairment (defined as at least a 25-dB hearing level (HL) loss in the better hearing ear over the 0.5, 1, 2 and 4 kHz octave bands) is estimated to be between 441 million and 580 million.
- In developed countries, noise is considered to be at least partially responsible for hearing impairment in over a third of all cases.
- In developing countries, occupational noise is an increasing risk factor for hearing impairment. There are limited epidemiological data on the prevalence of occupational noise in developing countries, but it is likely to be a substantial problem.
- In the European region, it is estimated that 25–35 million people work in potentially damaging noise environments.

NIHL is the fourth most frequently self-reported work-related illness in the United Kingdom (HSE, 2002).

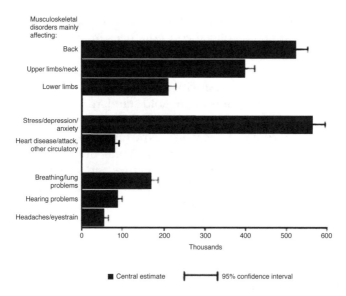

**Figure 10.1** Estimated prevalence of self-reported work-related illness in the UK, 2001–02. (From HSE, 2002, reproduced with kind permission.)

The findings of a recent large UK survey have estimated that the prevalence of hearing loss (moderate or worse) at least partially attributable to occupational noise in workers is 509 000 (Palmer et al., 2001). Despite the well-documented risks of exposure to loud noise at work (Health and Safety Executive or HSE, 1989), many UK workers continue to be exposed to potentially damaging levels of noise in the workplace. A 1995 UK survey found that 6% of male and 3% of female workers reported symptoms of tinnitus or hearing loss at the end of a work period at least once a week. Furthermore, 3% of male and 2% of female workers reported these symptoms as a daily occurrence (Jones et al., 1997).

A 1990 consensus statement by the US National Institutes of Health states that approximately 28 million US citizens have impaired hearing and noise exposure is at least partially attributable in 10 million of these cases (NIH, 1990).

**Main occupational groups at risk of NIHL (Environmental Protection Agency or EPA, 1981; HSE, 2003):**

- manufacturing;
- construction;
- military;
- transportation;
- mining;
- agriculture.

The responsibility for diagnosing NIHL lies with the clinician and there are often significant medicolegal consequences in making the diagnosis. There are a number of reasons why diagnosis can prove difficult. First, there are no symptoms, signs or investigations that, alone or in combination, will provide 100% sensitivity and 100% specificity in diagnosing the condition. Therefore, there is no 'gold standard' diagnostic tool at the clinician's disposal. Second, the effects of pathological changes in the cochlea that arise from chronic noise exposure are similar to those that arise from most other causes of sensorineural hearing loss (Michaels, 2003). Disruption of sensory hair cell structure and function is one of the principal endpoints of many different pathological processes that can affect the cochlea. This hair cell loss causes impairment of both hearing sensitivity and selectivity (Pickles, 1988). Furthermore, the majority of these pathological processes, including noise-induced damage, have a predilection for damaging the basal region of the cochlea, and the resulting

**Table 10.1** Causes of sensorineural hearing loss

| Category | Causative condition or agent |
| --- | --- |
| Age | Presbyacusis |
| Pregnancy and birth factors | Maternal infections in pregnancy, prematurity, low birthweight, neonatal jaundice, hypoxia |
| Structural | Congenital malformations involving the inner ear. |
| Genetic | Autosomal dominant, autosomal recessive, X-linked, mitochondrial, syndromal, chromosomal |
| Infection | Bacterial, viral, fungal, treponemal, rickettsial. (labyrinthitis, neuritis, polyneuritis, polygangliositis, encephalitis, meningitis) |
| Inflammatory | Autoimmune diseases |
| Metabolic | Thyroid disorders, diabetes mellitus, hyper-lipidaemia, renal failure |
| Neoplasia | Primary and secondary malignancies, haematological malignancies, acoustic neuroma |
| Ototoxic agents | Salicylates, loop diuretics, aminoglycoside antibiotics, quinine, platinum chemotherapy, industrial solvents, radiotherapy |
| Trauma | Acoustic trauma, barometric trauma, head injury |
| Vascular | Atheromatous disease, coagulopathy, sickle cell disease |
| Otological | Ménière's disease, cochlear manifestations of middle-ear disease, otosclerosis |
| Other | Neurological disease, Paget's disease |

hearing impairment is therefore more severe in the higher frequencies. A patient suffering with NIHL will typically present with a high-frequency sensorineural hearing loss centred around the 4-kHz octave band. Any clinician who is likely to treat such a patient must be fully aware of the differential diagnosis of sensorineural hearing loss.

Many patients presenting with possible NIHL will have a multifactorial aetiology to their hearing loss and it is neither feasible nor practical for the clinician to simply arrive at a diagnosis of NIHL by excluding all the other causes of sensorineural hearing loss. In particular, age-related hearing loss (presbyacusis) is a common coexisting pathology in patients with NIHL (Pyykko et al., 1998) (see Chapter 4).

In assessing a patient who presents with the complaint of hearing loss that may be due to noise exposure, the clinician must apply diagnostic strategies that will help to place the patient into one of five categories:

1. those with normal hearing;
2. those with noise-induced hearing loss;
3. those with hearing loss due to other causes;
4. those with hearing loss of unknown cause;
5. those with hearing loss due to a combination of noise and other factors.

Noise-induced hearing loss is a medical problem and is therefore best diagnosed via the standard medical model of history, examination and investigation. This model should be applied by a suitably trained and experienced clinician who must possess an up-to-date and evidence-based knowledge of the subject.

# Measurement of noise

Noise is recorded as a sound pressure level (SPL), which is a measure of the amplitude of the air pressure changes that are caused by the sound waves. The human cochlea is an extremely sensitive receptor that is able to detect a vast range of sound pressure levels, ranging from $2–10^{-5}$ Pa at the threshold of hearing to 20 Pa at the threshold of pain (National Physical Laboratory or NPL, 2003a). In order to facilitate comparison of sounds within this large range, sound pressure levels are measured on a logarithmic scale (see Chapter 2). The unit of this scale is the decibel (dB). An additional advantage of the decibel scale is that it correlates closely with the human perception of change in sound pressure level (loudness). An increase in sound pressure level of 10 dB results in an approximate doubling of the loudness perception (Pickles, 1997).

The human perception of loudness also varies with respect to frequency (Moore, 1997). For example, a 100-Hz tone at 52 dB SPL, a 1000-Hz tone at 40 dB SPL and a 4000-Hz tone at 37 dB SPL are all perceived at equal loudness (Yost, 2000). To simplify the comparison of noise at different frequencies, sound level meters used to record industrial and other potentially hazardous noise utilize the A-weighted frequency network

(Dobie, 2001). This network mathematically models the human frequency response and therefore sounds of differing frequency that are recorded at the same dB (A) are perceived as having equal loudness.

# Mechanisms of NIHL

Noise can be damaging to the cochlea. If the exposure causes cochlear damage that is reversible, the hearing impairment is temporary. If the exposure causes damage that is irreversible and affects sound perception, the hearing impairment is permanent.

### Temporary threshold shift

The typical symptoms of a temporary threshold shift (TTS) after hazardous noise exposure are hearing loss and high-frequency tinnitus.

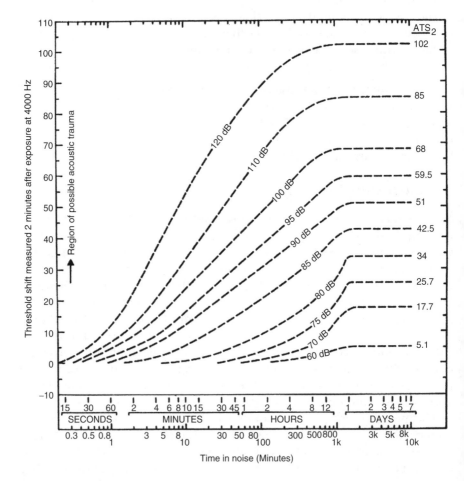

**Figure 10.2** Hypothetical growth of threshold shift measured 2 minutes after a single continuous exposure to noise. (From Miller, 1974, reproduced with kind permission.)

However, many patients will report a 'muffling' or 'dulling' of their hearing as opposed to a frank loss. The symptoms will completely resolve within a period of 48 hours of removal from noise.

The majority of experimental data on human TTS comes from studies that were performed prior to the proliferation in knowledge on the long-term effects of loud noise on hearing. In the light of this knowledge, such studies are no longer ethically acceptable. Miller's (1974) review of the effects of noise on people collated the evidence on TTS available at that time. The relationship between noise exposure and human TTS is demonstrated in Figure 10.2, taken from Miller's paper.

Some key concepts relating to TTS and its relationship to permanent hearing loss are listed below:

- For noise at a particular frequency, the greater the sound pressure level, the greater the resultant TTS. In addition, the greater the sound pressure level, the longer it will take for the TTS to recover (Miller, 1974).
- With continuing exposure to noise at a particular frequency, the degree of TTS increases steadily until it reaches a maximum level. This maximum level is referred to as the asymptotic threshold shift (ATS). Mills (1982) found that the ATS increased by 1.7 dB for every 1-dB increase in noise sound pressure level. The period of continuous noise required to produce the ATS is approximately 8 hours (Quaranta et al., 1998). Two important concepts relate the ATS to the risk of long-term NIHL: first, it is postulated that the permanent threshold shift produced by long-term, daily exposure to a noise is approximately equal to the ATS produced by a short-term exposure to the same noise (Melnick, 1991); secondly, it is suggested that the ATS produced by a noise represents the upper limit of any permanent threshold shift that arises from long-term exposure to the same noise (Mills, 1982). However, it is important to note that an individual's susceptibility to a TTS has not been proven to be predictive of that individual's risk of a permanent threshold shift (Melnick, 1991; Quaranta et al., 1998).
- There is a minimum safe level for noise at each frequency. Noise presented at a sound pressure level equal or less than this safe level will not cause a TTS. The safe level varies with frequency, with higher frequency sounds having a lower safe level. A large ($n = 300$) study by Mills (1982) demonstrated that the minimum safe levels for a 1-kHz noise, 2-kHz noise and 4-kHz noise were 82 dB, 78 dB and 74 dB respectively. It is generally accepted that prolonged exposure to a noise that cannot cause a TTS will not cause a permanent threshold shift. Long-term exposure to noise at a level less than 75 dB (A) is considered safe (NIH, 1990).
- The maximum TTS is observed at a frequency approximately 0.5–1 octave above the centre frequency of the noise (Alberti, 1987a). Industrial noise typically has a broadband frequency spectrum with a centre frequency of between 2 and 3 kHz (Feverstein, 2002). Broadband

noise with equal energies across all component frequencies has been shown to cause maximal TTS between 3 and 5 kHz, and particularly at 4 kHz (Quaranta et al., 1998). These attributes of TTS provide some explanation to the characteristic 4-kHz noise notch that arises from chronic noise exposure.

* There is good animal study evidence and some evidence from human studies that repeated exposure to a loud noise can lead to a progressive reduction in the TTS in response to the noise (Attanasio et al., 1998). This phenomenon is termed 'conditioning' or 'toughening' in the auditory system. Evidence from animal studies has indicated that the efferent olivocochlear nervous system plays an important role in conditioning (Henderson et al., 1993).

**Permanent threshold shift**

The main concern for the clinician is the patient who presents with a permanent threshold shift (PTS) that may be related to chronic noise exposure.

**Factors of relevance to NIHL**

* Intensity of noise exposure.
* Duration of noise exposure.
* Type of noise exposure
  o impulsive
  o continuous
  o intermittent
  o frequency.
* Susceptibility factors (Chapter 7).
* Personal/institutional protection (Chapters 29+30).
* Occupational/non-occupational exposure (Chapters 16,18–20,22).

It is known that long-term exposure to loud noise is associated with irreversible damage to cochlear structures including the outer and inner hair cells, stria vascularis and supporting cells (Alberti, 1998; Nordmann et al., 2000). These pathological changes manifest clinically as permanent hearing impairment. Permanent noise-induced threshold shifts are characteristically most severe at or around the 4-kHz frequency. This corresponds to structural damage to the organ of Corti at approximately 10 mm from the basal end (Igarashi et al., 1964).

In order to study the long-term effects of noise on hearing, researchers have concentrated on occupational groups known to have worked in noisy environments for many years. A typical study will establish the hearing status of such a group and then compare this to the hearing of matched controls who have not worked in noisy environments. Any observed difference in hearing thresholds between the two groups can then be ascribed to noise exposure. The definitive example is Taylor et al.'s (1965) study of jute weavers in Scotland.

The jute weavers were a good group to study because the investigators were able to obtain an unusually accurate measure of a worker's long-term noise exposure. This was due to the fact that the weaving machinery had remained essentially unchanged for many years and that much of the workforce had been employed at the same plant for a long period. The researchers were able to obtain comprehensive measurements of the weaving machinery noise output at the time of the study and therefore derive an accurate measure of an individual worker's exposure to noise, in terms of both level and duration of exposure.

It is important to note that there are some limitations in using this study as a model for other occupationally exposed groups. The jute weavers were predominantly female whereas most at-risk occupations have a predominantly male workforce. Furthermore, the noise produced by the weaving machinery differs slightly from typical broadband industrial noise. The noise exposure was unusually loud (99–102 dB SPL), the noise had an impact component and the peak levels in the noise frequency spectrum were at a lower frequency (1–2 kHz) than typical industrial noise (2–3 kHz). In recent years, occupational noise exposure at this high level is rare in the developed world but may be a common occurrence in developing industrial nations (WHO, 1997).

Despite these limitations, the jute weavers' study provides valid and useful information on the effects of chronic noise exposure on hearing. The main findings are demonstrated in Figure 10.3.

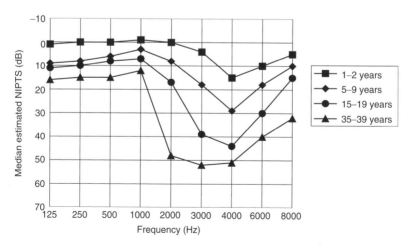

**Figure 10.3** Estimated noise-induced threshold shift for jute weavers as a function of frequency, for various durations of exposure. (From Taylor, 1965, reproduced with kind permission.)

Data from large studies of occupationally exposed workers form the basis of the International Organization for Standardization report on NIHL (ISO, 1990). This report provides formulae that can be used to generate an estimation of the degree of NIHL for a population based on the level and duration of noise exposure. Figures 10.4–10.7 display the relationship between noise exposure and PTS using data generated by the ISO formulae.

It is important to realize that the ISO data relate to populations and that there is considerable variation in susceptibility to NIHL between individuals (see under 'Susceptibility' and Chapter 7).

The typical pattern of hearing loss that results from chronic noise exposure starts at or around the 4-kHz frequency and, with continuing exposure, progresses at this frequency and then begins to involve the neighbouring frequencies.

The rate of progression is greater over the first 10–15 years of exposure, but ultimately begins to flatten out.

The pattern of hearing loss due to long-term noise exposure is also demonstrated by pure-tone audiogram (PTA) findings and is therefore discussed in detail under 'Audiological investigations'.

## Acute acoustic trauma

Acute acoustic trauma from a loud impulsive sound, such as a gunshot, with peak sound pressure levels of 120 dB SPL or greater may also cause

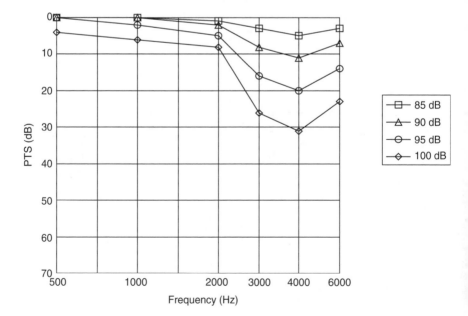

**Figure 10.4** Median noise-induced permanent threshold shift (PTS) after 10 years of exposure at varying noise exposure levels ($L_{EX, 8h}$). (Source: ISO, 1990. After Dobie, 2001.)

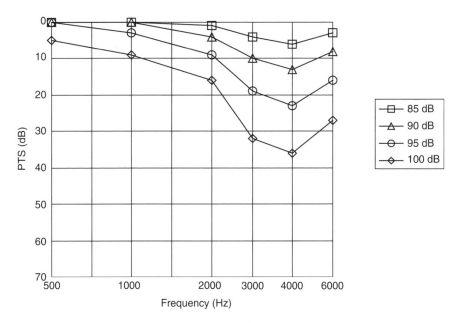

**Figure 10.5** Median noise-induced permanent threshold shift (PTS) after 20 years of exposure at varying noise exposure levels (L$_{EX, 8h}$). (Source: ISO, 1990. After Dobie, 2001.)

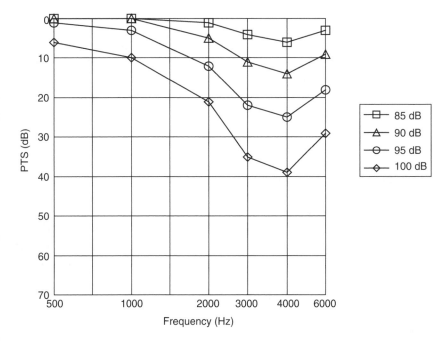

**Figure 10.6** Median noise-induced permanent threshold shift (PTS) after 30 years of exposure at varying noise exposure levels (L$_{EX, 8h}$). (Source: ISO, 1990. After Dobie, 2001.)

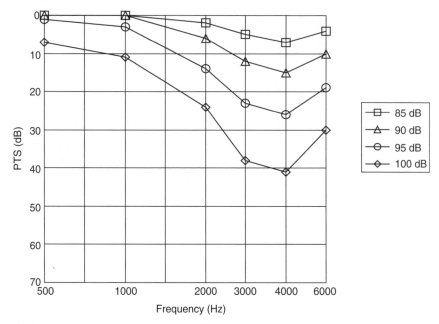

**Figure 10.7** Median noise-induced permanent threshold shift (PTS) after 40 years of exposure at varying noise exposure levels ($L_{EX, 8h}$). (Source: ISO, 1990. After Dobie, 2001.)

auditory damage (Chapter 17). The characteristic feature of impulsive sound is an initial rapid rise in sound pressure (rise time < 200 ms) and the damage is greater with higher peak pressures, steeper rises in sound pressure level and longer duration of sound (Kersebaum and Bennett, 1998).

More severe acute acoustic trauma arises from blast injuries, such as those associated with a bomb explosion (Chapter 13). A blast will typically result in an impulse sound, which is often extremely loud (peaks pressure greater than 160 dB SPL) and associated with significant movement of air and combustion products (Garth, 1994). Loud impulse noises and blasts can cause temporary and permanent cochlear damage. Patients will report symptoms of sudden onset hearing loss, often with concomitant tinnitus, loudness sensitivity and otalgia. The hearing impairment is typically a high-frequency sensorineural loss but it is important for the clinician to be aware that the 4-kHz notch is not characteristic of acute acoustic trauma (Garth, 1994). Vestibular symptoms are rarely reported as a consequence of acute acoustic trauma.

Van Campen et al. (1999) followed up 83 people who had been in the vicinity of the 1995 Oklahoma City bombing (Figure 10.8). These people had all been exposed to very high peak SPL impulse noise (> 160 dB SPL). The study found that 66 (80%) of the group had hearing loss (as defined as an age-corrected PTA threshold, averaged over the 1-kHz, 2-kHz and 4-kHz frequencies, of > 22.5 dB HL for one or both ears). An important

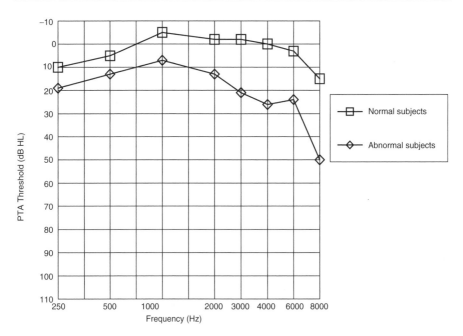

**Figure 10.8** Mean age-corrected pure-tone audiogram (PTA) thresholds (dB HL) for 66 people exposed to the 1995 Oklahoma City bombing. Squares represent blast-exposed subjects with thresholds < 22.5 dB HL bilaterally (*n* = 12). Diamonds represent blast-exposed subjects with one or more threshold(s) ≥ 22.5 dB HL (*n* = 44). (From Van Campen et al., 1999, reproduced by kind permission.)

finding was the observation that the hearing loss remained stable over a 1-year follow-up period and did not show any significant recovery.

Blast injuries frequently cause middle-ear pathology, resulting in a conductive component to the hearing impairment. The injuries predominantly involve varying degrees of tympanic membrane perforation and, less commonly, disruptions or fractures of the ossicular chain (Roberto et al., 1989). It has been suggested that patients with middle-ear blast injuries may be predisposed to cholesteatoma formation (Cripps et al., 1999). The proposed mechanism involves fragments of keratinizing squamous epithelium being seeded throughout the middle ear and mastoid cavity as a result of rapid inward movement of air and tympanic membrane perforation.

# What levels of occupation noise are dangerous?

The principal UK and USA occupational health bodies both specify 85 dB (A) as the minimum level of occupational noise that will present a significant risk of causing permanent NIHL (HSE, 1989; NIOSH, 1998). Employers therefore have a legal responsibility to take measures to protect their employees' hearing if they are exposed to occupational noise at or above this level.

One of the key difficulties in assessing the risk of occupational noise is the variability in types of exposure. An individual worker's noise exposure is rarely continuous and may be fluctuating, impulsive, interrupted or irregular.

Burns and Robinson (1970) addressed the variability in noise exposure in their seminal work on occupational hearing loss. They proposed that it is the acoustic energy that is damaging to the cochlea and that different noises will be equally damaging provided that they contain the same amount of total acoustic energy. This is known as the 'equal energy concept'.

Burns and Robinson used this concept as the scientific basis for a method by which the varying intensity and duration of noise exposure experienced by an individual worker could be converted into a single, comparable variable. This variable is expressed as the equivalent averaged continuous noise level and was termed the 'noise immission level'.

Following its inception, the equal energy concept was widely adopted in the analysis of occupational noise. For example, the ISO report on NIHL measures a worker's risk in terms of their averaged equivalent continuous exposure in decibels (A) over an 8-hour period (ISO, 1990). This report used the term $L_{EX,8h}$ to represent this averaged continuous exposure.

The US National Institute for Occupational Safety and Health (NIOSH) applied the equal energy concept in its guidance on safe durations of noise exposure. It specifies that the maximum safe period of daily exposure to an 85 dB (A) noise is 8 hours. It is known that a 3-dB rise in sound pressure level represents a doubling in acoustic energy. Therefore, according to the equal energy concept, the maximum safe period while exposed to an 88-dB (A) noise is 4 hours and similar safe periods could be calculated for noise exposure at different levels (Table 10.2).

It is generally accepted that the equal energy concept is a valid tool in helping to assess a worker's short-term noise exposure (for example, during the 8-hour working day). However, there is no good evidence to support the use of the concept in predicting the effects of long-term noise exposure (for example, over years) (Robinson, 1987).

Moreover, there is evidence from animal studies that also proposes that the equal energy concept may be invalid for certain types of impact and impulse noises. The concept states that the amount of hearing impairment is proportional to the acoustic energy contained within the noise, but studies have demonstrated that the temporal pattern and peak sound pressure levels also have a significant effect. Lataye and Campo (1996) exposed guinea pigs to a variety of noise exposures that had an identical acoustic spectrum and energy content, but differing temporal patterns. All the noise exposures had an equivalent averaged continuous noise level of 92 dB over 8 hours. Their results indicated that the equal energy concept was valid for moderate-intensity (95 dB) 4-hour noise and for 101-dB impulse noise. However, the equal energy model overestimated the amount of PTS produced by intermittent noise. Intermittence of noise exposure has been shown by Ward (1991) to reduce the amount of PTS. In his study, using chinchillas, dividing a continuous

**Table 10.2** Combinations of noise exposure levels and durations that no worker exposure should equal or exceed

| Exposure level dB (A) | Duration | | |
|:---:|:---:|:---:|:---:|
| | Hours | Minutes | Seconds |
| 80 | 25 | 24 | – |
| 81 | 20 | 10 | – |
| 82 | 16 | – | – |
| 83 | 12 | 42 | – |
| 84 | 10 | 5 | – |
| 85 | 8 | – | – |
| 86 | 6 | 21 | – |
| 87 | 5 | 2 | – |
| 88 | 4 | – | – |
| 89 | 3 | 10 | – |
| 90 | 2 | 31 | – |
| 91 | 2 | – | – |
| 92 | 1 | 35 | – |
| 93 | 1 | 16 | – |
| 94 | 1 | – | – |
| 95 | – | 47 | 37 |
| 96 | – | 37 | 48 |
| 97 | – | 30 | – |
| 98 | – | 23 | 49 |
| 99 | – | 18 | 59 |
| 100 | – | 15 | – |
| 101 | – | 11 | 54 |
| 102 | – | 9 | 27 |
| 103 | – | 7 | 30 |
| 104 | – | 4 | 57 |
| 105 | – | 4 | 43 |

From National Institute for Occupational Safety and Health (1998), reproduced with kind permission.

noise exposure into many discrete exposure periods resulted in a significant reduction in the degree of PTS. He pointed out that the equal energy concept would have predicted no change in the PTS with this change in noise exposure timing. The protective role of intermittency may be related to the phenomenon of 'conditioning' that is seen in respect of TTSs (see 'Mechanisms of NIHL').

There is also evidence to suggest that impulse noise with a peak sound pressure above a certain critical level will result in hearing impairment that is more severe than predicted by the equal energy concept (Henderson et al., 1993). This critical level probably varies in relation to the acoustic spectrum of the noise. Henderson's study using chinchillas estimated that the critical level is reached at approximately 125 dB peak equivalent SPL. It is postulated that the critical level represents a point where the stresses being placed on the cochlea change from being predominantly metabolic to predominantly mechanical. There are a number of additional animal studies that support the critical level hypothesis (Clark, 1991; Danielson et al., 1991; Lataye and Campo, 1996).

When relating these studies to human occupational noise exposure, it is important to realize that the study noise exposures are short term and controlled in comparison to the type of exposure that is typically experienced by a worker who may have worked in a noisy environment for many years.

The US NIOSH document on NIHL (NIOSH, 1998) reviews the human studies that have examined whether the 'equal energy concept' is a valid predictor of long-term PTS. The document cites a number of studies that support the concept and a number that suggest that impulse noise is more harmful than predicted by the equal energy concept.

# Evidence-based resources available to estimate the noise-induced threshold shift for populations

Over the years, a number of researchers and organizations have produced resources that can be used to generate an estimation of the noise-induced permanent threshold shift (NIPTS) for populations (Table 10.3).

**Table 10.3** Evidence-based resources that can be used to predict hearing loss from long-term noise exposure in populations

| Title | Organization | Reference |
|---|---|---|
| Public health and welfare criteria for noise | Environmental Protection Agency (USA) | EPA (1973) |
| Tables for the estimation of noise-induced hearing loss | National Physical Laboratory (UK) | Robinson, Shipton (1977) |
| Tables for the estimation of hearing impairment due to noise for otologically normal persons and for a typically unscreened population, as a function of age and duration of exposure | Health and Safety Executive (UK) | Robinson (1988) |
| Acoustics – determination of noise exposure and estimation of noise-induced hearing impairment | International Organization for Standardization (Europe) | ISO (1990) |
| Occupational noise and demographic factors in hearing  (a study based on data from the National Survey of Hearing) | Based on the National Survey of Hearing (UK) data | Lutman and Spencer (1991) |
| A re-examination of risk estimates from the NIOSH Occupational Noise and Hearing Survey (ONHS) | National Institute for Occupational Safety and Health (USA) | Prince et al. (1997) |

These resources differ in their methodology but all require two key variables in their calculation of the threshold shift:

1. equivalent averaged daily continuous noise exposure (defined in the previous section);
2. number of years of exposure.

All the resources include a method by which the expected age-related hearing loss (presbyacusis) is taken into account when estimating the effects of noise.

Given that there is significant variability in individual NIPTS, these resources are intended only to provide a valid estimation of the average NIPTS experienced by a population of people exposed to noise. However, they are useful in the clinical assessment of a patient who may have NIHL. If the clinician is able to ascertain the above two variables for his patient, he can then utilize these resources to estimate the theoretical NIPTS for a population exposed to the same noise stimulus. Diagnostically useful information may be obtained by observing the concordance or discordance between the estimated NIPTS and the patient's actual audiometric status.

The principal limitation of these resources relates to assessment of the noise exposure. Many patients with NIHL will present many years after the exposure to noise has ended (for example, during retirement) and obtaining an accurate measure of the noise exposure is not feasible. In this situation, the clinician will have to use the history of noise exposure to make an estimation of the equivalent averaged daily continuous noise exposure variable.

Occasionally the noise conditions that are implicated in a patient's NIHL are still in place (as was the case in Taylor's 1965 jute weavers' study described in 'Mechanisms of NIHL'). Published guidelines for the measurement of noise are available (HSE, 1990; ISO, 1990) and accurate measurement may be required, particularly if the case has medicolegal consequences. Detailed noise measurement will allow for an accurate estimation of the equivalent averaged continuous noise exposure variable.

Another limitation of these resources relates to the equal energy concept. By requiring the use of the equivalent averaged continuous noise exposure variable, the resources are utilizing a noise figure that is based on the equal energy concept. As discussed in the previous section, the equal energy concept is now not considered to be valid for certain types of noise exposure. A clinician using these resources must be aware that the equal energy concept may lead to an underestimation of the effects of impulse noise and over-estimation in situations where noise is intermittent. ISO 1999 (ISO, 1990) does provide an option to treat impulse noise as more damaging than other types of noise exposure.

It is beyond the scope of this chapter to discuss all the resources in detail. However, the ISO resource (ISO 1999 – ISO, 1990) will be discussed as it remains the most widely used and accepted resource for predicting NIPTS in populations. In addition, this chapter summarizes the Health and Safety Executive document as this has been generated from a comprehensive re-analysis of all the principal epidemiological studies of occupational hearing loss. This document also provides a comprehensive set of tables for ease of use.

## ISO 1999: Acoustics – Determination of occupational noise exposure and estimation of noise-induced hearing impairment

The ISO report on NIHL (ISO, 1990) is the most widely used resource to estimate occupational hearing loss for populations. Furthermore, the ISO methodology has also been incorporated into the equivalent American National Standard resource (American Standards Institute or ANSI, 1996).

The report enables the clinician to generate an estimation of the NIPTS (averaged between the two ears) at the frequencies 0.5, 1, 2, 3, 4 and 6 kHz. The NIPTS is obtained by referring to tables within the report (Table 10.4).

**Table 10.4** Example table from ISO 1999 demonstrating noise-induced permanent threshold shift (NIPTS) as a function of exposure time, in years, and a noise exposure level, $L_{EX,8h}$ of 95 dB for six frequencies and three fractiles (0.1, 0.5, 0.9)

| Frequency (Hz) | NIPTS (dB) | | | | | | | | | | | |
|---|---|---|---|---|---|---|---|---|---|---|---|---|
| | Exposure time (years) | | | | | | | | | | | |
| | 10 | | | 20 | | | 30 | | | 40 | | |
| | Fractiles | | | | | | | | | | | |
| | 0.9 | 0.5 | 0.1 | 0.9 | 0.5 | 0.1 | 0.9 | 0.5 | 0.1 | 0.9 | 0.5 | 0.1 |
| 500 | 0 | 0 | 1 | 0 | 0 | 1 | 0 | 1 | 1 | 0 | 1 | 1 |
| 1000 | 1 | 2 | 4 | 2 | 3 | 5 | 2 | 3 | 5 | 2 | 3 | 6 |
| 2000 | 0 | 5 | 13 | 5 | 9 | 17 | 7 | 12 | 20 | 9 | 14 | 22 |
| 3000 | 8 | 16 | 25 | 13 | 19 | 31 | 16 | 22 | 34 | 18 | 23 | 37 |
| 4000 | 13 | 20 | 27 | 16 | 23 | 32 | 18 | 25 | 34 | 19 | 26 | 36 |
| 6000 | 5 | 14 | 23 | 8 | 16 | 26 | 10 | 18 | 28 | 12 | 19 | 29 |

Table E.3 from ISO 1999 (ISO, 1990) is reproduced with the permission of the British Standards Institution on behalf of ISO under licence number 2003SK/105. BSI and ISO publications can be obtained from BSI Customer Services, 389 Chiswick High Road, London W4 4AL. United Kingdom. Tel. + 44 (0) 20 8996 9001. Email cservices@bsi-global.com.

To use the tables, the clinician must have the two key variables:

1. Equivalent averaged 8-hour continuous noise exposure ($L_{EX,8h}$): the report provides the mathematical formula that can be used to generate the $L_{EX,8h}$ from actual measures of occupational noise (using the

equal energy concept). The ISO accepts that there is some evidence that impulse noise may not conform to the equal energy concept and therefore provide the option to add 5 dB to any measure of impulse noise when calculating the $L_{EX,8h}$. The range of $L_{EX,8h}$ values of that can be used in the tables is between 85 dB and 100 dB (in 5-dB steps).

2. Duration of exposure: the range of values that can be used with the tables is between 10 and 40 years (in 10-year steps).

As the ISO report relates to populations, the tables generate three figures for the NIPTS: the median, 10th percentile and 90th percentile values. For example, using the ISO 1999 tables, the estimated NIPTS at 4 kHz for a population of workers exposed to a $L_{EX,8h}$ of 95 dB for 30 years is as follows:

- the median NIPTS is 25 dB;
- 90% of the exposed population would have a NIPTS of 18 dB or greater;
- 10% of the exposed population would have a NIPTS of 34 dB or greater.

Figures 10.4–10.7 demonstrate the NIPTS data generated by ISO 1999.

ISO 1999 accepts that many patients will have age-related hearing loss (presbyacusis) in addition to any NIPTS. Therefore a simple formula is provided that will generate the threshold level associated with age and noise for each frequency. The report uses data from the ISO 7029 report on age-related hearing loss as the age component in this formula (ISO, 1984).

ISO 7029 is based on the study of people who were screened for additional otological pathology and excluded if an additional cause of hearing loss was identified. ISO 1999 recognizes that clinicians using the resource may not be relating the findings to a population that has been similarly screened. It therefore provides the opportunity to substitute the ISO 7029 age-related hearing loss data with a different source of age-related hearing loss data of the clinician's choosing. This data source should reflect the otological status of the population in whom the effects of noise are being examined.

ISO 1999 is based on analysis of the data from a number of large studies that have examined the hearing of occupationally exposed workers, including Baughn's (1973) report on the hearing of 6835 workers in the automotive component industry and Burns and Robinson's (1970) study on 759 UK workers. A criticism of the report is that it does not provide information on how the data from these studies was analysed and utilized in the ISO formulae.

ISO report on NIHL (ISO, 1990) is the most widely used resource to estimate occupational hearing loss for populations. The ISO methodology has also been incorporated into the equivalent American National Standard resource (ANSI, 1996).

## UK Health and Safety Executive contract research reports 1987:001 (Robinson, 1987) and 1998:002 (Robinson, 1988)

Professor Robinson of the University of Southampton was one of the leading authorities in the field of NIHL. In 1987, he was commissioned by the UK Health and Safety Executive to re-examine the numerous studies on NIHL and to provide an updated method of estimating noise exposure risk. The re-examination was necessary because most of the principal studies of occupationally exposed workers were undertaken in the 1960s and 1970s, and much had been learnt about NIHL since that period.

The resultant 1987 report provides a detailed description of Robinson's re-analysis of these original studies and how the data were used to generate a new model to predict NIHL in populations. This model is based on data from testing of more than 13,000 ears and does not utilize the equal energy concept, which is not considered to be valid in the calculation of long-term NIPTSs. The 1988 report provides a comprehensive set of tables based on the model that can be used by the clinician as an easy method to estimate the NIHL in a population.

As in ISO 1999, Robinson's model incorporates ISO 7029 data to take into account the normal age-related hearing loss that is expected in older workers. Furthermore, separate sets of tables are provided for populations that have been screened to exclude other otological pathology and unscreened populations.

The input variables are similar to those used in all the resources:

- Equivalent averaged 8-hour continuous noise exposure: Robinson's reports do not provide information on noise measurement and how to derive this variable from separate measures of noise. Therefore a clinician will have to use other guidance (such as ISO 1999) to generate this variable. The range of exposure levels that can be used in the tables is between 83 dB and 102 dB (in 1-dB steps).
- Duration of exposure: the range of duration time that can be used with the tables is between 0 and 40 years (in 1-year intervals).

The 1998 report provides two types of table (A and B) for both screened and unscreened populations.

The A tables are used to generate an estimation of the hearing threshold level for different exposure times and levels. The value generated is the averaged threshold level at 1, 2 and 3 kHz across both ears and incorporates the NIPTS and the age-related hearing loss. As with ISO 1999, the data relate to populations and the threshold values are given for population percentiles (ranging from the 5th to 95th percentile, in 5% bands). An example of part of the 92 dB Table A is shown in Table 10.5.

The B tables generate a percentage figure in relation to the level and duration of noise exposure. This figure is the percentage of a population that would have hearing threshold levels (using the 1, 2, 3 kHz average)

**Table 10.5** Sample table for 92 dB (A) noise exposure

| | Hearing threshold level (dB) | | | | | | | | | |
|---|---|---|---|---|---|---|---|---|---|---|
| Exposure duration (years) | Percentile | | | | | | | | | Age (years) |
| | 50 | 55 | 60 | 65 | 70 | 75 | 80 | 85 | 90 | |
| 30 | 19.4 | 18.2 | 17.0 | 15.8 | 14.6 | 13.3 | 11.9 | 10.4 | 8.6 | 50 |
| 31 | 20.0 | 18.8 | 17.6 | 16.4 | 15.1 | 13.8 | 12.4 | 10.9 | 9.0 | 51 |
| 32 | 20.5 | 19.3 | 18.1 | 16.9 | 15.7 | 14.4 | 13.0 | 11.4 | 9.5 | 52 |
| 33 | 21.1 | 19.9 | 18.6 | 17.4 | 16.2 | 14.9 | 13.5 | 11.9 | 10.0 | 53 |
| 34 | 21.6 | 20.4 | 19.2 | 18.0 | 16.7 | 15.4 | 14.0 | 12.4 | 10.5 | 54 |

From the A tables from Robinson (1988). Hearing threshold levels (averaged over the 1-, 2- and 3-kHz frequencies across both ears and incorporating expected age-related hearing loss) for an otologically normal population with exposure durations between 30 and 34 years. The 50th to 90th percentile data are shown. (© Crown copyright material is reproduced with the permission of the Controller of HMSO and Queen's Printer for Scotland.)

over a designated level or 'fence'. Tables are provided in relation to a 30 dB and a 50 dB low 'fence'. An example of part of the 30 dB low 'fence' table is shown in Table 10.6.

**Table 10.6** Sample table for 30-dB low 'fence'

| | Noise level (dB (A)) | | | | | | | | | | |
|---|---|---|---|---|---|---|---|---|---|---|---|
| Exposure duration (years) | 83 | 84 | 85 | 86 | 87 | 88 | 89 | 90 | 91 | 92 | Age (years) |
| 31 | 7 | 8 | 10 | 12 | 14 | 16 | 19 | 22 | 24 | 28 | 50 |
| 32 | 8 | 9 | 11 | 13 | 15 | 18 | 20 | 23 | 26 | 29 | 51 |
| 33 | 9 | 10 | 12 | 14 | 16 | 19 | 22 | 25 | 28 | 31 | 52 |
| 34 | 10 | 12 | 13 | 16 | 18 | 21 | 23 | 27 | 30 | 33 | 53 |
| 35 | 11 | 13 | 15 | 17 | 19 | 22 | 25 | 28 | 32 | 35 | 54 |

From the B tables from Robinson (1988). The percentage of a typical unscreened population who will have hearing threshold levels (averaged over the 1-, 2- and 3-kHz frequencies across both ears and incorporating expected age-related hearing loss) exceeding 30 dB HL, for varying levels of noise exposure and duration (© Crown copyright material is reproduced with the permission of the Controller of HMSO and Queen's Printer for Scotland.)

# Susceptibility

It is well recognized that there is significant variability in the hearing loss experienced by groups of workers exposed to similar levels and types of noise. There is a concept that, in respect of NIHL, some people may have a 'tough' or 'vulnerable' auditory system (Chapter 7).

This has led researchers to try to identify intrinsic or extrinsic factors that are associated with an increased or decreased risk of NIHL. A number of potential risk factors have been reported in the literature.

**Potential factors affecting susceptibility to NIHL**

- gender;
- age;
- genetic predisposition;
- pre-existing sensorineural hearing loss;
- susceptibility to temporary threshold shift;
- vascular risk factors (blood pressure, blood lipid levels, smoking, diabetes mellitus);
- degree of pigmentation;
- ototoxic medications;
- exposure to industrial chemicals;
- hand–arm vibration syndrome;
- acoustic reflex and middle-ear status.

## Gender

It is known that male hearing sensitivity declines at more than twice the rate of that in females at most ages and frequencies (Pearson et al., 1995). It is not clear whether this difference is a result of differing risk factor profiles (for example, social noise, high blood pressure) in males and females or whether there is an intrinsic weakness of the male cochlea (Rosenhall, 1995).

Early epidemiological studies suggested a male predisposition to NIHL but these studies were not well controlled for confounding factors (Henderson et al., 1993). There is no clear evidence that male gender is a proven risk factor for NIHL.

## Age

Both extremes of age have been studied as a potential risk factor for NIHL. Henderson et al. (1993) have reviewed the literature on *in utero* and neonatal risk and they discuss animal studies that have demonstrated an increased risk of NIHL at these developmental stages. A further review by Hepper et al. (1994) considers the two human studies that have suggested an increased risk of sensorineural hearing loss in children born to mothers who have worked in noisy environments during their pregnancy. These studies are criticized for poor methodology and the reviewers state that no conclusions can be drawn on the risks of noise to the fetus with the current level of available research. The review authors suggest that the mechanism of any adverse effect of noise on the fetus is likely to be indirect and mediated via direct adverse effects on the mother during pregnancy. They therefore recommend that hearing protection guidelines must be strictly observed in pregnancy.

There is some concern that children may be at an increased risk of NIHL. This concern is particularly relevant given that there is evidence that some children's toys can generate potentially harmful levels of noise (Axelsson et al., 1991; Yaremchuk et al., 1997). Furthermore, some workers have suggested that children may be at risk from noise sources that do not present a risk to adults (Hellstrom et al., 1992). This is because the child's shorter external auditory canal will resonate at higher frequencies compared with the longer adult canal.

Ageing is well known to be associated with sensorineural hearing loss (presbyacusis). Many patients who present with NIHL are older and are likely to have an element of presbyacusis in addition to any NIHL. In humans, attempting to separate the effects of age and noise on hearing has presented one of the most significant challenges in the study and clinical assessment of NIHL. This is partly due to the fact that an ageing population will have many other confounding potential risk factors for hearing loss, such as ototoxic medication use, cardiovascular factors and military noise exposure. A recent well-controlled study estimates that ageing could account for up to 10% of the variability seen in NIHL thresholds (Pyykko, 1998).

Both age and noise affect similar regions of the cochlea and, given that age-related pathological changes are a ubiquitous finding in the older cochlea, some workers have speculated that 'presbyacusis eventually catches up with NIHL' (Rosenhall, 1998).

This concept is further explained by a quotation from Baughn's (1973) epidemiological study of occupational hearing loss:

> In a number of years, however, the noise induced component decreases and is lost and the age component – which has been steadily progressing at an accelerating rate – begins to catch up . . . our figures indicate that if a whole population could be kept alive to age 86 it would make no difference what the (noise) exposure history of the members of that population had been . . .

As described above, resources such as ISO 1999 take age-related hearing loss into account when considering NIHL. In generating an estimate of hearing thresholds, ISO 1999 treats presbyacusis and NIHL as having a simple additive effect on the final threshold value. There are some animal studies that suggest that this additive approach is valid only for long-term exposures and may lead to overestimations of hearing loss with short-term exposures to noise (Mills et al., 1998).

Another question that has been raised in relation to age and NIHL is whether a cochlea with presbyacusis is at increased risk from noise compared with the young, healthy cochlea. Boettcher et al. (1995) have reviewed this subject and note that laboratory data on this subject are minimal. They report animal studies that have shown equal susceptibility and other studies that have suggested that the auditory system in older animals is less at risk from noise. However, mice with a genetic predisposition to age-related hearing loss have been shown to be at increased risk of NIHL with short-term exposure (Davis et al., 2001).

At this stage, one cannot say that there is conclusive evidence that advancing age and presbyacusis are either protective against or risk factors for NIHL. However, a clinician must take into account the expected age-related hearing loss of any patient who presents with possible NIHL.

## Genetic predisposition

Recent years have seen a proliferation of knowledge in regard to the genetics of hearing loss. Currently 35 genes and 75 genetic loci have been implicated in non-syndromal hearing impairment, and many causative genes have been identified in syndromes that are associated with hearing impairment (Van Camp and Smith, 2003). There are no studies that have examined whether humans with a proven genetic risk factor for hearing loss have increased susceptibility to NIHL.

Animal studies have been undertaken to examine this question of genetic susceptibility. Kozel et al. (2002) demonstrated that mice that are heterozygous for a mutation in the *PMCA2* gene have increased susceptibility to NIHL. This gene encodes for a calcium pump located in the plasma membrane of the outer hair cell stereocilia. Mice that are homozygous for this mutation are deaf. This study raises the question of whether humans who are heterozygous for genetic mutations associated with autosomal recessive hearing loss, such as connexin 26 mutations, may be at increased risk of NIHL. Humans with autosomal dominant, progressive hearing losses could also theoretically have an increased susceptibility to NIHL.

As discussed above, a recessive gene in the mouse, associated with age-related hearing loss, has also been shown to be a risk factor for NIHL (Davis, 2001). Furthermore, mice that have been bred to lack a gene that encodes for an antioxidant enzyme have been demonstrated to be more susceptible to damage from short-term loud noise exposure (Ohlemiller et al., 1999).

More work is needed to examine the role of genetic factors in human susceptibility to NIHL but it is likely to be an important issue. It is quite possible that as yet unspecified genetic factors account for much of the variability in hearing loss observed between individuals who have similar noise exposures. Certainly, a clinician must consider genetic risks and obtain a comprehensive family history when assessing a patient who presents with possible NIHL.

## Pre-existing sensorineural hearing loss

When assessing a patient who presents with possible NIHL, the clinician must look for evidence of any pre-existing sensorineural hearing impairment, as this will have an impact on the patient's audiometric status.

Many patients will have additional presbyacusis and the clinician should have access to data that provide an estimation of the expected age-related hearing loss for the populations whom they are treating (for example, ISO 1984). In addition, patients who have been exposed to noise are no more or less likely to have any of the other causes of sensorineural hearing impairment listed in Table 10.1.

The effect of pre-existing sensorineural hearing loss on susceptibility to NIHL is not well understood. A clinical concern is that the previously damaged cochlea may be more vulnerable to the pathological effects of noise. However, it has been argued that, if a patient's cochlea has pre-existing basal pathology (for instance, as a result of presbyacusis), there is less potentially damageable tissue. Ward (1995) in his review on susceptibility discusses the theory that 'the less there is to lose, the less will be lost' and backs this up by pointing out that the hearing loss progression in long-term noise exposure is not linear and tends to diminish with time. He goes on to discuss animal studies that support this theory but also emphasizes that, if the noise stimulus affects a previously undamaged part of the cochlea, any pre-existing pathology does not influence the current risk.

### Susceptibility to temporary threshold shift

As with PTSs, there is much variation between individuals in TTS response to noise exposure. Therefore, an obvious clinical question arises as to whether individuals' susceptibility to permanent noise damage can be predicted by their susceptibility to TTSs. The various work undertaken to answer this question has been reviewed by Quaranta et al. (1998) and they conclude that: 'A global evaluation of the literature does not consider temporary threshold shift as an effective test for permanent threshold prediction.'

### Vascular risk factors

There is an increasing body of evidence to suggest that risk factors for atheromatous disease may also be risk factors for NIHL. Exposure to loud noise has been demonstrated to cause reduced cochlear blood flow (Attanasio et al., 2001). It is therefore reasonable to assume that a cochlea with an atheromatous vasculature will be more vulnerable to ischaemic damage as a result of a noise-mediated reduction in blood flow. Established atheromatous disease has been indirectly associated with sensorineural hearing loss by Susmano and Rosenbush (1988). This study examined the prevalence of sensorineural hearing loss in patients with proven ischaemic heart disease compared with patients with organic heart disease but normal coronary arteries. It was demonstrated that hearing impairment was approximately three times more common in those patients with ischaemic heart disease.

Cigarette smoking has been implicated as an independent risk factor for hearing loss. Cruickshanks et al. (1999) found that smokers were 1.69 times more likely to have a significant hearing impairment than non-smokers. Smokers' averaged high frequency thresholds have been found to be approximately 7 dB HL higher than non-smokers (Cocchiarella et al., 1995). A number of studies have examined whether smokers are more at risk of NIHL but the results have been variable and, at this stage, one cannot say that there is conclusive evidence that smokers are at an increased risk (Barone et al., 1987; Henderson et al., 1993; Virokannas and Anttonen, 1995; Ward, 1995; Starck et al., 1999).

It has frequently been reported that there is a correlation between raised blood pressure and hearing loss in workers who have been exposed to chronic noise (Talbott et al., 1985; Milkovi-Kraus, 1990; Sokas et al., 1995). However, there is debate as to whether the raised blood pressure increases noise susceptibility. It may be that the two conditions have unrelated pathological mechanisms and that they are both separate consequences of long-term noise exposure. One study of noise-exposed workers found that there was some relationship between hypertension and hearing loss, but only in older workers with severe losses (Talbott et al., 1990). Tarter and Robins (1990) found a relationship between blood pressure and high-frequency hearing loss in black workers, but no evidence of this relationship for white workers in the same occupational environment.

Other studies have suggested that raised low-density lipoprotein (LDL) cholesterol blood levels and type 2 diabetes mellitus are risk factors for NIHL (Axelsson and Lindgren, 1985; Ishii et al., 1992). In contrast, a recent, large ($n = 1490$), retrospective study found that raised cholesterol levels were associated with significantly better hearing (Jones and Davis, 2000).

When considered *in toto*, the evidence on atheromatous risk factors and hearing loss suggests that there is some relationship. However, these risk factors have not been proved to increase the risk of NIHL and, if present, the effects on hearing are likely to be minimal. A clinician should bear in mind the possibility that a patient with significant atheromatous risk factors may be at increased risk of sensorineural hearing impairment.

### Degree of pigmentation

Melanin-containing cells are found in the stria vascularis and many other areas of the auditory apparatus and they appear to have an influence on susceptibility to NIHL, although the mechanism is unclear. There is good evidence from the study of mouse models of the human Waardenburg's syndrome that the strial melanocytes are involved in generating the endo-cochlear potential (Holme and Steel, 1999).

People with blue eyes have been shown to have an increased suscepti-bility to a temporary threshold shift when compared with people with brown eyes (Barrenas and Lindgren, 1991). Furthermore, there is a good body of epidemiological evidence to suggest that white workers are more susceptible to occupational NIHL than black workers (Barrenas, 1998), and that this can lead to significant differences in the averaged thresholds, particularly in the higher frequencies (Figure 10.9). A recent study found that the average hearing thresholds (averaged across the 1-, 2-, 3-, and 5-kHz bands) for black workers in a metal fabricating plant was 18 dB HL compared with 26 dB HL for white workers at the same plant (Ishii and Talbott, 1998).

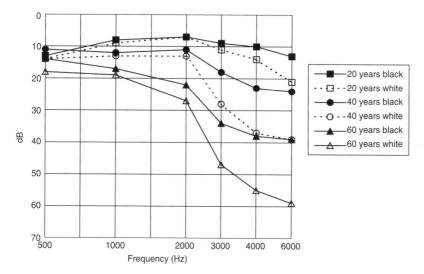

**Figure 10.9** Mean hearing thresholds in white and black male workers in North Carolina industry, aged 20, 40 and 60 years. (From Royster et al., 1980; reproduced with kind permission.)

## Ototoxic medications

There are five main classes of drug that are known to be ototoxic: amino-glycoside antibiotics, platinum-containing chemotherapy, loop diuretics, salicylates and quinine-based drugs.

A number of animal studies have shown that both aminoglycoside antibiotics and platinum-containing chemotherapy drugs can potentiate the effects of noise on hearing (Henderson et al., 1993). A recent study has found that hearing recovery from noise exposure may be impaired by levels of aminoglycoside antibiotics that are below the levels known to cause permanent cochlear damage (Tan et al., 2001).

The numerous studies on the combined effects of aspirin and noise have produced conflicting results (McFadden et al., 1984; Lambert et al., 1986; Bancroft et al., 1991; Henderson et al., 1993). There is no conclusive evidence of a clinically significant synergistic effect of aspirin and chronic noise exposure in humans. This is certainly an area that requires further study given that many people with long-term noise exposure will be prescribed regular aspirin because of the drug's preventive role in cardiovascular disease.

There are no data to provide comprehensive information on the combined effects of noise and loop diuretics or quinine-based drugs on hearing.

With the exception of aspirin and loop diuretics, it is unlikely that people with long-term noise exposure will be prescribed regular ototoxic medications. However, clinicians must obtain a full drug history from their patients. Patients must be directly questioned on whether they have ever been prescribed ototoxic medications, particularly during periods of noise exposure.

## Industrial chemicals

There is a significant body of evidence from animal and human studies to suggest that exposure to organic solvents can cause sensorineural hearing impairments (Chapter 21). Furthermore, there appears to be a synergistic effect of organic solvent exposure and noise exposure increasing the risk of a worker having a hearing loss (Johnson and Nylen, 1995; Frenkel, 1998; Morata, 1998). The organic solvents that are implicated in hearing impairment are toluene, styrene and xylene. There is also evidence of hearing loss with combined exposure to noise and carbon disulphide (Morata, 1989).

The clinician must therefore enquire about the possibility of exposure to industrial chemicals at any stage during the patient's working lifetime.

## Hand–arm vibration syndrome

Hand–arm vibration syndrome (HAVS) (previously known as vibration white finger syndrome) is a common occupational disease which occurs in workers who regularly use vibrating tools. It is characterized by episodic blanching of the fingers, particularly when the patient is in the cold. The condition is the most common occupational disease assessed by the UK Department of Social Services and it is estimated that over 1 million UK workers are at risk of developing HAVS (Shelmerdine, 1999).

A number of studies have found that workers with HAVS have greater susceptibility to NIHL (Pekkarinen, 1995). The thresholds in these workers have been observed to be approximately 10 dB worse than workers without HAVS who have had similar noise exposure. The mechanism underlying HAVS and the association with hearing loss is not known, but it has been proposed that the common factor is vasoconstriction and this may reflect underlying autonomic nervous system dysfunction. A recent epidemiological study has suggested that patients who report finger blanching have worse hearing than those without this symptom, irrespective of a history of noise exposure (Palmer et al., 2002).

**Acoustic reflex and middle-ear factors**

Evidence exists that the stapedial reflex is at least partially protective against temporary and permanent noise-induced threshold shifts (Dobie, 2001). Furthermore, it is logical to assume that a person with a significant pre-existing conductive hearing loss (an air-bone gap of greater than 30 dB HL) will have a degree of 'built-in' hearing protection. However, patients presenting with NIHL and known long-term loss of stapedial reflex (not due to significant hearing loss) or chronic conductive losses are rare and therefore middle-ear factors are of limited practical diagnostic significance. Obviously, concomitant middle-ear disease at the time of presentation will probably influence the picture of hearing loss.

# History

Noise-induced hearing loss is a medical problem and, therefore, as with the majority of other medical problems, accurate history taking remains one of the most sensitive diagnostic tools. A full medical and audiological history should be elicited, with attention paid to particular points that are relevant to noise exposure and sensorineural hearing loss. An outline of this history is provided below.

*History of hearing loss*

* Onset, duration, symmetry, functional impairment, disability and handicap.
* Associated tinnitus.
* Any associated otalgia, otorrhoea, vertigo.
* Medicolegal setting (compensation issues).

*Occupational history*

* Where the patient has worked.
* Details of any sources of noise (type of machinery).
* Details of nature of noise (level, frequency, duration, continuous or interrupted, impulsive).
* Availability of objective measures of noise in the workplace.
* Position of patient in relation to noise source.
* Use of hearing protection measures.
* Presence of industrial chemicals and solvents.
* Prevalence of hearing impairment in co-workers.

*Military history*

* Exposure to firearms and explosions.

*Social history*

* Social noise exposure (music concerts, music clubs, shooting sports).
* Tobacco and alcohol consumption.

A full past medical history must be obtained – points of particular relevance include:

- medical history of the patient's mother's pregnancy (infection);
- neonatal and childhood health (prematurity, low birthweight, jaundice, hypoxia, infections);
- full ear, nose and throat history;
- head injury;
- history of serious infection (meningitis, malaria, TB);
- history of vascular disease.

*Family history*

- History of any hearing or balance disorders in the family.
- Any known or suspected inherited conditions in the family.

*Drug history*

- Current or previous ototoxic medication use (aminoglycosides, salicylates, loop diuretics, chemotherapy).

The symptoms of NIHL are not significantly different from those of other causes of sensorineural hearing loss and the UK Industrial Injuries Advisory Council have stated that 'there are no signs or symptoms that are specific to noise induced deafness' (Industrial Injuries Advisory Council or IIAC, 1973).

The symptoms reported by the patient will typically be those of a gradual, onset-bilateral, progressive, sensorineural hearing loss. Deviation in symptoms from this pattern should raise a clinical suspicion of alternative or concomitant pathology (Sataloff and Sataloff, 2001).

There should be an obvious history of long-term noise exposure and, with the exception of acute acoustic trauma, the hearing loss should be gradually progressive. The onset of permanent symptoms is typically first noticed many years after noise exposure has commenced. The hearing loss is generally symmetrical and the severity ranges from mild to severe. A history suggestive of a markedly asymmetrical or profound loss is the exception.

Hétu et al. (1988) specifically questioned a group of 61 workers with NIHL and their spouses about the type of problems caused by their hearing loss. The reported disabilities are summarized in Table 10.7. This work highlights the fact that the clinician must assess the disabilities and handicaps that can arise as a result of any hearing impairment.

The clinician must also be aware that workers with NIHL will commonly have a reluctance to acknowledge their hearing problems (Hétu et al., 1990). This is mainly due to a fear of being stigmatized as a person who is 'deaf'. Many workers will deny that they have symptoms of hearing impairment and will minimize any symptoms to which they admit. In this situation, obtaining a history from a spouse or relative will often be very helpful. The effects of a worker's NIHL on the spouse and family are well documented (Hétu et al., 1987; Hallberg and Barrenas, 1993; Hétu et al., 1993). Table 10.8 details some of the problems reported by the spouses of workers with NIHL.

**Table 10.7** Categorization of permanent hearing disabilities associated with occupational hearing loss

## Listening problems

Environmental awareness
  Monitoring warning sounds:
  • The hearing-impaired person (HIP) does not always hear the doorbell or the telephone ringing
  • The HIP does not hear the telephone ringing in another room
  Being aware of sounds that are familiar:
  • The HIP cannot hear the birds singing

## Listening to speech

  During social or cultural activities:
  • The HIP does not hear as well if there is background noise
  • The HIP is unable to hear certain speech sounds
  • The HIP does not always understand when first spoken to
  • The HIP experiences listening problems in large rooms or halls:
    – evening courses
    – cinemas
    – church

  Television viewing:
  • The HIP is unable to hear the television at a normal volume if others are around talking
  • The HIP turns up the television loud
  • The HIP is unable to hear the television at normal volume

  Listening to car radio:
  • The HIP plays the radio loud
  • The HIP is unable to hear the radio at normal volume

## Verbal communication problems

During social or cultural activities:
  Communication problems in non-ideal situations:
  • At parties
  • In groups
  • In bars
  • In the car
  • In the car with the radio on
  • With someone in a another room
  • In meetings
  • With background noise
  • With the noise of television

  On the telephone:
  • Problems in communicating
  • Problems in communicating if there is background noise

From Hétu et al. (1988), reproduced with kind permission.

**Table 10.8** Repetoire of handicaps reported by the wives of male workers affected by occupational hearing loss

**Effort/irritation**
Having to repeat herself often
Having to act as an interpreter for her husband with others
Having to tolerate the loud sound of the television
Having to limit children's activities to prevent annoying noise for her husband
Having always to answer the telephone

**Stress and anxiety**
Not being able to rely on her husband any more in dangerous situations
Traumatizing experiences due to the impossibility of communication

**Restriction of social life as a couple**
Being isolated as a couple at parties
Always having to leave groups early when going out as a couple
Being deprived of opportunities to go out

**Negative self-image as a spouse**
Ill at ease in public because of her husband's loud voice
Feeling the weight of her husband's stigma

**Negative impact of the hearing loss on the family life**
The hearing disability

- Limits companionship
- Limits intimate communication
- Blocks communication
- Creates tension in the couple
- Makes the children feel uneasy

Sorrow, disappointment because of being isolated in the family

From Hétu et al. (1993), reproduced with kind permission.

It must also be remembered that some workers seeking compensation claims for NIHL may deliberately exaggerate the severity of their symptoms in order to attempt to further their claim (see 'diagnostic difficulties').

Tinnitus is often reported as a symptom in the history of the noise-exposed individual. In a study of 90 patients with clinically significant tinnitus, 40 (46%) were considered to have noise exposure as the causative factor (Penner, 1990). Analysis of the UK National Study of Hearing data demonstrated that a positive history of occupational noise exposure led to an increased risk of 70% of reporting tinnitus (Coles and Mason, 1984).

In a large study ($n = 110\ 647$) of noise-exposed (but not necessarily compensation-seeking) workers in Austria, 6.7% of the study population complained of tinnitus on direct questioning compared with a prevalence of 0.8% in the general Austrian population (Neuberger et al., 1992). In this study the median daily averaged sound pressure level was 90.5 dB (A) and

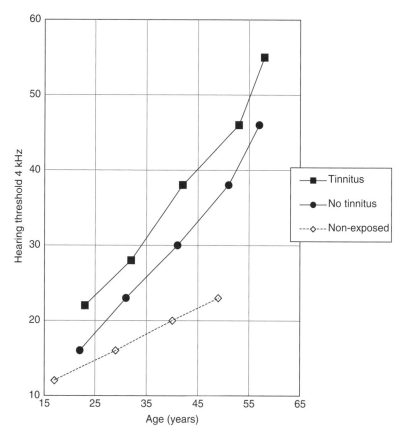

**Figure 10.10** Hearing thresholds at 4 kHz for male noise-exposed workers, as a function of age. Data separated for workers complaining of tinnitus, workers who do not complain of tinnitus and a non-noise-exposed control group not complaining of tinnitus. (From Neuberger et al. (1992), reproduced with kind permission.)

the median exposure time was 12.1 years. A similar prevalence was found in a large study of Canadian noise-exposed workers (Chung et al., 1984).

In workers claiming compensation for NIHL, the prevalence of tinnitus has been reported as being between 50% and 64% (Alberti, 1987b; McShane et al., 1988; Daniell et al., 1998). Tinnitus is also experienced by the majority of patients who have suffered acute acoustic trauma (Mrena et al., 2002).

As with other causes of sensorineural hearing loss, there is evidence that the presence of tinnitus has a correlation with the severity of the hearing loss (Phoon et al., 1993).

It has also been suggested that the presence of tinnitus in noise-exposed workers may be predictive of greater future threshold shifts with continuing exposure (Griest and Bishop, 1998). This theory requires further study but if proven has implications for both diagnosing and screening for NIHL.

# Clinical examination

The clinician must undertake a comprehensive otological examination including otoscopy. With the exception of acoustic trauma, there are no signs of NIHL but examination may identify outer- and middle-ear disease that may have an impact on the patient's symptoms and tests of hearing.

# Investigations

### Pure-tone audiometry

Pure-tone audiometry is the most important and widely used test when diagnosing hearing loss in adults. There is a large body of published work on the PTA results of people exposed to pathological noise and this provides a good evidence base for the diagnosing clinician.

It is vital that this test be performed under the correct conditions. The test should be administered by suitably trained professionals using reliable and well-maintained equipment. The testing should be carried out in line with published standards (British Society of Audiology or BSA, 1981, 1985, 1986). Although NIHL is a sensorineural loss, bone-conduction thresholds should be obtained to rule out a conductive contribution to any detected hearing loss. Testing should be performed after the patient has been away from loud noise for at least 24 hours to rule out any TTS contribution to the test results (Arslan and Orzan, 1998).

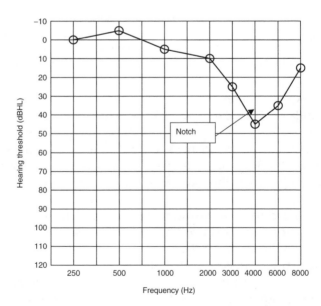

**Figure 10.11** A high-frequency notch in the audiogram, typical of noise-induced hearing loss. (From Coles et al. (2000), reproduced with kind permission.)

The characteristic audiometric pattern of chronic noise exposure is a high-frequency notch centred around the 4-kHz frequency. It is likely that the loss can in fact begin at any point between 3 and 6 kHz, but 6-kHz losses must be viewed with caution given that there are a number of recognized causes of an artefactual loss at this frequency (see 'Diagnostic difficulties').

Coles and his co-workers (2000) have utilized their extensive collective experience in assessing noise-exposed patients to provide guidelines on the diagnosis of NIHL. Their paper includes practically useful definitions of the PTA findings in NIHL. They define the high-frequency notch as 'where the hearing threshold level at 3 and/or 4 and/or 6 kHz, after due correction for headphone type, is at least 10 dB greater than at 1 or 2 kHz and at 6 or 8 kHz'. The reference to correction for headphone type is in relation to a particular audiometric calibration artefact at 6 kHz that can occur when TDH-39 headphones are used for testing. This point is discussed in detail under 'Diagnostic difficulties'.

With continuing exposure the loss progresses at the starting frequency and spreads to involve neighbouring frequencies. This can lead to flattening out of the notch that may be then visible only as a high-frequency bulge. Coles et al. define the high frequency bulge as being present 'if the hearing threshold levels at 3 and/or 4 and/or 6 kHz, after any due correction for earphone type, is at least 10 dB greater relative to the comparison

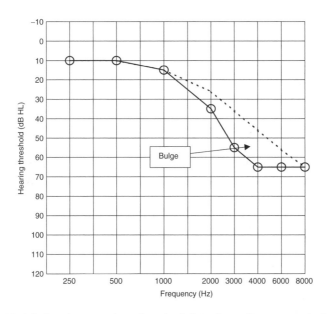

**Figure 10.12** A bulge downwards and to the left in the audiogram, typical of noise-induced hearing loss plus presumed age-associated hearing loss. Dashed line indicates mean age-induced hearing loss for men aged 70. (From Coles et al. (2000), reproduced with kind permission.)

values for age related hearing loss'. Their paper cites ISO 7029 (ISO, 1984) as the reference values for age-related hearing loss, but it is important for the clinician to be aware that the ISO generated these reference values from studies of populations carefully screened to rule out causes of hearing loss other than age. The clinician may wish to utilize less highly screened reference data that may be more relevant to the population from which their patient originates.

The position statement of the American College of Occupational Medicine (ACOM) defines features of occupational NIHL (ACOM, 1989).

### Key points relevant to the PTA in NIHL

1. The loss is almost always bilateral. Audiometric patterns are usually similar bilaterally.
2. It almost never produces a profound hearing loss. Usually, low-frequency limits are about 40 dB and high-frequency limits about 75 dB.
3. The earliest damage to the inner ears reflects a loss at 3000, 4000 and 6000 Hz. There is always far more loss at 3000, 4000 and 6000 Hz than at 500, 1000, and 2000 Hz. The greatest loss usually occurs at 4000 Hz. The higher and lower frequencies take longer to be affected than the 3000- to 6000-Hz range.
4. Given stable exposure conditions, losses at 3000, 4000 and 6000 Hz will usually reach a maximal level in about 10–15 years.

It is important for the diagnosing clinician to appreciate that NIHL is generally a symmetrical loss. Some minimal asymmetry (i.e. <10 dB HL between left and right thresholds at the same frequency) is often found and can be accepted as being within allowable limits. Studies of normal populations have demonstrated a general finding of slight left-ear inferiority on tests of hearing (Pirila et al., 1992). However, this inferiority is slight and is of a measure of up to 4 dB HL only.

Job et al. (1998) examined the effects of predominantly unilateral chronic noise exposure by testing the hearing of French army shooters. In the French army, eye preference (as opposed to hand preference) determines the side of the body that the weapon is fired from. Therefore, their sample of 644 soldiers included many left-eyed and right-eyed shooters. They found that the majority of soldiers demonstrated greater NIHL in the left ear, irrespective of the side of shooting. This study supports the general notion that any protective effect of the 'head shadow' is minimal with respect to loud noise.

It is recommended that patients with noise-exposure who demonstrate an asymmetry of thresholds greater than 10 dB at any frequency should be investigated to exclude retrocochlear pathology and other causes of hearing loss (Cox and Ford, 1995).

Obviously, the clinical picture as a whole must be taken into account, and other patients will be similarly investigated for clinical suspicion of retrocochlear pathology that arises separate to the pure tone audiogram.

## Acoustic impedance measures

Tympanometry and stapedial reflex threshold measurements should be recorded in all patients. Tympanometry will help to exclude or diagnose middle-ear disorders. Stapedial reflex threshold measurements provide objective information that will help to confirm the subjective hearing tests and aid the differentiation between cochlear and retrocochlear pathology. These tests will also help in the identification of disorders that predominantly affect the middle ear, but are also known to affect the cochlear in some cases (e.g. otosclerosis, chronic suppurative otitis media, trauma).

## Otoacoustic emissions

Chronic noise exposure causes a sensorineural hearing loss due to cochlear pathology that includes damage to the outer hair cells. The outer hair cell dysfunction can be objectively analysed by recording otoacoustic emissions.

It is known that click-evoked or transient evoked otoacoustic emissions (TEOAEs) are stable and repeatable over time for any individual and therefore they have been suggested as a suitable screening test for people at risk for cochlear pathology, such as those exposed to noise (Hall and Lutman, 1999). Furthermore, there is evidence that TEOAEs are more sensitive to early noise-induced cochlear damage than the pure-tone audiogram and therefore abnormalities may be predictive of future threshold changes with continued noise exposure (Xu et al., 1998). TEOAEs are sensitive enough to detect a 5-dB threshold shift in comparison to standard audiometric techniques that tend to detect threshold shifts of only 10 dB or greater (Lutman and Hall, 2000). Frequency-specific analysis of TEOAE in NIHL has shown poor correlation with behavioural tests and therefore the test cannot be reliably used to delineate the pattern of hearing loss (Tognola et al., 1999). No large-scale prospective trials using TEOAEs as a screening test for NIHL have been undertaken and therefore there is no conclusive evidence base to advocate such use for this test.

Distortion product otoacoustic emissions (DPOAEs) have similarly been found to be predictive of noise-induced hearing threshold change in some patients (Kowalska and Sulkowski, 1998). However, there is significant variability in the levels of DPOAEs, as exemplified by some patients with severe loss on pure-tone audiograms demonstrating normal DPOAEs. The test cannot be advocated as suitable for screening for NIHL (Attias et al., 1998). It is accepted that, unlike TEOAEs, DPOAEs do provide frequency-specific information in regard to hearing loss. This has been shown to be the case in NIHL (Oeken, 1999). However, the DPOAE results have not been proved reliable enough to be considered as the ideal objective audiogram and cannot replace the pure-tone audiogram/evoked response audiometry combination as the most accurate and objective technique to assess NIHL.

There is certainly a role for TEOAEs as a quick and easy objective method of confirming that the degree of hearing loss is genuine. Pure-tone audiogram thresholds greater that 40 dB HL due to outer hair cell dysfunction (as in NIHL) will result in significantly reduced TEOAEs at the corresponding frequencies. If the TEOAEs are within normal range, a high clinical suspicion of psychological overlay is raised and this can be investigated further.

### Cortical evoked response audiometry

Due to the relatively high incidence of deliberately exaggerated hearing thresholds in patients being assessed for NIHL, some objective measure of hearing thresholds should be undertaken. Otoacoustic emissions are useful but do not provide reliable frequency-specific information. Cortical evoked response audiometry has been proved a useful objective neurophysiological technique to assess hearing thresholds reliably (Prasher et al., 1993) and it has been proposed as the definitive test of auditory function in the face of subjective audiometric variability (King et al., 1992). A large study examining PTA and cortical evoked response audiometry in NIHL found a close correlation between the two tests with only 4.4% of individual ear tests showing an averaged frequency discrepancy exceeding 7.5 dB (Coles and Mason, 1984).

# Diagnostic difficulties

### PTA calibration/standardization

Clinicians must be aware of the limitations of PTA. In the UK, pure-tone audiometers are calibrated according to international standards under the guidance of the NPL. The NPL website provides an up-to-date summary of the international standards relevant to audiometric testing and calibration (NPL, 2003b). The 0 dB HL SPL for each frequency was designated as the modal value of the minimal audible threshold for pure tones in a healthy young population who were highly screened to exclude any auditory pathology. Thus if a patient has a PTA threshold at 0 dB HL at any frequency, this should be considered as 'perfect' hearing and thresholds equal to or less than 20 dB HL are generally accepted clinically as being within normal limits. Furthermore, the current standard accepts some deviation in the zero reference for individual audiometers. Deviations of ± 3 dB are accepted over the frequency range of 250–4 kHz and deviations of ± 5 dB are allowed for the remaining frequencies.

It is accepted that, even with trained personnel, there are often appreciable differences in PTA results when different audiologists test an individual. These variations can arise from differing technique between the testers or from changes in the individual's subjective response to the test, despite stable audiological function. These factors can lead to threshold variations in the range 6–11 dB (Fearn and Harrison, 1983).

Patients with noise exposure who have mild losses or minimal variations in their PTA results must be assessed bearing in mind the above factors.

## The 4-kHz notches

The 4-kHz notch is the characteristic PTA finding in NIHL. However, there are many patients with a 4-kHz notch who have not had significant noise exposure and some patients with NIHL who do not demonstrate the 4-kHz notch on their audiograms (McBride and Williams, 2001).

Many patients with a 4-kHz notch and no history of significant noise exposure have a history of hearing problems in the family (Murai, 1997; Berlin et al., 1999). Klockhoff and Lyttkens (1982) found that 76% of children with 4-kHz notches and no noise exposure had a family history of hearing loss. Genetic factors are therefore important but it is not known whether the notch arises as a result of directly genetically mediated cochlear pathology or indirectly via an increased genetic predisposition to NIHL.

Other documented causes of a 4-kHz notch include barotrauma (Molvaer and Natrud, 1979), closed head injury (Bergemalm and Borg, 2001) and labyrinthitis (Luxon, 1998). In addition, there are a number of patients with unexplained 4-kHz notches.

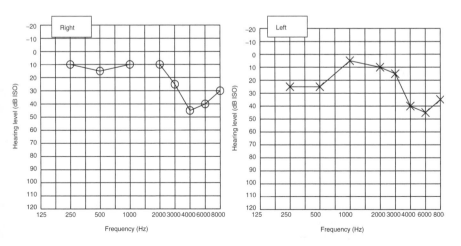

**Figure 10.13** Pure-tone audiogram of a 57-year-old man with a single acute episode of labyrinthitis with no history of hearing problems. (From Luxon (1998), reproduced with kind permission.)

There are no known audiometric characteristics of the NIHL-related 4-kHz notch that enable it to be distinguished from other causes of the 4-kHz notch (Murai, 1997). The clinician must interpret the 4-kHz notch in relation to the full clinical picture as obtained on history and examination.

## The 6-kHz notches

Audiometric notches at 6 kHz are often ascribed to noise exposure but caution must be observed as the 6-kHz notch is a frequent finding in general populations. Indeed, the UK National Study of Hearing found that a 6-kHz notch is characteristic of the UK population (Davis, 1995). Axelsson et al. (1994) tested the hearing of 500 randomly selected 18-year-old male military conscripts and observed that a 6-kHz notch was a common finding.

There has been debate as to whether this notch reflects true pathology or a recording/calibration error. Some have argued that the notch may reflect a history childhood noise exposure or social noise exposures that have not been picked up on the retrospective questioning that is often employed by large-scale epidemiological studies of hearing. The NPL has concluded that the ISO's level for audiometric zero at 6 kHz (ISO, 1998) is set too low (Robinson et al., 1981). Analysis of the National Study of Hearing data indicates that this error amounts to 9 dB (Lutman and Davis, 1994).

A recent study has found that a calibration factor can lead to an artifactual 6-kHz notch in patients tested with TDH-39 headphones (Lutman and Quasar, 1998). The notch is observed only if the headphone/audiometer equipment is calibrated using the IEC 303 coupler. The same patients demonstrate normal PTA results if the equipment is calibrated using the IEC 318 coupler.

Other causes of a 6-kHz notch include ear canal collapse, cerumen impaction, head injury and acute acoustic trauma (Stephens, 1981; O'Mahoney and Luxon, 1996). The clinician must be aware that there are many proposed reasons, other than noise, to account for the high prevalence of 6-kHz notches.

## Additional auditory pathology

Many patients with NIHL will also have additional medical problems that can affect the outer, middle and inner ears with consequent effects on the hearing tests. The clinical problem of additional pathology in NIHL was emphasized by Alberti (1987a):

> The most widespread error and one that is frequently made by those dealing with occupational noise induced hearing loss in an epidemiological context is to suggest that because hearing loss is present and there has been adequate noise exposure that [sic] the two are causally related. To believe this is to believe that working in noise protects the ear from all other forms of disease which cause hearing loss.

In particular a degree of age-related hearing loss is likely to be a factor in older patients presenting with NIHL. As mentioned earlier, this age effect has been taken into account in the different published guides that can be used to work out predicted NIHL for populations. Separate to these, many studies have been published that provide data on the expected hearing loss caused by age alone, including the UK National Study of Hearing (Davis, 1995) and the ISO document 7029 (ISO, 1984). If possible, the clinician should have access to normative age-related hearing loss data for the population from which his patient comes. The expected age-related loss can then be compared with the patient's audiometric status to help differentiate those losses that may be attributable to noise.

Age-related hearing loss data are generally presented in percentiles at certain frequencies. For example, using the age-associated hearing loss data tables presented in the paper by Coles et al. (2000), the predicted hearing threshold level for 70-year-old men at 4 kHz is 33 dB for the 75th percentile, 49 dB for the 50th percentile and 70 dB for the 25th percentile. The clinician can compare his patient's thresholds at each frequency with these expected population thresholds. If the patient's threshold at 4 kHz is in a significantly lower percentile than at other frequencies, NIHL is potentially implicated.

Other potentially confounding causes of outer-, middle- and inner-ear pathology are best detected by comprehensive history taking, examination and investigation of any patient presenting with possible NIHL.

**Exaggerated hearing loss**

Unfortunately, as with any medical problem with compensation issues, the deliberate exaggeration of symptoms is a common problem in patients presenting with possible NIHL. In an Australian study of 333 workers claiming compensation for NIHL, objective testing identified that 17.7% of claimants had exaggerated their hearing loss (Richards and De Vida, 1995). An American study of 246 claimants for NIHL reported that 9% of the claimants were proven to be malingering (Bars et al., 1994).

The prevalence of deliberately exaggerated hearing loss is certainly high enough to recommend that all patients who present with possible NIHL should be assessed to rule out deliberate exaggeration of symptoms.

Accurate history taking and audiological testing by experienced clinicians will often raise the suspicion of malingering. However, objective confirmation of the subjective hearing tests (PTA) is mandatory. Simple measures to identify major discrepancies include stapedial reflex measurements and TEOAEs. Cortical electric response audiometry remains the most accurate and reliable objective test of hearing thresholds in adults and therefore should be performed on all patients presenting with NIHL with compensation issues (Figure 10.14).

A diagnosis of malingering is an extremely sensitive and difficult diagnosis, which should be made only by an experienced clinician, and only after comprehensive audiological assessment.

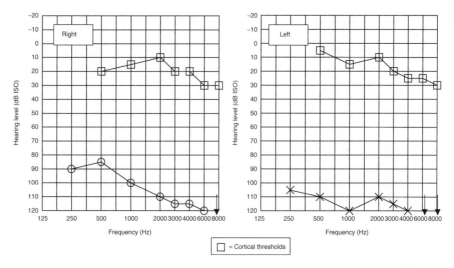

**Figure 10.14** A 59-year-old man with a 3-year history of hearing impairment and tinnitus and a 27-year history of exposure to noise in workshops at British Rail. (From Luxon (1998), reproduced with kind permission.)

The clinician must also be aware that some patients may unintentionally exaggerate their hearing loss. Factors such as patient anxiety, poor understanding of instructions (for example, because of language difficulties) and concurrent illness can lead to unintentional exaggeration of hearing thresholds on pure-tone audiogram testing.

## Conclusion

Noise-induced hearing loss is a common problem but it can be a difficult diagnosis to make. Furthermore there are often significant compensation issues that are dependent on the clinician's opinion as to whether noise is implicated in the causality of a person's hearing loss. There are no simple diagnostic tests for NIHL. The diagnosis is best achieved by:

- Assessment by suitably trained clinicians who possess evidence-based knowledge on the subject of NIHL.
- Comprehensive history taking which must include points relevant to noise exposure and sensorineural hearing loss.
- Careful examination of the patient.
- Appropriate subjective and objective testing of the patient's hearing. A typical battery of tests would include: PTA, tympanometry, stapedial reflex measurement, TEOAEs and cortical evoked response audiometry. The clinician must be fully aware of the strengths and limitations of particular audiological tests.
- Comparison of the patient's audiometric status with published evidence-based data on the degree of expected NIHL with varying noise exposures.

Despite these measures, there are many situations when it is difficult to achieve diagnostic certainty. The UK legal requirement in defining likelihood is that the cause should be 'more probable than not' (Coles et al., 2000) and even this is often a difficult diagnostic level to achieve.

# References

Alberti PW (1987a) Noise and the ear. In SDG Stephens (ed.) Scott-Brown's Otolaryngology – Adult Audiology, 5th edn. London: Butterworth-Heinemann.

Alberti PW (1987b) Tinnitus in occupational hearing loss: nosological aspects. Journal of Otolaryngology 16: 34–5.

Alberti PW (1998) Traumatic sensorineural hearing loss. In H Ludman, T Wright (eds) Diseases of the Ear, 6th edn. London: Arnold, pp. 483–94.

American College of Occupational Medicine (1989) Noise and Hearing Conservation Committee. Committee Report. Journal of Occupation Medicine 31: 996.

American National Standards Institute (1996) American national standard determination of occupational noise exposure and estimation of noise-induced hearing impairment. S3.44-1996. New York: ANSI.

Arslan E, Orzan E (1988) Audiological management of noise induced hearing loss. Scandinavian Audiology Supplementum 48: 131–45.

Attanasio G, Quaranta N, Sallustio V (1998) Development of resistance to noise. Scandinavian Audiology Supplementum 48: 45–52.

Attanasio G, Buongiorno G, Piccoli F, Mafera B, Cordier A, Barbara M et al. (2001) Laser Doppler measurement of cochlear blood flow changes during conditioning noise exposure. Acta Oto-Laryngologica 121: 465–9.

Attias J, Bresloff I, Reshef I, Horowitz G, Furman V (1998) Evaluating noise induced hearing loss with distortion product otoacoustic emissions. British Journal of Audiology 32: 39–46.

Axelsson A, Lindgren F (1985) Is there a relationship between hypercholesterolaemia and noise-induced hearing loss? Acta Oto-Laryngologica 100: 379–86.

Axelsson A, Hellstrom PA, Altschuler R, Miller JM (1991) Inner ear damage from toy cap pistols and fire-crackers. International Journal of Pediatric Otolaryngology 21: 143–8.

Axelsson A, Rosenhall U, Zachau G (1994) Hearing in 18-year-old Swedish males. Scandinavian Audiology 23: 129–34.

Bancroft BR, Boettcher FA, Salvi RJ, Wu J (1991) Effects of noise and salicylates on auditory evoked-response thresholds in the chinchilla. Hearing Research 54(1): 20–8.

Barone JA, Peters JM, Garabrant DH, Bernstein L, Krebsbach R (1987) Smoking as a risk factor in noise-induced hearing loss. Journal of Occupational Medicine 29(9): 741–5.

Barrenas ML (1998) Pigmentation and noise-induced hearing loss: is the relationship between pigmentation and noise-induced hearing loss due to an ototoxic pheomelanin interaction or to otoprotective eumelanin effects? In L Luxon, D Prasher (eds) Advances in Noise Research, Volume 1: Biological Effects of Noise. London: Whurr, pp. 59–70.

Barrenas ML, Lindgren F (1991) The influence of eye colour on susceptibility to temporary threshold shift in humans. British Journal of Audiology 25: 303–7.

Barrs DM, Althoff LK, Krueger WW, Olsson JE (1994) Work-related, noise-induced hearing loss: evaluation including evoked potential audiometry. Otolaryngology – Head and Neck Surgery 110: 177–84.

Baughn WL (1973) Relation between daily noise exposure and hearing loss as based on the evaluation of 6835 industrial noise exposure cases. AMRL-TR-73-53(AF 767 204): Aerospace Medical Research Laboratory, Wright-Patterson Airforce Base, OH.

Bergemalm PO, Borg E (2001) Long-term objective and subjective audiological consequences of closed head injury. Acta Oto-Laryngologica 121: 724–34.

Berlin M, Legum C, Muchnik C, Hildesheimer M (1999) Subclinical audiological findings in carriers of recessive genes for deafness. Journal of Basic and Clinical Physiology and Pharmacology 10: 201–8.

Boettcher FA, Gratton MA, Schmiedt RA (1995) Effects of noise and age on the auditory system. Occupational Medicine 10: 577–91.

British Society of Audiology (1981) Recommended procedures for pure-tone audiometry using a manually operated instrument. British Journal of Audiology 15: 213–16.

British Society of Audiology (1985) Recommended procedure for pure-tone bone-conduction audiometry without masking using a manually operated instrument. British Journal of Audiology 19: 281–2.

British Society of Audiology (1986) Recommendations for masking in pure-tone threshold audiometry. British Journal of Audiology 20: 307–14.

Burns W, Robinson DW (1970) Hearing and Noise in Industry. London: HMSO.

Chung DY, Gannon RP, Mason K (1984) Factors affecting the prevalence of tinnitus. Audiology 23: 441–52.

Clark WW (1991) Recent studies of temporary threshold shift (TTS) and permanent threshold shift (PTS) in animals. Journal of the Acoustical Society of America 80: 1350–7.

Cocchiarella LA, Sharp DS, Persky VW (1995) Hearing threshold shifts, white-cell count and smoking status in working men. Occupational Medicine 45: 179–85.

Coles RRA (1984) Epidemiology of tinnitus: (2) demographic and clinical features. Journal of Laryngology and Otology 9(suppl): 195–202.

Coles RRA, Mason SM (1984) The results of cortical electric response audiometry in medico-legal evaluations. British Journal of Audiology 18: 71–8.

Coles RRA, Lutman ME, Buffin JT (2000) Guidelines on the diagnosis of noise-induced hearing loss for medicolegal purposes. Clinical Otolaryngology and Allied Sciences 25: 264–73.

Cox HJ, Ford GR (1995) Hearing loss associated with weapons noise exposure: when to investigate an asymmetrical loss. Journal of Laryngology and Otology 109: 291–5.

Cripps NP, Glover MA, Guy RJ (1999) The pathophysiology of primary blast injury and its implications for treatment. Part II: The auditory structures and abdomen. Journal of the Royal Naval Medical Service 85(1): 13–24.

Cruickshanks KJ, Klein R, Klein BE, Wiley TL, Nondahl DM, Tweed TS (1999) Cigarette smoking and hearing loss: the epidemiology of hearing loss study. Journal of the American Medical Association 279: 1715–19.

Daniell WE, Fulton-Kehoe D, Smith-Weller T, Franklin GM (1998) Occupational hearing loss in Washington state, 1984–1991: II Morbidity and associated costs. American Journal of Industrial Medicine 33: 529–36.

Danielson R, Henderson D, Gratton MA, Bianchi L, Salvi R (1991) The importance of 'temporal pattern' in traumatic impulse noise exposures. Journal of the Acoustical Society of America 90(1): 209–18.

Davis A (1995) Hearing in Adults. London: Whurr.

Davis RR, Newlander JK, Ling X, Cortopassi GA, Krieg EF, Erway LC (2001) Genetic basis for susceptibility to noise-induced hearing loss in mice. Hearing Research 155(1–2): 82–90.

Dobie RA (2001) Medical-legal Evaluation of Hearing Loss, 2nd edn. San Diego, CA: Singular Press.

Environmental Protection Agency (1973) Public Health and Welfare Criteria for Noise. EPA Report 550/9-73-002. Washington DC: US Environmental Protection Agency.

Environmental Protection Agency (1981) Noise in America: The extent of the noise problem. EPA Report No. 550/9-81-101. Washington DC: US Environmental Protection Agency.

Fearn RW, Harrison DR (1983) Audiometric zero for air conduction using manual audiometry. British Journal of Audiology 17: 87–9.

Fechter LD (1995) Combined effects of noise and chemicals. Occupational Medicine 10: 609–21.

Feverstein JF (2002) Occupational hearing conservation. In J Katz (ed.) Handbook of Clinical Audiology, 5th edn. Baltimore, MD: Lippincott, Williams & Wilkins, pp. 567–83.

Frenkel A (1998) A review of the synergistic damage to hearing due to combined exposure to industrial noise and otoneurotoxic materials. In L Luxon, D Prasher (eds) Advances in Noise Research, Volume 1: Biological Effects of Noise. London: Whurr, pp. 295–9.

Garth RJ (1994) Blast injury of the auditory system: a review of the mechanisms and pathology. Journal of Laryngology and Otology 108: 925–9.

Griest SE, Bishop PM (1998) Tinnitus as an early indicator of permanent hearing loss. A 15 year longitudinal study of noise exposed workers. American Academy of Occupational Health Nurses Journal 46: 325–9.

Hall AJ, Lutman ME (1999) Methods for early identification of noise-induced hearing loss. Audiology 38: 277–80.

Hallberg LRM, Barrenas M-L (1993) Living with a male with noise-induced hearing loss: experience from the perspective of spouses. British Journal of Audiology 27: 255–61.

Health and Safety Executive (1989) Noise at Work: Guidelines on regulations. London: HMSO.

Health and Safety Executive (1990) Noise at Work: Noise Assessment, Information and Control. Noise Guides 3 to 8. London: HMSO.

Health and Safety Executive (2002) Health and Safety Statistics Highlights 2001/02. Suffolk: HSE Books.

Health and Safety Executive (2003) Noise induced deafness, www.hse.gov.uk/statistics/causdis/noise.htm (accessed on 22/06/2003).

Hellstrom PA, Dengerink HA, Axelsson A (1992) Noise levels from toys and recreational articles for children and teenagers. British Journal of Audiology 26: 267–70.

Henderson D, Subramaniam M, Boettcher FA (1993) Individual susceptibility to noise-induced hearing loss: an old topic revisited. Ear and Hearing 14: 152–68.

Hepper PG, Shahidullah S (1994) Noise and the Foetus: A critical review of the literature. Health and Safety Executive contract research report no. 63. London: HMSO.

Hétu R, Lalande M, Getty L (1987) Psychosocial disadvantages associated with occupational hearing loss as experienced in the family. Audiology 26: 141–52.

Hétu R, Riverin L, Lalande N, Getty L, St-Cyr C (1988) Qualitative analysis of the handicap associated with occupational hearing loss. British Journal of Audiology 22: 251–64.

Hétu R, Riverin L, Getty N, Lalande NM, St-Cyr C (1990) The reluctance to acknowledge hearing difficulties among hearing-impaired workers. British Journal of Audiology 24: 265–76.

Hétu R, Jones L, Getty L (1993) The impact of acquired hearing impairments on intimate relationships: implications for rehabilitation. Audiology 32: 363–81.

Holme RH, Steel KP (1999) Genes involved in deafness. Current Opinion in Genetics and Development 9: 309–14.

Igarashi M, Schuknecht HF, Myers EN (1964) Cochlear pathology in humans with stimulation deafness. Journal of Laryngology and Otology 78: 115–23.

Industrial Injuries Advisory Council (1973) Occupational Deafness. London: HMSO.

International Organization for Standardization (1984) ISO 7029: Acoustics – Threshold of hearing by air conduction as a function of age and sex for otologically normal persons. Geneva: ISO.

International Organization for Standardization (1990) ISO 1999: Acoustics – Determination of occupational noise exposure and estimation of noise-induced hearing impairment. 2 edn. Geneva: ISO.

International Organization for Standardization (1998) ISO 389-1: Acoustics – Reference zero for the calibration of audiometric equipment – Part 1: Reference equivalent threshold sound pressure levels for pure tones and supra-aural earphones. Geneva: ISO.

Ishii EK, Talbott EO (1998) Race/ethnicity differences in the prevalence of noise-induced hearing loss in a group of metal fabricating workers. Journal of Occupational and Environmental Medicine 40: 661–6.

Ishii EK, Talbott EO, Findlay RC, D'Antonio JA, Kuller LH (1992) Is NIDDM a risk factor for noise-induced hearing loss in an occupationally noise exposed cohort? Science of the Total Environment 127: 155–65.

Job A, Grateau P, Picard J (1998) Intrinsic differences in hearing performances between ears revealed by the asymmetrical shooting posture in the army. Hearing Research 122: 119–24.

Johnson AC, Nylen PR (1995) Effects of industrial solvents on hearing. Occupational Medicine 10: 623–40.

Jones JR, Hodgson JT, Osman J (1997) Self-reported working conditions in 1995: Results from a household survery. Health and Safety Executive Report. Norwich: HMSO.

Jones NS, Davis A (2000) A retrospective case-controlled study of 1490 consecutive patients presenting to a neuro-otology clinic to examine the relationship between blood lipid levels and sensorineural hearing loss. Clinical Otolaryngology and Allied Sciences 25: 511–17.

Kersebaum M, Bennett JD (1998) Acute acoustic trauma – its features and management. Journal of the Royal Army Medical Corps 144: 156-8.

King PF, Coles RRA, Lutman ME, Robinson DW (1992) Assessment of Hearing Disability. Guidelines for Medico-legal Practice. London: Whurr.

Klockhoff I, Lyttkens L (1982) Hearing defects of noise trauma type with lack of noise exposure. Scandinavian Audiology 11: 257–60.

Kowalska S, Sulkowski W (1998) Measurements of distortion product otoacoustic emissions in industrial workers with noise-induced hearing loss. In L Luxon, D Prasher (eds) Advances in Noise Research, Volume 1: Biological Effects of Noise. London: Whurr, pp. 205–12.

Kozel PJ, Davis RR, Krieg EF, Shull GE, Erway LC (2002) Deficiency in plasma membrane calcium ATPase isoform 2 increases susceptibility to noise-induced hearing loss in mice. Hearing Research 164: 231–9.

Lambert PR, Palmer PE, Rubel EW (1986) The interaction of noise and aspirin in the chick basal papilla. Noise and aspirin toxicity. Archives of Otolaryngology – Head and Neck Surgery 112: 1043–9.

Lataye R, Campo P (1996) Applicability of the L(eq) as a damage-risk criterion: an animal experiment. Journal of the Acoustical Society of America 99: 1621–32.

Lutman ME, Davis AC (1994) The distribution of hearing threshold levels in the general population aged 18–30 years. Audiology 33: 327–50.

Lutman ME, Hall AJ (2000) Novel Methods for Early Identification of Noise-induced Hearing Loss. Health and Safety Executive Contract Research Report 261. London: HMSO.

Lutman ME, Quasem HYN (1998) A source of audiometric notch at 6 kHz. In L Luxon, D Prasher (eds) Advances in Noise Research, Volume 1: Biological Effects of Noise. London: Whurr, pp. 170–6.

Lutman ME, Spencer HS (1991) Occupational noise and demographic factors in hearing. Acta Otolaryngologica Supplementum 476: 74–84.

Luxon LM (1998) The clinical diagnosis of noise-induced hearing loss. In L Luxon, D Prasher (eds) Advances in Noise Research, Volume 1: Biological Effects of Noise. London: Whurr, pp. 83–113.

McBride DI, Williams S (2001) Audiometric notch as a sign of noise induced hearing loss. Occupational and Environmental Medicine 58: 46–51.

McFadden D, Palttsmier HS, Pasanen EG (1984) Temporary hearing loss induced by combinations of intense sounds and non steroidal anti-inflammatory drugs. American Journal of Otology 5: 235–41.

McShane DP, Hyde ML, Alberti PW (1988) Tinnitus prevalence in industrial hearing loss compensation claimants. Clinical Otolaryngology and Allied Sciences 13(5): 323–30.

Melnick W (1991) Human temporary threshold shift (TTS) and damage risk. Journal of the Acoustical Society of America 90: 147–54.

Michaels L (2003) Pathology of the ear. In L Luxon (ed.) Textbook of Audiological Medicine – Clinical aspects of hearing and balance. London: Martin Dunitz.

Milkovi-Kraus S (1990) Noise-induced hearing loss and blood pressure. International Archives of Occupational and Environmental Health 62: 259–60.

Miller JD (1974) Effects of noise on people. Journal of the Acoustic Society of America 56: 729–64.

Mills JH (1982) Effects of noise on auditory sensitivity, psychophysical tuning curves and suppression. In RP Hamernik, D Henderson, R Salvi (eds) New Perspectives on Noise-induced Hearing Loss. New York: Raven Press, pp. 249–62.

Mills JH, Clark WW, Dobie RA, Humes LE, Johnson DL, Liberman MC et al. (1993) Hazardous Exposure to Steady-state and Intermittent Noise. Working group report. Washington DC: National Academic Press.

Mills JH, Dubno JR, Boettcher FA (1998) Interaction of noise-induced hearing loss and presbyacusis. Scandinavian Audiology Supplementum 48: 117–22.

Molvaer OI, Natrud E (1979) Ear damage due to diving. Acta Oto-Laryngologica Supplement 360: 187–9.

Moore BCJ (1997) The perception of sound. In M Gleeson (ed.) Scott-Brown's Otolaryngology: Basic Sciences, 6th edn. Oxford: Butterworth Heinemann.

Morata TC (1989) Study of the effects of simultaeneous exposure to noise and carbon disulphide on workers' hearing. Scandinavian Audiology 18: 53–8.

Morata TC (1998) Assessing occupational hearing loss: beyond noise exposure. Scandinavian Audiology Supplementum 48: 111–16.

Mrena R, Savolainen S, Kuokkanen JT, Ylikoski J (2002) Characteristics of tinnitus induced by acute acoustic trauma: a long-term follow up. Audiology and Neuro-Otology 7: 122–30.

Murai K (1997) Investigation of the 4,000 Hertz dip by detailed audiometry. Annals of Otology, Rhinology and Laryngology 106: 408–13.

National Institute of Health (NIH) (1990) Noise and Hearing Loss. NIH Consensus Statement 8(1): 1–24.

National Institute for Occupational Safety and Health (NIOSH) (1998) Criteria for a recommended standard. Occupational noise exposure. Revised Criteria 1998. DHSS (NIOSH) publication no. 98–126. Centers for Disease Control and Prevention: www.cdc.gov/niosh/98-126.html (accessed on 22/2/2003).

National Physical Laboratory (NPL) (2003a) What is Acoustics? www.npl.co.uk/npl/acoustics/publications/beginnersguide (accessed on 3/2/2003).

National Physical Laboratory (NPL) (2003b) Audiometric Calibration and Standards: www.npl.co.uk/npl/acoustics/techguides/audiometry (accessed on 01/04/2003).

Neuberger M, Korpert K, Raber A, Schwetz F, Bauer P (1992) Hearing loss from industrial noise, head injury and disease. A multivariate analysis on audiometric examinations of 111,647 workers. Audiology 31: 45–57.

Nordmann AS, Bohne BA, Harding GW (2000) Histopathological differences between temporary and permanent threshold shift. Hearing Research 139(1–2): 13–30.

Oeken J (1999) Topodiagnostic assessment of occupational noise-induced hearing loss using distortion product otoacoustic emissions compared to the short increment sensitivity index test. European Archives of Oto-Rhino-Laryngology 256: 115–21.

Ohlemiller KK, McFadden SL, Ding DL, Flood DG, Reaume AG, Hoffman EK et al. (1999) Targeted deletion of the cytosolic Cu/Zn-superoxide dismutase gene (Sod1) increases susceptibility to noise-induced hearing loss. Audiology and Neuro-Otology 4: 237–46.

O'Mahoney CF, Luxon LM (1996) Misdiagnosis of hearing loss due to ear canal collapse: a report of two cases. Journal of Laryngology and Otology 110: 561–6.

Palmer KT, Coggon D, Syddall HE, Pannett B, Griffin MJ (2001) Occupational Exposure to Noise and Hearing Difficulties in Great Britain. Health and Safety Executive Contract Research Report 361/2001. London: HMSO.

Palmer KT, Griffin MJ, Syddall HE, Pannett B, Cooper C, Coggon D (2002) Raynaud's phenomenon, vibration induced white finger, and difficulties in hearing. Occupational and Environmental Medicine 59: 640–2.

Pearson JD, Morrell CH, Gordon-Salant S, Brant LJ, Metter EJ, Klein LL et al. (1995) Gender differences in a longitudinal study of age-associated hearing loss. Journal of the Acoustical Society of America 97: 1196–205.

Pekkarinen J (1995) Noise, impulse noise and other physical factors: combined effects on hearing. Occupational Medicine 10: 545–59.

Penner MJ (1990) An estimate of the prevalence of tinnitus caused by spontaneous otoacoustic emissions. Archives of Otolaryngology and Head and Neck Surgery 116: 418–23.

Phoon WH, Lee HS, Chia SE (1993) Tinnitus in noise-exposed workers. Occupational Medicine 43: 35–8.

Pickles JO (1988) An Introduction to the Physiology of Hearing, 2nd edn. London: Academic Press.

Pickles JO (1997) Physiology of hearing. In M Gleeson (ed.) Scott-Brown's Otolaryngology: Basic Sciences, 6th edn. Oxford: Butterworth-Heinemann.

Pirila T, Jounio-Ervasti K, Sorri M (1992) Left-right asymmetries in hearing threshold levels in three age groups of a random population. Audiology 31: 150–61.

Prasher DK, Mula M, Luxon LM (1993) Cortical evoked potential criteria in the objective assessment of auditory threshold: a comparison of noise induced hearing loss with Meniere's disease. Journal of Laryngology and Otology 107: 780–6.

Prince MM, Stayner LT, Smith RJ, Gilbert SJ (1997) A re-examination of risk estimates from the NIOSH Occupational Noise and Hearing Survey (ONHS). Journal of the Acoustical Society of America 101(2): 950–63.

Pyykko I, Starck J, Toppila E, Kaksonen R (1998) Ageing as a major confounding factor in noise-induced hearing loss. In DK Prasher, LM Luxon (eds) Advances in Noise Research, Volume 1: Biological Effects of Noise. London: Whurr, pp. 215–225.

Quaranta A, Portalatini P, Henderson D (1998) Temporary and permanent threshold shift: an overview. Scandinavian Audiology Supplementum 48: 75–86.

Rickards FW, De Vidi S (1995) Exaggerated hearing loss in noise induced hearing loss compensation claims in Victoria. Medical Journal of Australia 163: 360–3.

Roberto M, Hamernik RP, Turrentine GA (1989) Damage of the auditory system associated with blast trauma. Annals of Otology, Rhinology and Laryngology – Supplement 140: 23–34.

Robinson DW (1987) Noise Exposure and Hearing: A New Look at the Experimental Data. Health and Safety Executive contract research report 1997:001. London: HMSO.

Robinson DW (1988) Tables for the Estimation of Hearing Impairment due to Noise for Otologically Normal Persons and for a Typically Unscreened Population, as a Function of Age and Duration of Exposure. Health and Safety Executive contract research report 1998: 002. London: HMSO.

Robinson DW, Shipton MS (1977) Tables for the Estimation of Noise-induced Hearing Loss. NPL Acoustics Report Ac 61, 2nd edn. Teddington: National Physical Laboratory.

Robinson DW, Shipton MS, Hinchcliffe R (1981) Audiometric zero for air conduction – a verification and critique of international standards. Audiology 20: 409–31.

Rosenhall U (1998) Presbyacusis related to exposure to occupational noise and other ototraumatic factors. In L Luxon, D Prasher (eds) Advances in Noise Research, Volume 1: Biological Effects of Noise. London: Whurr, pp. 164–9.

Rosenhall U, Pedersen KE (1995) Presbyacusis and occupational hearing loss. Occupational Medicine 10: 593–607.

Royster LH, Royster JD, Thomas WG (1980) Representative hearing levels by race and sex in North Carolina industry. Journal of the Acoustical Society of America 68: 551–66.

Sataloff RT, Sataloff J (2001) Differential diagnosis of occupational hearing loss. Occupational Health and Safety 70: 126–9.

Shelmerdine L (1999) Hand-arm vibration syndrome: a guide for nurses. Nursing Standard 13(22): 45–7.

Sokas RK, Moussa MA, Gomes J, Anderson JA, Achuthan KK, Thain AB et al. (1995) Noise-induced hearing loss, nationality and blood pressure. Americal Journal of Industrial Medicine 28: 281–8.

Starck J, Toppila E, Pyykko I (1999) Smoking as a risk factor in sensorineural hearing loss among workers exposed to occupational noise. Acta Oto-Laryngologica 119: 302–5.

Stephens SDG (1981) Clinical audiometry. In HA Beagley (ed.) Audiology and Audiological Medicine. Oxford: Oxford University Press.

Susmano A, Rosenbush SW (1988) Hearing loss and ischaemic heart disease. American Journal of Otology 9: 403–8.

Talbott E, Helmkamp J, Matthews K, Kuller L, Cottington E, Redmond G (1985) Occupational noise exposure, noise-induced hearing loss, and the epidemiology of high blood pressure. American Journal of Epidemiology 121: 501–14.

Talbott E, Findlay RC, Kuller LH, Lenkner LA, Matthews KA, Day RD et al. (1990) Noise-induced hearing loss: a possible marker for high blood pressure in older noise-exposed populations. Journal of Occupational Medicine 32: 690–7.

Tan CT, Hsu CJ, Lee SY, Liu SH, Lin-Shiau SY (2001) Potentiation of noise-induced hearing loss by amikacin in guinea pigs. Hearing Research 161(1–2): 72–80.

Tarter SK, Robins TG (1990) Chronic noise exposure, high-frequency hearing loss, and hypertension among automotive assembly workers. Journal of Occupational Medicine 32: 685–9.

Taylor W, Pearson J, Mair A, Burns W (1965) Study of noise and hearing in jute weaving. Journal of the Acoustical Society of America 38: 113–20.

Tognola G, Grandori F, Avan P, Ravanazzi P, Bonfils P (1999) Frequency-specific information from click evoked otoacoustic emissions in noise-induced hearing loss. Audiology 38: 243–50.

Van Camp G, Smith R (2003) Hereditary Hearing Loss Homepage, University of Antwerp: www.uia.ac.be/dnalab/hhh (accessed on 15/3/2003).

Van Campen LE, Dennis JM, Hanlin RC, King SB, Velderman AM (1999) One-year audiologic monitoring of individuals exposed to the 1995 Oklahoma City bombing. Journal of the American Academy of Audiology 10: 231–47.

Virokannas H, Anttonen H (1995) Dose-response relationship between smoking and impairment of hearing acuity in workers exposed to noise. Scandinavian Audiology 24: 211–6.

Ward WD (1991) The role of intermittence in PTS. Journal of the Acoustical Society of America 99: 164–9.

Ward WD (1995) Endogenous factors related to susceptibility to damage from noise. Occupational Medicine 10: 561–75.

WHO (World Health Organization) (1997) Prevention of Noise-induced hearing loss. Report of an informal consultation – held at the WHO, Geneva, 28–30

October 1997: www.who.int/pbd/pdh/Docs/NOISE_Cover_sum.htm (accessed 19/1/2003).

Yaremchuk K, Dickson L, Burk K, Shivapuja BG (1997) Noise level analysis of commercially available toys. International Journal of Pediatric Otolaryngology 41: 187–97.

Yost WA (2000) Fundamentals of Hearing: An introduction. 4th edn. San Diego, CA: Academic Press.

Xu ZM, Van Cauwenberge P, Vinck B, De Vel E (1998) Sensitive detection of noise-induced damage in human subjects using transiently evoked otoacoustic emissions. Acta Oto-Rhino-Laryngologica Belgica 52(1): 19–24.

# CHAPTER 11

# Disability assessment in noise-induced hearing loss

*Noise and Its Effects:* Edited by Linda Luxon and Deepak Prasher © 2007 John Wiley & Sons Ltd.

PHILIP H JONES

## Introduction

Most doctors first really encounter noise-induced hearing loss (NIHL) in the medicolegal context and their main concern when starting in this field is often how to assess disability. Experience, however, shows that this is much less important than obtaining a validated accurate pure-tone audiogram and a thorough history, and making a logical diagnosis. In the UK many cases were settled in the past by disability assessments already agreed between insurers and trade unions; currently most cases are settled, with or without compensation, before reaching court and in other cases the court will make its own judgment and award compensation influenced by awards made in comparable cases but allowing for the court's view of how the claimant's hearing loss has influenced his life for the worse. It will often have little interest in a percentage assessment by the medical expert.

This is expedient as there have been several methods used in the UK but none has persisted long and there is currently no recommended method. The *Black Book* (King et al., 1992), while containing much invaluable information, has not been formally endorsed as a method of disability assessment by any of its sponsoring bodies. This difficulty in assessing disability is not confined to the beginner. The *Black Book* has a low fence of −20 dB but, only a few years before its publication, one of its authors, the internationally recognized expert in NIHL in the UK, Professor DW Robinson, had proposed one of +30 dB (Robinson et al., 1984): a difference of just over 30 times in subjective loudness.

Therefore there is no method of disability assessment to recommend. This chapter covers some topics that the author feels may be of use to the medical examiner in assessing disability and attempts to correct some common errors. While a percentage disability assessment may be unrealistic, it is very often possible to provide a realistic estimate for the court of the loss in decibels due to noise at each different frequency. This is often smaller than is usually thought but industrial noise is, by comparison with age, a minor influence on the hearing. The National Study of Hearing found that a working lifetime at 90–100 dB (probably averaging a little below 95 dB) gave a loss maximum at 4 kHz, which averaged 12 dB at that frequency (Lutman and Spencer, 1991).

An accurate diagnosis and pure-tone audiogram are far more important in the medicolegal assessment of hearing loss than a disability assessment for which no good method exists.

## What type of audiometry measures disability best?

We seldom hear pure tones so it may seem that pure-tone audiometry is far removed from everyday life, but in practice this is not the case. Pure-tone audiometry shows whether the subject has a middle- or inner-ear loss and how the hearing compares with that of others of the same or of different age. The pattern and extent of the loss on a pure-tone audiogram compared with the extent and duration of the noise exposure are the crucial factors in the diagnosis of NIHL.

The hearing threshold levels indicate the extent of the loss and it is not difficult to predict from the pure-tone audiogram what difficulties the subject is likely to experience in real life. There is no other easily performed audiometric measurement with standards agreed worldwide that gives a more accurate assessment of hearing disability. It is much better than self-assessment of hearing disability, which is notoriously inaccurate (Robinson et al., 1984; King et al., 1992). Some with poor hearing deny problems and others with good, normal or even above-average hearing report difficulties. A high percentage of the normally hearing young adults in the recent National Study of Hearing reported excessive difficulty in distinguishing speech in a noisy background (Davis, 1997).

There are more subtle factors in the functions of the inner ear and subjects with the same pure-tone audiogram may have different abilities in frequency discrimination and temporal resolution. However, these differences will not be marked if the pure-tone audiograms are the same and noise exposure does not have an effect on these more subtle factors without affecting the pure-tone audiogram. In general, any effect that noise has on hearing disability is proportionate to its effect on the pure-tone audiogram (Robinson et al., 1984; Lutman, 1997).

Hearing ability is best assessed by pure-tone audiometry which is by far the best surrogate for hearing disability.

## Inconsistency in pure-tone audiometry

Volunteered pure-tone audiometry is the backbone of disability assessment in NIHL so the first question in assessing disability must always be:

'Is the audiogram accurate?' Consistent responses are often claimed to show that the volunteered pure-tone audiogram is accurate. This is not correct (King et al., 1992). Consistent audiograms tend to be accurate and inconsistent ones to be inaccurate but in one study about half the cases shown by a cortical electric response audiogram (CERA) to have an exaggerated loss on volunteered pure-tone audiometry were consistent in their responses (Robinson, 1990).

Consistency of pure-tone audiograms does not guarantee accuracy. Inconsistency arouses suspicion of inaccuracy.

The effect of gross exaggeration is often to produce an audiogram with a hearing loss that cannot be due to noise exposure because it is too severe, in the wrong frequencies and of the wrong pattern because exaggeration usually affects the lower frequencies more than the higher frequencies (Robinson 1990; King et al., 1992; Alberti, 1997). In a subject with a marked loss it is not sufficient to say that the loss cannot be due to noise exposure – one must consider whether the loss is real or not.

If the volunteered thresholds are close to 0 dB it is unlikely that exaggeration is present. If there is a marked loss at frequencies unlikely to be affected by noise exposure, for example 0.5 kHz, then exaggeration may be present. If the threshold is 25 dB or worse at 0.5 kHz the audiogram should be checked. The subject may volunteer an audiogram that shows a loss which if real would cause difficulty in conversation even with a hearing aid, but manages conversation easily with no aid and without lip reading. Similarly the stapedial reflex threshold may be close to the volunteered threshold.

A reverse air–bone gap with bone-conduction thresholds consistently worse than the air are an indication of inaccurate pure-tone audiometry. Although some think it theoretically impossible, a bone-conduction threshold worse than the air conduction will occur from time to time because

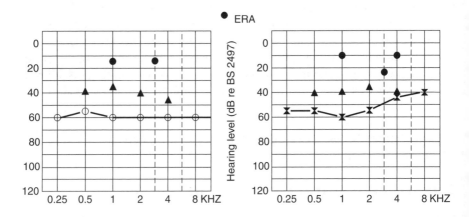

**Figure 11.1** Non-organic hearing loss in a young man aged 15. (From Lightfoot and Mason, 1989.)

of audiometric variability and error including the variability in calibration but one should not occur across a range of frequencies. Conversely, and more frequently, bone-conduction thresholds are often volunteered at a more accurate level than air conduction and in an inconsistent subject an air–bone gap may appear due to inconsistency.

Speech audiometry is a relatively simple way of checking the accuracy of the volunteered pure-tone audiogram (Robinson 1990), but does not give diagnostic or frequency-specific information. If there is a marked discrepancy between the actual speech audiogram and that predicted from the volunteered thresholds a CERA must be obtained.

Check the pure-tone audiogram for features of non-organic loss and with a speech audiogram. Obtain a CERA from an expert in any case in doubt.

# Cortical electric response audiometry

As accurate pure-tone audiometry is the mainstay of disability assessment in NIHL, if an accurate volunteered pure-tone audiogram cannot be obtained then a CERA, a technique that does not depend upon the subject's active cooperation, is needed. CERA testing provides a frequency-specific estimate of the true hearing thresholds that is objective, in that it does not rely on the subject's own volunteered responses, although it is subjective in that it relies upon the tester to decide what is the minimum level of stimulation at which a definite response can be seen.

Electric response audiometry performed by different machinery and different techniques can give different results and even in the best of hands the ERA is still only an estimate of the true hearing thresholds and is not a guaranteed method of measuring them exactly. In less than expert hands a CERA may be markedly inaccurate. In good hands it is stated that 90% of ERA estimates lie within 10 dB of the true thresholds. One unit of excellent reputation has found its CERA estimates of pure-tone thresholds to be about 4 dB worse on average than the true hearing threshold at 1, 2 and 3 kHz and more at the higher frequencies (GR Lightfoot, personal communication, 1992).

As audiometry is an inexact science, there is always some degree of variation in the results of different tests. However, as it is not possible to respond consistently to a stimulus that is not heard and, as virtually all audiological error tends to exaggerate a hearing loss (Lawton, 1991), the better of two results is almost always likely to be more correct and this applies to ERA testing. When reviewing ERA and multiple audiology tests in markedly inconsistent subjects, it is reasonable to assume that the best response obtained at any particular frequency is the most accurate and that when this is an ERA result some decibels should be subtracted from the result to allow for the known error rate of ERA testing.

Even in consistent subjects, repeated audiometry will tend to lower thresholds if this technique is used because of audiometric variability and in more consistent subjects it may be more accurate to use the best overall audiogram, provided that no individual threshold is an outlier. Another reasonable suggestion is to use the best threshold, provided that it has been repeated on at least one occasion or, if it has not, to use the second best threshold or the best plus 5 dB.

Audiometric variability is skewed to showing worse hearing than truly exists (Lawton, 1991). The true pure-tone threshold is, or lies close to, the best threshold in good audiometric subjects.

## The National Physical Laboratory tables for the estimation of NIHL

These tables have been the mainstay of diagnosis in the UK for many years. The second edition was published in 1977 (Robinson and Shipton, 1977). The tables derive from studies of industrial workers who were in general exposed to high noise levels for long periods of time. They enable one to predict for any particular frequency between 0.5 and 6 kHz what range of hearing thresholds will be obtained in a population at a given age after a set amount of noise exposure. They enable this prediction for men and women. The values are given in percentiles, the first percentile having the worst hearing and the 99th percentile the best hearing. The National Physical Laboratory (NPL) tables do not give individual audiograms – they give the range obtained in a population. As there is no evidence of any correlation between sensitivity to the effects of noise and sensitivity to the effects of ageing, two individuals of the same age, sex, duration and extent of noise exposure and with identical hearing threshold levels at a particular frequency may have differing degrees of NIHL. In one the loss at that frequency may be largely due to ageing and in the other largely due to noise.

The NPL tables come with a warning that they cannot be used to predict at an individual level. As we do not know before the individual has been subjected to noise what his sensitivity to the permanent effects of noise is, one cannot tell until after the event what size of loss will result from a given noise exposure. One can, however, use the tables to predict retrospectively – to take an audiogram after noise exposure and state whether its resemblance to the average is sufficiently strong to make it likely the loss is due to noise or whether its differences are so extreme that some factor other than noise exposure is present.

The NPL tables use the hypothesis, also used in the Code of Practice of 1978, that the extent of the loss will be in proportion to the noise dose, the noise dose will increase linearly with the duration of exposure and will double for each 3 dB in intensity, that is 93 dB for 1 year is equivalent to 90 dB for 2 years. The NPL tables therefore express the noise dose as a noise immission level (NIL). This equates the individual's total noise dose to the amount of noise that would be required to equal that noise dose calculated on the above basis in 1 year's exposure. As the male ear is more sensitive to the effects of noise and ageing than the female, for the male ear 1.5 dB is added to this level and for the female ear 1.5 dB is subtracted. One of the NPL tables allows noise exposures of varying durations and levels to be added to obtain a final NIL. Another set allows the NIL to be calculated if the duration of exposure and extent of exposure are known. The next gives the different frequencies at different ages an age correction factor $F$, which is not presbycusis. The NPL tables can be used only to reconstruct an average audiogram and factor $F$ cannot be considered in isolation from factor $H$. This is derived from the next set of tables, which, at various NILs, at various percentiles of the population, give the expected hearing loss $H$; $F$ and $H$ are added to give $H'$, which is the average hearing threshold level in the population under consideration. $H$ is not the noise-induced component of the loss. It includes some degree of presbycusis and, obviously, the variation of presbycusis between one individual and another and between the two sexes.

At the 99th percentile of the NPL tables, which must include those whose ears are most resistant to the effects of noise and ageing, a noise-induced effect is still present because there is a small notch at 4 kHz. The reason for this is simple: variability in the sensitivity to ageing effects is much greater than variability in the sensitivity to noise-induced loss (Dobie, 1993). Most of the subjects at the 99th percentile therefore were highly resistant to the effects of ageing. Some, however, were not wholly insensitive to the effects of noise. Therefore the average audiogram of all individuals at the 99th percentile will reflect an amount of noise-induced loss. This, of course, does not mean that all, or even most, individuals in that population had a noise-induced loss.

If, at a given NIL, expected hearing loss $H$ exceeds 0 dB at the 50th percentile, it may be thought that the average man exposed to such noise would have a noise-induced loss and therefore more probably than not that there is a noise-induced loss present in an individual. This argument might seem to be capable of extension into an assessment of the probable extent of the NIHL and hence disability. However, it is not valid and betrays a fundamental misunderstanding of the structure of the NPL tables. That the average man exposed to a certain level of noise would have an NIHL does not prove the individual has one. The NPL tables themselves state they cannot be used to predict for the individual.

Finally, the point is not whether $H$ is greater than 0 dB but whether $F$ plus $H$, which gives the average hearing threshold level in that population, is greater than the hearing threshold level that would be obtained in an identical population not exposed to noise. Even so this does not mean that the individual has a noise-induced loss. If $H'$ ($H' = H + F$) is greater than the average hearing threshold level in a noise-free population then the noise level concerned would have an influence in some but not all or even the majority of that population. Conversely, however, if $H'$ is equal to or less than the average hearing threshold levels (average HTLs) in a noise-free population then that NIL would have had no influence on the average HTLs in the population concerned and would be very unlikely therefore to have affected the individual. An analogy is to consider a possibly fatal factor (X) with a danger that depends on dose. If a set dose does not alter mortality rates then it is unlikely that it will kill any individual. If it does alter mortality rates that does not mean that it is the most probable cause of death in a particular individual. When it more than doubles the number of deaths in the population, it does become the most probable cause but only if we know nothing else about the individual. If, for example, we know that X always causes the body to turn green but never yellow, then any dead yellow body cannot have died of X whatever the dose to which they were subjected but a dead green body may have died of X provided that the dose of X was at a potentially fatal level and that there is no other more likely cause of death also causing green discoloration.

A drawback of the NPL tables is the concept of the NIL itself. Because they were derived from the audiograms of individuals with many years' exposure to high levels of noise, the differential effect of noise and different times at different frequencies is not allowed for. It is allowed for in ISO 1999 (National Organization for Standardization or ISO, 1990), the international standard for the diagnosis of NIHL.

> The NPL tables for NIHL are essential for the medicolegal expert but must be used carefully. They do not separate hearing loss into age-associated and noise-induced components.

## Presbycusis

However extensive the history and investigation, and a thorough investigation is more than a history, examination of the eardrums and pure-tone audiometry, in the majority of cases of hearing loss no certain cause can be found (Browning, 1986). Hearing loss is common at all ages and becomes increasingly common with age (Davis, 1997). Age-associated loss is known as presbycusis. Presbycusis is not due solely to the direct effects of ageing. The longer the life the more likely it is that damage to the hearing will occur from unknown causes and appear as an age-associated effect – that is, presbycusis may be divided into two parts: pathological and physiological but, because we do not know the cause of most pathological presbycusis, we cannot distinguish between the two. Individual variability in sensitivity to ageing effects is much greater than the variation in sensitivity to the effects of noise (Dobie, 1993). Hence, it is important to have tables showing the variation in HTLs with age in a population free of noise exposure and conductive hearing loss but matched for age, sex and occupational status with the subject.

It is likely that presbycusis in a population already complaining of hearing loss will be more marked than in the average population. A population claiming for industrial NIHL has been pre-selected for hearing loss in advance of presbycusis as the claimant population should contain few or no subjects whose hearing loss is due solely to presbycusis of less than average extent but is likely to contain many whose loss is due solely to presbycusis of more than average extent.

It is not logical to argue that a subject has a hearing loss due to a factor other than ageing because the loss is worse than average. Fifty per cent of the population by definition has worse than average hearing. If the audiogram is similar in thresholds and pattern to that seen in those of the noise-free population of the same age exhibiting more marked ageing effects than average then there is no reason to diagnose anything other than age-associated loss particularly if there is a loss in the lower frequencies, which are seldom affected by noise.

> Hearing loss that is worse than average for the subject's age is most usually due to more advanced than average presbycusis which is only to be expected in a subject complaining of hearing loss.

## Tables for presbycusis

Many tables exist for presbycusis. In the UK it has been traditional to use the NPL tables relating pure-tone audiometric thresholds to age (Shipton, 1979). These values were adopted by the ISO as ISO 7029 (ISO, 1984). It is often assumed that the values given in the tables are HTLs, they are not: they are shifts with age from the HTLs of otologically normal 18-year-olds. They are not audiometer dial readings. They would be so only if 0 dB, as given in ISO 389 (ISO, 1991), represented average HTLs in otologically normal 18-year-olds. However, it is known that average human hearing is actually worse than 0 dB, even in otologically normal 18-year-olds and this difference is particularly marked at 6 kHz.

The value 0 dB is defined by an international standard ISO 389 so that, worldwide, all audiometers are calibrated in the same way. ISO 389 is theoretically related to normal young human hearing and was originally based upon a series of papers published between 1933 and 1960. The present version of ISO 389 does not mention its derivation or refer to normal hearing. Two of the papers that went to make up ISO 389 (Dadson and King, 1952; Wheeler and Dickson, 1952) are from the British literature and those papers selected the test population by methods that biased the results in favour of what might be called normal, good, young, human hearing. As equipment used for calibration has altered over the years so ISO 389 has been updated and the current edition of ISO 389 gives what are called RETSPLs or reference equivalent threshold sound pressure levels.

The major determinant of human hearing is, of course, age and a number of surveys of the changes in hearing with age have been published. In 1978 Robinson and Sutton developed the equations used to generate the NPL tables from a number of surveys from the 1930s to the 1970s and they were then adopted as an international standard (ISO 7029 – ISO,

1984). They made clear in their report that the data used were not ideal but were all that was available. The surveys were unrepresentative of the general population and overweighted towards non-manual workers. Most of the surveys do not give full details of their methods and those that do would now be regarded as scientifically suspect. Most did not give the HTLs measured in their baseline young population but only the variation or shift with age from that baseline. In the surveys that did, the hearing levels found in the young population, particularly at 6 kHz, were not 0 dB. Hence, ISO 7029 does not represent the HTLs measured, but those measured altered by a number of factors, one of which is the difference between 0 dB and normal young human hearing. It is logical, if one is trying to measure hearing threshold shifts with age, to measure only the shifts with age compared with the levels in the normal young population so that all factors unrelated to ageing are taken out of account. Unfortunately, this means that ISO 7029 figures can be read only as HTLs if normal young human hearing is assumed to be 0 dB.

The NPL tables 94 (Shipton, 1979, p. 2) state: 'The tables do not strictly give the absolute hearing threshold level.'

Robinson (1988 p 6) stated the following on typical populations

> There is strong evidence that the conventional audiometric zero does not correspond exactly to the median threshold of young normal hearing. In the case of S individuals the ARHL data are presented in ISO 7029 as hearing levels relative to median values for age 18 years for the same sex. These values are not exact HTLs relative to ISO 389; the above mentioned difficulties were side stepped. (S equals screened individuals, ARHL equal age-related hearing loss, HTL equals hearing threshold level)

Hinchcliffe (1997 p iv) wrote in his obituary to 'Dix' (Wallace Dixon Ward) in the *Journal of Audiological Medicine*:

> In . . . 1986 Dix made a statement . . . 'All actual field studies of non-industrial-noise-exposed 20-years-olds have found median HTLs of at least 3–5 dB at most test frequencies . . . tables or graphs that purport to show realistic HTLs to be expected in a group of workers at a particular age if their industrial noise exposures have had no effect must consist of age corrections added to the actual HTLs of the 20-year-olds.

Robinson and Sutton argued that the difference was due to the screening of the population – that the worse hearing in the typical population data was derived because known causes of hearing loss were screened out of the databases that went to make up ISO 7029, by the application of the concept of otological normality, but it has been shown that screening cannot make such a difference because most causes of hearing loss are unknown.

The Medical Research Council Institute of Hearing Research National Study of Hearing found that normal young human hearing is not 0 dB at any frequency and that the discrepancy at 6 kHz is larger than was previously thought (Lutman and Spencer, 1991; Davis, 1995).

ISO 7029 data are generated from the equations derived from the survey by Robinson and Sutton in 1978, which showed that in the median normal young population of the ISO 7029 series, the hearing was not actually 0 dB and the discrepancy was most marked at 6 kHz where it was 11.9 dB in men and 7.3 dB in women. As they were assessing hearing threshold shifts they reduced all their figures by the shifts compared with median 18-year-old values and so this discrepancy disappeared – in their survey young hearing was not 0 dB but they assumed that it should have been and called the discrepancy the 'calibration factor', which does not appear in the actual NPL tables or ISO 7029.

The National Study of Hearing was a survey performed by the MRC's (Medical Research Council's) Institute of Hearing Research during the early 1980s. The figures published include those for a population screened for any noise exposure and for any air–bone gap (Davis, 1995). The reasons for the discrepancy between ISO 7029 and the National Study of Hearing have been discussed in a number of papers and the 6-kHz notch effect has now been explained (Lutman and Qasem, 1997). A notch at 6 kHz does not represent a hearing loss; it occurs in people who have normal hearing. It represents a deficiency in ISO 389 if it is regarded as a measure of normal young human hearing.

ISO 7029 and the National Study of Hearing figures can be reconciled, provided that either the former are regarded as hearing threshold shifts with age and the latter are used to provide the levels of hearing in the average youth or the processing of the figures in ISO 7029 is reversed. The relevant factors are the following:

- The difference between 0 dB and normal young human hearing.
- The step (also known as the quantization) factor (Leijon A 1992). In the past it was usual to deduct 2.5 dB or half the step size from the measured threshold.
- The NPL tables do not distinguish between manual and non-manual workers but the National Study of Hearing does.
- There are small effects arising from the slightly different definitions of the young population and the use of mean, modal and median figures.

If an examiner holds that ISO 7029 gives accurate HTLs for the otologically normal population then, as the average population does not hear as well as ISO 7029, he must hold that screening makes a difference and the majority of subjects examined should therefore be compared not with otologically normal data but with typical population data. One cannot argue that, although the subject has abnormal eardrums, middle-ear function is normal and the scarring has had no effect on the hearing and so the subject is otologically normal. This argument implicitly accepts that screening for otological normality makes no difference and therefore the difference between ISO 7029 and typical population data and the National Study of Hearing must arise for other reasons.

Until ISO 7029 is revised, use typical population data for estimating hearing thresholds in a noise-free population. In the UK, and perhaps elsewhere also, the best figures are from the National Study of Hearing (Davis, 1995). A notch at 6 kHz is normal and not due to hearing loss.

# Otological normality

The document on which the NPL tables is based (Robinson and Sutton, 1978, p. 8) reads in part: 'The annotation R is added where the description implies rigorous selection, for example.' ISO R 389 1964 defined otological normality as: 'free from all signs or symptoms of ear disease.'

The reviews that were incorporated into ISO 7029 or the NPL tables all defined otological normality in different ways (Lawton, 1991). By the strictest criteria any abnormality of the eardrum, any history of ear disease past or present or any history of a condition thought to be perhaps associated with hearing loss (for example, head injury; noise exposure; military service; ototoxic drug administration; excess alcohol or smoking; cardiac, metabolic, renal or vascular disease and other ill-health) would cause the subject to be classed as other than otologically normal. It must be doubtful whether there is any individual in Western society who has not been treated with a drug that has been reported somewhere as being potentially ototoxic, for example aspirin or non-steroidal anti-inflammatory drugs. If not so strictly applied in borderline cases the argument that the subject's hearing was unaffected so that he or she was otologically normal, and its converse, must have been tempting – one sees it advanced in medicolegal reports today – but would inevitably bias the results. It is not possible to tell if this was so.

The National Study of Hearing results are more valid than the NPL tables. One reason is that the HTLs in individuals exposed to noise at frequencies unaffected by noise exposure (Bauer et al., 1991) are much closer to the predictions of the National Study of Hearing than the values given in ISO 7029 if these are regarded as HTLs. The hearing threshold shifts given in ISO 7029 are not inaccurate and if ISO 7029 is added to the actual HTLs of normally hearing, young 18-year-olds the results parallel those of the National Study of Hearing.

The median audiogram in a man or woman of a given age after a given amount of noise exposure predicted by the NPL tables and the National Study of Hearing is very similar. This shows that the estimated NILs of subjects in the National Study of Hearing must be as accurate as those for subjects in the NPL tables. ISO 1999 for the estimation of NIHL refers to ISO 7029 as database A and specifically allows the application of any other more appropriate database for age-associated hearing loss as database B.

Otological normality is an outdated and invalid concept devised to account for the difference between so-called screened and typical populations. The true explanation is that normal young human hearing is not 0 dB.

## Problems with otological normality

- Many of the conditions excluded have not been shown to influence hearing threshold levels (Brant et al., 1996; Blakley and Kim, 1998). The statistical effect of those that have is often not marked. Most cases of sensorineural hearing loss (94% according to Browning, 1986) have no known cause.
- Applying such screening to later databases has not resulted in improved threshold levels in the screened population.
- Abnormalities of the eardrums are common now and more common in older populations, as is childhood middle-ear disease but there is no good evidence that sensory thresholds are affected by such disease.
- Assessing the ear drums for abnormality is a subjective test and influenced by technique – for example, whether a microscope or an auriscope is used, and by the experience of the observer.
- It is not clear if the screening was blinded to the results of audiometry.
- The screening process was not the same in all surveys.
- If strict screening was correctly applied it is likely that very few subjects would have passed screening.

# Noise-induced hearing loss and presbycusis

It is often assumed that these two factors are additive and an NIHL once present is permanent, but this is not so as the two overlap. When both are small the overlap can be ignored and the two treated as additive. Consider a set of 100 sensory cells subjected to two harmful influences, both causing a 1% loss; the overall loss will be 1.99% or effectively 2%. If we consider the same population exposed to two harmful influences, one causing a 90% loss and the other a 1% loss, then the end result whichever comes first is loss of 90.1%, effectively 90%.

As the prime influence on hearing is age this means that as ageing proceeds NIHL disappears. Noise-induced loss progresses most rapidly in the earlier years of exposure; age-associated loss increases more rapidly with increasing age. In an individual exposed to noise for a working lifetime who develops an NIHL as a result, the noise-induced component to the HTLs will be near maximum by the onset of middle age or earlier.

At this stage the inner-ear sensory elements may be considered to fall into two groups – those working and those not working – and those not working into three groups: those damaged by age alone, those damaged by noise alone and those initially damaged by noise but which by the subject's present age would have fallen victim to ageing in any case. As ageing proceeds so the first and third of these subgroups increase and the second, those damaged by noise alone, falls and the NIHL disappears.

By the age of 70 years in women and 80 years in men, noise exposure has no influence upon the HTLs of a population and any subject whose hearing is at the level of the average 70-year-old in women or 80-year-old in men is on the balance of probabilities unlikely to have a noise-induced component to their hearing loss whether they did have a noise-induced loss in the past or not. While this probability should be borne in mind, obviously each individual case should be considered on its own merits (Rosenhall et al., 1990; Robinson, 1991).

Noise-induced hearing loss, if defined as the difference between the hearing as it now is and as it would have been without noise exposure, decreases as presbycusis increases and eventually disappears.

## Sensitivity to the effects of noise and ageing

It may seem fair and simple to assume that an individual susceptible to the effects of ageing is likely to be equally susceptible to the effects of noise on the basis that both influence the same cells in the inner ear. This is unlikely on theoretical grounds. NIHL is a fairly pure form of damage. Ageing has effects not only on every aspect of cochlear function but throughout the peripheral and central auditory systems (Willott, 1991; see also Chapters 3 and 4). Older people with the same inner-ear function, as shown by the pure-tone audiogram, as younger people have more difficulty in hearing in a background of noise due to ageing affecting the central nervous system (Davis, 1987; Willott, 1991). Most of the factors involved in pathological presbycusis are unknown, but they are diverse.

Age-associated hearing loss therefore consists of a very large number of factors influencing the whole of the inner ear. Noise-induced loss has its primary effect upon the outer hair cells in the 4-kHz region. The major effect of age on the hair cells is at the highest frequencies and while, on a pure-tone audiogram, this appears to be 8 kHz, this is only because hearing is not routinely measured at higher frequencies but it is the hearing above 8 kHz that is initially affected by age.

The outer hair cells at different points along the length of the cochlear duct are not the same but vary in their structure (Wright, 1997). It seems that the main effect of noise exposure is on the stereocilia of the 4-kHz outer hair cells (Alberti, 1997) but the outer hair cell is itself a very complicated structure. It is as such highly unlikely that the sensitivity to noise of the stereocilia of the 4-kHz outer hair cells of a particular individual is the same as the average sensitivity to the many factors involved in ageing of all the individual components of the auditory system in the same individual.

This theory is confirmed by fact. The variability in HTLs due to variation in the sensitivity to the effects of ageing is much greater than the variability due to variation in the susceptibility to the effects of noise (Davis, 1989; Dobie, 1993). This is evident from a consideration of the various databases giving hearing threshold variation with noise exposure and with ageing (for example, the NPL tables, ISO 1999, the National Study of Hearing). Hence the two sensitivities cannot be the same. In those individuals in the NPL tables with the best HTLs there were still quite clearly some individuals sensitive to the effects of noise, even though all those individuals must have been highly insensitive to the effects of ageing. Dobie's median allocation method assumes that the sensitivity to the two factors is equal but that does not prove that they are and Dobie clearly states that they are not.

Assuming equal sensitivity to noise and age is perhaps equitable when allocating disability but is not justifiable in diagnosis.

## Dobie's median-based allocation method

With more severe degrees of loss the patterns of average presbycusis and of noise-induced loss may be similar and the important diagnostic factor is whether the noise does make it likely that the loss is due to noise exposure as well as ageing or solely to ageing. The sensitivities needed to the effects of noise and ageing, to arrive at the given degree of loss, must be calculated to see which is the more likely cause. In these circumstances it may be more equitable to conclude that there is a portion of noise-induced loss and age-induced loss present, particularly if the noise exposure was such as to be likely to damage the hearing of the average person and if the degree of loss is not totally disproportionate to the degree of noise exposure. In these circumstances, not only will high noise levels and a sensitive ear be required but many decades of noise exposure as it is only after about 25 years that 2 kHz begins to shift to a significant extent.

Dobie (1993) suggested that an individual exposed for decades to levels of noise high enough to have damaged the inner ear of the average individual, and who has a hearing loss that is not markedly disproportionate to that expected for the noise exposure experienced but whose loss is too severe to be due to noise exposure and average ageing alone, probably has a loss due to above-average sensitivity both to noise exposure and to presbycusis.

He suggests that it is incorrect to assume that these subjects have average presbycusis and that the excess is due to noise exposure, and equally incorrect to assume that they have an average degree of noise-induced loss and that the excess is due to increased ageing. They are probably more sensitive to the effects of both noise and ageing than average. He suggests a compromise method, which is to assume that the two sensitivities are similar. As the variability in the sensitivity to ageing effects is greater than that to the effects of noise this will, as he states, indicate a larger noise-induced component than is actually the case.

Dobie also suggests that such an individual allocation is median based, by which he means that the allocation of this excess loss is made in proportion to the losses that would occur in the median individual with average sensitivity to the effects of both noise and ageing subjected to the same noise level.

The procedure, therefore, depends on knowing the NIL and calculating the HTLs that would occur in the median individual exposed to such noise and comparing those with the hearing loss that occurred due to ageing in the median identical individual not exposed to noise. The difference between the two is the noise-induced loss, and the loss in the individual not exposed to noise is the age-associated loss. The loss in the highly sensitive individual under consideration is then allocated according to the ratio of the two losses that would occur in the median individual.

## Hearing losses and hearing threshold levels

In addition to the variability in hearing loss associated with age, not all human beings are born hearing at the same level. The normal range of human hearing is generally stated to be −10 to +20 dB (Stephens and Rendell, 1988; Arlinger, 1991; International Association of Physicians in Audiology or IAPA, 1992). A healthy young adult with no history of hearing loss who has hearing threshold levels at 15 dB does not have a hearing loss of 15 dB. There is no evidence that he ever heard at 0 dB. The evidence is that his natural HTLs lie at a normal level of 15 dB. Nor, if the average for his age is 5 dB, does he necessarily have a loss of 10 dB – merely a 15-dB HTL. Variation in thresholds from the average is not in itself proof of loss.

An HTL is not the same as a hearing loss.

## Obscure auditory dysfunction syndrome or auditory dysfunction with normal hearing

Patients may present complaining of hearing difficulties with pure-tone audiometry within normal limits, usually defined as better than 20 or 25 dB between, say, 0.25 or 0.5 kHz and 4 or 8 kHz (Stephens and Rendell, 1988). Extensive investigation of such individuals essentially shows that the hearing abilities are in the normal range. There are a number of possible factors but a major one seems to be a loss of auditory confidence that the individual is worried that his hearing is not normal when, in fact, it is (Hinchcliffe, 1992). In the recent National Study of Hearing, 26% of adults complained of difficulty hearing speech in a background of noise (Davis, 1989), which perhaps reflects the fact that human hearing is not perfect.

Comparison of the normally hearing with and without this complaint results in two groups, which are never fully comparable because the control group will, by definition, have average hearing whereas the test group will, also by definition, contain a disproportionate number of individuals whose hearing, although within the normal range, is at the worse end of the normal range and minor differences will therefore always occur between the control and the subject group. Similarly, although major problems with inner-ear function do not occur in the absence of changes in the pure-tone audiogram, there are other factors involved in hearing including temporal resolution, frequency discrimination, central auditory processing, linguistic ability and lip reading. Again those with obscure auditory dysfunction syndrome will tend to have slightly worse abilities, whichever parameter is measured, than the control group.

It has been argued that noise exposure may have an effect on hearing ability in the absence of an effect upon the pure-tone audiogram. This is not so. Such a hypothetical individual would by definition suffer from obscure auditory dysfunction syndrome but noise exposure is not associated with this syndrome (Hinchcliffe, 1992). The first change is a dip at about 4 kHz (Robinson, 1976; American College of Occupational and Environmental Medicine or ACOEM, 1997).

Noise exposure does not cause hearing difficulty without influencing the pure-tone audiogram.

## Disability resulting from hearing loss

Impairment may be defined as a loss of some function previously possessed. In terms of hearing, therefore, a permanent loss involves an increase in the HTLs at a particular frequency or frequencies.

Disability may be defined as a departure of ability from the normal range. It is therefore possible for a subject to have an impairment but no disability if the impairment has not taken hearing outside the normal range and by normal we may understand normal for age. This, of course, does raise questions. By normal do we mean perfect, average or a range centred upon the average and, if a range, what range is included. Often the 5th to 95th percentiles are accepted as the normal range. Sometimes the 25th to the 75th percentiles are used as a range that is certainly 'within normal limits'. In statistics two standard deviations are used, which is approximately the 2nd to the 98th percentiles.

The handicap is whatever cannot be done because of the disability, that is the non-auditory consequences (Stephens and Hetu, 1991; King et al., 1992; Hinchcliffe, 1994).

## Assessing disability

The simplest method of judging a disability or handicap is to ask the subject. However, it is impossible to do so with hearing loss because many individuals, even with quite marked loss, will deny any problems and some individuals with normal hearing feel that they have hearing difficulties. The self-assessment of hearing disability is therefore without great value. The medical examiner should ask the individual what problems they feel arise from their hearing loss and include this in the report. One reason is respect for the subject who expects to be asked such questions. The inaccuracy of the self-assessment of hearing disability is not a feature of the claimant population in particular but of humankind in general. However, the descriptions given often will not match an objective assessment and description. This is not surprising as any individual who believes that he has an impairment of any physiological function will ascribe any difficulty experienced to that impairment even if such difficulties arise on occasion in the normal population. For example, we all occasionally mishear on the telephone, miss telephone or door bells ringing, and have increased difficulty in hearing in noisy places. Conversely those who mistakenly feel that their hearing is normal will blame genuine hearing difficulties on factors other than their hearing loss, such as the poor diction of modern actors compared with the golden age of the past.

It is always of value to know when a subject with a marked degree of loss took specific steps to remedy a hearing problem, such as fitting a loud doorbell or telephone bell, fitting an amplifier on the telephone, obtaining a TV listening device or a hearing aid, as this enables a more objective assessment of the date of onset of hearing disability than the individual human memory.

If a sufficiently large sample is questioned about hearing ability and their audiograms compared with their complaints, the results, while showing a wide scatter, will show a relationship between the reported disabilities and the HTL. Therefore all methods of disability assessment have been based on accurate pure-tone audiometry. A good discussion of this point is contained in the *Black Book* (King et al., 1992).

> Disability assessment in hearing loss can be rationally based only upon an accurate pure-tone audiogram.

## Which frequencies and HTLs should be used?

The next step is to decide which frequencies and threshold levels should be used in the assessment of disability. Disability assessments should be made relatively simple and involve as few frequencies as necessary to achieve reasonable accuracy. Human hearing is used for the perception of speech that contains a wide range of frequencies. The highest frequencies are used by animals to detect the direction of sound but frequencies above 4 kHz do not contribute to the ability to hear speech. Telecommunications engineers generally broadcast between 0.3 kHz and 3.4 kHz for this reason. It is not necessary to hear the whole range of frequencies contained in speech in order to understand it. The resonances on the fundamental frequency give meaning to speech. The fundamental frequency is around 70–280 Hz so the relevant thresholds are between 0.5 and 4 kHz. Some consonants have a significant part of their energy spectrum in the higher frequencies but a high-frequency hearing loss does not mean that these consonants cannot be heard as there will also be a lower-frequency component and as there is a large element of redundancy in speech perception, which is essential to any efficient means of communication.

Disability might be assessed using all the frequencies measured but not all frequencies are equally important in speech perception and so, if fewer frequencies are used, the assessment not only is simpler but may be more accurate. The frequency that best predicts disability is not necessarily the frequency that contributes most to hearing ability and the frequency most affected by noise is neither. The frequency that best predicts disability is 2 kHz (Acton, 1970), which, as one of the speech frequencies, lies intermediate between the high and low frequencies. Thus the threshold level at 2 kHz correlates with the threshold levels at other frequencies in a way that, for example, the threshold at 0.5 kHz cannot. This does not necessarily mean that 2 kHz is more important in speech perception than 1 kHz.

This leaves 0.5, 1, 2, 3 and 4 kHz as possible frequencies to consider in disability assessment. Including both 3 and 4 kHz gives an undue bias to one octave. Noise exposure has little detectable effect below 3 kHz in the average population so using 0.5, 1 and 2 kHz means that the disability assessment will be at frequencies unaffected by noise and will not vary with the degree of noise-induced loss present. The lower two of these frequencies usually lie at much the same level. The use of four rather than three frequencies adds nothing to the accuracy of the assessment. The frequencies 0.5 and 4 kHz are more variable when tested than 1, 2 and 3 kHz (Lawton, 1991; King et al., 1992). Noise affects 4 kHz most but 4 kHz is not a frequency that contributes greatly to the ability to hear speech, although there are some sounds at that frequency and a loss at this frequency does seem to cause problems in distinguishing speech against a background of noise. The 1983 British Association of Otolarynogologists/British Society of Audiology's *Blue Book* method used 1, 2 and 4 kHz, 4 kHz presumably being included because it is the frequency most affected by noise. The *Blue Book* has long had its recognition withdrawn. The report of the Inter-Society Working Group or *Black Book* used 1, 2 and 3 kHz, as have most methods. The general consensus seems to be to use 1, 2 and 3 kHz. These are the most consistent frequencies in testing and their average correlates better with disability than estimates using more frequencies (King et al., 1992). Lawyers often ask for an estimate of the loss at 4 kHz, which is valid. However, in disability assessment only 1, 2, and 3 or 1, 2 and 4 kHz should be used and not 1, 2, 3 and 4 kHz. The next problem is what percentage disability should be ascribed to different degrees of loss. This depends on the scale used, whether it is linear or non-linear, and upon the high and low fences selected.

Disability assessment is simplest and most accurate using three frequencies only. These may be 1, 2 and 3 or 1, 2 and 4 kHz.

# High and low fences

The high fence is the level at which disability is rated at 100%. When hearing is at a threshold level beyond the sound levels encountered in everyday life it is of no effective use. A little hearing at 90 dB is perhaps better than none at all. Most methods assume that if an HTL is 100 dB or worse, the loss is effectively total.

The low fence occurs at the other end of the hearing range. Although the *Black Book* claims not to use a low fence it is, by definition, impossible not to do so because any scale must have a level of zero disability. The *Black Book* in practice abolishes the low fence by placing it at an average –20 dB at 1, 2 and 3 kHz, which is a level of hearing never encountered in humans. This has the illogical consequence of assessing an individual with no loss, and markedly better than average hearing for a normal 18-year-old, as disabled. Disability is not the converse of ability. That one individual is more able than the next does not mean that the less able individual has a disability.

The only logical low fence is the worse end of the normal range for young people. This value is a matter of debate. Social adequacy is usually defined as thresholds averaging 30 dB or better at 0.5, 1 and 2 kHz. The National Study of Hearing defined loss as HTLs greater than 25 dB between 0.5 and 4 kHz. Neither is the same as normal hearing in an 18-year-old. The higher end of the normal range is therefore perhaps either 15 dB or 20 dB, more probably the latter (Stephens and Rendell, 1988; Arlinger, 1991; IAPA, 1992).

If there is a normal range of HTLs there is a normal range of hearing ability and, if disability is a departure from that normal range, then someone whose hearing is within the normal range does not have a disability, although he may have an impairment. It is fair in reporting on such an individual to state that there is a hearing impairment due to noise and that, because of the noise exposure, the hearing is worse than it would otherwise have been, but that there is no hearing disability because the hearing is within the normal range. Whether an impairment that has not caused a disability merits compensation is a question for the court rather than for the medical examiner.

High and low fences are logical and unavoidable and lie at perhaps 20 and 100 dB respectively.

# What allowance should be made for ageing?

Most disability assessments assume that the HTLs would in normal circumstances have been average for age. This is the only reasonable method if a percentage disability is needed. If the actual loss due to noise at a particular frequency is needed, it is illogical to assume automatically that the hearing would in normal circumstances have been average unless it is impossible to judge those circumstances accurately or if near-average presbycusis obtains at frequencies unaffected by noise exposure. Some individuals could naturally have worse than average hearing for their age at the frequencies affected by noise, because their HTLs are poorer than average at those frequencies unaffected by noise exposure such as 0.5 kHz or, in a younger age group, 8 kHz where the recovery of hearing from the dip at 4 kHz can be dramatic. In such cases it is reasonable to presume that the noise-induced component of the hearing loss is less than the estimate achieved by assuming that the hearing would in normal circumstances be average for age.

In assessing disability assume average presbycusis unless there is clear evidence to the contrary.

## What allowance is made for asymmetry

Hearing loss may be asymmetrical. In noise-induced loss there should normally only be minor asymmetries present as industrial noise exposure is usually symmetrical and the two ears are similarly sensitive to the effects of noise (Robinson, 1984). A major asymmetry in the absence of asymmetrical noise exposure should be discounted. Minor asymmetries are probably not due to noise exposure but hardly matter. The better ear dominates hearing ability so most methods weight in favour of the better ear. A commonly used ratio is 4:1, that is 80% of the disability assessment depends on the better ear and 20% on the worse ear. This seldom results in a significant difference from an assessment based on the better ear alone.

If exposure was symmetrical ignore minor and discount major asymmetry.

## Published methods of assessing disability

The *Black Book* (King et al., 1992) was produced by a working group set up by four bodies: the British Association of Otolaryngologists (BAOL), the British Association of Audiological Scientists (BAAS) and the British Association of Audiological Physicians (BAAP), and the British Society of Audiology (BSA). One of the members of the group resigned before publication because he disagreed with its recommendations and none of the sponsoring bodies has formally endorsed it. A number of criticisms have been made (Dobie, 1993). A method that suggests that a subject with better-than-average young hearing has a hearing disability does seem flawed and a further problem is that the levels of presbycusis used by the tables in the

*Black Book* are based on the NPL tables or ISO 7029, which were known to be inaccurate at the time the *Black Book* was published.

The Coles–Worgan method (for which see Chuang, 1986) is sometimes described as outdated, but it is difficult to see how the verbal descriptions made 25 years ago of hearing problems expected from a given pure-tone audiogram could be so described. Although there will never be precise agreement about any method of assessing disability in percentage terms, it is the only method that gives a description of the hearing difficulties expected from the pure-tone audiogram.

Methods of disability assessment have come from, among others:

- DHSS(1973);
- Iron Trades/GMBATU Agreement (Neild, 1985);
- The *Blue Book* (BAO/BSA,1983);
- The *Black Book* (King, Coles, Lutmen and Robinson,1992);
- Coles–Worgan (Chuang,1986).

## What is a significant loss?

Does every decibel count? Certainly when the camel's back breaks every straw counts but the first straw is not significant until the last straw is added, and in reality any measurement must have a level of significance and therefore of insignificance. Pure-tone audiometry, like any scientific measurement, has errors, inaccuracies and variations. A variation in HTLs smaller than the degree of variation between one test and another in an accurate subject is not significant either in diagnosis or in disability assessment. The step size of manual pure-tone audiometry is 5 dB and ±3 dB is an acceptable level of calibration, so a 'loss' of this size is not significant and does not necessarily represent a hearing loss. Before a change is significant it must be a larger-than-average variation between one test and another, which in a reliable subject is about 5 dB in the lower tones and 10 dB in the higher tones (Lawton, 1991) so, with a manual pure-tone audiogram performed in 5-dB steps, a significant change must be no smaller than 10 dB at frequencies up to and including 2 kHz, and 15 dB at higher frequencies. At the very least a variation of 5 dB in the lower and 10 dB in the higher frequencies must be assessed as insignificant. The BAOL/BSA (1983) *Blue Book* method, for example, used a dip of 15 dB at 4 kHz compared with the values obtained at adjoining frequencies before allowing the application of the prognosis allowance – allowing a diagnosis of noise-induced loss because it took into account the above factors. Other writers have suggested that a significant variation must be 17 dB or more at one frequency or 10 dB or more at two adjacent frequencies. Individuals lose much more than this before they notice a problem with their hearing.

Consider inter-test variability when deciding whether or not a threshold variation is significant.

# Disability scales

The disability scale may be linear or non-linear between the low and high fences. The latter is more scientific but the former is easier and, in practice, there is usually no marked difference between the two as non-linear scales tend to be linear or close to linear across most of their range. Assessing hearing disability in percentage from a pure-tone audiogram is inherently illogical and any method must at times be arbitrary. There is no real advantage in using a non-linear scale.

A linear scale is simpler and, in practice, as accurate as a non-linear disability scale.

# Allocation of disability

Noise-induced loss increases most rapidly in the early years of exposure so, perhaps, when allocating disability to different periods of noise exposure the earlier exposure should rate higher. A counterargument is that noise-induced loss tends to spread to the frequencies that are more important for the perception of speech to a significant degree, only later in the course of noise exposure however, this requires prolonged exposure to generally high levels of noise and a sensitive ear. In medicolegal practice it is simpler and sufficiently accurate to assume that each period of noise exposure contributes to the disability in proportion to the noise level and its duration.

Allocate disability in proportion to the total noise dose.

# Conclusions

- An individual may have a noise-induced hearing impairment but no disability.
- Compensation for impairment is not a matter for the clinician.
- An individual hearing at 15–20 dB or better at 0.5, 1, 2 and 4 kHz has normal hearing and no disability.
- It is reasonable to omit 0.5 kHz and to substitute 3 kHz for 4 kHz in a disability formula but not to use both 3 and 4 kHz.
- A hearing threshold level at 90–100 dB or worse at any particular frequency is effectively a total (100%) loss.
- Changes must be greater than 10 dB at one frequency or at least 10 dB at two adjacent frequencies before they may be judged as significant.
- Asymmetry is generally slight in NIHL but a weighting of 4:1 in favour of the better ear in disability assessment is usual.
- Disability is attributed to individual periods of noise exposure in direct proportion to their durations and intensities, that is in proportion to their contributions to the total dose.
- In marked losses there may be no characteristic effect of noise in the audiogram and, if there is a strong history of noise exposure and the

loss is not disproportionate to the noise dose, the application of Dobie's median-based allocation method may be thought equitable.

- A subject with hearing at the level of the average 70-year-old woman or 80-year-old man is unlikely to have an NIHL.
- There is a little logic but no real merit in using a non-linear scale between 0% disability at the low fence and 100% disability at the high fence.
- There is no scientific logic in disability assessment but it is logical in legal terms as damage requires compensation, which can be judged only in monetary terms. The purpose of the law is to resolve disputes in society without bias and without force. In practice the court will decide on compensation without reference to a percentage disability assessment.
- Presbycusis should be assessed using the National Study of Hearing data. In a percentage disability assessment average presbycusis should be assumed in the absence of clear evidence to the contrary.
- To assess the actual loss in dB due to noise at particular frequencies, the percentile of presbycusis to be used may be assessed by examining the HTLs at those frequencies that are not affected by noise.

# Appendix 1: the Coles–Worgan classification

### Description of the handicaps associated with the auditory handicap groups

*Group 0*: no significant auditory handicap.

*Group I*: the hearing is not sufficiently impaired to affect the perception of speech, except for a slight (additional to normal) difficulty in noisy backgrounds.

*Groups II and III*: slight (II) to moderate (III) difficulty whenever listening to faint speech, but would usually understand normal speech. Would also have distinctly greater difficulty when trying to understand speech against a background of noise.

*Groups IV and V*: frequent difficulty with normal speech and would sometimes (IV) or often (V) have to ask people to 'speak up' in order to hear them, even in face-to-face conversation.

*Group VI*: marked difficulties in communication since he would sometimes be unable to clearly understand even loud speech. In noise he would find it impossible to distinguish speech.

*Groups VII and VIII*: would understand only shouted or amplified speech, and then only moderately well (VII) or poorly (VIII).

*Group IX*: minimal speech intelligibility even with well amplified speech.

*Group X*: virtually totally deaf with respect to understanding of speech.

Note: in Groups II–IX some benefit could potentially be gained from a suitable hearing aid.

# Appendix 2: disability ratings

| Sensorineural hearing level disability averaged over 500–1000 –2000 Hz (dB)[a] | Sensorineural hearing level at 4 kHz | Auditory group | Brief description of handicap | % |
|---|---|---|---|---|
| < 25 | < 25 | 0 | Not significant | 0 |
| < 25 | > 25, < 50 | I | Just significant | 5 |
| < 25 | > 55 | II | Very slight | 10 |
| >25, < 30 | n/a | II | Very slight | 10 |
| > 30, < 40 | n/a | III | Slight | 20 |
| > 40, < 50 | n/a | IV | Mild | 35 |
| > 50, < 60 | n/a | V | Moderate | 50 |
| > 60, < 70 | n/a | VI | Marked | 65 |
| > 70, < 80 | n/a | VII | Fairly severe | 80 |
| > 80, < 90 | n/a | VIII | Very severe | 90 |
| > 90, < 100 | n/a | IX | Extremely severe | 95 |
| > 100 | n/a | X | Total | 100 |

a Binaural assessment.
n/a, not applicable.

# References

Acton WI (1970) Speech intelligibility in background noise and noise-induced hearing loss. Ergonomics 13: 546–54.

Alberti PW (1997) Noise and the ear. In D Stephens (ed.) Adult Audiology. Volume 2. Scott-Brown's Otolaryngology, 6th edn. London: Butterworth Heinemann.

American College of Occupational and Environmental Medicine (1996) Occupational Noise-Induced Hearing Loss: Position Statement: http://acoem.org/04 StatementsGuides/PositionPapers/ps-nihl.html

Arlinger S (ed.) (1991) Manual of Practical Audiometry, Volume 2. London: Whurr.

Arnold P (1998) Guest editorial: is there still a consensus on impairment, disability and handicap in audiology? British Journal of Audiology 32: 265–71.

Bauer P, Korpert K, Neuberger M, Raber A, Schwetz F (1991) Risk factors for hearing loss at different frequencies in a population of 47,388 noise exposed workers. Journal of the Acoustical Society of America 90: 3086–98.

Blakley BW, Kim S (1998) Does chronic otitis media cause sensorineural hearing loss? Journal of Otolaryngology 27: 17–20.

Brant IJ, Gordon-Salant S, Pearson JD, Klein LL, Morrell CH, Metter EJ (1996) Risk factors related to age-associated hearing loss in the speech frequencies. Journal of the American Academy of Audiology 7: 152–60.

British Association of Otolaryngologists/British Society of Audiology (1983) Method of assessment of hearing disability. British Journal of Audiology 17: 203–12.

Browning GG (1986) Progressive sensorineural hearing impairments. In: Clinical Otology and Audiology. London: Butterworths.

Chuang WP (1986) Forensic audiology. Journal of Otology and Laryngology suppl 11: 1–57.

Dadson RS, King JH (1952) A determination of the normal standard of hearing and its relation to the standardisation of audiometers. Journal of Laryngology and Otology 66: 366–78.

Davis A (1983) Hearing disorders in the population: first phase findings of the MRC National Study of Hearing. In ME Lutman, MR Haggard (eds) Hearing Science and Hearing Disorders. London: Academic Press.

Davis A (1987) Epidemiology. In D Stephens (ed.) Adult Audiology, Volume 2. Scott-Brown's Otolaryngology, 5th edn. London: Butterworths.

Davis A (1989) The prevalence of hearing impairment and reported hearing disability among adults in Great Britain. International Journal of Epidemiology 18: 911–17.

Davis A (ed.) (1995) Hearing in Adults. London: Whurr.

Davis A (1997) Epidemiology. In D Stephens (ed.) Adult Audiology. Volume 2. Scott-Brown's Otolaryngology, 6th edn. London: Butterworth-Heinemann.

Department of Health and Social Security (1973) National Insurance (Industrial Injuries) Act 1965: Occupational Deafness. CMND 5461. London: HMSO.

Dobie RA (1993) Medical-Legal Evaluation of Hearing Loss. New York: Van Nostrand Reinhold.

Dobie RA (2001) Medical-Legal Evaluation of Hearing Loss, 2nd edn. San Diego, CA: Singular.

Health and Safety Executive (1978) Code of Practice for Reducing the Exposure of Employed Persons to Noise. London: HMSO.

Hinchcliffe R (1992) King–Kopetzky syndrome: an auditory stress disorder? Journal of Audiological Medicine 1: 89–98

Hinchcliffe R (1994) Sound, infrasound and ultrasound. In PAB Raffle, PH Adams, PJ Baxter, W Lee (eds) Hunter's Diseases of Occupations. London: Edward Arnold.

Hinchcliffe R (1997) Obituary to 'Dix' (Wallace Dixon Ward). Journal of Audiological Medicine 6: iii–vi.

International Association of Physicians in Audiology (1992) IAPA Bulletin 9: 10–11.

International Organization for Standardization (1984) ISO 7029: Acoustics – Threshold of hearing by air conduction as a function of age and sex for otologically normal persons. Geneva: ISO.

International Organization for Standardization (1990) ISO 1999: Acoustics – Determination of occupational noise exposure and estimation of noise induced hearing impairment. Geneva: ISO.

International Organization for Standardization (1991) ISO 389: Acoustics – Standard reference zero for the calibration of pure-tone audiometers, 3rd edn. Geneva: ISO.

King PF, Coles RRA, Lutman ME, Robinson DW (1992) Assessment of Hearing Disability. London: Whurr.

Lawton BW (1991) Perspectives on Normal and Near-normal Hearing. ISVR Technical Report No. 200, University of Southampton

Leijon A (1992) Quantization error in clinical pure-tone audiometry. Scandinavian Audiology 21: 103–8.

Lightfoot GR, Mason SM (1989) Course Notes – Electric Response Audiometry Principles, Techniques and Clinical Applications. University of Liverpool. U.K.

Lutman ME (1997) Diagnostic audiometry. In D Stephens (ed.) Adult Audiology, Volume 2. Scott-Brown's Otolaryngology. London Butterworth: Heinemann.

Lutman ME, Qasem HYN (1998) A source of audiometric notches at 6 kHz. In D Prasher, L Luxon (eds) Advances in Noise Research, Volume 1. London: Whurr, Chapter 16.

Lutman ME, Spencer HS (1991) Occupational noise and demographic factors in hearing. Acta Otolaryngologica Supplementum. 476: 74–84.

Neild P (1985) Occupational Deafness. London: The Chartered Insurance Institute, p50.

Robinson DW (1976) Characteristics of noise-induced hearing loss. In D Henderson, RP Hamernik, DS Dosanjih, JH Mills (eds) Effects of Noise on Hearing. New York: Raven.

Robinson DW (1984) Audiometric Configurations and Repeatability in Noise-induced Hearing Loss. ISVR Technical Report No. 123. University of Southampton.

Robinson DW (1988) Threshold of hearing as a function of age and sex for the typical unscreened population. British Journal of Audiology 22: 5–20.

Robinson DW (1990) Non-organic hearing loss. In DW Robinson (ed.) Clinical Audiology Course Notes. Southampton: Institute of Sound and Vibration Research, University of Southampton.

Robinson DW (1991) Relation between hearing threshold and its component parts. British Journal of Audiology 25: 93–103.

Robinson DW, Shipton MS (1979) Tables for the estimation of noise-induced hearing loss. NPL Acoustics Report Ac 61, 2nd edn. Teddington: National Physical Laboratory.

Robinson DW, Sutton GJ (1978) A comparative analysis of data on the relation of pure-tone audiometric thresholds to age. NPL Acoustics Report Ac 84. Teddington: National Physical Laboratory.

Robinson DW, Wilkins PA, Thyer NJ Lawes JF (1984) Auditory Impairment and the Onset of Disability and Handicap in Noise Induced Hearing Loss. ISVR Technical Report No. 126. University of Southampton.

Rosenhall U, Pedersen K, Svanborg A (1990) Presbycusis and noise-induced hearing loss. Ear and Hearing 11: 257–63.

Shipton MS (1979) Tables relating pure-tone audiometric threshold to age. Acoustics Report Ac 94. Teddington: National Physical Laboratory.

Stephens SDG, Hetu R (1991) Impairment, disability and handicap in audiology. Audiology 30: 185–200.

Stephens SDG, Rendell RJ (1988) Auditory disability with normal hearing. Quaderni di Audiologia 4: 233–8.

Wheeler IJ, Dickson EDD (1952) The determination of the threshold of hearing. Journal of Laryngology and Otology 66: 379–95.

Willott JF (1991) Aging and the Auditory System: Anatomy, physiology and psychophysics. London: Whurr.

Wright A (1997) Anatomy and ultrastructure of the human ear. In M Gleeson (ed.) Basic Sciences, Volume 1, Scott-Brown's Otolaryngology, 6th edn. London: Butterworth-Heinemann.

# CHAPTER 12

# Tinnitus and external sounds

*Noise and Its Effects:* Edited by Linda Luxon and Deepak Prasher © 2007
John Wiley & Sons Ltd.

BORKA CERANIC

## Introduction

The relevance of external sounds to tinnitus has been well recognized for a long time. Sound may cause tinnitus by 'excitement of the senses' (Ibn'i Sina, AD 980–1038) and cure tinnitus 'because a greater sound drives out less' (Hippocrates, 460–377 BC) (quoted by Vernon, 1981; Stephens, 1984).

The interaction between the auditory system and sounds is fundamental to the evaluation of the acoustic environment and the process of adaptation in general. Nevertheless, in some adverse circumstances, the combination of inherent characteristics of the auditory system of an individual, and particular physical properties of environmental sounds, may create a basis for the generation of tinnitus.

External sounds may interact with the auditory system in a way that leads to tinnitus, even when they are well below the known hazardous level. However, the effect of intense sounds, which exceed the physiological range of the auditory system and cause pathological alterations at different levels of the auditory system, leading to tinnitus, is much more common and well recognised.

This chapter will explore different ways by which sounds may interact with the auditory system, with tinnitus as a consequence. The generation of tinnitus will also be considered in the context of the complex feedback control mechanism of the auditory system.

## Pathogenesis of tinnitus – functional anatomy of the auditory system

The term 'tinnitus' encompasses a variety of auditory sensations, occurring as a consequence of altered spontaneous neural activity, due to aberrant

258

'stimulation' from within the auditory system, which differs from the baseline, unstimulated state.

It may also be assumed that tinnitus arises from an altered state of excitation and/or inhibition of the auditory system.

# The auditory system and its feedback control

The optimal operating status of the auditory system is maintained by a complex feedback mechanism, which involves the afferent, ascending, and the efferent, descending pathways, as illustrated schematically in Figure 12.1. The auditory pathway is also linked with other, extra-auditory structures, which support its integration with the central nervous system (CNS) network.

The afferent pathway, which provides an input to the proximal structures of the auditory system, facilitates predominantly excitatory processes, while the parallel efferent pathway, which modulates acoustic information, facilitates predominantly inhibitory processes.

## The auditory pathway

### The cochlea

The afferent system originates at the cochlear level, from the organ of Corti, which contains the outer (OHCs) and the inner (IHCs) hair cells (Figure 12.1). The OHCs are the principal elements of the active mechano-electrical transduction system (Brownell, 1990; Gale and Ashmore, 1997), with the capacity to amplify or attenuate the incoming acoustic signal. The OHCs feed controlled mechanical oscillation to the IHCs, which represent a true sensory receptor, transducing mechanical energy into neural activity.

The afferent pathway runs almost exclusively from the synapse with the IHCs, with glutamate, known to be a widespread excitatory neurotransmitter of the CNS, as the main neurotransmitter (Puel, 1995). The IHCs receive a small fraction of the efferent input, through the lateral olivocochlear fibres. In contrast, the OHCs receive the major portion of the efferent input predominantly via the medial olivocochlear fibres. Efferent activity is mediated by acetylcholine, which at the cochlear level acts as a fast inhibitory neurotransmitter, unlike its role in the CNS as an excitatory neurotransmitter (Oliver et al., 2000). Another efferent neurotransmitter is $\gamma$-aminobutyric acid (GABA) (Altschuler and Fex, 1986), which is the main inhibitory neurotransmitter of the CNS.

This distinctly different innervation pattern in the cochlea underpins the dual sensory system in the cochlea: the IHCs as a part of the afferent system and the OHCs as the effector organ of the efferent system, both controlled and modulated by the CNS.

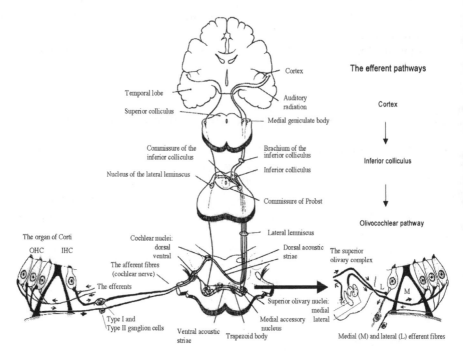

**Figure 12.1** The schematic view of the auditory system, including the efferent pathway. IHC, inner hair cell; OHC, outer hair cell.

## Retrocochlear afferent pathway

The *auditory nerve* enters the brain stem at the cerebellopontine angle and this point marks the beginning of the central auditory system. The auditory nerve branches into three major divisions, to the anteroventral, posteroventral and dorsal *cochlear nuclei* (CN), located on the posterolateral surface of the pontomedullary junction. The fibres from the CN project ipsilaterally and contralaterally to the *superior olivary complex* (SOC) and contralaterally to the lateral lemniscus (LL) and in to the inferior colliculus (IC).

The SOC is located in the pons and is composed of several nuclei, including the lateral superior olivary (LSO) and medial superior olivary (MSO) nuclei. Both of these structures receive bilateral innervation, and, therefore, provide the anatomical basis for binaural representation and integration of acoustic signals and reciprocal cochlear interaction, mediated by the olivocochlear (OC) system.

The next relay station is the *lateral lemniscus* (LL) and related nuclei, which receive inputs from the CN and the SOC, contra- and ipsilaterally. The LL is a major auditory tract containing afferent and efferent fibres. The LL on both sides communicates through the commissure of Probst or via the pontine reticular formation.

The next station is the inferior colliculus (IC), which receives the auditory fibres predominantly crossing from the opposite side. The central nucleus of the IC is composed purely of auditory fibres, while the pericentral nucleus, contains both auditory and somatosensory fibres. The IC is highly tonotopically organized and is characterized by extremely sharp tuning curves, suggesting a high degree of frequency resolution.

The next relay station is the *medial geniculate body* (MGB), which is located on the inferior, dorsolateral surface of the thalamus. From the MGB there are multiple and complex thalamocortical projections upon the tonotopically organized cortical fields. The major thalamo-cortical pathway projects to the primary auditory cortical area in Heschl's gyrus. Another thalamocortical pathway, containing auditory, somatic and, possibly, visual fibres, passes towards the secondary acoustic areas.

The *auditory cortical area* encompasses the posterior three-quarters of the Sylvian fissure. Heschl's gyrus (also termed the transverse gyrus) is considered the primary auditory cortical area (Brodmann's areas 41 and 42), which receives most of the thalamocortical projections and is tono-topically organized, suggesting that most of the auditory information is processed initially in this area. The secondary auditory cortical areas are responsible for a variety of complex auditory processing, including the analysis of complex sounds (for example, noise, music or speech decoding), short-term memory for comparison of tones, inhibition of unwanted motor responses and intent listening (attention).

The primary auditory area has intra- and interhemispheric connections to different parts of the brain, which enable activation of different specialized secondary areas, depending on the complexity of the auditory signals.

The *corpus callosum* (CC) contains interhemispheric auditory fibres, confined to the posterior half of the CC, which connect the cortices of each hemisphere. The presence of excitatory and inhibitory fibres, suggests a role of the CC in modulating the activity in both hemispheres, allowing optimal integration of cortical responses (Musiek, 1986).

## The efferent pathway

The efferent system runs in parallel to the afferent system, from the cortex to the cochlea, allowing multiple feedback loops (Suga et al., 2000), but it is less well defined than the afferent auditory system. It is thought that there is a pathway from the cortex to the MGB and another from the cortex to the different nuclei in the brain stem. The IC receives input from both the cortex and the MGB. From the IC, there are efferent connections to the SOC system and CN, and to the nuclei of the LL.

The best known part of the efferent system is the OC system, which was first described by Rassmusen in 1946 arises from the SOC (see Figure 12.1). The fibres from the lateral SO nucleus are arranged in the predominantly uncrossed, lateral (LOC) bundle that projects to afferent fibres of the IHCs. The fibres from the medial nucleus are arranged in the mainly crossed, medial (MOC) bundle and project directly on to the OHCs. During this course, the MOC bundle runs under the floor of the fourth ventricle. The olivocochlear bundle (OCB) fibres leave the brain stem and join the vestibular nerve trunk, which, together with the auditory nerve, travels towards the cochlea.

Although the MOC system has been the most studied part of the efferent system, its functional aspects are still not well understood. The MOC system is considered to be responsible for the control of the OHCs' motility (Zenner, 1986), by an inhibitory effect (Wiederhold, 1986), which has been demonstrated as reduced otoacoustic emission response amplitude, during contralateral acoustic stimulation (Collet et al., 1990; Ryan et al., 1991). However, there is evidence to suggest that the MOC system enhances transient stimuli if they are presented against background noise (Kavase et al., 1993).

Anatomical and physiological studies of the IC connections with the SOC system, and in particular the origin of stimulation of the OC neurons, allowing direct collicular influence on cochlear mechanics (Warr and Guinan, 1979; Dolan and Nuttall, 1988; Huffman and Henson, 1990), strongly suggest that the IC plays a role in the activity of the OC system.

Much less is known about the LOC system. It is believed that it may have a protective role against excessive noise and/or excitotoxicity (Pujol, 1994). It may also facilitate the excitatory effect of glutamate by modulation of sensitivity of glutamate-sensitive $N$-methyl-D-aspartate (NMDA) and non-NMDA receptors, and therefore, enhance neuronal activity and spontaneous discharge, through release of endogenous opioid peptides, the dynorphins (reviewed by Sahley et al., 1999).

The efferent auditory system probably controls the level of excitation within the auditory system and its assumed role is to facilitate and enhance the targeted acoustic signal and to inhibit unwanted signal, such as noise. It also mediates frequency-selective auditory attention.

## Extra-auditory neural connections

The auditory pathway has connections with other parts of the CNS, making the auditory system an integral part of the CNS and allowing direct and indirect effects of the CNS on auditory function.

The *reticular formation* appears to play a major role in auditory alertness, reflexes, sleep and habituation. Serotoninergic fibres and terminal endings are present in the cochlear nucleus, the IC, the nuclei of the LL, the SOC and the primary auditory cortex (Andorn et al., 1989; Thompson et al., 1994; Woods and Azeredo, 1999). A serotoninergic input to the lower brain stem may provide a basis for modulation of the acoustic reflexes, both olivocochlear and stapedial (Thompson and Thompson, 1995; Maison et al., 1999). The serotoninergic system appears to have a major role as a 'stabilizer' in the autoregulatory circuitry within the CNS (review by Simpson and Davies, 2000).

The auditory system also has connections with the *somatosensory system*, including the MGB (a multisensory thalamic area) and the IC which coordinates auditory, visual and somatic information (Hufmann and Henson, 1990).

Via the IC, the auditory pathway has input from the *hypothalamus* (Adams, 1980) – the principal organ of integration of the endocrine system and the control centre of all autonomic functions, including mechanisms of adaptation – response to stress and emotions.

The *limbic system*, which is the site of instinctive behaviour and emotions, receives projections from the MGB, and this link is hypothesized to serve in the attachment of emotional significance to perceived sounds (LeDoux et al., 1983).

# The relevance of the auditory feedback mechanism to tinnitus

The ascending, predominantly excitatory, and the efferent, predominantly inhibitory, pathways, interact through the feedback mechanism, thus creating a highly dynamic system in which pathological alteration at one level may have functional consequences at other level(s) of the auditory system. For instance, a noise-induced cochlear lesion with a resulting decrease in the auditory input, leads to compensatory disinhibition in the proximal auditory pathway and, in the long term, tonontopic reorganization, which could be a basis for tinnitus (see below).

A change in the equilibrium between the excitatory and inhibitory forces, regardless of the nature and site of the pathological abnormality within the auditory system, may alter spontaneous activity in the auditory cortex, with the perception of tinnitus as a consequence.

**Functional anatomy – summary points**
- The auditory system sets the 'scene' for the occurrence of tinnitus.
- With all its integral parts, each of them having some degree of autonomy and at the same time dependency, the auditory system creates a multitude of possibilities for generation of tinnitus.
- The links of the auditory system with other parts of the central nervous system allow the emergence of tinnitus-related activity even outside the auditory system and the extra-auditory connections increase the complexity of tinnitus.
- The afferent and efferent pathways create the highly dynamic system, with a hierarchy of the feedback auto-regulatory loops, due to which alterations in one part may have functional consequences in other parts of the auditory system.

# Tinnitus-related cortical activity

The recent emergence of functional imaging techniques has provided new insight into *spatial processing* of tinnitus-related signal. Single-proton emission computed tomography (SPECT), positron emission tomography (PET) and functional magnetic resonance imaging (fMRI) have demonstrated that the perception of tinnitus is associated with alterations in the cortical areas. Investigation is of particular value in those patients who are able to control their tinnitus – they can 'switch' it on and off by a voluntary act, such as change in gaze direction or jaw movement (Lockwood et al., 1998), with increased metabolic activity when subjects turn on their tinnitus. There is evidence that more auditory cortical areas are activated in patients with tinnitus than in control subjects, including the associative cortices, the left hypocampus, the right prefrontal–temporal network and the limbic areas (Shulman et al., 1995; Lockwood et al., 1998, 1999). The extent of the neuronal network involved is thought to influence the quality and attributes of tinnitus. The activation of cortical centres subserving emotions (the limbic system) may explain the emotional response to tinnitus.

Figure 12.2 illustrates the neural sites in the auditory cortex, that may mediate tinnitus (Lockwood et al., 2002).

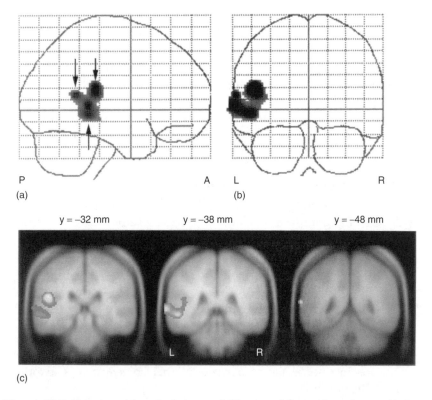

**Figure 12.2** Drawings (a) sagittal view and (b) coronal from (c) positron emission tomography (PET) scan indicating neural sites in the auditory cortex that mediate right-sided tinnitus, with the areas of activation in the left cortical sites: the unilaterality suggests that tinnitus (aberrant activity) is of central origin (as peripheral auditory stimulation is associated with bicortical sound representation); the $y$ values indicate the distance of each site from the plane of the anterior commissure. A= Anterior, P=Posterior, L=Left, R=Right (From Lockwood et al., 2002.)

The *temporal aspect* of neural activity (altered rate, temporal discharge pattern, and/or temporal correlation between the discharge patterns of different nerve fibres) may also be of relevance for tinnitus generation and have been subjects of interest of a number of authors. Bursts of neural activity after salicylate or noise exposure has been observed in the auditory nerve (Liberman and Kiang, 1978; Evans et al., 1981) and in the IC (Chen and Jastreboff, 1995), but not in the cortex (Ochi and Eggermont, 1997). However, the greater degree of synchronous firing in the cortical neurons of cats has been documented (Ochi and Eggermont, 1997).

**Tinnitus-related cortical activity – Summary points**

- Functional imaging techniques have allowed mapping of the neural sites, auditory and extra-auditory, that mediate the generation of tinnitus.
- Recording of tinnitus-related cortical activity provides the evidence of the 'physical' nature of tinnitus.

# The generation mechanisms of sound-related tinnitus

The empirical data suggest that a source of the alteration in spontaneous activity within the auditory system could be a lesion or dysfunction at any level of the auditory system, from the cochlea to its uppermost levels.

Among different causes, the exposure to intense sounds is reported to be a single most common cause of tinnitus (46%: Penner, 1990; 28%: Axelsson, 1992), although less commonly, tinnitus may arise from the interaction with sounds below the known hazardous level, as discussed below. In the general population, tinnitus is more common in those with a history of excessive noise exposure (20%) than those without (7.5%) (Davies and Rafaie, 2000).

# Pathophysiological mechanisms relevant to sound-induced tinnitus

## Abnormal afferent excitation at the cochlear level

### *'Mechanical' tinnitus related to spontaneous cochlear oscillations*

The discovery of the existence of spontaneous otoacoustic emissions (SOAEs) and their recording (Kemp, 1979) have led to the expectation that SOAEs might be an objective correlate of tinnitus. Although subsequent extensive studies have produced disappointing results (reviewed by Ceranic et al., 1995), it has been established that SOAEs could be a direct cause of tinnitus – SOAEs being audible to the patient, in a small number of individuals with tinnitus: the 95% confidence limits for the prevalence are 1% and 9.5% (Penner, 1990).

Spontaneous cochlear activity may be relevant to tinnitus, not necessarily as a direct cause of tinnitus. It is likely that the presence of spontaneous activity makes the cochlea, and therefore the auditory system, inherently unstable and sensitive to external sounds. Sound may act as a source of energy to set the cochlea into a state of mechanical instability and sustained oscillations (Kemp, 1981, 1982). Thus spontaneous cochlear activity could predispose to tinnitus, a concept that is supported by the finding of tinnitus more commonly in subjects with audiometrically normal hearing and recordable SOAEs than those without SOAEs (Duchamp et al., 1995). Whether tinnitus-related spontaneous activity is a result of changes within the cochlea, or a dysfunctional efferent system, is difficult to establish. Figure 12.3 illustrates SOAEs and transient evoked emissions of the high amplitude, as an expression of increased cochlear gain, thought to be due to efferent dysfunction and the subsequent disinhibition phenomenon, which has been suggested as a cause of tinnitus (Ceranic et al., 1998a). Tinnitus may also be due to

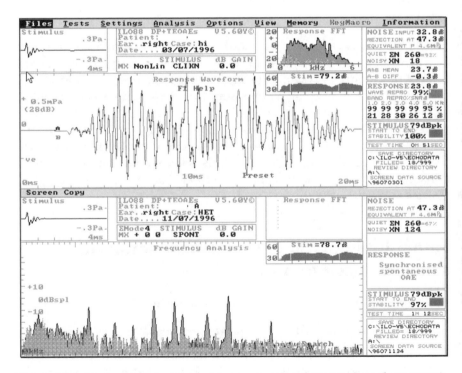

**Figure 12.3** 'Strong' transient evoked (upper trace) and spontaneous (lower trace) otoacoustic emissions in a 44-year-old man who complained of tinnitus, hyperacusis and difficulty in hearing, following a brain injury. He had normal pure-tone audiometric thresholds and the olivocochlear test indicated absence of suppression on the right (0 dB) and reduced suppression on the left (0.2 dB).

some instability between the excitation and inhibition within the auditory system, reflected by variable SOAEs (Ceranic et al., 1998b).

*Interaction of SOAEs and external sounds*

Spontaneous otoacoustic emissions may interact directly with external sounds, leading to different auditory perceptions.

The phenomenon of the interaction between external and hypothetical 'internal' sounds had been known long before SOAEs were demonstrated (Kemp, 1979).

In 1931, in his classic paper on tinnitus, following experiments on his own tinnitus, Wegel described a perceptual experience of 'beats' on the introduction of a test tone. Flottorp (1953) and Ward (1955) have also demonstrated that external pure tone can elicit sensation of 'beats' when a single tone near the frequency of the 'idiotone', presumably an SOAE, was presented, and that the beat rate depended on the intensity of the external tone. Flottorp, therefore, concluded that 'idiotone makes itself known by interfering with the stimulus tone'.

Following the introduction of otoacoustic emissions (OAEs), Zurek (1981) during his experiments, also experienced 'beats', but he was able to demonstrate acoustically the temporal variation of the 'beats', synchronized SOAE, by changing the sound pressure of the acoustic input at the frequency of his own SOAE.

Wilson (1980) and Wilson and Sutton (1981) have demonstrated that synchronization may occur following pure-tone, click or tone-burst stimuli, at a relatively low level of stimulation (around 25 dB sound level or SL) and that an SOAE 'would be forced to oscillate at the same frequency as the stimulus' – its frequency would be 'pulled in'. At a stimulus intensity level just below this, phase locking will occur for a certain period; then influences such as noise and change in sensitivity will allow the emission to escape control and to oscillate at its natural frequency until phases are sufficiently close for locking to be re-established. This process repeats in an irregular manner and explains why beats between tinnitus and an external tone are irregular and slower than would usually be expected for independent oscillations.

Flottorp (1953) and Ward (1955) have described a condition in which a pure tone does not sound 'pure', but elicits a sensation of multiple tones. This distortion was apparent at low sound pressures, but above an upper limit, which depended on the frequency of tone, the sensation was no longer distorted and was that of a pure tone. The multitonality that arises from single-tone stimulation (monaural diplacusis) can now be understood as being *combination tones* (distortion products), resulting from two tones, primaries, at closely spaced frequencies $f_1$ and $f_2$, one corresponding to the SOAE and the other to an external tone. Zurek (1981), again, in addition to his perceptual experience, was able to demonstrate this phenomenon acoustically, as distortion products, generated through the interaction of the external tone and his SOAE.

It is apparent that a multitude of possible interactions of 'overactive' cochlear elements (SOAEs) and external sound may occur. Binaural exposure to sounds in normal environmental conditions is assumed, and additional contralateral effects make the relationship between the external sounds and the sound emitted by the cochlea even more complex. It is also very likely that a perceptual experience corresponding to the interaction of external sounds and 'overactive' elements in tinnitus patients, in whom an altered spontaneous auditory activity and/or imbalance in inhibitory/excitatory mechanisms may exist, could be even more pronounced.

These phenomena may help to explain why some subjects are affected by environmental noise, well below a hazardous level, leading to the complaints such as induced or prolonged tinnitus, sound distortions or 'echoing' tinnitus. The results of OAEs in such a subject are illustrated in Figure 12.4.

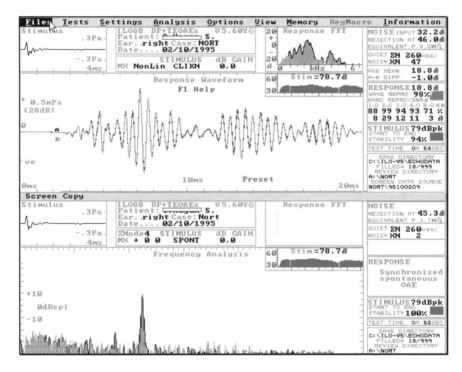

**Figure 12.4** Spontaneous otoacoustic emissions (lower trace) and sustained, 'oscillating' transient evoked otoacoustic emission responses (upper trace) in a 38-year-old male patient who complained of 'echoing' tinnitus in the presence of environmental sounds and who was tinnitus free in quiet conditions.

## Glutamate neuro-excitotoxicity

As outlined earlier in the section on functional anatomy, glutamate has been considered the main neurotransmitter of the cochlear afferents, released into the IHC synaptic region. Besides its potent excitatory effect, glutamate also displays a highly neurotoxic effect, observed in various pathological conditions, including acoustic trauma (Puel, 1995). Excessive noise exposure leads to excessive glutamate release and excitotoxic intracellular $Ca^{2+}$ overload, which could be a basis for tinnitus (Pujol, 1994). It has been reported that glutamate receptors, for example NMDA, can be selectively blocked by their agonist (for example, Caroverine), abolishing tinnitus in a significant number of patients (Brix et al., 1995; Denk et al., 1997).

### Modulation (enhanced sensitivity) of NMDA and non-NMDA receptors

The lateral olivocochlear efferents may play a role in modulating the sensitivity of the afferent receptors in the cochlea. It has been suggested that dopamine, as a neurotransmitter, may produce permanent gain control at the site of the action potential initiation (Puel et al., 2002). The application of dopamine agonist (Piribedil) has been found to have a protective action against glutamate-induced excitotoxicity, reducing the incidence of noise-induced tinnitus (D'Aldin et al., 1995).

It has also been suggested that endogenous opioid peptide dynorphins, released on to the IHC synaptic region by the lateral olivocochlear fibres as a part of the response to stress (Sahley et al., 1999), may enhance sensitivity of the NMDA and non-NMDA receptors and facilitate afferent excitation, thus providing a basis for stress-induced tinnitus.

### Efferent dysfunction/reduction of the GABA effect

As described in the section on functional anatomy, the efferent system acts as an inhibitory force within the auditory system and its malfunction may lead to disinhibition, which could be a basis for tinnitus. Following the introduction of OAE techniques and the olivocochlear suppression test (recording of OAEs under contralateral acoustic stimulation) (Collet et al., 1990), several studies have suggested dysfunction (a reduction in the suppressive effect) of the medial olivocochlear system, as the underlying mechanism of tinnitus (Veuillet et al, 1992; Chèry-Croze et al, 1994; Ceranic et al, 1998a). Furthermore, it has been suggested, from the data of recording event-related potentials, that this could be part of a global efferent dysfunction, involving other sensory modalities (Attias et al, 1996). A significant intra-subject variability of the medial olivocochlear suppressive effect may also be of relevance for tinnitus (Graham and Hazell, 1994).

Recent animal experiments (Maison et al, 2002), have indicated that surgical de-efferentation and reduced 'strength' of the medial olivocochlear reflex increase vulnerability to acoustic injury, and therefore tinnitus, implying a protective role of this system. Furthermore, the authors have demonstrated that deletion of the gene for the nicotinic $\alpha$-9-cholinergic receptor expressed in the OHCs makes experimental animals functionally de-efferented. The over-expression of this receptor enhances classic efferent effects on the cochlea, leading to resistance to acoustic injury. This implies genetically based susceptibility to noise damage and tinnitus.

Exposure to intense sounds, as well as ageing, may alter inhibitory amino acid neurotransmitter receptors in the central auditory pathways, particularly in the cochlear nucleus and inferior colliculus, and a down-regulation of GABA has been suspected to alter/reduce inhibitory function of the efferent system (Caspary et al., 2001).

## Alteration of spontaneous activity and tonotopic reorganization following intense sound exposure

Transient tinnitus as a result of excessive external sounds of short duration is a common phenomenon. In experiments with brief noise overexposure (16–30 s, 100–110 dB SPL), Kemp (1982) demonstrated a biphasic effect: first, the reduction of the cochlear echo was observed, followed by the enhancement of micromechanical cochlear activity (enhanced OAEs), coinciding with post-noise exposure tinnitus and consistent with a compensatory (disinhibitory) feedback response, with an 'overshoot'.

However, when the sound intensity exceeds the cochlear physiological working range, it leads to the structural damage of the cochlea. The resulting sound deprivation further leads to alteration of spontaneous activity in the proximal pathway and plastic transformations within the brain. These alterations may occur instantly or with a delay (Eggermont, 2000).

Electrophysiological studies have indicated that cochlear lesions alter activity in the auditory nerve and increase spontaneous activity of the dorsal cochlear nucleus (DCN), IC (Willot and Lu, 1982; Salvi and Ahroon, 1983; Salvi et al., 1996; Zacharek et al., 2002; Kaltenbach et al., 2004), MGB (Gerken, 1979) and cortical neurons (Komiya and Eggermont, 2000). This noise-induced neural hyperactivity, which is thought to be a neurophysiological correlate of tinnitus, has been demonstrated to be maintained independently of the cochlea, implying that hyperactivity, and therefore tinnitus, originate centrally (Zacharek et al., 2002). As the IC is the obligatory relay for the ascending auditory pathway (Huffman and Henson, 1990), this hyperactivity may cause an imbalance between excitatory and inhibitory mechanisms, mediated by the neurotransmitters of the auditory pathways, such as glutamate, glycine, acetylcholine or GABA. This is supported by the finding of an increase in DCN spontaneous activity, following intense tone exposure, which implies that hyperactive changes in the dorsal nucleus are due to changes in the cholinergic centrifugal pathways (Chang et al., 2002), whereas baclofen (GABA$_B$ agonist) reverses noise-induced hyperactivity of the IC (Szczepaniak and Møller, 1996). In addition to an increase in spontaneous neural rate, acute and chronic noise exposure also show functional reorganization at the IC level, with a significant expansion of the low-frequency tail of the tuning curve and a significant improvement in sensitivity in the tail of the tuning curve (Wang et al., 2002). These changes suggest heterogeneous disinhibition in the IC from the proximal pathway, as a result of acoustic trauma.

Studies of the auditory cortical neurons have indicated changes in their frequency selectivity. Reduced afferent input, due to cochlear lesions, initiates a sequence of changes in the relative levels of excitatory and inhibitory inputs to the primary auditory cortical neurons. This leads to expansion of the receptive field (located in the cochlea, adjacent to the damaged region) of the cortical neurons (Rajan et al., 1992), which in turn raises the threshold sensitivity and broadens frequency selectivity. Restricted damage to the cochlea also produces a tonotopic reorganization of the receptor surface in the primary auditory cortex. The area in the auditory cortex deprived of its characteristic frequency peripheral input acquires a new characteristic frequency – of that at the edge of the region of cochlear damage (Robertson and Irvine, 1989; Schwaber et al., 1993). In other words, the damage to the cochlea leads to an expansion of the cortical representation of a restricted frequency band adjacent to the region of the cochlear loss. Such plasticity of frequency selectivity and auditory maps may alter perceptual function and, therefore, may contribute to the emergence of tinnitus.

The findings from functional imaging (PET, fMRI) of expansion of the brain regions responsive to tones provide strong evidence for plastic tonotopic transformation of the brain in these patients (Møller, 2000). Similar observations have been made in experimental animals after damage to the cochlea (Recanzone et al., 1993). More recently, using EEG-mismatch negativity, abnormal auditory-mismatch responses, as lesion-edge-specific effects related to the slope of high-frequency hearing loss in tinnitus patients, were demonstrated, indicating complex reorganization of neural response properties in the auditory cortex following cochlear damage and suggesting objective evidence for tinnitus (Weisz et al., 2004). Moreover, enhancement of steady-state auditory evoked magnetic fields was found to be consistent with increased excitability of the frequency in the primary auditory cortex above the audiometric edge and the perception of tinnitus (Diesch et al., 2004).

Information processing in the CNS has also been shown to be affected in a patient with tinnitus following noise-induced hearing loss, as measured by auditory and visual event-related potentials (Attias et al., 1993, 1996; Attias and Bresloff, 1997), contingent negative variation (Hoke and Hoke, 1997) and neuromagnetic fields (Hoke et al., 1989; Shiomi et al., 1997).

These data imply that tinnitus may be due to altered spontaneous activity in the CNS and aberrant neural pathways formed during plastic transformation of the brain. The major role in mediating these alterations

has been attributed to serotoninergic system, which is thought to regu-
late/modulate the complex autoregulatory circuitry of a compensatory
mechanism, as a result of an auditory insult (Cransac et al., 1996).

Indeed, abnormal serotonin reuptake on SPECT was found to be associated with tinnitus and depression (Uusitalo et al., 2004).

**Stress and noise**

Circumstantial evidence exists that stress is of relevance in the generation
of tinnitus, particularly in individuals with negative psychological conditions or psychiatric disturbances (Lundberg, 1999). Moreover, in a recent
study (Hebert et al., 2004) it was demonstrated that elevated saliva cortisol levels are associated with high tinnitus-related distress. Stress may
activate various biological functions, including the sympathetic adrenal
medullary system, with secretion of catecholamines (adrenaline and noradrenaline), and the hypothalamic–pituitary–adrenocortical system, with
the secretion of glucocorticoids (such as cortisol). The response to stress
may not be sufficiently effective in maintaining homeostasis of the auditory system and, therefore, stress may provide a basis for the emergence
of tinnitus. Stress may also contribute to the generation of tinnitus
through the activity of the lateral olivocochlear system, which, as discussed earlier, may enhance the sensitivity of glutamate receptors by
release of the endogenous opioid peptide dynorphins onto the IHC
synaptic region. Chronic exposure to dynorphin may lead to neural excitotoxicity and possibly tinnitus (Sahley and Nodar, 2001), which would be
even more pronounced in the presence of intense noise and resulting
glutamate exitotoxicity.

Therefore, stress, in addition to sound exposure, increases the vulnerability of an individual to developing tinnitus.

# Psychological disorders/depression and dysfunction of monoamine neurotrasmitter circuits

Dysregulation of monoamine neurotransmitters, particularly serotonin
(6-hydroxytryptamine or 6-HT) and noradrenaline, as well as dopamine,
has been implicated in the pathophysiology of depression and mood disorders (Owens and Nemeroff, 1998; Ressler and Nemeroff, 1999; Meyer
et al., 2001). It has also been suggested that serotonin might play a role
in the generation of tinnitus (Simpson and Davies, 2000), which may
explain the well-recognized co-morbidity of tinnitus and depression
(Anderson and McKenna, 1998). This implies that individuals with such
disorders may be more susceptible to the development of sound–induced
tinnitus.

**The mechanisms of the generation of sound-related tinnitus – summary points**

- External noise is the single most common cause of tinnitus and it may alter spontaneous activity at different levels of the auditory system through various mechanisms.
- Abnormal afferent excitation at the cochlear level, as the external noise may:
  - influence cochlear mechanics
  - produce excessive release of glutamate, leading to excitotoxicity
  - modulate the sensitivity of glutamate receptors (NMDA and non-NMDA).
- Reduced efferent suppression is suspected to increase the vulnerability of the auditory system to external noise and could be a basis for tinnitus.
- Noise-induced structural damage of the cochlea may lead to compensatory hyperactivity in the proximal auditory pathway, with subsequent plastic transformation of the brain and tonotopic reorganization of the receptive fields.
- Stress and negative psychological conditions may predispose the emergence of tinnitus, the former through the release of sympathetic neuroactive substances and the latter through disregulation of monoamine and other neurotransmitter systems.

# Conclusion

A number of studies have demonstrated that sound exposure produces morphological and functional changes at different levels of the auditory system and, therefore, both 'peripheral' and 'central' mechanisms are intertwined in the generation of tinnitus. In the majority of cases of sound-related tinnitus, tinnitus is attributed to the excessive level of sound and, owing to the mechanical force of sound exposure, the most extensive morphological changes are expected to occur in the cochlea. However, tinnitus in some individuals may result from interaction between the auditory system and external sound, below the known hazardous level. It therefore appears that the mechanisms of tinnitus generation depend on structural integrity of the auditory system and other specific, inherent characteristics, which could make an individual susceptible to developing tinnitus, including genetic background, negative psychological conditions, reduced effectiveness of physiological protective mechanisms (the medial SOC and the stapedial reflex), the presence of SOAEs, and so forth.

Consideration of potential mechanism(s) involved in the generation of tinnitus in each individual is essential for adopting a rational approach in the management of this condition.

# References

Adams JC (1980) Crossed and descending projections to the inferior colliculus. Neuroscience Letters 19:1–5.

Andersson G, McKenna L (1998) Tinnitus masking and depression. Audiology 37:174–82.

Andorn AC, Vittorio JA, Bellflower J (1989). $^3$H-spiroperidol binding in human temporal cortex (Brodmann areas 41–42) occurs at multiple high affinity states with serotonergic selectivity. Psychopharmacology 99:520–5.

Altschuler RA, Fex J (1986) Efferent neurotransmitters. In RA Altschuler (ed.) Neurobiology of Hearing: The Cochlea. New York: Raven Press pp.383–96.

Attias J, Bresloff I (1997) Neurophysiology of tinnitus. In Book of Abstracts, 2nd European Conference on Protection Against Noise (PAN), London.

Attias J, Urbach D, Gold S, Shemesh Z ( 1993) Auditory event related potentials in chronic tinnitus with noise induced hearing loss. Hearing Research 71: 106–13.

Attias J, Furman V, Shemesh Z, Bresloff I (1996) Impaired brain processing in noise-induced tinnitus patients as measured by auditory and visual event-related potentials. Ear and Hearing 17:327–33.

Axelsson A (1992) Causes of tinnitus. In JM Aran, R Dauman (eds) Tinnitus 91. Proceedings of the IV International Tinnitus Seminar, Bordeaux. Amsterdam/ New York: Kugler Publications, pp.275–7.

Brix R, Denk DM, Ehrenberger K (1995) Neurophysiological control in therapy of tinnitus with cochlear disorders. In GE Reich, JA Vernon (eds) Proceedings of the V International Tinnitus Seminar 1995, Portland, Oregon, USA. American Tinnitus Association, pp.101–5.

Brownell WE (1990) Outer hair cell electromotility and otoacoustic emissions. Ear and Hearing 11:82–92.

Caspary DM, Salvi RJ, Helfert RH, Brozoski TJ, Bauer CA (2001) Neuropharmacology of noise iduced hearing loss in brainstem auditory structures. In D Henderson, D Prasher, R Kopke, R Salvi, R Hamernik (eds) Noise Induced Hearing Loss: Basic mechanisms, prevention and control. London: Noise Research Network Publications, pp.169–83.

Ceranic JB, Prasher DK, Luxon LM (1995) Tinnitus and otoacoustic emissions. Clinical Otolaryngology 20: 192–200.

Ceranic B, Prasher DK, Raglan E, Luxon LM (1998a) Tinnitus following head injury – Evidence from otoacoustic emissions. The Journal of Neurology Neurosurgery and Psychiatry 65:523–9.

Ceranic B, Prasher DK, Luxon LM ( 1998b) Presence of tinnitus indicated by variable spontaneous otoacoustic emissions. Audiology & Neuro-Otology 3:332–44.

Chang H, Chen K, Kaltenbach JA, Zhang J, Godfrey DA ( 2002) Effects of acoustic trauma on dorsal cochlear nucleus neuron activity in slices. Hearing Research 164:59–68.

Chen G, Jastreboff PJ (1995) Salicylate-induced abnormal activity in the inferior colliculus of rats. Hear Res 82: 158–78.

Chéry-Croze S, Moulin A, Collet L, Morgon A (1994 ) Is the test of medial efferent system function a relevant investigation in tinnitus? The British Journal of Audiology 28: 13–25.

Collet L, Kemp DT, Veuillet E, Duclaux R , Moulin A, Morgon A (1990) Effect of contralateral auditory stimuli on active cochlear micromechanical properties in human subjects. Hearing Research 43: 251–62.

Cransac H, Peyrin L, Cottet-Emard JM, Farhat F, Pequignot JM, Reber A (1996) Aging effects on monoamines in rat medial vestibular and cochlear nuclei. Hearing Research 100:150–6.

D'Aldin C, Eybalin M, Puel JL, Charachon G, Ladrech R, Renard N, Pujol R (1995) Synaptic connections and putative functions of the dopaminergic innervation of the guinea pig cochlea. European Archive of Oto-Rhino-Laryngology 252:270–4.

Davies A, Rafaie EA (2000) Epidemiology of tinnitus. In R Tyler (ed.) Tinnitus Handbook. San Diego: Singular. pp.1–23.

Denk DM, Heinzl H, Franz P, Ehrenberger K (1997) Caroverine in tinnitus treatment. A placebo-controlled blind study. Acta Otolaryngologica 117:825–30.

Diesch E, Struve M, Rupp A, Ritter S, Hulse M, Flor H (2004) Enhancement of steady-state auditory evoked magnetic fields in tinnitus. The European Journal of Neuroscience 19: 1093–104.

Dolan DF, Nuttall AL (1988) Masked cochlear whole-nerve response intensity functions altered by electrical stimulation of the crossed olivocochlear bundle. The Journal of the Acoustical Society of America 83:1081–6.

Duchamp C, Morgon A, Chéry-Croze S (1995)Tinnitus sufferers without hearing loss. In GE Reich, JA Vernon, (eds) Proceedings of the V International Tinnitus Seminar 1995, Portland, Oregon, USA. American Tinnitus Association, pp.266–9.

Eggermont JJ (2000) Physiological mechanisms and neural models. In R Tyler (ed.) Tinnitus Handbook. San Diego: Singular, pp.85–122.

Evans EF, Borerwe TA (1982) Ototoxic effects of salicylates on the responses of single cochlear nerve fibres and on cochlead potentials. Br J Audiol 16:101–8.

Flottorp G (1953) Pure-tone tinnitus evoked by acoustic stimulation: idiophonic effect. Acta Otolaryngologica 43: 395–415.

Gale JE, Ashmore JF (1997) An intrinsic frequency limit to the cochlear amplifier. Nature 389:63–6.

Gerken GM (1979) Central denervation hypersensitivity in the auditory system of the cat. The Journal of the Acoustical Society of America 66: 721–7.

Graham RL, Hazell JW (1994) Contralateral suppression of transient evoked otoacoustic emissions: intra-individual variability in tinnitus and normal subjects. The British Journal of Audiology 29: 235–45.

Hebert S, Paiement P, Lupien SJ (2004) A physiological correlate for the intolerance to both internal an external sounds. Hearing Research 190: 1–9.

Hoke M, Hoke ES (1997) Tinnitus and event-related activity of the auditory cortex. In Book of Abstracts, 2nd Eurpean Conference on Protection Against Noise (PAN), London

Hoke M, Feldmann H, Pantev C, Lütkenhöner B, Lehnertz K (1989) Objective evidence of tinnitus in auditory evoked magnetic fields. Hearing Research 37: 281–6.

Huffman RF, Henson Jr OW. (1990) The descending auditory pathway and acousticomotor system: connections with the inferior colliculus. Brain Research Review 15: 295–323.

Kaltenbach JA, Zacharek MA, Zhang J, Frederick S (2004) Activity in the dorsal cochlear nucleus of hamsters previously tested for tinnitus following intense tone exposure. Neuroscience Letters 23:121–5.

Kawase B, Delgutte, Liberman MC (1993) Antimasking effects of the olivocochlear reflex. II. Enhancement of auditory-nerve response to masked tones. The Journal of Neurophysiology 70: 2533–49.

Kemp DT (1978) Stimulated acoustic emissions from within the human auditory system. The Journal of the Acoustical Society of America 64: 1386–91.

Kemp DT (1979) Evidence of mechanical nonlinearity and frequency selective wave amplification in the cochlea. Archives of Oto-rhino-laryngology 224: 37–45.

Kemp DT (1981) Physiologically active cochlear micromechanisms-one source of tinnitus. In D Evered, G Lawrenson (eds.) Tinnitus. CIBA Foundation Symposium 85, London: Pitman Books Ltd. pp.54–81.

Kemp DT (1982) Cochlear echoes: implication for noise-induced hearing loss. In RP Hamernik, D Henderson, R Salvi (eds.) New Perspectives on Noise-induced Hearing Loss. New York: Raven Press, pp.189–206.

Komiya H, Eggermont JJ ( 2000) Spontaneous firing activity of cortical neurons in adult cats with reorganised tonotopic map following pure-tone trauma. Acta Otolayngologica 120:750–6.

LeDoux JE, Sakaguchi A, Reis DJ (1983) Subcortical efferent projections of the medial geniculate nucleus mediate emotional responses conditioned to acoustic stimuli. The Journal of Neuroscience 4: 683–98.

Liberman MC, Kiang NYS (1978) Acoustic trauma in cats. Cochlear pathology and auditory nerve activity. Acta Otolaryngol Suppl 358: 1–63.

Lockwood AH, Salvi RJ, Coad ML, Towsley ML, Wack DS, Murphy BW (1998) The functional neuroanatomy of tinnitus: evidence from limbic system links and neuronal plasticity. Neurology 50: 114–20.

Lockwood AH, Salvi RJ, Burkard RF, Galantowicz PJ, Coad ML, Wack DS (1999) Neuroanatomy of tinnitus. Scandinavian Audiology Suppl 51: 47–52.

Lockwood AH, Salvi RJ, Burkard RF (2002) Tinnitus. The New England Journal of Medicine 347: 904–10.

Lundberg U (1999) Coping with stress: neuroendocrine reactions and implications on health. Noise & Health 4: 67–74.

Maison SF, Liberman MC (2000) Predicting vulnerability to acoustic injury with non-invasive assay of olivochlear reflex strength. The Journal of Neuroscience 20: 4701–7.

Maison S, Micheyl C, Collet L (1999) The medial olivocochlear efferent system in in humans: structure and function. Scandinavian Audiology Suppl 51:77–84.

Maison SF, Luebke AE, Liberman MC, Zuo J (2002) Efferent protection from acoustic injury is mediated via alpha9 nicotinic acetylcholine receptors on outer hair cells. The Journal of Neuroscience 15:10838–46.

Meyer JH, Kruger S, Wilson AA, Christensen BK, Goulding VS, Schaffer A, Minifie C, Houle S, Hussey D, Kennedy SH (2001) Lower dopamine transporter binding potentials in striatum during depression. Neuroreport 12:4121–5.

Møller AR (2000) Similarities between severe tinnitus and chronic pain. Journal of the American Acdemy of Audiology 11: 115–24.

Musiek FE (1986) Neuroanatomy, neurophysiology and central auditory assessment. Part II: the cerebrum. Ear and Hearing 7:283–94.

Ochi K, Eggermont JJ (1997) Effects of quinine on neutral activity in cat primary auditory cortex. Hear Res 105: 105–118.

Oliver D, Klöcker N, Schuck J, Baukrowitz T, Ruppersberg JP, Fakler B (2000) Gating of $Ca^+$-activated; $k^+$ channels controls fast inhibitory synaptic transmission of auditory outer hair cells. Neuron 26:595–601.

Owens MJ, Nemeroff CB (1998) The serotonin transporer and depression. Depression and Anxiety 8:5–12.

Penner MJ (1990) An estimate of the prevalence of tinnitus caused by spontaneous otoacoustic emissions. Archives of Otolaryngology Head & Neck Surgery
116: 418–23

Penner MJ (1992) Linking spontaneous acoustic emissions and tinnitus. British
Journal of Audiology 26: 115–23.

Puel JL (1995) Chemical synaptic transmission in the cochlea. Progress in
Neurobiology 47: 449–76.

Puel JL, Ruel J, Guitton M, Wang J, Pujol R (2002) The inner hair cell synaptic
complex: physiology, pharmacology and new therapeutic strategies. Audiol
& Neuro-otology 7: 49–54.

Pujol R (1994) Lateral and medial efferents: a double neurochemical mechanism
to protect and regulate inner and outer hair cell function in the cochlea.
British Journal of Audiology 28: 185–91.

Rajan R, Irvine DRF, Calford MB, Wise LZ (1992) Effects of frequency-specific
losses in cochlear neural activity on the processing and representation of frequency in primary auditory cortex. In AL Dancer, D Henderson, RJ Salvi, RP
Hamernik (eds.) Noise Induced Hearing Loss. St. Louis: Mosby Year Book,
pp.119–29.

Rasmussen G (1946) The olivary peduncle and other fibre projections of the
superior olivary complex. The Journal of Comparative Neurology 84: 141–219.

Recanzone GH, Schreiner CE, Merzenich MM (1993) Plasticity in the frequency
representation of primary auditory cortex following discrimination training in
adult owl monkeys. The Journal of Neuroscience 13: 87–103.

Ressler KJ, Nemeroff CB (1999) Role of epinephrine in the pathophysiology and
treatment of mood disorders. Biological Psychiatry 46: 1219–33.

Robertson D, Irvine DR (1989) Plasticity of frequency organisation in auditory
cortex of guinea pigs with partial unilateral deafness. The Journal of
Comparative Neurology 282: 456–71.

Ryan S, Kemp DT, Hinchcliffe R (1991) The influence of contralateral acoustic
stimulation on click-evoked otoacoustic emissions in humans. British Journal
of Audiology 25: 391–7.

Sahley TL, Nodar RH.(2001) A biochemical model of peripheral tinnitus. Hearing
Research 152:43–54.

Sahley TL, Nodar RH, Musiek FE (1999) Endogenous dynorphins: possible role in
peripheral tinnitus. International Tinnitus Journal 5: 76–91.

Salvi RJ, Ahroon WA (1983) Tinnitus and neural activity. J Speech Hearing
Research 26: 629–32.

Schwaber MK, Garraghty PE, Kaas JH (1993) Neuroplasticity of the adult primate auditory cortex following cochlear hearing loss. American Journal of Otology 3: 252–8.

Shiomi Y, Nagamine T, Fujiki N, Hirano S, Naito Y, Shibasaki H, Hanjo I (1997)
Tinnitus remission by lidocaine demonstrated by auditory evoked magnetoen-
cephalogram. Acta Otolaryngol (Stockh) 117: 31–34.

Shulman A, Strashun AM, Afriyie M, Aronson F, Abel W, Goldstein B (1995) SPECT
imaging of brain and tinnitus – neurotologic/neurologic implications. Int
Tinnitus J 1: 13–29.

Simpson JJ, Davies WE (2000) A review of evidence in support of a role for 5-HT
in the perception of tints. Hear Res 145: 1–7.

Stephens SDG (1984) The treatments of tinnitus – A historical perspective. J
Laryngol Otol 98: 936–72.

Suga N, Gao E, Zhang Y, Ma Y, Olsen JF (2000) The corticofugal system for hearing recent progress. Proc Nadl Acad Sci USA 97: 11807–14.

Szczepaniak WS, Moller AR (1996) Effects of baslofen, clonazepam and diazepam on tone exposure-induced hyperexcitability of the inferior colliculus in rat: possible therapeutic implications for pharmacological management of tinnitus and hyperacusis. Hear Res 97: 46–53.

Thompson AM, Thompson GC (1995) Light microscopic evidence of serotoninergic projections to olivo cochlear neurones in the bush baby otolemur garnetti. Brain Res 695: 263–6.

Thompson GC, Thompson AM, Garrett KM, Britton BH (1994) Serotoniu and serotonin receptors in the central auditory system. Otolaryngol Head Neck Surg 110: 93–102.

Uusitalo AL, Valkonen-Korhonen M, Helenius P, Vanninen E, Bergstrom KA, Kuikka JT (2004). Int J Sports Med 25:150–3.

Vernan J (1981) The history of masking as applied to tinnitus. J Laryngol Otol 4: 76–79.

Veuillet E, Collet L, Disant F, Morgon A (1992) Tinnitus and medical cochlear efferent system. In JM Aran, R Dauman, (eds.) Tunnitus 91. Proceedings of IV International Tunnitus Seminal, Bordeaux. Amsterdam/New York: Kugle Publications, pp.205–9.

Ward WD (1955) Tonal monoaural diplacusis. J Acoust Soc Am 27: 365–72.

Wang J, Ding D, Salvi RJ (2002) Functional reorganisation in chinchilla inferior colliculus associated with chronic and acute cochlear changes. Hear Res 168:238–49.

Warr WB, Guinan JG (1979) Efferent innervation of the organ of corti: Two Separate Systems. Brain Res 173: 152–5.

Wegel RLA (1931) A study of tinnitus. Archives of Otolaryngology Head & Neck Surgery 14: 160–5.

Weisz N, Voss S, Berg P, Elbert T (2004) Abnormal auditory mismatch response in tinnitus sufferers with high-frequency hearing loss is associated with subjective distress. BMC Neuroscience 5: 8.

Wiederhold ML (1986) Physiology of the olivocochlear system. In R Altschuler, R Bobin, D Hoffman (eds.) Neurobiology of hearing. The Cochlea. New York: Raven Press, pp. 349–70.

Willot JF, Lu S-V (1982) Noise-induced hearing loss can alter neutral coding and increase excitability in the central nervous system. Science 216: 1331–2.

Wilson JP (1980) Evidence for a cochlear origin for acoustic re-emissions, threshold fine-structure and tonal tinnitus. Hearing Research 2: 233–52.

Wilson JP, Sutton GJ (1981) Acoustic correlates of tonal tinnitus. In D Evered, G Lawrenson, (eds.) Tinnitus (CIBA Foundation Symposium). London: Pitman Books Ltd. 82–107.

Woods CI, Azeredo WJ (1981) Noradrenergic and serotonergic projections to the superior olive: potential for modulation of olivocochlear neurons. Brain Research 1999; 836:9–18.

Zacharek MA, Kaltenbach JA.Mathog TA, Zhang J (2002) Effects of cochlear ablation on noise induced hyperactivity in the hamster dorsal cochlear nucleus: implication for the origin of noise induced tinnitus. Hearing Research 172:137–44.

Zenner HP (1986) Motile responses in outer hair cells. Hearing Research 22: 83–90.

Zurek PM (1981) Spontaneous narrowband acoustic signals emitted from human ears. The Journal of the Acoustical Society of America 69: 514–3.

CHAPTER 13
# The effects of blast on the ear

*Noise and Its Effects:* Edited by Linda Luxon and Deepak Prasher © 2007
John Wiley & Sons Ltd.

ALAN G KERR

## Introduction

The ear can detect signals with a pressure level of one five-billionth of an atmosphere, causing an excursion of the tympanic membrane of the order of the diameter of a hydrogen atom. At the same time it can withstand, without damage, energy levels millions of times greater than this. Charles Dickens described in the *Pickwick Papers*, in 1824, temporary hearing loss following exposure to gunfire and both temporary and permanent hearing loss has been part of everyday military life for over two centuries. Despite this Hirsch (1968) reported that there were only 13 published papers in the medical literature by 1900.

Sadly there have been many occasions to publish further papers since then and modern-day terrorism has led to the exposure of civilians to blast injuries. Consequently, this subject is now of interest to all in the medical profession.

## The nature of blast

A blast wave occurs when, in an explosion, solid, liquid or gaseous material, is suddenly increased in volume. The uncomplicated wave has three components: the shock front, the positive pressure phase and the negative pressure phase (Figure 13.1).

The shock front results from the rapid build-up of pressure, which may be very high, although often with very little energy. Initially this travels supersonically. The damage caused by the shock front is usually much less than that from the following positive pressure wave with which it soon becomes amalgamated because the shock front slows down quite quickly.

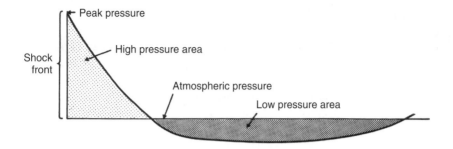

**Figure 13.1** Friedlander curve illustrating the shock front, and the positive and negative phases of the blast wave.

The duration of the positive phase depends on the amount and type of explosive but in conventional materials is usually of the order of milliseconds. The amount of energy is related to the nature of the explosive materials and depends on the speed of the build-up of pressure, the height of the peak pressure and the duration of the wave. Most of the damage from an explosion occurs as the result of this positive pressure wave. Finally there is the following negative pressure phase. This cannot be greater than atmospheric pressure and is usually of the order of tens of milliseconds, and the amount of energy is roughly equal to that in the positive pressure phase.

However, it is only rarely in clinical practice that one comes across a patient who was exposed to an uncomplicated blast wave. Usually the blast is complicated by the positions of other objects, especially when it occurs within a building or building complex. There will then be deflections of the waves, with shadow areas, and reflections of waves from walls and other objects. The positive phase may be augmented and the negative phase entirely cancelled by these deflections and reflections.

This chapter will deal only with damage to the person although that will, of course, be complicated by damage to surrounding structures.

**Damage from blast is categorized into primary, secondary and tertiary:**

- Primary damage results from the blast wave itself.
- Secondary damage is usually the most serious and results from the impact of damaged structures or flying debris.
- Tertiary damage occurs when the subject himself is propelled by the wave and actually becomes part of the flying debris.

It is the air-containing organs of the body that suffer most from primary damage. The ear is the organ most commonly affected but ear damage is rarely of any life-threatening significance and therefore is often either ignored or undetected. A paper by Hadden, Rutherford and Merrett (1978) reported 15 perforated tympanic membranes in 1535 victims of terrorist explosions. This certainly suggests underdetection, especially in the light of the Abercorn explosion where there were 60 perforations, among about 100 victims, from one 5-lb (2-kg) bomb. However, as tympanic membrane damage occurs only in a small proportion of those with ear damage, the study by Hadden et al. illustrates the serious under-detection that occurs.

Almost everyone close to an explosion suffers from some short-lived hearing impairment with tinnitus. Happily in the vast majority this damage *is* only temporary, similar to temporary threshold shift from noise.

The second organ most often subject to primary damage is the lung. This is not common but can be fatal; patients may die without any outwardly visible injury. Damage to the bowel may also occur but is very rare. However, there is one exceptional situation and that is where the blast occurs under water and the pressure wave is transmitted to the subject actually in the water. A blast wave through fluid is more intense, as it is almost incompressible and, in that situation, thoracic and abdominal injury may be more common than ear damage.

# Airborne stimulation deafness

**There are essentially three types of airborne stimulation deafness:**

1. The most common is noise-induced deafness. This affects only the cochlea and one does not expect to see either vestibular or middle-ear damage. Noise does not rupture the tympanic membrane or dislocate the ossicles.
2. There is report trauma, which occurs in those exposed to gunfire where there are usually repeated stimuli and the duration of the positive pressure wave is less than 1.5 ms. Middle-ear or vestibular damage is very rare.
3. There is blast, which usually is a single stimulus, where the duration of the positive pressure phase is greater than 1.5 ms.

In the first two the damage tends to be at the high frequencies whereas in blast trauma all frequencies may be affected. In blast the main pathological changes occur in the cochlea but there may also be middle-ear and vestibular damage.

# Factors influencing ear damage from blast

**These are:**

- nature of the explosive;
- amount of explosive;
- duration of blast wave;
- location of explosion;
- relation of ear to explosion;
- state of ear canal;
- health of tympanic membrane;
- noise level of environment.

The most important components in whether or not there will be damage from blast are the nature and amount of explosive. These influence the rise time or speed with which the pressure builds up, the height or intensity of the peak pressure and also the third constituent, the duration of the blast wave, all of which are factors in the amount of energy released. The location of the explosion is a fourth factor. A confined space, or even an adjacent building or wall, may result in reflection of the wave and consequent additional build-up of pressure.

When considering the specific damage to the ear, there is a fifth factor and that is the relationship of the ear to the explosion. The effects of blast often appear to be capricious because of the deflections or reflections that can occur from even quite narrow objects. Usually when one ear is in direct line with the blast wave there is some protection of the other ear unless reflection occurs (Figure 13.2). When the blast wave is not in direct line with the ear canal some attenuation is afforded to the ear simply by the obliquity. The greatest attenuation occurs when the bomb is directly behind the patient as the auricles provide some protection.

A sixth factor is the state of the ear canal. A narrow or blocked outer-ear canal attenuates the blast. The amount and position of any wax are important. Wax that is insufficient to occlude the canal provides very little protection. However, when it occludes the canal with a pocket of air between it and the tympanic membrane, much of the blast energy is absorbed by the wax. On the other hand, when hard wax is in contact with the tympanic membrane it may be driven through it and result in rupture of the drum and damage to the ossicles. Golden and Clare (1965), cited by Hirsch, have shown that a normal, wax-free ear canal itself produces an increase in sound pressure of the order of 20% compared with any other point at the same distance from the explosion.

A seventh factor is the health of the tympanic membrane. A thin atrophic membrane will rupture more easily than a thick tympanosclerotic one. The tympanic membranes of the young tend to be more resistant to blast damage than those of the elderly. Finally it has been suggested that

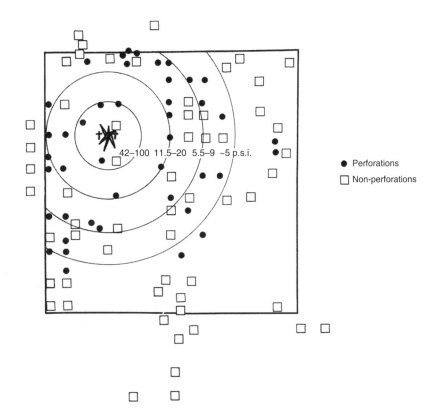

**Figure 13.2** Estimated pressures in pounds per square inch (p.s.i.) from a 5-lb (2-kg) explosion, without any consideration of augmentation due to reflection. This augmentation probably accounted for the two perforations on the extreme right of the figure. Abercorn explosion (1 p.s.i. is equivalent to 6.9 kPa). (Reproduced with the kind permission of the editor of *The Practitioner* from Kerr, 1978).

a very noisy environment gives protection to the ear because the stapedius muscle may be in a state of tension.

# The effect of blast on the ear

One does not expect to see damage to the auricle or outer-ear canal from primary blast damage. This may, of course, occur as a result of secondary or tertiary damage. The most commonly damaged part of the ear is the cochlea but middle-ear damage is also common.

## Middle ear

Occasionally one sees nothing more than a little bleeding into the tympanic membrane (Figure 13.3)

If the energy reaching the ear is sufficiently high, rupture of the tympanic membrane is likely to occur. Various workers have estimated the pressures required to rupture the tympanic membranes of animals and humans, starting with Zalewski in 1906 who was over 40 years ahead of all other researchers in this field. Zalewski (1906), cited by Hirsch (1968), used static overpressures on fresh human cadavers and found that the range required for rupture was 37–304 kPa (5.4–44.1 p.s.i.). He also found that the pressures required in the first decade of life were much higher than in older age groups, being 228 kPa compared with 138 kPa.

Other workers later measured dynamic pressures and confirmed that fast-rising pressure waves were more traumatic than slow-rising waves. They also found that the pinna and ear canal made a difference but that this also varied, depending on their size and whether the wave was direct or coming at an angle. In their dynamic studies James et al. (1982) concluded that pressures at the tympanic membrane needed to be of the order of 50 kPa for rupture to begin to occur. As we have seen, the deflections and reflections that occur with blast waves result in apparently capricious damage and the outcomes look even more unpredictable because of these other factors. Richmond et al. (1989) produced similar figures in their comprehensive studies and the extensive work of White, Bowen and

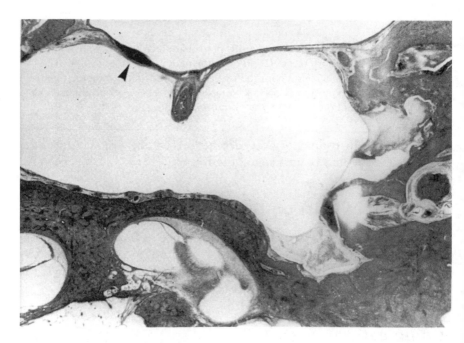

**Figure 13.3** Bleeding into the tympanic membrane. (Reproduced with the kind permission of the editor of the *Journal of Laryngology and Otology* from Kerr and Byrne, 1975).

Richmond (1970) in animals has contributed to the understanding of this problem.

There have been discussions in the past about which phase of the blast wave causes the rupture of the tympanic membrane. There is little doubt that the negative phase is capable of causing rupture and the everted edges, which are often seen, have been cited as support for this case. However, once a drum has been ruptured, the negative phase is always likely to cause eversion of the edges. The following facts suggest that the positive phase causes the rupture: inversion of the edges of the perforations has been seen; squamous epithelium from the tympanic membrane has been seen histologically in the middle ears of patients who died following explosions (Figure 13.4); squamous epithelial cysts have also developed later in the middle ear, suggesting implantation of epithelium at the time of the explosion; and, in addition, wax and other debris have also been found in the middle ear, suggesting that the positive phase caused the rupture and also carried material from the external ear canal onward into the middle ear. Kerr and Byrne (1975), in the light of these findings, concluded that most perforations are caused by the positive phase of the blast wave.

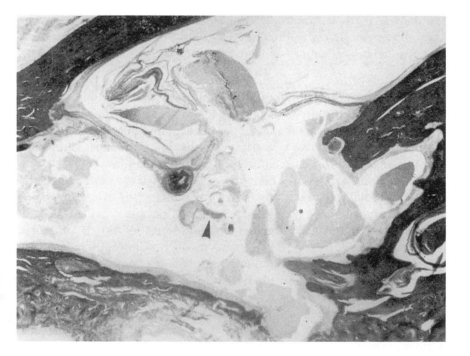

**Figure 13.4** Squamous epithelium and keratin in the middle ear cleft. (Reproduced with the kind permission of the editor of the *Journal of Laryngology and Otology* from Kerr and Byrne, 1975).

# Dislocation

Dislocation of the ossicles as a result of primary blast injury is uncommon and does not occur in the absence of rupture of the tympanic membrane. In the Abercorn explosion, which resulted in 60 perforations, Kerr and Byrne (1975) did not see one case of ossicular damage. There have been some reports suggesting quite a high incidence of ossicluar damage (Sudderth, 1974), but these have been in series specially selected for surgery and do not reflect the true incidence of dislocation. The most common lesions involve the incus, which may be subluxated or dislocated. Fracture of the stapes superstructure has also been reported.

# The inner ear

The inner ear may be affected at pressures well below those required to rupture the tympanic membrane. Pressures as low as 7 kPa (1 p.s.i.) can cause temporary damage.

A good rule of thumb about the likelihood of a given blast having caused ear damage is the surrounding windows. Generally speaking, if the blast is insufficiently strong to break nearby domestic windows it is unlikely to be sufficiently strong to damage the inner ear.

There is always the problem, in assessing ear damage due to any particular blast, that the previous hearing levels are usually not known. It is common knowledge that many people believe their hearing to be normal when, in fact, it is not. However, it seems that blast can affect all frequencies although high tones are affected more often than low.

The initial damage from a bomb may be such that the patient feels that he or she is totally deaf. It is common for patients to say that, immediately after the explosion, they could see the lips of people moving but could not hear anything. This suggests hearing levels of 80 dB or worse. However, there is usually quick initial recovery. Figure 13.5 shows the recovery over 12 days in a young man exposed to a bomb. He had already noticed an improvement in his hearing before the first audiogram was taken at 2 hours. There may be continued recovery over the first few months after an explosion but thereafter the sensorineural hearing loss tends to be permanent (Figure 13.6). It is doubtful if total sensorineural deafness ever occurs as a result of primary blast injury.

It has been said that rupture of the tympanic membrane provides protection for the inner ear. However, in the Abercorn explosion, those with the most severe inner-ear hearing loss had all had rupture of the tympanic

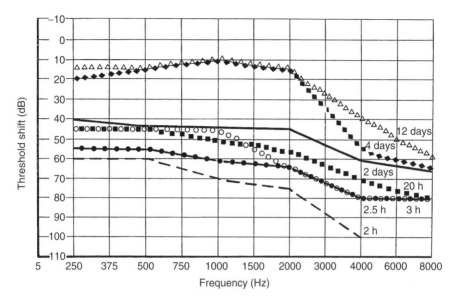

**Figure 13.5** Serial audiograms in a young man whose only injury was to the inner ears. He was lost to follow-up after 12 days but probably recovered normal hearing (see Figure 13.6). (Reproduced with the kind permission of the editor of *The Practitioner* from Kerr, 1978).

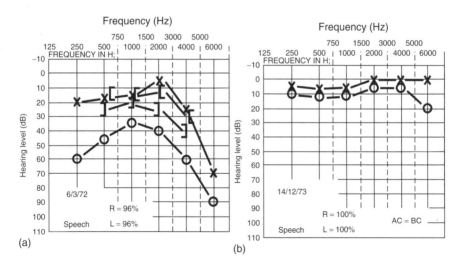

**Figures 13.6** Audiograms of the same patient (a) 2 days and (b) 18 months after an explosion. This was a 21-year-old woman who had been sitting two tables away from the Abercorn bomb. She had already experienced a considerable improvement in her hearing before the first audiogram was taken. She had bilateral perforations, one small and one subtotal. She did not receive any active treatment for her ears. Both perforations healed and her hearing recovered to normal. (Reproduced with the kind permission of the editor of the *Journal of Laryngology and Otology* from Kerr and Byrne, 1975).

membrane, suggesting that any protection afforded by ear-drum failure is minimal.

Tinnitus is a common accompaniment of blast injury. Indeed this may occur even in the absence of any detectable hearing loss, although the severity is generally related to the severity of the deafness. There are often strong psychological overtones in many of those suffering from tinnitus and blast-induced cases are no different. Resentment against the source of the explosion and prolonged litigation are, as always, bad prognostic factors.

Vertigo is not common following primary blast injury but two types must be considered. Benign positional vertigo is sometimes seen and the clinical course is similar to other cases of this type. Perilymph fistulae are rare but, once again, the possibility must be kept in mind because otherwise they may be missed.

# Pathology of inner-ear damage

The exact pathology of damage to the cochlea is not entirely clear but Patterson and Hamernik (1997) have helped clarify this. They postulated that the temporary deafness is due to changes in the integrity of the tight cell junctions of the reticular lamina, possibly with changes in permeability or development of holes, allowing mixing of perilymph and endolymph.

They also reported animal experiments where sections of the organ of Corti were torn off the basilar membrane, resulting in permanent damage to the hearing. In other areas there was more specific damage to the hair cells themselves or to Hensen's cells. Generally speaking the outer hair cells were damaged more than the inner ones.

# Treatment

## Prevention

Common sense is one of the most important measures to prevent blast injury. However, it is quite surprising how the public's curiosity overcomes the self-preservation instinct so that they stand and watch while the police or army deals with a suspect device. Sometimes the suspected bomb proves to be just that and explodes causing unnecessary injury to the general public.

Protection of the ears is possible simply by using ear muffs or occluding plugs. However, these interfere with communication so that their use is limited. The best inexpensive compromise is a rubber plug with a built- in, finely perforated, metal plate which allows normal passage of speech sounds but which attenuates blast waves. A more expensive, and at times less practical, although efficient, alternative is ear muffs with a built-in radio receiver that protects against blast waves but allows easy communication.

## General

Blast victims usually suffer a marked emotional shock and this needs to be borne in mind when treating their acute injuries. In addition there may be other life-threatening general injuries that require immediate action so that the auditory system is sometimes overlooked.

## Middle ear

Simple contusion of the tympanic membrane does not require any treatment. Most perforations will heal spontaneously and are best left untouched. However, if there is an indriven part of the drum head in the middle ear, careful elevation of this may be of benefit, providing the operator has experience with ear surgery and access to a microscope. Similarly, if there is debris lying in the meatus or middle ear this is better removed by an experienced operator. If the operator does not have any experience with ear surgery, it is probably better to leave the ear untouched. There is no place for routine antibiotic/steroid ear drops in the absence of an infection. Indeed, in the absence of infection, the potential ototoxic effects of these drops can increase the inner-ear damage that may already have occurred.

If the perforation is still present at 6 months surgery should be considered to close this, although the usual indications and contraindications for ear surgery must be kept in mind. For example, a dry central perforation that is giving no trouble apart from a minimal degree of hearing impairment and occurring in an only hearing ear should not be closed surgically because of the remote risk of causing sensorineural deafness.

Those rare cases of ossicular damage should, again, be dealt with according to the principles of middle-ear surgery. There should be realism about the likelihood of success, with special reference to the hearing level in the other ear in terms both of the dangers of operating on better or only hearing ears and of operating on ears with marked sensorineural damage when there is a normal hearing ear on the other side.

## Inner ear

It is almost impossible to make any assessment of the efficacy of treatment of blast injury to the inner ear. Initial recovery occurs so quickly that a controlled trial is almost impossible. This is compounded by the fact that there is so much spontaneous recovery that one cannot really assess the effect of treatment.

Consequently there are many uncontrolled and anecdotal accounts of inner-ear damage being reversed by various treatments such as bed rest, vasodilators, steroids and intravenous low-molecular-weight dextran. It seems likely that treatment does not influence the outcome in terms of hearing recovery although it may affect the patient's attitude to the final hearing situation. Consequently, there will be situations where some form of treatment is indicated, such as when severe deafness occurs in an only hearing ear and where to withhold all treatment, just because there is limited evidence of benefit, might result in severe psychological trauma.

The author has never seen permanent profound bilateral deafness from primary blast injury but when there is already a problem in one ear this must be a possibility. Secondary and tertiary damage, of course, carry these risks. Post-injury psychological care will be important in such cases and deafness rehabilitation may be required. Fortunately, in most cases the final outcome is good because of the ear's natural tendency to recovery.

# References

Golden R, Clare PM (1965) The hazards to the human ear from shock waves produced by high energy electrical discharge. UK Atomic Energy Authority Weapons Group, Atomic Weapons Research Establishment, Report AWRE-E-1, Aldermaston, Berkshire, England, August.

Hadden WA, Rutherford WH, Merrett JD (1978) The injuries of terrorist bombing: a study of 1532 consecutive patients. British Journal of Surgery 65: 525–31.

Hirsch FG (1968) Effects of overpressure on the ear – a review. Annals of the New York Academy of Sciences 152: 147–62.

James DJ, Pickett VC, Burdett KJ, Cheeseman A (1982) The response of the human ear to blast. Joint Atomic Weapons Research Establishment, Aldermarston, Berkshire England/CDE Report No 04/82.

Kerr AG (1978) Blast injuries of the ear. Practitioner 221: 677–82.

Kerr AG, Byrne JET (1975) Concussive effects of bomb blast on the ear. Journal of Laryngology and Otology 89: 131–43.

Patterson JH, Hamernik RP (1997) Blast overpressure induced structural and functional changes in the auditory system. Toxicology 121: 29–40.

Richmond DR, Yelverton JT, Fletcher ER, Phillips YY (1989) Physical correlates of ear drum rupture. Annals of Otology, Rhinology and Laryngology Supplement 140: 35–41.

Sudderth ME (1974) Tympanoplasty in blast-induced perforation. Archives of Otolaryngology 99: 157–9.

White CS, Bowen IG, Richmond DR (1970) The relation between eardrum failure and blast induced pressure variations. Space Life Sciences 2: 158–205.

Zalewski T (1906) Experimentelle untersuchungen ueber die resistheitsfaehigkeit des trommelfells. Zeitschrift für Ohren 52: 109–28.

# CHAPTER 14

# Interaction of noise, general medical disorders and state of health with hearing

*Noise and Its Effects:* Edited by Linda Luxon and Deepak Prasher © 2007
John Wiley & Sons Ltd.

ULF ROSENHALL

## Introduction

Sensorineural hearing loss is often the result of a multifactorial process involving more than one causative factor. Some factors are intrinsic, caused by biological processes within the individual. Others are extrinsic, caused by environmental influence. Noise-induced hearing loss (NIHL) belongs to the group of extrinsically caused hearing impairments and is by far the most common entity within this domain. It might interact with other factors causing hearing loss, both intrinsic and extrinsic. In numerous studies the additive effect of exposure to both noise and ototoxic drugs or organic solvents has been described in both research animals and humans. Exposure to noise might influence health without causing hearing loss. One well-known example is hypertension. It has been discussed for a long time whether disturbing (but not ototraumatic) noise might be so stressful as to cause hypertension. The purpose of this chapter is to review the scientific literature regarding possible interactions between NIHL and various health factors, and to discuss the relevance of the reported interactions. The subject is difficult to study. Many reports present controversial results, which are difficult to amalgamate into a distinct pattern. However, there are advantages if it is possible to calculate possible additional risks of the development of hearing loss due to noise exposure in conjunction with different medical conditions. Unnecessary hearing loss can possibly be avoided, and the patients' right to information can be met.

# Noise-induced hearing loss and cardiovascular disease

**Possible vascular risk factors in development of NIHL**

Arterial hypertension
Atherosclerosis
Hyperlipidaemia
Hypercholesterolaemia
Hyperlipoproteinaemia
Increased blood viscosity
Diabetes mellitus

## Cardiovascular disease and hearing loss

Cardiovascular disease (CVD) is one of the major causes of morbidity and mortality in all societies. There are numerous manifestations of CVD, some representing initial, subclinical stages. Examples are arterial hypertension, atherosclerosis, and increased levels of blood lipids such as hyperlipidemia, hyperlipoproteinemia and hypercholesterolemia, and alterations of blood viscosity. Coronary heart disease is a very common and serious manifestation of CVD, often resulting in myocardial infarction and cardiac arrhythmia. Cardiac insufficiency/ischaemic heart disease can be caused by coronary heart disease, valvular dysfunction, conduction abnormalities, pulmonary diseases, myocarditis/pericarditis and congenital heart malformations. Other manifestations of CVD are cerebrovascular disease such as stroke and brain infarction, intermittent claudication and arterial hypotension. Diabetes mellitus causes microvascular disease, and periarteritis is a rare condition seen in conjunction with autoimmune disease. Lifestyle factors have also been discussed in relation to CVD, the most important being smoking.

The literature relating hearing loss (most often presbyacusis) and cardiovascular disease/risk factors is not extensive and the results are often difficult to interpret or even contradictory. In a critical review of the earlier literature it was concluded that the evidence supporting a relationship between presbyacusis and hyperlipoproteinaemia remained questionable (Ray, 1991). In the more recent literature, some reports favour a relationship (Susmano and Rosenbuch, 1988; Gatehouse and Lowe, 1991; Gates et al., 1993; Toppila et al., 2000; Rosenhall and Sundh, 2005). Parving et al. (1993) described a correlation between hearing problems and parameters reflecting mild CVD, but not with robust CVD-factors like hypertension, angina pectoris and previous myocardial infarction. Jones and Davis (2000) could not find any significant association between hearing and a number of cardiovascular risk factors in a large group of patients.

## Early epidemiological studies

A relationship of CVD, dietary factors, exposure to noise and presbyacusis was proposed in 1962 by Rosen and his collaborators in a series of studies involving populations from different parts of the world (Rosen et al., 1962, 1970; Rosen and Olin, 1965).

There are relatively few studies in which the complex interactions of hearing loss, exposure to noise and CVD have been studied. In a large epidemiological study of middle-aged men, no correlation between hearing and cardiovascular risk factors was found (Drettner et al., 1975). In their study heavy smoking tended to be correlated to hearing loss, but no synergistic effect of smoking and noise exposure was observed.

## Hypertension and exposure to noise – animal experiments

Borg and collaborators have performed a series of important animal studies. They reported that genetically hypertensive rats were more susceptible to NIHL than normotensive rats (Borg, 1982b). However, animals with induced hypertension showed no correlation between hearing loss and systolic blood pressure (Borg, 1982a; Borg and Viberg, 1987). This observation does not support the hypothesis that hypertension directly interacts with noise exposure. The observed correlation between sensitivity to noise and hypertension seemed to have a common genetic cause. Another interesting animal study was performed by Pillsbury (1986). In a carefully designed study he studied the effects of noise, atherogenic diet, and hyperlipoproteinaemia spontaneously on hypertensive rats and normotensive rats. He described synergistic effects of genetically determined hypertension and atherogenic diet in the pathogenesis of NIHL.

## Blood lipids, hypertension and NIHL in humans

Axelsson and Lindgren (1985) studied two groups of 50-year-old men, one with high serum cholesterol levels and another that was randomly selected. They reported a slightly increased risk of acquiring high-frequency loss in the combination of work in noisy environments and high cholesterol levels.

Talbott et al. (1985, 1990) reported that severe NIHL was an independent predictor of hypertension in retired metal assembly workers aged 64 years or older. Milkovic-Kraus (1990) found that systolic and diastolic blood pressure were increased in noise-exposed workers, who also had hearing loss. Tarter and Robins (1990) studied industrial workers exposed to noise and reported that hearing loss at 4 kHz was significantly associated with blood pressure and hypertension among black workers but not among white workers. Nieminen et al. (1993) reported an association between serum cholesterol levels and blood pressure for the development of NIHL. Fourtes et al. (1995) performed a prospective epidemiological study including CVD factors and exposure to noise. They found that systolic blood pressure and cholesterol level were independently associated with a decline in auditory sensitivity.

## Exposure to noise as a cause of hypertension

An important issue is whether long-lasting noise exposure causes hypertension (Andrén et al., 1980; for a review see also Babisch, 1998). One example is the report of an increased risk for hypertension in men (but not women) with high noise annoyance (Belojevic and Saric-Tanaskovic, 2002). This effect is different from the hypothesis that hypertension has a synergistic effect together with noise exposure for the development of NIHL, but a combination of both effects is also plausible. Tomei et al. (2000) studied three groups of workers, one with hearing loss, exposed to occupational noise exceeding 90 dB (A), one group with less intense exposure to noise and a third without significant exposure. The most exposed group had the highest diastolic blood pressure and the highest prevalence of hypertension. They concluded that noise is a cardiovascular risk factor and that CVD often accompanies auditory damage. Since high noise levels might cause NIHL, there might be an interaction of exposure to noise, stress, NIHL and hypertension. One hypothesis is that there may be a population at increased risk for both hearing loss and high blood pressure, which is in accordance with the animal findings presented by Borg et al. (Borg, 1982a,b; Borg and Viberg, 1987).

## Cerebrovascular disease and hearing loss

A distinct entity, separate from the reports described above, is hearing loss seen in connection to cerebrovascular disorder. It is well known that lesions affecting the central auditory system (CAS) cause auditory dysfunction, in most cases a central auditory processing disorder (Musiek and Oxholm, 2003). The diagnosis of these lesions includes the use of a central auditory test battery, which is beyond the scope of this communication. Cerebrovascular lesions affecting the brain stem can cause sensorineural hearing loss, which tend to be slight to moderate (Luxon, 1980; Cohen et al., 1996). It can be speculated that brain-stem lesions, as well as retrocochlear lesions, might be more sensitive to exposure to noise because of increased loudness tolerance, abolished stapedius reflexes and dysfunction of the efferent olivocochlear systems. This proposed interaction with noise could be caused not only by cerebrovascular disease, but also by a variety of other diseases, such as multiple sclerosis and tumours in the cerebellopontine angle and the posterior fossa. However, it must be emphasized that there are no studies confirming this hypothesis.

### Cerbrovascular disease and NIHL – conclusions

Exposure to noise adds another parameter into a complicated, multifactorial situation.

Most studies that include exposure to noise favour the concept of an association between NIHL and cardiovascular factors. However, there is no general consensus regarding this issue: Drettner et al. (1975) and Hirai et al. (1991) could not demonstrate any significant relationship. Moreover, in many of the studies cited, the level of evidence connecting NIHL/exposure to noise to CVD is generally low. Only few animal studies have been performed, but they have a high level of evidence. The results of Borg (1982a,b) tend to favour the concept of parallel events rather than a direct influence of hypertension on the development of NIHL. Pillsbury (1986) favoured a synergistic model including diet as well as exposure to noise and hypertension. In both studies the importance of genetic factors were emphasized. A cautious conclusion is that a relationship between cardiovascular factors and NIHL is possible but more research is needed to establish such a link. In summary:

- Most (but not all) studies favour a correlation between CVD and hearing loss.
- There are indications that CVD sensitizes the cochlea to noise, but the level of evidence is moderate to low.
- Genetic factors are suspected to be of importance in the interactive processes of CVD and NIHL.

# Noise-induced hearing loss and other health disorders

### NIHL and diabetes mellitus

Duck et al. (1997) investigated interactions between diabetes and auditory function in both clinical and animal studies. Type 1 diabetes and hypertension were found to have a synergistic effect on high-frequency hearing loss. Diabetic end-organ damage was intensified by concomitant hypertension. There are also numerous other studies showing a connection between hearing loss and diabetes mellitus. The proposed cause is diabetic microangiopathy in the inner ear. Not much is known about the possible effect of exposure to noise on diabetic hearing loss. Hodgeson et al. (1987) examined the relationship of diabetes, noise exposure and hearing loss, and reported that noise and diabetes together did not appear to produce higher hearing thresholds than either insult alone.

### NIHL, vibration and Raynaud's phenomenon

It has been suggested in the literature that vibration may potentiate the effect of noise and may increase the risk of NIHL (Iki et al., 1986;

Pyykkö et al., 1988; Hamernik et al., 1989; Iki, 1994). An association between vibration-induced white fingers and hearing loss has been proposed, and the mechanism causing the hearing loss could be sympathetic vasoconstriction in the cochlea. Starck et al. (1999) described an interaction of smoking, hypertension and occupational Raynaud's phenomenon, resulting in worsened NIHL in noise-exposed workers. Raynaud's phenomenon, without correlation to occupational vibration, is also correlated with hearing difficulty (Palmer et al., 2002).

# Noise-induced hearing loss, physical fitness and lifestyle factors

**Lifestyle factors and NIHL**

Physical fitness
Physical stress
Body temperature
Smoking
Excessive alcohol consumption

Cardiovascular health does not only implicate CVD. Lifestyle factors are of great importance to maintain good health and to counteract the development of CVD and other medical disorders. Such factors are physical fitness, dietary habits and abstention from smoking.

### Physical fitness and exposure to noise

Manson et al. (1994) and Christell et al. (1998) studied hearing after noise exposure, exercise and a combination of both. A very fit group had better hearing compared with an unfit group in all conditions. According to the authors cardiovascular health was associated with hearing sensitivity, and they suggested a cardiovascular health–hearing synergism. Kolkhorst et al. (1998) studied normally hearing women of various fitness levels. They found a moderate association of physical fitness and diminished temporary threshold shift (TTS) after noise exposure.

### Physical exercise and simultaneous exposure to noise

Lindgren and Axelsson (1988) studied the effect of physical exercise on the susceptibility of TTS. They compared the hearing sensitivity after combined physical exercise with exposure to noise, and exposure to noise only. Their results indicated that noise with simultaneous exercise increased the TTS susceptibility. The same research group that proposed the cardiovascular health–hearing synergism studied the hearing sensitivity after submaximal exercise (Alessio and Hutchinson, 1991; Hutchinson et al., 1991). They had three test situations: exercise and noise, exercise only and noise only. They found that TTS occurred only after noise exposure; exercise did not enhance the hearing loss. According to them, TTS was driven by noise only, not exercise. Vittitow et al. (1994) studied the effects of loud music and exercise on hearing function. They found that music plus exercise caused statistically greater TTS than each one of these conditions separately. Nassar (2001) measured the hearing function in an aerobic class. One group, with high noise levels during the exercise, demonstrated TTS. A second group without exposure to noise had no TTS.

The interactions between physical fitness and hearing, and between simultaneous physical exercise and exposure to noise, have been described in a limited number of scientific reports. The design and performance of these studies are, in general, of a high quality, even if the numbers of participants are often somewhat small. A review of the literature shows that there seems to be a moderate cardiovascular health–hearing synergism. A high level of physical fitness can diminish the sensitivity to NIHL. There are rather strong indications that intense physical exercise sensitizes the cochlea to NIHL, even if the results of different studies are not in total accordance. A possible explanation for this interaction is that the body temperature is somewhat increased during intense exercise. A very positive trend among many people, not only young ones, is to attend aerobic classes and to exercise in gyms. However, it is currently popular to listen to high-volume music presented by loudspeakers or personal music systems during exercise to promote optimal effort. A recommendation of caution is well founded. Listening to very loud music should be avoided while performing maximal physical exercise.

## Body temperature and exposure to noise

It has been known for a long time that changes of body temperature have an influence on auditory function. Hypothermia prolongs the latencies of the later auditory brain-stem response (ABR) waves, and below the temperature of 25°C the waves disappear (Stockard et al., 1978; Kaga et al., 1979). When the body temperature is raised, the ABR waves reappear. Hyperthermia shortens the latencies of all ABR waves, up to a certain limit. This finding was regarded as a sign of permanent auditory damage (Katbamna et al., 1993). Temperature mechanisms, both hypothermia and hyperthermia, influence the generation of otoacoustic emissions (Ferber-Viart et al., 1995; Seifert et al., 2001). The efferent median olivocochlear (MOC) system is also affected by hypothermia. Animal studies have shown that hypothermia protects the cochlea from noise damage and hyperthermia increases NIHL (Henry and Chole, 1984;

Henry, 2003). These conditions are valid when the noise exposure occurs during the body temperature alteration. An interesting observation is that heat stress administered before exposure to noise protects research animals from acoustic injury, probably by an upregulation of heat shock proteins (Yoshida et al., 1999).

There are a number of studies with high-grade evidence that body temperature has an influence on auditory function. This observation can possibly explain the observed interaction between noise exposure and extreme physical exercise. It is also sensible to recommend the avoidance of exposure to high-intensity noise for people with fever, if such a situation were to arise.

## NIHL and smoking

Smoking has been studied regarding possible effects on hearing function. The results of most studies indicate a relationship between smoking and hearing loss, which in most cases represents presbyacusis (Drettner et al., 1975; Rosenhall et al., 1993; Noorhassim and Rampal, 1998; Cruickshanks et al., 1998; Itoh et al., 2001). Barone et al. (1987) found a significantly elevated risk for smokers to develop hearing loss. Their findings suggested that smokers are at increased risk of NIHL. A Finnish research group found that smoking did not increase the risk of hearing loss (Pyykkö et al., 1988). However, smoking in combination with elevated blood pressure and occupational Raynaud's phenomenon increased the risk for heavily noise-exposed workers to develop hearing loss (Starck et al., 1999). In another Finnish study an interaction between exposure to noise and heavy smoking was reported (Virokannas and Anttonen, 1995).

In two recent investigations comprising very large populations possible effects of smoking and hearing have been described. Sharabi et al. (2002) studied more than 13 000 Israelis with regard to smoking. Audiograms were available for all participants. A significantly higher incidence of all types of hearing loss was found in current and past smokers compared with non-smokers. The risk was especially high for young adults (< 35 years old). It should be noticed that NIHL was not included in their study. Palmer et al. (2004) have published a very large questionnaire study from the UK, including more than 10 000 participants. They reported a small extra risk to hearing incurred by smoking in high noise levels. The risk was, however, small relative to that from the noise itself.

Dengerink et al. (1987, 1992) reported an intriguing finding regarding TTS and cigarette smoking. Smokers had consistently smaller TTSs than non-smokers in a number of test situations. According to the authors, the results indicated that both acute and chronic effects of smoking, attributable to carbon monoxide, caused the diminished TTS.

Smoking seems to increase the risk of developing permanent hearing loss somewhat. This risk includes an interaction with noise exposure, with a possible aggravation of NIHL. The mechanisms of smoking-induced permanent hearing loss, and the effects of smoking on TTS, seem to be different.

**Effect of lifestyle on NIHL**

- There is rather robust evidence that some health factors protect from or sensitize to NIHL.
- A protective factor is a high level of physical fitness.
- Negative factors are increased body temperature and extreme physical exercise together with exposure to noise.
- One important negative lifestyle factor is smoking, which has a probable sensitizing effect on NIHL.

# Noise-induced hearing loss and ageing/age-related hearing loss

Age-related hearing loss (ARHL), or presbyacusis, has a complex aetiology including both intrinsic and extrinsic factors. Among the latter factors the influence of noise exposure has long been regarded as important. An influence of noise on presbyacusis has been postulated in numerous reports for almost a century. However, it is difficult to identify one single factor, such as the effects of prolonged noise exposure, with a duration of many decades. The effect of noise is equivocal. The interactions of NIHL and ARHL are complex, difficult to determine and poorly understood. One major problem is that ARHL is highly multifactorial. ARHL is a sensorineural hearing loss affecting both ears. The audiometric configuration of ARHL is gently sloping, steeply sloping, or more or less flat over the entire frequency range. In most cases there is a high-frequency hearing loss, often resembling that of NIHL.

### Epidemiological investigations – pure-tone audiometry

Important information about ARHL can be found in a number of important epidemiological investigations, performed in different countries: in Europe, the USA and Australia. Data from six different epidemiological investigations regarding pure-tone thresholds from male populations aged 75 years, or for the age stratum 70–80 years, are shown in Figure 14.1. These investigations were chosen because study groups and pure-tone audiometic data were presented in a way that allowed a comparison. In four of these investigations data from unscreened populations were presented (Gates et al., 1990, the Framingham cohort; Davis, 1995, the MRC National Study of Hearing; Jönsson and Rosenhall, 1998, Gothenburg gerontological and geriatric population study; Cruickshanks et al., 1998, Epidemiology of Hearing Loss Study, Beaver Dam). The results of these investigations were in fairly good agreement (Figure 14.1, grey lines). Three populations were screened regarding exposure to noise (the most important being occupational noise), but not regarding otological diseases and other causes of hearing loss (Rosenhall et al., 1990, Gothenburg gerontological and geriatric population study; Davis, 1995, the MRC, National Study of Hearing; Johansson, 2003). Again, the pure-tone thresholds of these three populations were in fairly good agreement (Figure 14.1, thick, black lines). The pure-tone thresholds of the noise-screened populations were slightly better than those of the unscreened populations, but the difference was small and not only confined to the high frequencies. The sixth study comprised predominantly white, well-educated, relatively affluent men participating in the Baltimore Longitudinal Study of Aging (Pearson et al., 1995). The participants were carefully screened for otological disease, unilateral hearing loss and NIHL (defined as an audiometric notch at 3–6 kHz). The results of this investigation (Figure 14.1, thin black line) deviated considerably from those of the other studies, especially the unscreened ones. The screened population had better thresholds not only within the typical NIHL area (3–6 kHz), but also over the entire frequency range. This indicates that not only exposure to noise, but also the influence

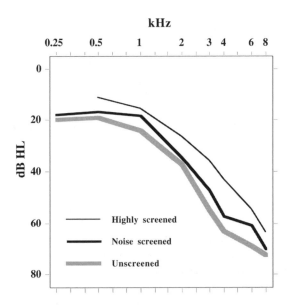

**Figure 14.1** Audiometric results from seven relatively recent epidemiological investigations. All populations represent men aged 75 years, or the age stratum 70–80 years. Thin black line (top): a population of predominantly well educated, financially well-off men, screened regarding otological diseases, evidence of NIHL (presence of high-frequency notches) or unilateral hearing loss (Pearson et al., 1995). Thick, black line (middle): mean pure-tone thresholds from three populations screened for noise exposure, especially occupational noise, but otherwise not screened (Rosenhall et al., 1990; Davis, 1995; Johansson, 2003). Grey line (bottom): mean pure-tone thresholds from four unscreened populations (Gates et al., 1990; Cruickshanks et al., 1998; Davis, 1995; Jönsson and Rosenhall, 1998).

of other extrinsic, and possibly also intrinsic, factors are of importance to explain the development of ARHL.

A comparison between unscreened populations and populations screened only for noise exposure indicates that the noise effect is minor and not unequivocally convincing. One explanation could be that it is problematic to compare different studies. However, three investigations included data of both unscreened and noise-screened populations (Rosenhall et al., 1990; Davis 1995; Jönsson and Rosenhall, 1998). Both studies reported threshold differences between the populations, but the differences were minute. A comparison has been performed between two screened subgroups of two cohorts of 70-year-old men in the Gothenburg study (Rosenhall, 2003). One subgroup included men without exposure to occupational noise, and the other included men with heavy occupational noise exposure, for 15 years or more (Figure 14.2). In this study a clear difference between the two subgroups can be discerned.

In summary, poorer hearing has been reported in noise-exposed elderly men than in those not exposed to occupational noise. This tendency is generally accepted, but there is no agreement on how strong it is. A mild-to-moderate influence of noise on hearing in old age is accepted. Most epidemiological investigations take occupational noise exposure into consideration, but the influence of everyday and leisure-time noise exposure for many decades is not known.

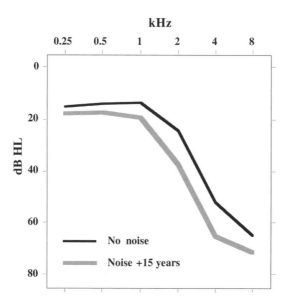

**Figure 14.2** Audiometric results from one population study of 70-year-old men (Rosenhall, 2003). Two screened groups are presented. Black line (top): 137 men with no occupational noise. Grey line (bottom): 100 men exposed for occupational noise for 15 years or more.

## ARHL: predictive factors

Stephens (1982) and Lim and Stephens (1991) studied elderly patients with hearing problems attending a rehabilitation clinic. About 17–19% of these patients were considered to have ARHL only. One-third had a history of vascular disease, 14%–33% had chronic otitis media, 12–15% had noise-induced or traumatic hearing loss, 6–9% had familial/genetic background factors, and 3–5% had a possible metabolic influence. These elderly people with hearing loss were at a greater risk of having vascular or biochemical abnormalities than participants of an age-matched control group. In this clinical material exposure to noise appears as one among many other factors.

Preliminary results from a study of male twins (Karlsson et al., 1997) show that environmental effects on hearing function become more important with age. These effects are of the non-shared type, not related to shared family environments, but explained by different exposures for the twins of each pair.

A recent very large epidemiological study, the North-Trøndelag Hearing Loss Study (Tambs et al., 2003), contains important information regarding NIHL in various ages. The questionnaire contained a detailed history of noise exposure, both occupational and leisure time. The effects from occupational noise and impulse noise exposure were apparent among middle-aged and old men. Only moderate effects of noise could be detected among women. No significant effects of frequent exposure to music were found.

## Influence of noise on ARHL – is there a simple addition, or an increased or decreased sensitivity to noise with age?

The most commonly accepted assumption is a simple, accumulative effect of noise and ageing on the hearing, the *additive model*. The traditional model to assess NIHL in older people assumes that presbyacusis adds to the permanent noise-induced threshold shift (NIPTS). This model was accepted in the original version of ISO 1999 (Burns and Robinson, 1970; Welleschick and Raber, 1978; Robinson and Sutton, 1979). A basically additive model, with some modification, is embraced by the current version of ISO 1999 (Robinson, 1988; International Organization for Standardization or ISO, 1990). The formula accepted by ISO 1999 has the implication that the total hearing loss is the sum of age-related hearing loss and NIPTS minus a compression factor, which is used when threshold shifts exceeds 20–25 dB. The additive model is favoured in a recent animal study (Fraenkel et al., 2003). In this study old and young adult rats were equally susceptible to the effect of noise exposure. According to this study there appeared to be a linear addition of presbyacusis and NIHL.

Willott et al. (1994) studied noise-induced central auditory damage in mice of different ages. They found little influence of the age of the mice when they were exposed to noise, or how long NIHL was present prior to old age. The only exception was very intense noise exposure, in which case the older auditory system seemed to be more vulnerable than the young one.

The validity of the additive model has been challenged (Bies and Hansen, 1990; Macrae, 1991; Mills et al., 1997, 1998). Mills and collaborators reported that a *less-than additive model (subadditivity)* was in agreement with their findings in gerbils. They exposed gerbils to intense short-term noise at a young age. The animals were tested with ABR at old age, and a comparison was done with non-exposed old gerbils. According to them, the additive model greatly overestimates the interaction between noise and ageing. The subadditive model means that the deterioration caused by presbyacusis is reduced within the noise frequencies in noise-damaged ears. According to Mills, the subadditive model is valid for intense, short noise exposure. The additive model is more accurate for moderate, long noise exposure.

Other, contradictory results have been published, favouring a *more than additive model (superadditivity)*. According to Henry (1982a,b) older mice without presbyacusis have a slightly increased susceptibility to noise overstimulation, compared with young adult mice. Miller et al. (1998) studied different strains of mice (CBA/Ca and C57/BL/6). They found that ageing, with or without hearing loss, increased the sensitivity to NIHL. It was speculated that other factors, most likely genetic disposition, might contribute to NIHL.

### Is there a progression of hearing loss after noise exposure?

Gates et al. (2000) have described an interesting and intriguing finding in elderly men with noise notches in their audiograms. In these subjects they found a reduced progress of hearing loss over time at 3, 4 and 6 kHz, and an accelerated hearing loss in frequency areas adjacent to noise-damaged frequencies, especially 2 kHz. In men without typical noise notches this pattern was reversed. These data suggest that the ageing process is different in a noise-damaged cochlea than in a 'pristine' one. The deterioration is less in the NIHL frequencies in a noise-damaged ear than in an ear not influenced by noise, but increases in adjacent frequencies, corresponding to an increased vulnerability of the regions on the basilar membrane bordering the NIHL region.

Gates et al. (2000) have described a continued loss of hearing in individuals with noise notches at frequencies adjacent to noise frequencies, especially at 2 kHz. This accelerated loss of hearing in noise-exposed individuals was also accompanied by a decreased loss at the noise frequencies, compared with a contrast without noise notches. Data from the Gothenburg gerontological and geriatric population study, Sweden, include longitudinal data of both audiometry and information about occupational data. A reanalysis of these data support the model described by Gates et al. – an accelerated hearing loss at frequencies adjacent to NIHL frequencies in noise-exposed elderly men (Rosenhall, 2003).

## NIHL, ARHL and genetic vulnerability

Erway et al. (1993) and Johnson et al. (1997) identified and mapped the first putative gene for presbyacusis in the C57 mice, the *Ahl* (age-related hearing loss) gene, on the proximal end of chromosome 10. The *Ahl* gene causes progressive cochlear damage irrespective of exposure to noise. Noise damage is not the basic mechanism causing ARHL in these mice. However, young mice with the *Ahl* gene suffered more severe NIHL, before the gene had an effect on hearing (Erway and Willott, 1996). This finding is in accordance to the study on different strains of mice, performed by Miller et al. (1988).

## Histopathology of ARHL and NIHL

Degenerative changes, affecting the cochlea, start relatively early in life, and increase with age. There is a difference of the degenerative patterns of inner hair cells (IHCs) and outer hair cells (OHCs) with age. The OHCs show a patchy degeneration most pronounced in the apical and basal coils (Bredberg, 1968). The degeneration of IHCs, and also the nerve fibres, is predominantly confined to the basal coil. Over the age of 50 the degeneration of OHCs is more severe than the degeneration of IHCs. The most pronounced degeneration of both OHCs and IHCs is found in the basal coil (Sousec et al., 1987). Johnsson and Hawkins (1972) described severe degeneration of OHCs in the apical region, but only mild nerve degeneration. Other histopathological findings related to ARHL are atrophy of the spiral ganglion and the nerves in the osseous spiral lamina, and ultrastructural changes such as accumulation of intracellular inclusions and alterations of stereocilia.

A wealth of information about inner-ear changes caused by exposure to noise is available (see Chapter 5). The most noise-susceptible sensory cells in the organ of Corti are, in decreasing order: OHCs of the first, second and third row and IHCs (Hunter and Willott, 1987). There are some resemblances between age-related degenerative patterns and noise-induced cochlear damage, but there are also pronounced differences.

Schuknecht has described four predominant pathological types of presbyacusis, and two mixed or intermediate types. The basis of this classification is a large investigation of archival human temporal bones, some of them from individuals with audiometric data (Schuknecht and Gacek, 1993). Sloping types of audiograms were the most common pattern regularly seen in many of the types. One important exception is strial presbyacusis, with a clinical feature of flat or slightly descending pure-tone audiometric pattern associated with excellent word discrimination scores. There was a patchy atrophy of the stria vascularis in the middle and apical turns of the cochlea (Schuknecht, 1964; Schuknecht and Gacek, 1993). Age-related histopathological changes of the stria vascularis has been reported in research animals (C57 mice) (Di Girolamo et al., 2001). Schuknecht and Gacek concluded that elderly individuals with abrupt high-tone hearing loss ('sensory presbyacusis') have inner-ear pathology that cannot be differentiated from NIHL. It has been proposed that strial degeneration is the typical histopathological finding of 'true' presbyacusis. However, in a recent study of human temporal bones (Nelson and Hinojosa, 2003) stria vascularis atrophy was only an infrequent finding in individuals with presbyacusis and flat hearing loss. OHC loss alone, or in combination with IHC or ganglion cell loss, was a more common finding in their study.

## Conclusions

Exposure to different types of noise for many decades is likely to have negative effects on the hearing. There is unanimous acceptance of an interaction between NIHL and ARHL, but its extent and appearance are difficult to determine, and are also discussed. A basically additive model is favoured by ISO 1999, but a subadditive effect has been proposed, as well as a superadditive effect. A combination of both these models has also been described: a reduced effect of ageing and noise at noise-associated frequencies, but an accelerated effect in adjacent frequencies. These various models are probably valid in different situations, depending on, for example, the initial state of the cochlea, other interactive factors, genetic mechanisms, and possibly the age at exposure. Other very important factors are certainty noise levels, duration of exposure and type of noise exposure. Animal models are important to study, but the interpretation of the results related to humans must be done with caution.

### Interaction between noise and age on hearing

* An interaction between NIHL and ARHL exists.
* The extent of this interaction is difficult to determine, and remains to be established.
* Different models to explain the interaction between ageing and noise exposure exist.
* The interaction between noise exposure and ageing is probably different depending on a number of factors, such as state of hearing, genetic susceptibility, age, and properties of noise exposure.

# References

Alessio HM, Hutchinson KM (1991) Effects of submaximal exercise and noise exposure on hearing loss. Research Quarterly for Exercise and Sport 62 413–419.

Andrén L, Hansson L, Björkman M, Jonsson A (1980) Noise as a contributory factor in the development of elevated arterial pressure. Acta Medica Scandinavica 207: 493–8.

Axelsson A, Lindgren F (1985) Is there a relationship between hypercholesterolemia and noise-induced hearing loss? Acta Otolaryngologica 100 379–86.

Babisch W (1998) Epidemiological studies of cardiovascular effects of traffic noise. In N Carter, SRF Jd (eds) Noise Effects '98. Proceedings of the 7th International Congress on Noise as a Public Health Problem. Noise Effects, vol. I, pp. 221–9. PTY Ltd, Sydney, Australia.

Barone JA, Peters JM, Garabrant DH, Bernstein L, Krebsbach R (1987) Smoking as a risk factor in noise-induced hearing loss. Journal of Occupational Medicine 29: 741–5.

Belojevic G, Saric-Tanasovic M (2002) Prevalence of arterial hypertension and myocardial infarction in relation to subjective ratings of traffic noise exposure. Noise & Health 4: 33–7.

Bies DA, Hansen CH (1990) An alternative mathematical description of the relationship between noise exposure and hearing loss. The Journal of the Acoustical Society of America 88: 2743–54.

Borg E (1982a) Noise-induced hearing loss in rats with renal hypertension. Hearing Research 8:93–9.

Borg E (1982b) Noise-induced hearing loss in normotensive and spontaneously hypertensive rats. Hearing Research 8: 117–30.

Borg E Viberg A (1987) Age-related hair cell loss in spontaneously hypertensive and normotensive rats. Hearing Research 30: 111–18.

Bredberg G (1968) Cellular pattern and nerve supply of the human organ of Corti. Acta Otolaryngologica Supplement 236: 1–135.

Burns W, Robinson DW (1970) Hearing and noise in industry. London: HMSO, Appendix 10.

Cohen M, Luxon L, Rudge P (1996). Auditory deficits and hearing loss associated with focal brainstem haemorrhage. Scandinavian Audiology 25: 133–41.

Cristell M, Hutchinson KM, Alessio HM (1998) Effects of exercise training on hearing ability. Scandinavian Audiology 27: 219–24.

Cruickshanks KJ, Klein R, Klein BE, Wiley TL, Nondahl DM, Tweed TS (1998a) Cigarette smoking and hearing loss: the epidemiology of hearing loss study. The Journal of the American Medical Association 279: 1715–19.

Cruickshanks KJ, Wiley TL, Tweed TS, Klein BE, Klein R, Mares-Perlman JA, Nondahl DM (1998b) Prevalence of hearing loss in older adults in Beaver Dam, Wisconsin. The epidemiology of hearing loss. American Journal of Epidemiology 148: 879–86.

Davis AC (1995) Hearing in adults. The prevalence and distribution of hearing impairment and reported hearing disability in the MRC Institute of Hearing Research's National Study of Hearing. London: Whurr Publishers.

Dengerink HA, Lindgren F, Axelsson A, Dengerink JE (1987) The effects of smoking and physical exercise on temporary threshold shifts. Scandinavian Audiology 16 131–6.

Dengerink HA, Lindgren F, Axelsson A (1992) The interaction of smoking and noise on temporary threshold shifts. Acta Otolaryngologica 112: 932–8.

Di Girolamo S, Quaranta N, Picciotti P, Torsello A, Wolf F (2001) Age-related histopathological changes of the stria vascularis: an experimental model. Audiology 40: 322–6.

Drettner B, Hedstrand H, Klockhoff I, Svedberg A (1975) Cardiovascular risk factors and hearing loss. A study of 1000 fifty-year-old men. Acta Otolaryngologica 79: 366–71.

Duck SW, Prazma J, Bennett S, Pillsbury HC (1997) Interactions between hypertension and diabetes mellitus in the pathogenesis of sensorineural hearing loss. Laryngoscope 107: 1596–605.

Erway LC, Willott JF (1996) Genetic susceptibility to noise-induced hearing loss in mice. In A Axelsson, HM Borchgrevink, RP Hamernik, P-A Hellström, D Henderson, RJ Salvi (eds) Scientific Basis of Noise-Induced Hearing Loss. New York: Thieme, 56–64.

Erway LC, Willott JF, Archer JR, Harrison D (1993) Genetics of age-related hearing loss in mice. I. Inbred and F1 hybrid strains. Hearing Research 65: 125-32.

Ferber-Viart C, Savourey G, Garcia C, Duclaux R, Bittel J, Collet L. (1995). Influence of hyperthermia on cochlear micromechanical properties in human. Hearing Research 91: 2002–207

Fourtes LJ, Tang S, Pomrehn P, Anderson C (1995) Prospective evaluation of associations between hearing sensitivity and selected cardiovascular risk factors. American Journal of Industrial Medicine 28: 275–80.

Fraenkel R, Freeman S, Sohmer H (2003) Susceptibility of young adult and old rats to noise-induced hearing loss. Audiology & Neuro-otology 8: 129–39.

Gatehouse S, Lowe GDO (1991) Whole blood viscosity and red cell filterability as factors in sensorineural hearing impairment in the elderly. Acta Otolaryngologica, Supplement 476: 37–43.

Gates GA, Cooper JC, Kannel WB, Miller NJ (1990) Hearing in the elderly: the Framingham cohort, 1983-1985. Part I. Basic audiometric test results. Ear and Hearing 11: 247–56.

Gates GA, Cobb JL, D'Agostino RB, Wolf PA (1993) The relation of hearing in the elderly to the presence of cardiovascular disease and cardiovascular risk factors. Arch Otolaryngol Head Neck Surg 119: 156–61.

Gates AG, Schmid P, Kujawa SG, Nam B, D'Agostino R (2000) Longitudinal threshold changes in older men with audiometric notches. Hearing Research 141: 220–8.

Hamernik RP, Ahroon WA, Davis RI, Axelsson A (1989) Noise and vibration interactions: effects on hearing. The Journal of the Acoustical Society of America 86: 2129–37.

Henry KR (1982a) Age related changes in the sensitivity of the post-pubertal ear to acoustic trauma. Hearing Research 8: 285–94.

Henry KR (1982b) Influence of genotype and age on noise-induced auditory losses. Behavior Genetics 12: 563–73.

Henry KR (2003) Hyperthermia exacerbates and hypothermia protects from noise-induced threshold elevation of the cochlear nerve envelope response in the C57BL/6J mouse. Hearing Research 179: 88–96.

Henry KR, Chole RA. (1984). Hypothermia protects the cochlea from noise damage. Hearing Research 16: 225–30.

Hirai A, Takata M, Mikawa M, Yasumoto K, Iida H, Sasayama S, Kagamimori S (1991) Prolonged exposure to industrial noise causes hearing loss but not high blood pressure: a study of 2124 factory laborers in Japan. Journal of Hypertension 9: 1069–73.

Hodgeson MJ, Talbott E, Helmkamp JC, Kuller LH (1987) Diabetes, noise exposure, and hearing loss. Journal of Occupational and Environmental Medicine 29: 576–9.

Hunter KP, Willott JF (1987) Aging and the auditory brainstem response in mice with severe or minimal presbycusis. Hearing Research 30 207–18.

Hutchinson KM, Alessio HM, Spadafore M, Adair RC (1991) Effects of low-intensity exercise and noise exposure on temporary threshold shift. Scandinavian Audiology 20: 121–7.

Iki M. (1994). Vibration-induced white finger as risk factor for hearing loss and postural instability. Nagoya Journal of Medical Science 57, Supplement: 137–45.

Iki M, Kurumatani N, Hirata K, Moriyama T, Satoh M, Arai T (1986) Association between vibration-induced white finger and hearing loss in forestry workers. Scandinavian Journal of Work, Environment & Health 12: 365–70.

ISO 1999 (1990) Acoustics - Determination of occupational noise exposure and estimation of noise-induced hearing impairment. International Standard. Geneva: International Organization for Standardization, second edition.

Itoh A, Nakashima T, Arao H, Wakai K, Tamakoshi A, Kawamura T, Ohno Y (2001) Smoking and drinking habits as risk factors for hearing loss in the elderly: epidemiological study of subjects undergoing routine health checks in Aichi,1 japan. Public Health 115: 192–6.

Johansson M (2003) On noise and hearing loss. Prevalence and reference data. Linköping University Medical Dissertation, Appendix II, p 82.

Johnson KR, Erway LC, Cook SA, Willott JF, Zheng QY (1997) A major gene affecting age-related hearing loss in C57BL/2J mice. Hearing Research 114: 83-92.

Johnsson L-G, Hawkins JE Jr (1972) Sensory and neural degeneration with aging, as seen in microdissection of the human inner ear. The Annals of Otology, Rhinology, and Laryngology Supplement 470: 88–96.

Jones NS, Davis A. (2000). A retrospective case-controlled study of 1490 consecutive patients presenting to a neuro-otologic clinic to examine the relationship between blood lipid levels and sensorineural hearing loss. Clinical Otolaryngology 25 511–17.

Jönsson R, Rosenhall U (1998) Hearing in advanced age. A study of presbyacusis in 85-, 88- and 90-year-old people. Audiology 37: 207–18.

Kaga K, Takigushi T, Myokai K, Shiode A (1979) Effects of deep hypothermia and circulatory arrest on the auditory brain stem responses. Archives of Otolaryngology 225: 199–205.

Karlsson KK, Harris JR, Svartengren M (1997) Description and primary results from an audiometric study of male twins. Ear and Hearing 18: 114–20.

Katbamna B, Bankaitis AE, Metz DA, Fisher LE (1993) Effects of hyperthermia on the auditory-evoked brainstem responses in mice. Audiology 32: 344–55.

Kolkhorst FW, Smaldino JJ, Wolf SC, Battani LR, Plakke BL, Huddleston S, Hensley LD (1998) Influence of fitness on susceptibility to noise-induced temporary threshold shift. Medicine and Science in Sports and Exercise 30 289–93.

Lim DP, Stephens SDG (1991) Clinical investigation of hearing loss in the elderly. Clinical Otolaryngology 16 288–93.

Lindgren F, Axelsson A (1988) The influence of physical exercise on susceptibility to noise-induced temporary threshold shift. Scandinavian Audiology 17: 11–17.

Luxon LM (1980). Hearing loss in brainstem disorders. Journal of Neurosurgery and Psychiatry 43: 510–15.

Macrae JH (1991) Presbycusis and noise-induced permanent threshold shift. The Journal of the Acoustical Society of America 90: 2513–16.

Manson J, Alessio HM, Cristell M, Hutchinson KM (1994) Does cardiovascular health mediate hearing ability? Medicine and Science in Sports and Exercise 26: 866–71.

Mikovic-Kraus S (1990) Noise-induced hearing loss and blood pressure. International Archives of Occupational and Environmental Health 62: 259–60.

Miller JM, Dolan DF, Raphael Y, Altschuler RA. (1988) Interactive effects of ageing with noise induced hearing loss. Scandinavian Audiology 27, Supplement 48: 53–61.

Mills JH, Boettcher FA, Dubno JR (1997) Interaction of noise-induced permanent threshold shift and age-related threshold shift. The Journal of the Acoustical Society of America 101: 1681–6.

Mills JH, Dubno JR, Boettcher FA (1998) Interaction of noise-induced hearing loss and presbyacusis. Scandinavian Audiology, Supplement 48: 117–22.

Musiek FE, Oxholm VB (2003) Central auditory anatomy and function. In L Luxon (ed) Textbook of Audiological Medicine. Clinical Aspects of Hearing and Balance London: Martin Dunitz, Taylor & Francis Group, pp. 179–200.

Nassar G (2001) The human temporary threshold shift after exposure to 60 minutes' noise in aerobics class. British Journal of Audiology 35: 99–101.

Nelson EG, Hinojosa R (2003) Presbycusis: a human temporal bone study of individuals with flat audiometric patterns of hearing loss using a new method to quantify stria vascularis volume. Laryngoscope 113 1672–86.

Nieminen O, Pyykkö I, Starck J, Toppila E, Iki M (1993) Serum cholesterol and blood pressure in the genesis of noise induced hearing loss. Transactions of the XXV Congress of the Scandinavian Oto-Laryngological Society, Bergen. pp. 48–50.

Noorhassim I, Rampal KG (1998) Multiplicative effect of smoking and age on hearing impairment. The American Journal of Otology 19: 240–3.

Palmer KT, Griffin MJ, Syddall HE, Pannett B, Cooper C, Coggon D (2002) Raunaud's phenomenon, vibration induced white finger, and difficulties in hearing. Occupational and Environmental Medicine 59: 640–2.

Palmer KT, Griffin MJ, Syddall HE, Coggon D (2004) Cigarette smoking, occupational exposure to noise, and self reported hearing difficulties. Occupational and Environmental Medicine 61: 340–4.

Parving A, Hein HO, Suadicani P, Ostri B, Gyntelberg F (1993) Epidemiology of hearing disorders. Some factos affecting hearing. The Copenhagen Male Study. Scandinavian Audiology 2: 101–7.

Pearson JD, Morrell CH, Gordon-Salant S, Brant LJ, Metter EJ, Klein LL, Fozard JL (1995) Gender differences in a longitudinal study of age-associated hearing loss. The Journal of the Acoustical Society of America 97: 1196–205.

Pillsbury HC (1986) Hypertension, hyperlipoproteinemia, chronic noise exposure: is there synergism in cochlear pathology? Laryngoscope 96: 1112–38.

Pyykkö I, Koskimies K, Starck J, Pekkarinen J, Inaba R (1988) Evaluation of factors affecting sensory neural hearing loss. Acta Otolaryngologica 449: 155–8.

Ray J (1991) Is there a relationship between presbyacusis and hyperlipoproteinemia? A literature review. Journal of Otolaryngology 20: 336–41.

Robinson D (1988) Threshold of hearing as a function of age and sex for the typical unscreened population. British Journal of Audiology 22: 5–20.

Robinson D, Sutton G (1979) Age effect in hearing. A comparative analysis of published threshold data. Audiology 18: 320–34.

Rosen S, Olin P (1965) Hearing loss and coronary heart disease. Archives of Otolaryngology 82:236–43.

Rosen S, Bergman M, Plester D, El-Mofty A, Satty M (1962) Presbycusis study of a relatively noise-free population in the Sudan. The Annals of Otology, Rhinology and Laryngology 71: 727–42.

Rosen S, Preobrajensky N, Khechinashvili T, Glazunoc I, Kipshidze N, Rosen HV (1970) Epidemiologic hearing studies in the USSR. Archives of Otolaryngology 91: 424–8.

Rosenhall U (2003) The influence of ageing on noise-induced hearing loss. Noise & Health 5: 47–53.

Rosenhall U, Sundh V (2004) Age-related hearing loss and blood pressure. Noise & Health

Rosenhall U, Pedersen K, Svanborg A (1990) Presbycusis and noise-induced hearing loss. Ear and Hearing 11: 257–63.

Rosenhall U, Sixt E, Sundh V, Svanborg A (1993) Correlations between presbyacusis and extrinsic noxious factors. Audiology 32 234–43.

Schuknecht HF (1964) Further observation on the pathology of presbycusis. Archives of Otolaryngology 80 369–82.

Schuknecht HF, Gacek MR (1993) Cochlear pathology in presbyacusis. The Annals of Otology, Rhinology and Laryngology 102: 1–16.

Seifert E, Brand K, van de Flierdt K, Hahn M, Riebandt M, Lamprecht-Dinnesen A. (2001) The influence of hypothermia on outer hair cells of the cochlea and its efferents. British Journal of Audiology 35: 87–98.

Sharabi Y, Reshef-Haran I, Burstein M, Eldad A (2002) Cigarette smoking and hearing loss: lessons from the young adult periodic examinations in Israel (YAPEIS) database. The Israel Medical Association Journal 4: 1118–20.

Soucek S, Michaels L, Frohlich A (1987) Pathological changes in the organ of Corti in presbycusis as revealed by microslicing and staining. Acta Otolaryngologica Supplement 436:93–102.

Starck J, Toppila E, Pyykkö I (1999) Smoking as a risk factor in sensory neural hearing loss among workers exposed to occupational noise. Acta Otolaryngologica 119: 302–5.

Stephens SDG (1982) What is aquired hearing loss in the elderly? In F Glennerding (ed) Aquired Hearing Loss and Elderly People. Stoke on Tent: Beth Johnson Foundation Publications, pp. 9–26.

Stockard JJ, Sharborough FW, Tinker JA (1978) Effect of hypothermia on the human brainstem auditory response. Annals of Neurology 3: 368–70.

Susmano A, Rosenbush SW (1988) Hearing loss and ischemic heart disease. The American Journal of Otology 9: 403-8.

Talbott E, Helmkamp J, Matthews K, Kuller L, Cottington E, Redmond (1985) Occupational noise exposure, noise induced hearing loss, and the epidemiology of high blood pressure. American Journal of Epidemiology 121: 501–14.

Talbott EO, Findlay RC, Kullert LH, Lenkner LA, Matthews KA, Day RD, Ishii EK (1990) Noise-induced hearing loss: a possible marker for high blood pressure in older noise-exposed populations. Journal of Occupational and Environmental Medicine 32: 690–7.

Tambs K, Hoffman HJ, Borchgrevink HM, Holmen J, Samuelsen SO (2003) Hearing loss induced by noise, ear infections, and head injuries: results from the North-Trøndelag Hearing Loss Study. Int J Audiol 42: 89–105.

Tarter SK, Robins TG (1990) Chronic noise exposure, high-frequency hearing loss, and hypertension among automobile assembly workers. Journal of Occupational and Environmental Medicine 32: 685–9.

Tomei F, Fantini S, Tomao E, Baccolo TP, Rosati MV (2000) Hypertension and chronic exposure to noise. Archives of Environmental Health 55: 319–25.

Toppila E, Pyykkö I, Starck J, Kaksonen R, Ishizaki H (2000) Individual risk factors in the development of noise-induced hearing loss. Noise & Health 2: 59–70.

Virokannas H, Anttonen H (1995) Dose-response relationship between smoking and impairment of hearing acuity in workers expoed to noise. Scandinavian Audiology 24: 211–16.

Vittitow M, Windmill IM, Yates JW, Cunningham DR (1994) Effect of simultaneous exercise and noise exposure (music) on hearing. Journal of the American Academy of Audiology 5: 343–8.

Welleschick B, Raber A (1978) Einfluss von Expositionszeit und Alter auf den Larmbedingten Hörverlust. Laryngo-rhino-otologie 57: 1037–48.

Willott JF, Bross LS, McFadden SL (1994) Morphology of the cochlear nucleus in CBA/J mice with chronic severe sensorineural cochlear pathology induced during adulthood. Hearing Research 74: 1–21.

Yoshida N, Kristiansen A, Liberman MC (1999). Heat stress and protection from permanent acoustic injury in mice. Journal of Neuroscience 19: 10116–24.

# CHAPTER 15

# Methodology and value of databases: an individual hearing conservation programme

*Noise and Its Effects:* Edited by Linda Luxon and Deepak Prasher © 2007 John Wiley & Sons Ltd.

ESKO TOPPILA, ILMARI PYYKKÖ, JUKKA STARCK, ANN-CHRISTIN JOHNSON, MARTTI JUHOLA

## Introduction

In Europe, around 50 million individuals are exposed to hazardous levels of environmental noise, with a risk of noise-induced hearing loss (NIHL) and tinnitus. The loss in economic terms is substantial: at a minimum level of 0.2% of national net income. This equals about 400 billion euros annually and includes direct and indirect costs, although the indirect costs do not include factors related to reduced quality of life. These factors include social isolation, increased unemployment and difficulties in family life due to communication difficulties caused by hearing handicap. NIHL remains one of the leading health-related problems in industrialized countries.

There are no global or European Community figures available for the prevalence of NIHL. Data from two neighbouring countries with similar economic structures indicate substantial differences in the number of subjects, with annual reports of occupational NIHL (Figure 15.1). Even though these member states represent the most advanced states of occupational health care in the EU, the data on NIHL is subject to political and economic decisions. Prevalence figures, if they did exist, would provide data that would allow focused control methods to reduce the risk at national levels.

The ultimate goal of development of a database and prevention of noise damage to the ear is to develop an individual hearing conservation programme (IHCP) that determines total environmental exposure to noise, and takes into consideration individual susceptibility due to genetic inheritance, biological and other environmental factors.

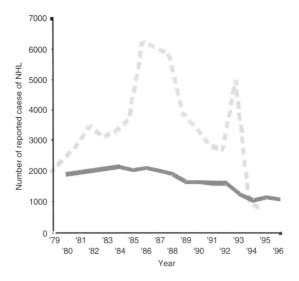

**Figure 15.1** Incidence of noise-induced hearing loss in two neighbouring industrialized countries of EU: ▬ ▬ Number of cases in the first country ▬▬Number of cases in the second country.

# Objectives of databases

## Demands set by new EU directives

The EU has set a directive for the protection of workers from occupational hazards (European Commission, 1989). Based on this framework, a new Directive (2003/10/EEC) for the protection of workers against harmful effects of noise was published in 2003. In this directive, the need to evaluate all factors affecting the development of NIHL is recognized. The employer must pay particular attention when carrying out risk assessment in workers belonging to particularly sensitive groups throughout their whole working career, provided that no sensitive data are transferred. However, the Directive does not define the contents of the record or how the record should be organized. A database should, therefore, include all environmental and health-related factors that may be involved in NIHL

Noise-induced hearing loss is defined by changes seen in the audiogram; its handicapping influence is seen by changes across the speech frequencies (0.5–4 kHz). Threshold shifts in hearing show great variability across noise-exposed subjects, indicating differences in susceptibility to the harmful effects of noise (see Chapter 7). This variation has been generalized by using statistical models, which include age, gender and noise exposure, and these are used to explain changes in hearing threshold of industrial populations (ISO 1999 – International Organization for Standardization or ISO, 1975, 1990). However, because the individual susceptibility for NIHL shows great variability, a statistical model is not useful in the prediction of NIHL at an individual level. Significant contributions to NIHL are linked to human factors such as blood pressure, lipids, smoking habit, use of analgesics, exposure to vibrations, solvents and genetic background.

### Composition of the database

The approach used in a database should be multidisciplinary, and the extent of hearing loss should be studied as a function of environmental noise exposure, individual sensitivity factors, interacting diseases and genetic background. In the assessment of these factors, artificial intelligence may be used to create a hearing conservation programme (HCP) valid for individual subjects. The database is usually composed of three parts based on static, semi-static and dynamic data. The static data are constant, for example gender or eye colour. The semi-static data normally hold their values, but the values can be changed; for example, in the case of ear surgery, new values will pertain postoperatively. The dynamic data vary with time, for example weight, noise dose and usage rate of hearing protector devices (HPD).

**Components in a database:**

- information about separate and combined exposures for occupational noise;
- information about use and type of HPD;
- information about separate and combined effects of non-occupational noise;
- information about human (risk) factors for hearing impairment;
- information about interaction of diseases for hearing impairment;
- information about hereditary factors in the aetiology of hearing impairment;
- relevant audiological test results;
- otological history and examination;
- the impact of hearing impairment on quality of life.

Noise-induced hearing loss is insidious and progressive in nature, and it is invisible. At no time is there a sudden noticeable change in hearing. The loss of frequency resolution passes unnoticed by most people. Affected workers attribute their difficulties to fatigue, lack of interest or concentration, poor articulation of speakers and excessive background noise. Interaction with hearing-impaired people reveals inconsistent behaviour and is attributed to an unwillingness to communicate. The awareness of hearing difficulties is further hampered by the stigma associated with deafness. The experience of hearing difficulties has a strong negative impact on self-image, which manifests itself as a sense of being incompetent, and perceiving oneself as abnormal, physically diminished, prematurely old or having a defect. Any sign of impairment is seen as a sign of weakness, and thus concealment is adopted as a strategy. When NIHL is moderate to severe it leads to speech distortion, reduced word discrimination, noise intolerance and tinnitus. Reduced oral communication is a social handicap. NIHL also reduces the perception of warning signals, environmental sounds and music. Consequently, NIHL may lead to social isolation, decreased worker productivity and morale, and an increase in job-related accidents. It may limit quality of life. Therefore a database should also record factors related to quality of life. In Europe, an instrument, which is relatively simple to use and only requires answers to a few questions, is E-QoL 5D. The 5 item – environmental quality of life questionaire (E-QoL 5D) is more tuned towards population studies and has a limited capability to resolve the effect of diseases. The QoL 15 D has 15 questions each with five choices, and is better suited for evaluation of the effect of hearing loss on quality of life.

# Historical databases used in evaluation of NIHL

One of the first sets of damage-risk criteria based on exposure to steady-state noise was proposed by Kryter (1965). The damage-risk criteria were composed from a group of curves, which were based on laboratory experiments on the development of temporary threshold shift (TTS). Data collected in 1955–6 on permanent threshold shifts (PTSs) in workers exposed to industrial noise were also included. The Committee on Hearing, Bioacoustics and Biomechanics (CHABA) (Kryter, 1965) used these data to explore hearing loss contours as a function of exposure. This was the first norm proposed for evaluation of hazardous noise.

Baughn (1973) made the first large epidemiological study on the relationship between noise exposure and hearing loss. His studies from the early 1960s involved a large worker population ($N = 6835$) working in stable locations and under conditions with stable noise exposure (Baughn, 1966, 1973). The duration of exposure extended to 45 years with average noise exposure levels of 78, 86 and 92 dB. Baughn (1973) recommended that the hearing loss of subjects exposed to the 78 dB (A) noise would be considered as representing typical non-noise-exposed males. According to his data, it is possible that factory workers suffer more socioacusis and nosoacusis than the general population.

Burns and Robinson studied 759 subjects, of whom 422 males were exposed to four classes of noise ranging from 87 dB (A) to 97 dB (A) (Burns and Robinson, 1970). The maximum exposure was about 49 years. As controls, 97 subjects not exposed to noise were included in the study. The population was screened to be otologically normal. The authors developed a mathematical generalization of the predicted hearing loss (Robinson, 1968; Robinson and Shipton, 1977). This model introduced the energy principle to enable the combination of different sound levels (Burns 1973). Hearing loss was divided into two parts: age-dependent hearing loss (presbycusis) and NIHL. After correcting the model for age and gender, the distribution of hearing loss can be calculated by using the given formulae. The separation of presbycusis from NIHL leads to a predicted hearing loss that is smaller than that found in other models, partly because the material was rigorously and otologically screened (Suter, 1994).

Passchier-Vermeer (1974) summarized the results of 19 smaller studies, 12 of which have 50 or fewer cases. The data agree well with the Robinson's data at some frequencies, but at other frequencies large differences were found. One reason was the deviation in the definition of the audiometer zero level used in some of the studies (Glorig and Nixon, 1960).

## Historical datasets

| 1965 | Kryter | Damage-risk criteria |
|------|--------|----------------------|
| 1973 | Baughn | Epidemiological study ($n = 6835$) |
| 1970 | Burns and Robinson | Epidemiological study ($n = 759$) |
| 1974 | Passchier-Vermeer | Review of 19 studies |
| 1977 | Robinson and Shipton | Mathematical formula for predicted hearing loss secondary to noise |
| 1974 | NIOSH | Table of NIHL ($n = 792$) |
| 1975 | ISO 1999 (ISO 1975) | Standard for hearing conservation |
| 1990 | ISO 1999 (ISO 1990) | Standard mathematical model |

Johnson (1973) prepared a report for the US Environmental Protection Agency (EPA) on the prediction of noise-induced permanent threshold shift (NIPTS) from exposure to continuous noise. This report is based on the data of Burns and Robinson (1970) and of Passhier-Vermeer (1974). The data of Baughn (1966, 1973) were also used in the evaluation of the hearing loss of the non-exposed population. For this reason the hearing loss of the non-exposed population is somewhat less in this report than in the works by Burns and Robinson (1970) or Passchier-Vermeer (1974).

The National Institute for Occupational Safety and Health (NIOSH) in the USA conducted a study on industrial workers exposed to noise levels of approximately 85, 90 and 95 dB (A) and control subjects exposed to levels below 80 dB (A) (NIOSH, 1974). The study consisted of an otologically screened population of 792 noise-exposed subjects and 380 controls. Hearing loss was tabulated by a function determined by exposure level and duration. Using these tables, the occurrence of NIHL could be calculated by subtracting the control values from hearing threshold values measured in noise-exposed subjects.

The ISO, in 1975, provided a standard for assessing occupational noise exposure for hearing conservation. The information on which the standard is based is not identified, but according to Suter (1994), the data of Baughn (1966, 1973) form its basis. The ISO standard adopted the equal energy principle for the combination of different sound exposures from the Robinson model. According to ISO tables, 50% of non-noise-exposed people have a hearing loss, whereas Robinson and Sutton (1979) demonstrated a figure of 10%, and a US public health services study (Glorig and Roberts, 1965; Rowland, 1980) demonstrated a 20% prevalence of hearing loss for non-noise-exposed people. The ISO model was later corrected, and a mathematical form for the hearing loss was given in order to produce the present standard model (ISO, 1990).

The problem with the historical data is that they were not screened for hereditary factors, and with few exceptions the workers were exposed to noise of the same character. In today's society, the noise exposure sources vary, and leisure noise exposure has become an important source of NIHL.

# Construction of a modern database program

## Interface

**A functionally 'customer friendly' database includes:**

- the database;
- an interference engine;
- an interface.

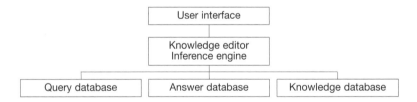

**Figure 15.2** Structure of a database program.

The purpose of the *interface* is to provide the user with easy access to both existing data and the inclusion of new cases. The *inference engine* assists the user to combine different noise sources into a single value for the exposure, and to determine the efficacy of hearing protective devices (HPDs) against noise. It should also present warnings of excessive noise, hearing protective devices' sensitivity, and print out the risk factors for NIHL in individual cases.

The inference engine is based on knowledge and decision-making rules. Usually the executive part is composed from abstract grammar or algorithms (genetic algorithms, neural networks and decision trees among others). The engine calculates constantly different possible ways of classification of the data, and its 'knowledge' is based on previously 'learned' examples. The risk models should preferably be based on the ISO 1999 model and secondarily on risk models designed by the analysis. A sophisticated database is the basis for an individual hearing conservation programme (IHCP). In real life all data are not available (typically exposure data or ear diseases at a younger age). To overcome this problem the database has to accept uncertain answers and have the capability to handle them, for example using fuzzy logics

The interface between the subject and the database may be remote, as was previously common when the occupational hygienist determined the exposure history. It may be based on questionnaires, which can be scanned into the database, on an interview with a professional with direct access to the database, or on an interactive method whereby the subject completes the database from the computer by himself (Auramo et al., 1995). The direct data input is useful in large-scale surveys, e.g. in recruiting people in a military base or in assessing hearing loss in factories. The interactive questioning with direct access into the database is most commonly used by medium-sized and small industries where the occupational nurse will feed the data into the system from case histories. The paper-based questionnaire is mostly used in field studies and in cross-sectional studies. Commonly, the questionnaires are scanned in with a text scanner and screened for possible errors. The authors have experience of all these models.

**Table 15.1** Selected software for database and individual hearing conservation programmes (IHCPs)[a]

| Name | Industrial noise data | IHCP characteristics | Hereditary factors | Risk factors | Audiometric analysis |
|------|------------------------|----------------------|--------------------|--------------|----------------------|
| NoiseScan 4.0 | Yes | Yes | Yes | Yes | Yes |
| NoiseCalc | Yes | Yes | No | No | No |
| ADAM 2.5 | No | No | No | No | Yes |
| Hearing Conservation Manager | No | No | No | No | Yes |
| Audiograf 3.0 | No | No | No | No | Yes |
| HEARSAF2000 | Yes | Yes | No | No | Yes |
| Hear/Track | No | Yes | No | No | Yes |

[a] Their ability to handle confounding factors and estimated threshold shifts based on audiometry are shown.

At present there are several commercial and non-commercial databases available on the market (Table 15.1). Most of these are aimed at special tasks, such as collecting data from industries for hazard prevention, evaluation of the success of preventive measures and, for research purposes. Some of them, such as NoiseScan and NoiseCalc, are developed partly to fill the gap between individual and group noise exposure evaluation. Both these programs are able to predict, based on occupational noise exposure and the development of hearing loss, and show the respective ISO 1999 curve family. NoiseScan is aimed at industrial use and has data collection routines fulfilling the demands of the proposed EU Directive

(2003/10/EEC) for protection of individual workers against noise. Furthermore, NoiseScan has a database that is used to create a risk model for NIHL, in which different confounding factors are included. The risk model can be used to predict individual hearing loss.

In the following section the structure of the database program NoiseScan 4.0 is provided.

### Subject selection

When a database program is opened, a subject selection button is provided in the bar on the left-hand side of the screen. The subject can be new, or an existing subject can be examined. The search of existing cases works incrementally, indicating that either a part of the name or a part of the ID can be the input. When the first feasible case is found, it is provided to the user. It can be accepted or the search can be continued (Figure 15.3). After accepting a name, all the main buttons are activated on the left-hand bar.

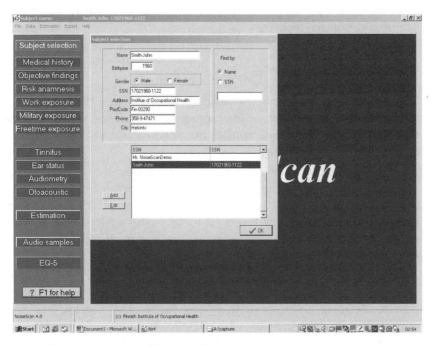

**Figure 15.3** Main screen and buttons for NoiseScan 4.0.

By looking at existing cases, new data can be added, audiograms may be revised or added, and medical history can be supplemented. Each subject has his or her individual ID, which is most commonly the social security number. The program includes routines for scrambling the IDs when the data are exported or joined to another database, to ensure privacy of the data of the workers.

## Medical history

In the medical history, several questions are activated. The first group is linked to questions on:

- *Ear diseases,* to exclude inflammatory ear disease, which may confound NIHL.
- *Ear operations* are reported separately. All the major ear operations are included so that the specialist may decide whether the hearing loss can be linked to the ear pathology or to surgery. These questions are paged so that, if the answer is yes, a new screen is opened and details of the type of ear disease or operation are requested.
- *Neurological diseases* and possible central nervous system infections are reported, and if the history is positive a screen with detailed questions is provided.
- *Explosions or head trauma* may explain hearing loss, and these are also noted. In a previous version we tried to classify the duration and severity of head trauma but returned to the present non-detailed version, since the duration of unconsciousness did not provide additional information on hearing loss.
- *Vertigo* is an indication of an inner-ear disease, which is often linked to sensorineural hearing loss, independent of NIHL. Vertigo should be included in the database as an exclusion criterion.
- *Tinnitus* may or may not be present, and may increase the handicap of NIHL. In assessing quality of life among noise-exposed workers, tinnitus may be more of a handicap than hearing loss and should, therefore, be included in the database.
- *Skin pigmentation* seems to affect vulnerability to NIHL. A study among African–Americans showed a somewhat better average in hearing threshold levels than white people (Royster et al., 1980). This has been attributed to higher levels of melanocytes and their protective capability in the inner ear against noise damage (Barrenäs and Lindgren, 1991; Barrenäs, 1998).
- A significant part of the unexplained hearing loss seems to be linked to *genetic inheritance.* The database therefore also includes a question on possible hearing impairment in the pedigree. The hearing loss may appear in a syndromic form, with specific symptoms or signs that are relatively easy to detect (Morton, 1991). It may also appear in non-syndromic form, without specific symptoms or signs, and is often difficult to separate from NIHL. The non-syndromic form often increases with ageing. The genetic background of non-syndromic hearing loss is quite heterogeneous and, to date, 41 different genes for non-syndromic hearing loss have been localized (19 autosomal-recessive hearing loss, 21 autosomal-dominant hearing loss, 1 X-linked hearing loss and 7 mitochondrial mutations) (Smith and Van Camp, 2005). From these gene mutations, the connexin 26 (*Cx26*) mutation is most frequent, and can

be observed in 3% of the population (Green et al., 1999). In the recessive form, the *Cx26* mutation is observed in 50% of the population (Green et al., 1999). In the extension of the Framingham study, a good correlation was found with early onset of hearing loss and extent of presbycusis within the family (Gates et al., 1999). In males the relationship was not as evident as in females, which could be linked to environmental noise as a confounding factor (Gates et al., 1999). There are insufficient data available on the relationship between NIHL and genetic background. Such data could be crucial in explaining the great variability of noise vulnerability in population studies. In the future, subjects with indications of genetically induced hearing loss might be tested for a possible defect in the *Cx26* gene and possibly also for some mitochondrial defects. The number of new known gene mutations is constantly increasing, and the current situation can be verified by looking at the home page for Hereditary Hearing Loss (www.uia.ac.be/ dnatab/hhh).

- *Vibration-induced white finger syndrome* is a risk factor that would cause about 10-dB greater hearing loss than if this syndrome were not present (Pyykkö et al., 1986). The effect of vibration-induced white finger and noise seems to be synergistic. The mechanism of increased vulnerability to noise in conjunction with vibration-induced white finger is not known. It may be linked to activation of the sympathetic nervous system or act directly on the cochlear compartments in susceptible people. In recent animal experiments after vibration of the temporal bone, two characteristic things were observed: hearing loss with moderate hair cell loss and prominent expression of tumour necrosis factor $\alpha$ (TNF-$\alpha$) with upregulation of P75 receptors (Jing et al., 2002). In experiments using magnetic resonance imaging (MRI), leakage of gadolinium in the scala media was also observed (Jing et al., 2002). The hearing loss was irreversible and could not prevented with antioxidant treatment but could be alleviated with neurotrophic factors (Jing et al., 2001). It is possible that the cochlear system (stria vascularis and upregulation of mediators) can be influenced by vibration, especially in sensitive people.

- Finally, *exposure to aminoglycoside antibiotics* is sought. Aminoglycoside antibiotics are still widely used and are ototoxic in conjunction with noise. They can produce significant hearing loss and potentiate the effect of noise on hearing (Mäkitie et al., 2002).

## Objective findings

**'Objective findings'**

- cholesterol;
- blood pressure;
- weight;
- gender;
- height.

The role of several biological factors in exacerbating NIHL has been studied. In population surveys, severe hearing loss in non-exposed populations has been attributed to biological and environmental factors (Hinchcliffe, 1973). Nevertheless, the data on NIHL in carefully controlled studies show considerable case-to-case variation, indicating that individual susceptibility also plays a significant role (Chung et al., 1982; Pyykkö et al., 1989). Factors such as elevated blood pressure (McCormic et al., 1982; Pyykkö et al., 1989) and altered lipid metabolism (Rosen and Olin, 1965) are believed to contribute to NIHL. Animal studies have indicated that arterial hypertension accelerates age-related hearing loss (Borg, 1982; McCormic et al., 1982). An antihypertensive medication may partly mask the effect of elevated blood pressure on NIHL (Pyykkö et al., 1989). The effect of hypertension on hearing may be promoted by other factors, but there is not sufficient evidence to show whether the effects of noise and hypertension are additive or synergistic.

The cholesterol level is correlated with hearing loss and, when combined with noise exposure and hypertension, produces a significantly more prominent hearing loss than each factor alone (Pyykkö et al., 1988; Toppila et al., 2000; Toppila et al., 2001). Depending on the age group the importance of cholesterol in NIHL varies (Table 15.2). We have calculated that an elevated cholesterol level alone explains about 2–4 dB of hearing loss at different audiometric frequencies (Pyykkö et al., 1989). This cholesterol-linked hearing loss is age dependent and is observed in subjects aged 40 years or over (Nieminen et al., 2000).

Many authors have found a significant and relatively large difference in vulnerability for NIHL between men and women (Berger et al., 1978; ISO, 1990). These results may be explained by women's smaller exposure to leisure noise, especially to gunfire. In a recent study, where these factors were controlled more accurately, no difference was found (Davis et al., 1998).

**Table 15.2** Logistics regression analysis results in four different age percentile groups

| Percentile of age | Mean age | Range | 4-kHz hearing loss (dB) | Risk factor (OR) | Risk factor (OR) | Risk factor (OR) | Power (%) |
|---|---|---|---|---|---|---|---|
| 0–25 | 28 | 19–32 | 9.4 | Cholesterol (7.2) | | | 83.3 |
| 26–50 | 36 | 33–38 | 13.7 | Cholesterol (2.6) | | | 67.7 |
| 51–75 | 44 | 39–44 | 19.1 | Analgesics (5.8) | Cholesterol (1.8) | | 65.4 |
| 76–100 | 49 | 45–62 | 31.5 | Cholesterol (1.8) | LANI (1.2) | Blood press (1.1) | 80.2 |

Mean age, range, mean HL at 4 kHz, and odds ratios for factors causing HL are given with explanatory power of the regression model. LANI is the total noise exposure inside the hearing protector.

### Risk history

The 'risk history' contains factors such as smoking, and use of painkillers with and without prescription. When the case history is indicative, a detailed quantitative history for smoking is taken and a similar approach also allows painkillers to be quantified. Smoking, together with hypertension, heightens the role of smoking in causing NIHL (Starck et al., 1998).

Other factors are included as appropriate and there can be an unlimited amount of input data.

## Work history

Differing from previous databases (Royster and Royster, 1986; Franks et al., 1989) we decided to collect subjects' lifetime working history, which may contain different noise exposure profiles. A new data sheet (Figure 15.4) is provided for each work task, noise exposure period or occupation. Thus, a subject may have an unlimited number of noise exposure data sheets. Each data sheet begins with a statement on the duration of the work period. It can be input, as in the data form, with information on the beginning and end of the job, or specify the duration of each job period in years and months. A job description is also required for the documentation. The noise exposure time is asked about with an accuracy of hours per day and days per week. The noise level is collected, as well as the frequency content of noise, which is divided into low–medium or high–medium frequency content. If the noise level is not measured or known, the program provides guestimates for noise level, based on occupation, work task, environment and machine type.

All the different occupational histories are shown in a table at the bottom of the screen.

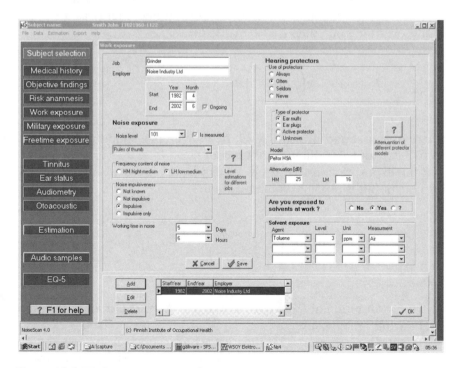

**Figure 15.4** Work noise exposure sheet.

The time domain characteristics of noise have been shown to affect the harmfulness of noise; the risk of NIHL is higher in those occupations where workers are exposed to impulse noise. In several occupations, the impulses are so rapid that they contribute only a minimal amount to the energy content of noise. For example, in impulsive noise among shipyard workers, there was a 10 dB higher hearing loss at 4 kHz than could be predicted by the model. The observed hearing levels were very consistent with the model for forest workers, where the noise was not impulsive (Starck et al., 1988). Pauses in exposure allow for some recovery, and the resulting hearing loss is not as great as is proposed by the equal energy principle in animal experiments (Campo and Lataye, 1992). Recently Suvorov et al. (2001) showed that, among the workers in a forge hammering plant with impulsive noise exposure, the observed hearing loss occurred on average about 3.5 years faster than predicted by the ISO model (ISO, 1990,1999). The mean exposure time in this factory was 8.9 years whereas based on calculations of steady-state noise the observed hearing should be attained in 12.4 years. The difference in exposure time was 30%.

As noise in the workplace tends to vary, and workers are often exposed to different tasks with different noise levels, a method is needed to combine the different levels to a single number that is related to risk of hearing impairment. The equivalent noise level ($L_{eq}$) is the most commonly used at present. It is the sound level that, when integrated over a specified period of time, would result in the same energy as a variable sound over the same time (Earshen, 1986):

$$L_{eq} = 10*\log\left(\frac{1}{T}\int_0^T \left(\frac{p(t)}{p_0}\right)^2 dt\right) \qquad [1]$$

where $p(t)$ = sound pressure level; $p_0$ = reference sound pressure level ($2 \times 10^{-5}$ Pa); and $T$ = duration of exposure.

If the exposure consists of several exposure periods using the following equation it is possible combine them:

$$L_{eq,\,tot} = 10*\log\left(\frac{\sum_i 10^{L_i/10}*T_i}{\sum_i T_i}\right) \qquad [2]$$

where $T_i$ = duration of $i$-th exposure; and $L_i$ = A-weighted sound pressure level during $i$-th exposure.

The total noise dose ($L_{Ex}$) is the total acoustical power that has entered the ear. It is calculated from the equivalent levels using the following equation:

$$L_{ex} = L_{eq} + 10 * \log\left(\frac{T}{T_0}\right) \hspace{2cm} [3]$$

where $L_{ex}$ = exposure; $L_{eq}$ = equivalent level; $T$ = length of exposure usually in years; and $T_0$ = reference time, usually 1 year.

## Hearing protection

The use of ear protectors is reported by evaluating the percentage of usage. The analysis of the usage rate as a percentage was changed to class mode in the current version, due to the inaccuracy of the retrieved history in percentages. The type and model of the HPDs used are inputs. Certified protectors commonly used in western Europe are included in the database with their attenuation efficacy. If the protector is known, the attenuation is automatically given on the screen for both low- and high-frequency noise. Otherwise, an estimation is provided that can be corrected or accepted. At the end of the exposure data sheet, there are buttons with which the previous or next exposure data screens can be retrieved. Among paper mill workers, the hearing loss of those who used HPDs on average 50% of the time was less than that among those who never used HPDs. The difference could not be explained by the change in exposure (Starck et al., 1996). The authors concluded that even temporary use of HPDs may provide protection against hearing loss.

Finally exposure and type of solvents used is noted. Synergism occurs also between noise and solvents. In animal experiments, noise combined with a high level of styrene (600 p.p.m./m$^2$) caused a threshold shift in hearing that is 30 dB greater than when the animals were exposed to noise or styrene alone (Mäkitie et al., 1997).

## Non-industrial (free time) noise exposure

The type, exposure duration and level of leisure noise are collected. Leisure noise is focused on four main topics: playing music, visiting discotheques and concerts, use of power tools and shooting or hunting. Noise from vehicles and from rock music is extremely common in an urban society, and represents a different kind of noise exposure that is almost impossible to quantify. Special attention is paid to shooting noise and to work with chain saws, both of which are common in the rural setting in Nordic countries. In the evaluation of shooting noise, the number of shots and the usage rate of HPDs are estimated (see 'Military noise' below). Exposure to power tool noise is also evaluated. In all of these noise sources, frequency of the noise exposure, loudness level, use of protectors and duration in years of exposure are noted. For these questions, 'yes/no' answers suffice.

**Table 15.3** Examples of commonly used hearing protectors and their attenuations

| Name | H | M | L |
|------|---|---|---|
| Peltor H6C | 27 | 18 | 11 |
| Peltor H9A | 33 | 25 | 16 |
| Peltor H9F | 27 | 23 | 14 |
| Peltor H7A | 37 | 30 | 21 |
| Peltor H3A | 36 | 29 | 20 |
| Peltor Blue | 28 | 23 | 21 |
| Peltor Bull's Eye 6 | 32 | 23 | 15 |
| Peltor Bull's Eye 9 | 33 | 25 | 16 |
| Peltor Tactical 7 | 29 | 26 | 19 |
| Peltor Hörskyddtelefon HTB7A | 29 | 26 | 17 |
| Peltor Headset MT7H7A | 31 | 28 | 20 |
| Peltor Aviation 7002 | 29 | 26 | 18 |
| Silenta Bell II | 25 | 18 | 12 |
| Silenta Bella | 28 | 20 | 13 |
| Silenta Ergo II | 30 | 26 | 17 |
| Silenta Super | 30 | 27 | 18 |
| Silenta Supermil | 31 | 22 | 14 |
| Silenta Sportmil | 28 | 19 | 11 |
| Silenta Universal | 31 | 24 | 15 |
| Bilsom 727 | 35 | 27 | 18 |
| Bilsom Loton 2401 | 29 | 24 | 16 |
| Bilsom Comfort 2420 OH | 35 | 24 | 15 |
| Bilsom Viking 2421 OH | 37 | 28 | 19 |
| Bilsom Pocket 2428 OH | 31 | 22 | 14 |
| Bilsom Original 2450 OH | 33 | 25 | 17 |
| Bilsom Marksman Pro 2902 | 33 | 28 | 19 |
| Bilsom Impact 707 | 31 | 27 | 19 |
| Bilsom FM Radio 797 | 31 | 27 | 19 |
| Bilsom Marksman Electronic 2905 | 27 | 24 | 17 |
| Bilsom PerFlex/PerFlex Det. OH | 24 | 21 | 20 |

The protectors are classified on the basis of attenuation H (high), M (medium) and L (low) frequency range protectors.

## Military noise

The program opens a new screen with a separate database file for military noise exposure (Figure 15.5). The type of service is selected as the first procedure. Thereafter, the number of shots with hand-held guns, heavy guns, and use of armoured vehicles and helicopters are noted. If the subject is exposed, then the type and use of HPDs is reported.

Exposure to gunfire noise is difficult to assess because there is no standard method available to evaluate its effect on the inner ear. The existing measurement methods can be divided into two categories: the peak level methods and energy methods. With the peak level methods (CHABA, 1968; Pfander, 1975; ACGIH, 1999) the risk for hearing loss is related to the peak level and duration. These methods do not provide a way of combining different gunfire exposures or gunfire exposure with work noise exposure into a single exposure index. The latest approach is to apply the energy attenuation of the impulse in risk assessment (Dancer et al., 1996; Patterson and Johnson, 1996; ANSI, 2000).

Exposure to attack rifle noise and bazookas often results in a deterioration of the hearing of military conscripts. It is noteworthy that a single shot at a noise level exceeding 140 dB can cause a measurable effect on hearing (Price, 1986). Even a few shots with bazookas or artillery, when the immission noise level exceeds 170 dB (in heavy bazookas 184 dB), may be detrimental to hearing (Pekkarinen et al., 1993). The military noise exposure of conscripts, especially during the handling of heavy weapons, causes an average of 5 dB hearing loss at 4000 Hz (Pekkarinen et al., 1993). Thus, exposure to military noise in a man may cause a significant threshold shift in hearing that is commonly disregarded when occupational NIHL is evaluated.

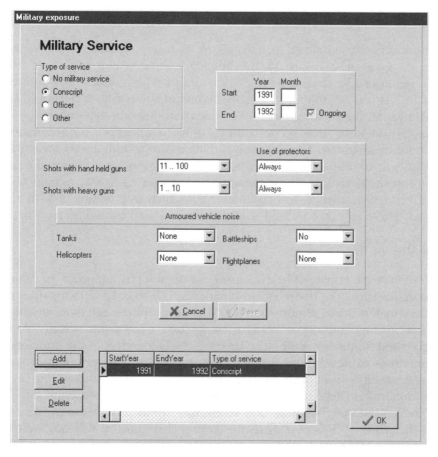

**Figure 15.5** Exposure to military service noise.

## Tinnitus

Information about tinnitus is recorded in a separate screen and file. If tinnitus is present, further questions open on the screen, and a more detailed analysis of the severity of tinnitus is determined. To date tinnitus is commonly noted with NIHL, but detailed measures are rarely recorded. As tinnitus reduces quality of life, it is a reason for benefits in some countries. It is therefore appropriate to determine the occurrence and severity of tinnitus.

## Ear status

The ears are inspected otoscopically and the tympanic membranes are described. If the status is not normal, a pop-up window appears, upon which the findings of the tympanic membrane are recorded. The questions address otorrhoea, tympanic membrane perforation or middle-ear conduction defect. Usually an ear with ongoing middle-ear disease does not qualify to be included in the database, as it biases the characteristics of NIHL.

## Audiometry

The audiograms are filled into the user's own screen and stored in separate database files (Figure 15.6). The examination year is recorded. Also the result of speech audiometry can be input. The number of audiometric inputs can be unlimited. Possible contamination with TTS should be included in the hearing threshold evaluation. Also the type of the audiometry: clinical, Békésy, screening, bone conduction or automated should be included. The rationale is that screening audiometry measures hearing at 20 dB hearing level, whereas other methods measure real hearing threshold values. The automated audiometer has a step accuracy of 1 dB in contrast to clinical audiometry in which step widths of 5 dB are used. These all cause variability in the database and should be recorded.

## Quality of life

To analyse the impact of hearing loss on a person it is important to distinguish impairment, disability and handicap (WHO, 1980). Impairment refers to functional abnormality. In NIHL, impairment refers to an alteration in the auditory system, such as loss of hearing sensitivity or decreased frequency resolution. Hearing disability refers to the functional limitations caused by impairment in everyday activities, primarily where communication is concerned. Handicap refers to the social consequences of impairment. In NIHL, handicap refers to the social consequences of communication difficulties, such as social isolation and unemployment.

The 'fitness' of a person in the twenty-first century will be, for the most part, defined in terms of his or her ability to communicate effectively. Societal self-interest will drive an increased allocation of resources to optimize the communication ability of its population, for this is how

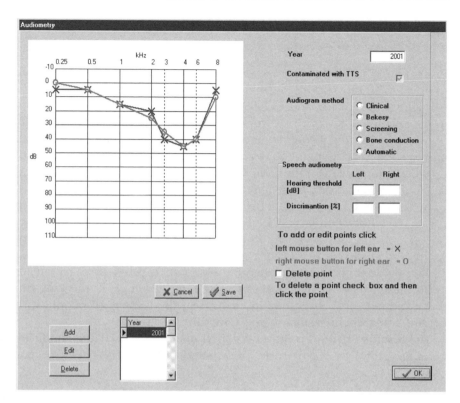

**Figure 15.6** Audiometric data sheet.

society prospers. A major challenge and underlying factor to the quality of life relate to hearing loss caused by environmental noise. As a person gets older, the auditory system will show the cumulative damage caused by noise, especially in susceptible people. It is the number one disability in Western countries (Rubens, 2000). During most of human history a person with a communication disorder was not thought of as being disabled. The shepherds, seamstresses, ploughmen and spinners of the past did not require optimal communication skills to be productive members of their society, as they primarily depended upon their manual abilities. Today a well-educated industrial worker who has no job and suffers from poor communication skills is not only unemployed, but, for the most part, unemployable (Rubens, 2000).

**Hearing impairment may comprise the following symptoms (Hétu et al., 1995):**

- The individual threshold of sound detection is decreased.
- The increase in loudness is distorted when the sound level increases.
- Difficulties in resolving neighbouring sounds.
- Ability to detect gaps in an ongoing sound is reduced.

- Ability to localize the sound sources is reduced.
- Persistent tinnitus.

In working conditions, workers with hearing impairment require a signal-to-noise (S/N) ratio up to 25 dB higher than those of normal listeners for detecting, recognizing and localizing the sound (Hétu et al., 1995). Due to the characteristics of the warning signals in industry, and the necessity of wearing hearing protection, workers with hearing impairment are more prone to accidents than workers with normal hearing. As a result of a loss of frequency resolution, the S/N ratio in communication must be up to 10 dB higher among hearing-impaired listeners (Plomp, 1986).

In daily communication, subjects with NIHL experience difficulty in communication when faced with less than ideal conditions – for example, on a telephone, and in varying levels of background noise, in reverberant rooms and group conversations (Hallberg and Barrenäs, 1993; Hétu et al., 1995). Because the onset of hearing loss is deceptive, people tend to avoid these situations, where they feel at a disadvantage. In the long run this avoidance process results in changes in the lifestyle of people with hearing impairment (Hallberg and Carlsson, 1991).

The resulting handicap caused by NIHL affects the social and family life in different ways. The partner of a person with NIHL needs to pay

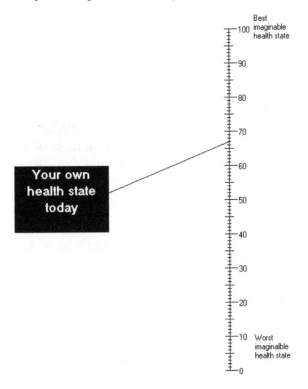

**Figure 15.7** The thermometer based on E-QoL 5D quality-of-life questionnaire.

attention when communicating with the impaired family member. Verbal contact should be performed under good visual conditions and the information content must be confirmed. The handicap affects the unimpaired family member by forcing him or her to keep conversations brief. Other consequences may include setting higher volumes when watching television or listening to music, loud speech and the increased social dependence of the impaired partner (Hétu et al., 1993). A handicap score based on E-QoL 5D is shown in Figure 15.7.

### Estimated hearing loss

When all the patient data have been input, they can be evaluated with two models: the ISO 1999 model and NoiseScan model for NIHL. The ISO 1999 model (Figure 15.8) is used for teaching purposes, and gives a good estimate of age-corrected hearing loss due to noise emission. The NoiseScan model may also have data on hearing protection and, thus, noise immission levels can be calculated. Both programs calculate the average hearing loss caused by occupational noise exposure. Medical factors and additional risk factors can explain the difference between measured and estimated hearing loss.

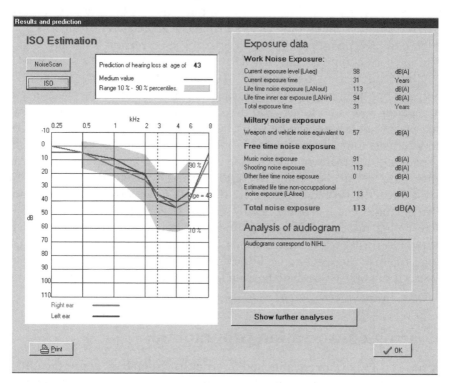

**Figure 15.8** Output of audiogram with exposure history and confounding factors. The ISO curves (10th and 90th percentiles) are shown as shadowed area for given noise exposure.

# The role of age

Age is one of the factors that emerges in risk analysis; in many cases it over-rides the exposure data (Pyykkö et al., 1986, 1989; Royster and Royster, 1986; Franks et al., 1989). This does not mean that age, in itself, would cause hearing loss (Robinson 1968; Robinson and Sutton 1979). Several factors have been suspected of underlying the development of presbycusis, such as hypertension, dietary habits, drugs and social noise exposure. For example, Rosen et al. (1965) and Hinchcliffe (1973) suggested that, if all environmental and disease processes could be controlled, no prominent age-related hearing impairment would be demonstrated. Driscol and Royster (1984) concluded in their study on the aetiology of sensorineural hearing loss (SNHL) and ageing that the existing databases are contaminated by environmental noise, and therefore there is an overestimation of the effect of age on hearing. Stephens (1982) examined consecutive presbycusis patients who were seeking rehabilitation, and found that in 93% of these cases there was an underlying cause for presbycusis. In a prospective study on the causes of hearing loss in the elderly, Lim and Stephens (1987) discovered that 83% of the cases had a disease condition that was associated with the hearing loss. About 30% of the subjects took medication that was known to be ototoxic. Humes (1984) made a critical review on the causes of hearing loss and discovered several confounding factors that affect age-related hearing loss.

To compare people of different ages, an age correction is usually made. The age correction according to ISO 1999 has some exceptions (case 5, ISO, 1990). If the hearing loss exceeds 40 dB at any frequency, the age correction will not be applied. Thus, at lower hearing thresholds the effect of age on hearing loss is no longer additive. The interaction of NIHL and presbycusis does not yet seem to be well established (Rössler, 1994). Selection of an internal control group might diminish the uncertainty of age correction. Usually a group that would be otologically screened and exposed to similar environmental stressors other than noise is not available. Robinson (1968) focused on the problem to evaluate the NIHL in an industrial population. He concludes that it is not generally realistic to compare such a population with an age-matched 'otologically normal' baseline, since a noise-exposed population will include adventitious hearing loss as well as noise-related components. The use of a well-documented baseline for data comparison makes it possible to estimate hearing loss in different geographical areas by using standard forms.

# Hearing conservation programme

Several HCPs have been launched in order to understand better the effect of occupational noise on the human ear (Royster et al., 1980; Melnik, 1984). Some recent HCPs utilize database analysis programs comparing data on the noise emission level, and including evaluation of factors other than workplace noise (Royster and Royster, 1986; Franks et al., 1989).

These programs may take into consideration, for instance, the association of ageing, non-occupational noise, and medical history (Franks et al., 1989). Other researchers use models based on risk analysis in which the relative importance of various factors, as well as workplace noise, is considered (Pyykkö et al., 1986, 1989).

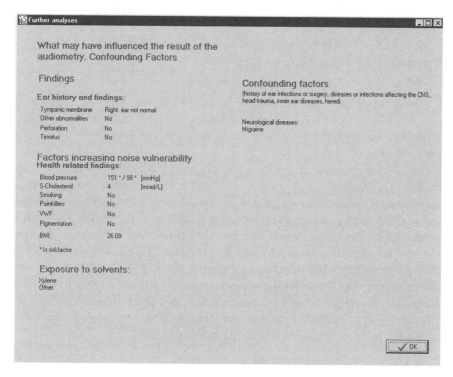

**Figure 15.9** Output of confounding factors in an individual hearing conservation programme.

Although individual models for the development of NIHL have been provided in a few of them (Royster et al. 1980; Royster and Royster, 1986) the studies have not been very successful so far. One reason may be the inaccuracies in the evaluation of the exposure data, in the usage rate of HPDs or in estimations of sociocusis and of nosocusis, especially in the detection of genetic factors.

The primary goal of a HCP must be the prevention, or at least limitation, of NIHL associated with exposure to industrial noise (Royster et al., 1980). Other goals may be formulated in addition to this primary goal, such as reduction of employees' stress and absenteeism, and reduction of work place accidents.

## Components of an effective HCP (Stewart, 1994)

- measurement of work-area noise levels;
- identification of over-exposed employees;

- reduction of hazardous noise exposure to the extent possible through engineering and administrative control;
- provision of HPDs if other controls are inadequate;
- initial and periodic education of workers and management;
- motivation of workers to comply with HCP policies;
- professional audiogram review and recommendations;
- follow-up for audiometric changes;
- detailed record-keeping system for the entire HCP;
- professional supervision of HCP.

One observes that many of these tasks are not well defined. The exposure evaluation is not a simple straightforward task, and the comparison of audiograms is not easy, due to large variations in NIHL and the strong effect of age.

One major problem in HCPs is establishing individual baseline values. Royster and Royster (1986) demonstrated a significant improvement of age-corrected audiograms when the subjects were annually tested over 6 years. The improvement was interpreted to be due to the training effect but depended on the noise emission level. Also, those with prominent hearing loss had less training effect. Royster and Royster (1986) proposed that the audiogram showing the best hearing at frequencies of 500–6000 Hz should form the baseline level. Thus any audiometric evaluation used in an HCP should be based on serial audiograms, and the database should include some expert programs to validate the data, in order to establish baseline values for hearing and also to calculate hearing loss.

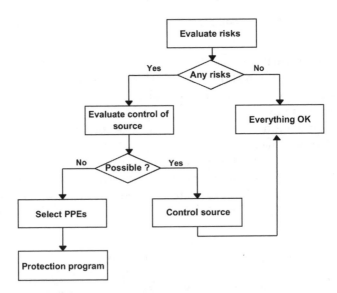

**Figure 15.10** General approach to the database and hearing protection programme for workers who are at risk of developing NIHL.

The data should preferably refer to a large international database of individual worker information to include the individual susceptibility factors and thereby provide a personalized HCP. The flow chart of the individual HCP may be as shown in Figure 15.10.

The approach to the protection of workers described in the Directive 86/188/EEC is based on the identification of the risks in the workplace. Risk assessment must be done by qualified personnel. If there is risk of NIHL, the employer must develop an HCP. In HCPs the first task is to evaluate the sources of noise and the possibilities of reducing the levels by technical means. If reduction of the noise source is not possible, the workers should be provided with HPDs and the workers should be informed about the risks and the correct use of the selected HPDs in an appropriate way.

These guidelines are not sufficient for practical purposes. The following problems must be solved:

• how to guarantee that the HPDs are used properly;
• how to discover risky workplaces or tasks;
• addressing the counter-measures against the relevant noise source, especially if the greatest exposure occurs in leisure, is difficult.

By solving these problems, the minimal legal requirements of an HCP will be achieved. A good HCP contains additional elements. These elements are added to increase the power of the HCP.

A new European Union Noise Directive 2003/10/EC will be brought into force by 2006. The new directive will fix the daily noise exposure levels and peak sound pressure for exposure limit value and exposure action values:

a) exposure limit values: LEX, 8h=87 dB(A) and Ppeak=200 Pa respectively
b) upper exposure action values: LEX, 8h=85 dB(A) and Ppeak=140 Pa respectively
c) lower action values: LEX, 8h=80 dB(A) and Ppeak=112 Pa respectively

When applying the exposure limit values, the determination of the worker's effective exposure shall take account of the attenuation provided by the individual HPDs worn by the worker. The exposure action values shall not take account of the effect of any such protection. In the risk assessment, the following factors have to be included:

a) exposure to impulse noise,
b) combined effects from the interactions between noise and ototoxic substances and between noise and vibrations,
c) any effects concerning the health and safety of workers belonging to particularly sensitive groups. When the noise exposure level exceeds the lower exposure action values, the employer shall make HPDs available to workers and in the case when noise exposure level matches or exceeds the upper action values, HPDs must be used. HPDs must be so selected as to eliminate the risk to hearing or to reduce the risk to a minimum.

# The motivation of workers to use HPDs

The use of HPDs gives best results with motivated users. Low motivation to wear HPDs is seen as low usage rates and low true attenuation values (Foreshaw and Cruchley, 1981). Successful motivation can be obtained via appropriate education and training. The users must be informed about the effects of noise and the risks at work (86/188/EEC). Best results are obtained if personal audiometric data are used (Lipscomb, 1994). This means that education must be given privately. Users need training in maintenance, installation and use of HPDs. The attenuation of protectors works well only if they are well maintained (EN 458-1993). Good maintenance consists of cleaning, changing of replaceable parts like cushions, and overall monitoring of the state of the HPD. Application must take place before entering the noisy area (EN 458-1993). If earplugs are used special attention must be paid to the proper installation technique (Foreshaw and Cruchley, 1981; Berger et al., 1983).

Although it is possible to obtain highly motivated users with proper education and training, motivation tends to decrease over time. To avoid this, education and training must be repeated consistently (Lipscomb, 1994).

## Factors affecting the selection of the type of hearing protector

| Earmuffs | Earplugs |
| --- | --- |
| May cause communication problems | May cause communication problems |
| Skin irritation in hot weather | Sometimes feeling of vertigo |
| High attenuation means high mass | May cause infections in ear canal |
| Need for maintenance | Often provides good attenuation |
| Highly frequency dependent | against low-frequency noise |
| attenuation | Poor insertion techniques result in |
| Loss of sound direction | poor attenuation |

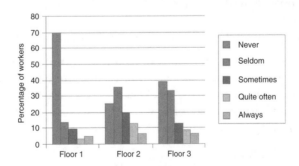

**Figure 15.11** Comparison of the use of hearing protection devices (HPDs) in three factory floors. The usage rate is indicated from 'never used' to 'always used'.

A simple measure of the motivation of the workers is the usage rate of HPDs. Figure 15.11 shows the situation in three factory floors having a noise level of 93–97 dB (A). On floor 1, use of HPDs is extremely poor, while it is relatively poor on floors 2 and 3. When a motivation

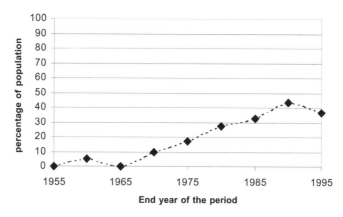

**Figure 15.12** The percentage of people always using hearing protection devices in a factory as a function of time.

programme is started its effect must be followed. Figure 15.12 shows a motivation programme with efficiency. Although the use of HPDs is increasing after 15 years the usage is still below 40%.

# Early detection of problems

The most prominent observation in NIHL is the large inter-individual variation. For example according to ISO 1999 (ISO, 1990), among men the difference between the 10th and 90th percentiles of hearing loss is 60 dB at 4 kHz when the subjects are exposed to a noise level of 100 dB (A) for 30 years. This large variation means that a large number of subjects are needed before any conclusions can be made. In order to reduce the number of subjects two possibilities exist:

1. Removal of subjects with non-NIHL from the data.
2. Taking into account the effect of individual risk factors of NIHL.

By taking a population with a similar risk profile, the variation of results is reduced. Figure 15.13 shows the effect of noise on hearing loss. In subjects

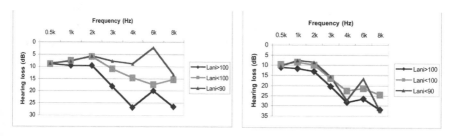

**Figure 15.13** Effect of individual risk factors on mean hearing loss. Left: subjects with 0–1 risk factor. Right: subjects with at least three risk factors. Lani is the noise immission level inside the hearing protector.

with several risk factors, the effect of noise may be masked by the risk factors. In subjects with practically no risk factors, the effect of noise on hearing is usually incontrovertible. In cases of interaction of a chemical and noise, this effect may easily be masked in small populations, unless the risk profile of the worker's exposure is taken into account.

# Expert systems for NIHL

By definition, an expert system is *a system that by internal rules assists in decision-making in a complex medical problem.* It differs from a traditional computer program in that the expert program generates its own decisions by learning and adapting to new rules to handle large amounts of medical data. Expert systems, on the other hand, work in disciplines where associations are not completely understood and in which associations are not linearly connected. They have proven efficacy in several fields of medicine, especially in very information-intensive fields and are extensively used in pharmacology (study of drug interactions, therapeutic drug monitoring), clinical chemistry, bacteriology and computer-assisted editing of genome sequences.

To convert the data on environmental, genetic and subject-linked factors into models, in addition to classic statistics, modern artificial intelligence-based computing techniques should be used. These techniques are well suited to analysis of complex data sets where relationships between the different parameters are not linear. They include data mining, decision trees, neural network computing and genetic algorithms (Goldberg, 1989; Quinlan, 1993; Swingler, 1996). Data mining looks for complex associations, neural networks compute the relationships between various factors, decision-tree making gives probabilities in nonlinear relationships, and genetic algorithms can search for a solution by creating mutations in the data and screening off springs for best solutions. They are the newest steps of decision-making in computer science, and have routines to handle incomplete data (missing values) and operate with fuzzy logic. Each one of these techniques has its strengths and limitations, but they should be able to complement each other.

Global modelling should facilitate the prediction of the development of a subject's NIHL. For the global modelling task artificial intelligence has several tools to model efficiently and classify complicated structures of data and information that seem to be inherent in NIHL. This includes neural networks, which can be applied to an area where the relationship cannot be mathematically described (Kentala et al., 1997). In addition, neural networks poorly tolerate missing data. Therefore, a large sample size is needed. Genetic algorithms are used to invoke thematic rules about the data (Kentala et al., 1999). Such rules reflect relationships between causal factors in the data, and they are used to build a rule-based classifier to show possible sources and causes of NIHLs. Missing data and fuzzy logic can be applied to genetic algorithms, but the reasoning for the end user is not as good as using the decision-tree (IBM CV) method where stem and leaves provide the information on decision-making (Laurikkala et al., 1999; Viikki et al., 1999). We have previously compared the accuracy of different methods in assessing vertigo and found that the decision tree is the easiest method for researchers to understand the decision-making (clustering) (Viikki et al., 2000).

Local pattern searching uses pattern recognition methods to find out 'peculiarities' from a subject's data. Unusual patterns are unexpected or unusual phenomena in a subject's data profile that may reveal some new, interesting and useful features related to NIHL, which may affect its prediction or may be interesting for research into NIHL. For the local pattern-searching task, we shall use several searching methods from the traditional types (such as clustering and nearest neighbour searching) with more recent techniques such as associative rules. For example, associative rules are efficient in searching for local relationships between cases and variables (input data) that can reveal useful features in the data. We have previously undertaken both theoretical and applied research on all the aforementioned methods and several others in the field of artificial intelligence are currently in the process of applying them to the NoiseScan program (Kentala et al., 1996).

# Conclusions

The risk of hearing loss in workers depends on several factors: work noise and its characteristics, leisure noise and its characteristics, exposure to ototoxic agents and individual susceptibility. All these factors should be recorded according to the newly adopted directive for noise (2003/10/EEC – EC, 2003). Unfortunately, there are no calculation rules available to combine the effect of all these factors. For example, interactions of impulsiveness of noise, genetic susceptibility, ototoxic chemicals and leisure noise cannot be modelled. Still, by using a properly designed database, information about their influence on NIHL can be evaluated using non-linear methods and comparison of the actual mean hearing loss to the prediction of, for example, ISO 1999 (ISO, 1990) for a group of workers in the same conditions. In addition, the database can be used to evaluate the success of preventive action such as the use of HPDs.

The value of databases further increases when individual factors are included in the database. Knowledge about the exposure pattern may facilitate the introduction of counter-measures against work noise as well as against leisure noise, particularly if the free-time noise exposure predominates. Motivation is the key factor for preventing NIHL. A database establishes the basis for a HCP, and the goal of a HCP is to provide individual hearing protection. Once there is a better grasp of the role of various confounding factors, the individual HCP may reduce the number of older people who are hard of hearing.

# References

American Conference of Governmental Industrial Hygienists (1999) Threshold Limit Values for Chemical Substances and Physical Agents. Cincinnati: ACGIH.

ANSI S12.9 –1999x – Part 4 Draft 2 (2000) Determination of the effects of impulse noise. New York: ANSI.

Auramo Y, Juhola M, Pyykko I, Nieminen O (1995) Graphical user interface for the analysis of noise induced hearing loss. J Med Syst 19: 323–32.

Barrenäs M (1998) Pigmentation and noise-induced hearing loss: is the relationship between pigmentation and noise-induced hearing loss due to an ototoxic pheolaminin interaction or to otoprotective eumelan effects. In D Prasher, L Luxon (eds) Advances in Noise Research, Vol. 1. Biological effects of noise. London: Whurr, pp. 59–70.

Barrenäs M, Lindgren F (1991) The influence of eye color on susceptibility to TTS in humans. Br J Audiol 25: 203–7.

Baughn W (1966) Noise control – percent of population protected. Int Audiol 5: 331–8.

Baughn W (1973) Relation between daily exposure and hearing loss based on evaluation of 6835 industrial noise exposure cases. Report AMRL-TR-7353. US Air Force.

Berger E, Royster L, Thomas W (1978) Presumed noise-induced permanent threshold shift resulting from exposure to an A-weighted Leq of 89 dB. J Acoust Soc Am 64: 192–7.

Berger E, Franks J, Lindgren F (1983) International review of field studies of hearing protector attenuation. In A Axelsson, H Borchgrevink, RP Hamenik, P Hellström, D Hendersson, RJ Salvi (eds) Scientific Basis of Noise-Induced Hearing Loss. New York: Thième.

Borg E (1982) Noise-induced hearing loss in normotensive and spontaneously hypertensive rats. Hear Res 8: 117.

Burns W (1973) Permanent effects of noise on hearing. In W Burns (ed.) Noise and Man, 2nd edn. London: John Murray.

Burns W, Robinson DW (1970) Hearing and Noise in Industry. London: HMSO.

Campo P, Lataye PR (1992) Intermittent noise and equal energy hypothesis. In AL Dancer (ed.) Noise-Induced Hearing Loss. St Louis, MO: Mosby, pp. 456–6.

CEN (1993) EN 458: Hearing Protectors – Recommendations for Selection, Use, Care and Maintenance – Guidance Document. Brussels: CEN.

Chung DY, Willson GN, Cannon RP, Mason K (1982) Individual susceptibility to noise. In RP Hammernik, D Henderson, R Salvi (eds) New Perspectives on Noise-induced Hearing Loss. New York: Raven Press, pp. 511–19.

Committee of Hearing, Bioacoustics and Biomechanics (CHABA) (1968) Proposed Damage-risk criterion for impulse noise (Gunfire) Report of working group 57. National Academy of Sciences National Research Council. Washington DC: CHABA.

Dancer AL, Franke R, Parmentier G, Buck K (1996) Hearing protector performance and NIHL in extreme environments: actual performance of hearing protectors in impulse noise/nonlinear behavior. In A Axelsson, H Borchgrevink, R Hamernik, PA Hellstrom, D Henderson, R Salvi (eds) Scientific Basis of Noise-induced Hearing Loss. New York: Thième.

Davis A, Smith P, Wade A (1998) A longitudinal study of hearing – effects of age, sex and noise. Proceedings of Nordics Noise, 12–15 March, Stockholm.

Driscoll DP, Royster L (1984) Comparisons between the median hearing threshold levels for a black non-industrial noise exposed population (NINEP) and four presbycusis data bases. Am Ind Hyg Assoc J 45: 577–93.

Earshen J (1986) Sound measurement: instrumentation and noise descriptors. In EH Berger, WD Ward, JC Morrill, LH Royster (eds) Noise and Hearing Conservation Manual.

European Commission (1986) 86/188/EEC. Council directive on the protection of workers from the risks related to exposure to noise at work. Brussels: European Commission.

European Commission (1989) 89/391/EEC. Council directive on the introduction of measures to encourage improvements in the safety and heath of workers at work. Brussels: European Commission.

European Commission (2003) 2003/10/EEC Directive 2003/10/EC of the European Parliament and of the Council of 6 February 2003 on the minimum health and safety requirements regarding the exposure of workers to the risks arising from physical agents (noise). Brussels: European Commission.

Foreshaw S, Cruchley J (1981) Hearing protector problems in military operations. In P Alberti (ed.) Personal Hearing Protection in Industry. New York: Raven Press.

Franks JR, Davis RR, Kreig EF (1989) Analysis of hearing conservation program data base: factors other than work place noise. Ear Hear 10: 273–80.

Gates GA, Couropmitree NN, Meyers RH (1999) Genetic associations in age-related hearing thresholds. Arch Otol Head Neck Surg 125: 654–9.

Glorig A, Nixon J (1960) Distribution of hearing loss in various populations. Ann Otol Rhinol Laryngol 69: 497–516.

Glorig A, Roberts JJ (1965) Hearing levels of adults by age and sex: United States 1960–1962, Rep. PHS-PUB-100-SER-11-11, National Center for Health Service Research and Development, October 1965.

Goldberg DE (1989) Genetic Algorithm in Search, Optimization and Machine Learning. Reading MA: Addison-Wesley.

Green GE, Scott DA, McDonald JM, Woodworth GG, Sheffield VC, Smith RJ (1999) Carrier rates in the mid western United States for GJB2 mutations causing inherited deafness. JAMA 281: 2211–16.

Hallberg LR, Barrenäs ML (1993) Living with a male with noise induced hearing loss: experiences from the perspective of the spouses. Br J Audiol 27: 255–62.

Hallberg LR, Carlsson SG (1991) A qualitative study of the strategies for managing a hearing impairment. Br J Audiol 25: 201–11.

Hétu R, Jones L, Getty L (1993) The impact of acquired hearing loss on intimate relationships: implications for rehabilitions. Audiology 32: 363–81.

Hétu R, Getty L, Hung TQ (1995) Impact of Occupational Hearing Loss on the Lives of the Workers in Occupational Medicine. State of the Art Reviews, Volume 10. Philadelphia, PA: Hanlay & Belfus Inc.

Hinchcliffe R (1973) Epidemiology of sensory-neural hearing loss. Audiology 12: 446–52.

Humes LE (1984) Noise-induced hearing loss as influenced by other agents and by some physical characteristics of the individual. J Acoust Soc Am 76: 1318–29.

International Organization for Standardization (1975) ISO 1999: Acoustics – Assessment of occupational noise exposure for hearing conservation purposes. Geneva: ISO.

International Organization for Standardization (1990) ISO 1999: Acoustics – Determination of occupational noise exposure and estimation of noise induced hearing impairment. Geneva: ISO.

Johnson D (1973) Prediction of NIPTS due to continuous noise exposure, Rep. No. AMRL-TR-73-91, US Air Force, July.

Kentala E, Pyykkö I, Auramo Y, Juhola M (1996) Otolaneurological expert system. Ann Otol Rhinol Laryngol 105: 658–954.

Kentala E, Pyykkö I, Auramo Y, Juhola M (1997) Neural networks in neurotologic expert systems. Acta Otolaryngol Suppl 529: 127–9.

Kentala E, Laurikkala J, Pyykkö I, Juhola M (1999) Discovering diagnostic rules from neurotologic database with genetic algorithm. Ann Otol Rhinol Laryngol 108: 948–52.

Kryter KD (1965) Damage risk criterion and contours based on permanent and temporary hearing loss data. J Am Ind Hyg Assoc 26: 34–44.

Laurikkala J, Kentala E, Juhola M, Pyykkö I (1999) Treatment of missing values with imputation for the analysis of otologic data. Stud Health Technol Inform. 68: 428–31.

Lim D, Stephens SGD (1987) Clinical investigation of hearing loss in the elderly. Paper read to the British Society of Audiology, Hull, 1985. Cited in J Irwin (1987) Causes of hearing loss in adults. In D Stephens (ed.) Adult Audiology. Scott-Brown's Otolaryngology. London: Butterworths, pp. 127–56.

Lipscomp DM (1994) The employee education program. In DM Lipscomb (ed.) Hearing Conservation in Industry, Schools and the Military. San Diego, CA: Singular, pp. 81–230.

McCormic G, Harris DT, Hartley CB, Lassiter RBH (1982) Spontaneous genetic hypertension in the rat and its relationship to reduce cochlear potentials: implications for preservation of human hearing. Proc Natl Acad Sci USA 79: 26–68.

Machlin PS, Dempsey J, Brooks J, Rand J (1991) Using neural network to diagnose cancer. J Med Syst 15: 11–19.

Mäkitie A (1997) The ototoxic effect of styrene and its interactions with an experimental study in rats. Academic dissertation, University of Helsinki, Helsinki University Hospital.

Melnick W (1984) Evaluation of industrial hearing conservation programs: a review and analysis. Am Ind Hyg Assoc J 45: 459–67.

Morton NE (1991) Genetic epidemiology of hearing impairment. Ann NY Acad Sci 630: 16–31.

National Institute for Occupational Safety and Health (1974) Occupational noise and hearing 1968–1972: NIOSH.

Nieminen O, Pyykkö I, Starck J, Toppila E, Iki M (2000) Serum cholesterol and blood pressure in the genesis of noise induced hearing loss. Transactions of the XXVth Congress of the Scandinavian Oto-Laryngological Society. Bergen: Daves Tryckeri Bergen, pp. 48–50.

Passchier-Vermeer W (1974) Hearing loss due to continuous exposure to steady-state broad-band noise. J Acoust Soc Am 46(5): 1585–93.

Patterson JH, Johnson DL (1996) Temporary threshold shifts produced by high intensity free-field impulse noise in humans wearing hearing protection. In A

Axelsson, H Borchgrevink, R Hamernik, PA Hellstrom, D Henderson, R Salvi (eds) Scientific Basis of Noise-induced Hearing Loss. New York: Thième, pp. 313–20.

Pekkarinen J, Iki M, Starck J, Pyykkö I (1993) Hearing loss risk from exposure to shooting impulses in workers exposed to occupational noise. Br J Audiol 27: 175–82.

Pfander F (1975) Das Knalltrauma. Berlin: Springer Verlag.

Plomp R (1986) A signal-to-noise ratio model for the speech-reception threshold of hearing-impaired. J Speech Hear Res 29: 146–54.

Price GR (1986) Hazard from intense low-frequency acoustic impulses. J Acoust Soc Am 80: 1076–86.

Pyykkö I, Pekkarinen J, Starck J (1986) Sensory-neural hearing loss in forest workers. An analysis of risk factor. Int Arch Occup Environ Health 59: 439–54.

Pyykkö I, Koskimies K, Starck J, Pekkarinen J, Inaba R (1988) Evaluation of factors affecting sensory neural hearing loss. Acta Otolaryngol Suppl 449: 155–60.

Pyykkö I, Koskimies K, Starck J, Pekkarinen J, Färkkilä M, Inaba R (1989) Risk factors in the genesis of sensorineural hearing loss in Finnish forestry workers. Br J Ind Med 46: 439–46.

Quinlan JR (1993) C4.5. Programs for Machine Learning. San Mateo, CA: Morgan Kaufman.

Robinson DB, Shipton MS (1977) Tables for the Estimation of Noise-induced Hearing Loss. National Physical Laboratory Acoustics Report Ac 61 (2nd). Teddington, Middlesex. National Physical Laboratory.

Robinson DW (1968) The Relationship between Hearing Loss and Noise Exposure. NPL Aero Report Ac 32 Teddington, National Physical Laboratory.

Robinson DW (1971) Estimating the risk of hearing loss due to continuous noise. In DW Robinson (ed.) Occupational Hearing Loss. London: Academic Press.

Robinson DW, Sutton GJ (1979) Age effects in hearing – a comparative analysis of published threshold data. Audiology 18: 320–34.

Rosen S, Olin P (1965) Hearing loss and coronary heart disease. Arch Otolaryngol 82: 236–43.

Rössler G (1994) Progression of hearing loss caused by occupational noise. Scand Audiol 23:13–37.

Rowland M (1980) Basic data on hearing levels of adults 25–74 years. DHEW Publ. no. (PHS) 80-1663, series 11, no 215 US Dep Health, Education and Welfare, January.

Royster JD, Royster LH (1986) Using audiometric data base analysis. J Occup Med 28: 1055–68.

Royster LH, Lilley LT, Thomas WG (1980) Recommended criteria for evaluating effectiveness of hearing conservation program. Am Ind Hyg Assoc 41: 40–8.

Rubens RJ (2000) Redefining the survival of the fittest: communication disorders in the 21st century. Laryngoscope 110: 241–5.

Smith RJH, Van Camp G (2005) Deafness and Hereditary Hearing Loss Overview http://www.geneclinics.org/profiles/deafness–overview/details.html.

Starck J, Pekkarinen J, Pyykkö I (1988) Impulse noise and hand-arm vibration in relation to sensory neural hearing loss. Scand J Environ Health 14: 265–71.

Starck J, Pyykkö I, Toppila E, Pekkarinen J (1996) Do the models assess noise-induced hearing loss correctly? ACES 7(3-4): 21–6.

Starck J, Toppila E, Pyykkö I (1999) Smoking as a risk factor in sensory neural hearing loss among workers exposed to occupational noise. Acta Otolaryngol 199: 302–5.

Stewart AP (1994) The comprehensive hearing conservation program. In DM Lipscomb (ed.) Hearing Conservation in Industry, Schools and the Military. San Diego, CA: Singular, pp. 81–230.

Suter A (1994) The development of federal noise standards and damage risk criteria. In D Lipscomb (ed.) Hearing Conservation in Industry, Schools and the Military. San Diego, CA: Singular.

Suvorov G, Denisov E, Antipin V, Haritonov V, Starck J, Pyykkö I et al. (2001) Effects of peak levels and number of impulses on hearing among forge hammering workers. Appl Occup Environ Hyg 16: 816–22.

Swingler K (1996) Applying Neural Networks. London: Academic Press.

Toppila E, Pyykkö I, Starck J, Kaksonen R. Ishizaki H (2000) Individual risk factors in the development of noise-induced hearing loss. Noise and Health.8: 59–70.

Toppila E, Pyykkö I, Starck J (2001) Age and noise-induced hearing loss. Scand J Audiol 30: 236–44.

Viikki K, Isotalo E, Juhola M, Pyykkö I (1999) Modelling oculomotor data with decision tree induction. Stud Health Technol Inform 68: 660–3.

World Health Organization (1980) International Classification of Impairments, Disabilities and Handicaps. Geneva: WHO.

# CHAPTER 16

# Environmental noise: a contextual public health perspective

*Noise and Its Effects:* Edited by Linda Luxon and Deepak Prasher © 2007
John Wiley & Sons Ltd.

PETER LERCHER MD, MPH
*Associate Professor*

## Introduction

The pollution of our environment by noise from a multitude of interfering sources is still increasing. Within a decade (early 1980 to early
1990), the percentage of the European population exposed to sound
levels above 65 dB $L_{Aeq,24h}$ (so-called 'black spots') increased from 15%
to 26% (Stanners and Bordeau, 1995). Transportation noise (mainly
road traffic) is responsible for 80% of this excess in noise exposure.
The additional rise in exposure to the 55–65 dB range (above levels
recommended for residential areas by the WHO guidelines) is attributed mainly to the growth in traffic volume and its spread to previously
quieter areas. In a report to the Administrative Conference of the
United States, Suter (1991) estimated a general increase in noise levels
of about 11% with a higher increase in noise from aircraft. A study of
urban areas in Bavaria showed a 3.3 dB (A) increase in night-time levels between 1976 and 1991, thus reducing the proportion of people
with exposure of less than 45 dB (A) from 74% to 51% (Leuner, 1992).
The Noise Incidence Study (NIS) in the UK revealed some indication of
a slight worsening of background levels at night also between 1990 and
2000 (Department for Environment, Food and Rural Affairs or DEFRA,
2002). Therefore, it is not surprising that noise is the only environmental factor for which public complaints have increased since 1992 in
the EU (European Report No. 2173, 9 November 1996). Furthermore,
most 'driving force' indicators in the transportation area (car use,
freight transport and so forth) show that the upwards trend is continuing (European Environment Agency or EEA, 2000, 2002).

**Noise levels increase**

Although the database across countries is small, a general increase in noise levels during the last 20 years is evident. Most worrying is the general spread to previously quieter areas and the silent increase of background levels, especially during night.

These data are not quoted to downplay the potentially intrusive, *intermittent* effect of other sources of noise annoyance such as neighbours, barking dogs, construction noise, industrial and certain recreational activities or more recent activities such as imposed cellular phone conversations in public spaces. The acute impact of such noise sources is easier to recognize, to remember and to communicate. Typically, neighbour and construction noise ranks top in the list of spontaneous complaints to health authorities – but due to the typical time restrictions of these sources the potential adverse effects in terms of population coverage are limited. The description and treatment of these sources need a special framework. Noise from neighbours (including cellular phone communication and barking dogs) should be viewed as a special case. First, there is considerable variability in importance among countries in spite of comparatively little difference in legislation across EU-member states. However, essential differences exist in law enforcement and in standards of thermal and noise insulation between countries. Second, due to its individual origin, noise from neighbours falls into the rubric of 'daily hassles' and – *sensu strictu* – not under the heading 'ambient stressors'. This important distinction was made by Campbell (1983) to characterize the chronic, perceivable, non-urgent, intractable nature of environmental stressors such as transportation noise, air pollution or crowding.

It is the insidious, latent nature of the prevalent *chronic* noise exposure through transportation sources that matters most in terms of environmental quality of life, health and economic loss at the population level and which requires prioritization.

Accumulating evidence shows that the traditional *emission*-oriented approaches used in the assessment and management of noise are inefficient in terms of economic and social costs (Sandberg, 1995; CEC, 1996; Staples, 1997; WHO, 2000, Sandberg, 2001a, b). Therefore, a short outline of the capability and limits of the existing approaches is a necessary starting point to a better understanding of the problem and the most effective road to the prevention of adverse effects of environmental noise.

# Conceptual approaches to environmental noise

## Classic approaches

### *The engineering approach*

This physical approach to noise was very successful in the 'early' years of noise research and prevention, when standardized measurement procedures were needed. Engineers successfully established industry standards for *noise emissions* from machines, automobiles, airplanes and so forth. Typically, average noise levels, expressed in A-weighted decibels, were used. Although the limitations of this approach were recognized early – by experts, administrators and exposed alike – the fast administration and the lack of easy alternatives kept it running. Only in the 1990s has the large discrepancy found between expected theoretical reductions based on more stringent standards in engine noise and actual sound levels led to the recognition of the failure of this narrow approach (Sandberg 1995, 2001a,b; Commission of the European Community CEC, 1996; WHO, 2000).

## The failure of noise reduction policy

It has been recognized that the traditional **emission** oriented approaches used in the assessment and management of noise are inefficient both in terms of economic and social costs. The expected reductions based on more stringent standards in engine noise have never been met.

On the *imission or receptor* side, the assessment of community noise problems by a simple summary indicator ($L_{Aeq}$) was a problem from the very beginning. In an attempt to bring in the subjective perspective of the noise exposed annoyance surveys were added and normative dose–response curves were created. The highly influential dose–response curve of Schultz (1978) even claimed to be valid for all kinds of noise. This belief was criticized and nowadays separate dose–response curves are available for aircraft, road traffic, rail and impulse noise, derived by meta-analyses from large data archives (Fidell et al., 1991; Miedema and Vos, 1998; Miedema and Oudshoorn, 2001). Their normative character, however, is still retained, as the new EU Environmental Noise Directive (2002/49/EC) relies fully on these curves.

## One size does not fit all: Limits of the Environmental Noise Directive

The normative use of an aggregated database (TNO-database is dominated by surveys from the 1970s and 1980s) in estimating exposure–response relationships runs the risk of neglecting the considerable variation known to exist due to factors that vary a lot within the European countries (see Table 16.1)

By linking the existing annoyance database with actual calculated (or measured) sound data ('noise mapping') from the concerned area via a geographical information system (GIS) an assessment of the size of the problem is made (Hinton, 2002, or www.defra.gov.uk/environment/noise/birmingham/report/index.htm; Knauss, 2002). This normative use of an aggregated database (dominated by surveys from the 1970s and 1980s) means applying a 'one size fits all' approach – although the exact relationship between sound and annoyance is known to vary considerably from area to area (Table 16.1) depending on geography, meteorology, building structure, land use, lifestyle, culture, and the mix of attitudinal and health factors (Jonsson et al., 1969; Job 1988; Fields, 1993; Porter et al., 1993; Lercher, 1996, 1998a, 2001; Staples, 1997; Gjestland, 1998; Miedema and Vos, 1999, Pesonen, 2000; Diaz et al., 2001; Job and Hatfield, 2001; Botteldooren et al., 2002; Sato et al., 2002; Yano et al., 2002).

**Table 16.1** Effect size of moderator variables

| Moderator | Decibel equivalent |
| --- | --- |
| Fear of crashes | 6 |
| Noise sensitivity | 9 |
| Belief: noise harms health | 14 |
| Satisfaction with life | 10 |
| Attitude to the source | 8–15 |
| Neighbourhood has complained | 9 |
| Satisfaction with neighbourhood | 13 |
| Reduction in rates | 15 |
| Sight of the noise source | 10 |
| Dust, air pollution, loss of privacy | 26 |

Source: Job (1991) (based on various sources).

Specific problems exist with the assessment of sound sources that contain strong low-frequency components such as diesel cars, trucks, ventilation or air-conditioning systems (Persson and Rylander, 1988; Berglund et al., 1996; Mirowska, 1998; Van den Berg, 1998; Persson Waye et al., 2001, 2002).

Moreover, acousticians themselves are concerned whether sound propagation models are sufficiently accurate for the main sources in difficult terrain and building structures, at greater distances and under non-standard meteorological conditions (Embleton, 1996; Van den Berg and Gerretsen, 1996; Heimann and Gross, 1999; Sutherland, 2000; Kragh, 2001; Alberola et al., 2002; Blumrich and Heimann, 2002; Iu and Li, 2002). The existing experience with the models rests on the traditional approach of dealing with each sound source in isolation. For the community noise-mapping exercise, however, a valid integration of all existing sound sources is needed. Although helpful, even the most perfect acoustic risk assessment will fail when risk characterization is not pertinent to the population at risk and takes into account such issues as community needs and environmental justice, as experience with other environmental hazards indicates (Goldstein, 1995).

Without knowledge of the determining factors 'behind' the dose–response curves the decision process to 'action plans' is narrowed down and alternative courses of action to handle the noise problem cannot be sufficiently considered (Wright and Grimwood, 1999; Flindell and Porter, 2000). Only through the understanding of the pathways in the exposure will chain preventive action be effective and efficient (Goldstein, 1995; Staples, 1997).

## The medical and psychological approach

Basically, two different approaches can be distinguished (Taylor and Wilkins, 1986; Van Kamp, 1990; Lercher, 1996; Stansfeld et al., 2000). A 'direct effects model' (black box approach) links average noise levels (provided by engineers) with physical health or psychological outcome measures. This model treats noise as a physical factor, just like particles or radiation in other pollution research. Taking into account the shortcomings of this model, an adjustment for medical history, current health status and personality traits such as noise sensitivity is made in epidemiological studies. The second approach uses an 'indirect effects model' acknowledging the potential moderation of the noise response through personal and environmental factors. The most comprehensive studies of this approach use an interactional perspective with statistical modelling (regression or path analysis) to address the joint influence of all these factors.

Unfortunately, most of the evidence is available from research using the direct effects model with personality variables adjusted in psychological investigations and demographic and health variables adjusted in medical studies (Lercher, 1998a; Stansfeld et al., 2000; Van Kempen et al., 2002). Several major limitations arise. The excessive emphasis on individual determinants (medical or psychological) neglects situational constraints and other contextual determinants such as the presence of other stressors in either the social or physical environment that could be the target of policy interventions. Second, by the use of *severe* and *specific* morbidity indicators like hypertension, coronary heart disease or psychiatric admissions noise has to compete with many other and more easily measurable somatic risk factors, which makes it difficult to detect the assumed direct effect of noise. Such analytical strategies do not address indirect effects of noise (via negative appraisals or inadequate coping strategies) which in theory enhance the susceptibility to a wider range of diseases (Cohen et al., 1986; Staples, 1996; Lercher, 1998a; Evans, 2001).

**Noise health risk assessment neglects the broader impact of noise**

The focus in risk assessment on *severe* and *specific* morbidity indicators, like hypertension, coronary heart disease or psychiatric admissions, does neglect the much broader 'invisible' iceberg of smaller effects such as cumulative fatigue, reading and memory impairments in children, social impacts or other signs of early health burden (increase in stress hormones) that may surface only later at the health care level.

Finally, the shortcomings and the ambiguity of many study results in this area, together with the lack of clear policy advice, may have been an obstacle to a precautionary policy approach over the years (Staples, 1996; De Hollander et al., 1999).

## Modern approaches

### Psychoacoustics, soundscape and sound design

One of the basic requirements of a noise measurement method is its validity and reliability. Over the years, psychoacousticians have provided many examples to show how the loudness of single sound sources can be underestimated or how differences in loudness between several sources are overestimated by the use of the A-weighted sound level in decibels as criterion metric (Zwicker and Fastl, 1986, 1999). An impressive example is the case of a motorbike that peaked in loudness but received a 'green label', because it did better in terms of the established dB (A) criterion (Zwicker, 1982).

With the development of further assessment criteria – like sharpness, roughness – fluctuation strength and the introduction of binaural measurements, complex sound environments can be further analysed and intervention measures specifically tailored to reduce the most annoying frequencies of the individual sound spectra.

Unfortunately, this analytical potential has been almost exclusively used for consumer and industrial products or for closed spatial units such as cars, trains, aeroplanes and workplaces. Applications within the field of community annoyance remain rare, partly because a sound propagation model for loudness does not yet exist and the expense of the currently required measurements is prohibitive for standard application. Schomer (2000) and Schomer et al. (2001) have recently proposed an approximate method (loudness-level weighting) that is easier to implement for environmental noise assessment.

The engineering approach of the sound design community has considerable overlap with psychoacoustics (Genuit, 2002). The emphasis is more on auditory system quality (Hempel and Blauert, 1999; Hempel, 2001). The range of contributions goes from product sound quality (Blauert and Jekosch, 1998), virtual simulations of noise exposure, improvement of the human–environment interaction to sound quality assessment (Blauert and Jekosch, 1996; Susini et al., 1999). The sound design of indoor and outdoor spaces is a specialized branch of these activities (Namba, 1994; Ando, 1998).

A further contribution for a better assessment of environmental noise can be expected by adopting the approach of acoustic ecology. In this young field a broad variety of approaches exist (for example, ecological, sociological, phenomenological, semiotic).

The main aim of this approach is the study and the improvement of the relationship between the 'aural space' and the living environment – the 'soundscape' (Wrightson, 2000). Sounds are seen here as mediators between humans, their activities and the environment. Depending on 'acoustic col-oration' from the larger environment (geography, climate, wind, water, people, buildings, animals and so forth) sound sources create 'meanings' to those exposed to them and block or enable human activities, thoughts, feelings. Therefore, sound quality assessment is based on both the acoustic dimensions and other dimensions such as visual, aesthetic, geographical, social and cultural modalities in the context of human activity in space and time. Some work in environmental psychology and sociology is related to this approach (Kastka and Noack, 1987; Carles et al., 1992; Tamura, 1997; Maffiolo et al., 1999; Suzuki et al., 2000; Berglund and Nilsson, 2001; Schulte-Fortkamp, 2002; Viollon et al., 2002) and should receive more attention. Acoustic ecologists have developed descriptive and analytical techniques, such as 'participatory sound and listening walks', 'écoute réactivée', 'cognitive maps', 'acoustical spectrographic maps', 'soundscapeg-raphy' (Amphoux, 1993, 1995; Truax, 1999; Augoyard, 1999; Hiramatsu, 1999a, 2001). Architectural groups within this very heterogeneous approach (Karlsson, 1999) have a strong emphasis on urban planning, make heavy use of GISs by adding layers of other modalities to implement innovative procedures into architecture and sound design (Grosjean and Thibaud, 2001) – for example, visit their web pages (Cresson, CERMA, Acroe/ICA). In Japan, soundscape activities have focused mainly on inter-disciplinary research, the sonic design and conservation of public spaces (Hiramatsu, 1999b). An outstanding part of the last activity is a huge con-servation programme of 100 diverse soundscapes across the country (Torigoe, 1999; Hiramatsu, 1999b).

## *The environmental stress approach*

In most general terms stress can be defined as an imbalance between environmental demands and response capabilities of the subject involved in this interaction. With their transactional stress model, Lazarus and Folkman (1984), Folkman et al. (1986), Folkman and Moskowitz (2000) and Lazarus (1991, 1993, 2000) have provided a helpful framework for analysing and understanding the processes involved in the mutual inter-actions (transactions) between the environment and human beings. According to their theory, the wide individual variation of the human response to a stressor can be explained by two major moderation pro-cesses: differences in the cognitive and emotional appraisal of the stressor and differences in coping with the stressor.

Environmental noise can affect this process both directly and indirectly. If annoying noise makes you feel angry because this is the only room where you can do your work and there is a deadline tomorrow then the emotional response triggered by the inescapable situational constraints will clearly have an impact on your coping abilities and drain your ener-gy while you try hard (adaptive response) to meet the deadline. Clearly, both the negative effect and the adaptive response to the challenge will make an impact on the neuroendocrine and cardiovascular systems and will possibly affect your behaviour and attitudes towards the people who intend to interrupt you working. If you have a quiet room where you can go this makes a big difference.

To make this psychological concept an effective framework for the assessment and prevention of adverse effects of environmental noise (Lercher, 1996), it has to be placed into an ecological and contextual research perspective (Cohen et al., 1986; Stokols, 1987; Staples, 1997; Stallen, 1999). This perspective directs attention to the many social and environmental factors (Table 16.2) that may influence both the appraisal and coping capabilities. Moreover, it opens the way to possible mediation processes where the social and physical environment and psychological or biological traits and dispositions interact. The insight you gain from the transactional analyses can be used to develop public health strategies which may later impact at the individual, social and/or environmental level (Cohen et al., 1986; Staples, 1997; Lercher, 2001).

**Table 16.2** Selected examples of contextual factors known to influence response to noise

| Climate | Geography/ architecture | Environment | Social ecology | Culture |
|---|---|---|---|---|
| Cold, hot or moderate Seasons Prevailing winds | Nature/topography: flat, hilly, valley, lake, sea Area layout: the built environment Housing: type of house, common green, garden | Vibration: air pollution, odours Visual appearance Density, room design | Land use: residential mixed Neighbour-hood relationships Access to services Recreation, safety | Habits and life-style Meaning of living attitudes Meaning of place |

After-effects, cumulative fatigue, helplessness and overgeneralization of learned coping strategies to other life domains are known costs to humans of trying to adapt to chronic ambient stressors (Cohen et al., 1986; Dougall and Baum, 2001; Evans, 2001).

On the positive side, the appraisal of a stressor is re-evaluated all the time. This means that it is open to modification if something important has changed (for example, if a night curfew on aircraft has been set into force).

From the environmental stress approach and existing empirical evidence we can formulate some core hypotheses that can guide further research and management of environmental noise:

1.  Environmental noise acts as a chronic ambient stressor. It affects health and well-being in a specific and non-specific way (Figure 16.1)

through a mix of both direct and indirect pathways (Lercher, 1996; Ising and Braun, 2000; Evans, 2001; Babisch, 2002). Noise cannot therefore be studied or treated like an infection or a toxic chemical with a specific and direct pathway to the health effect (classic medical approach).

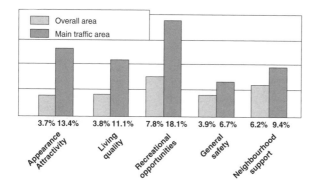

**Figure 16.1** Dissatisfaction with residential area: rather or very much dissatisfied.

2. The total context is responsible for the effects at both the individual and the population level. This requires the examination of the total stressor load. Monosensory viewpoints that treat noise in isolation from its context – neglecting vibration, air pollution, environmental degradation and social severances accompanied by transportation – are obsolete and tell only part of the story that you need if you are to intervene efficiently (Figure 16.2).
3. Moderation of the potential effects (higher or lower) is to be expected by individual, psychosocial, cultural and environmental factors (Evans and Lepore, 1997). Depending on the population distribution of these factors, complex interactions and transactions can build up further.
4. The actual total context (2) and the possible effects of moderation (3) can produce large differences in both individual and population response to a similar noise exposure (Lercher, 1998 a and b). This means that different results from effect studies should be expected and lead to a more sensitive interpretation of 'obviously discrepant' results. A thorough investigation should be made into (2) and (3) before discarding the results as inconsistent. Likewise, the average view resulting from aggregate responses (normative dose–response curves) should be handled cautiously.

Empirical examples of this approach can be found in environmental noise research (Cohen et al., 1986; Pulles et al., 1990; Van Kamp, 1990; TOI, 1991; Lercher et al., 1993, 1998b, 2002; Evans et al., 1995, 1998; Lercher, 1996; Lercher and Kofler, 1996; Job and Hatfield, 2001; Klæboe,

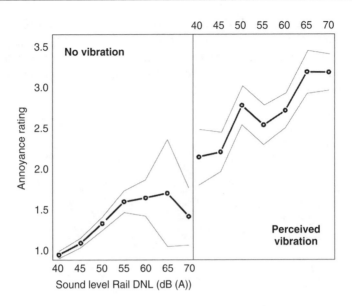

**Figure 16.2** Interaction between exposure to noise and vibration.

2001; Yano et al., 2002). Some noise policy oriented publications also use implicitly this perspective (TOI, 1991; Passchier-Vermeer, 1997; Passchier-Vermeer et al., 2000; NEHAP – Austria 1999; NEHAP – Switzerland, 2000).

# Integrated assessment of impact

## Personal and public impact

People exposed to environmental noise elicit responses at various levels of health and well-being and report decrements in quality of life (Halpern, 1995; Carter, 1996; Lercher et al., 1998; Babisch, 2000; Stansfeld et al., 2000; Neus and Boikat, 2000; WHO, 2000; Evans, 2001; van Kempen et al., 2002; see also Chapter 25). Over decades, judgments of overall noise annoyance have been used to characterize the individual and public impact from the most prevalent noise sources. Archival databases on noise annoyance from surveys around the globe are the central source for administrators. An analysis of de Hollander et al. (1999) has indicated a significant contribution of noise annoyance to the disease burden in terms of DALYs (disability-adjusted life years). Very late, however, a standardization of the central annoyance question has been accomplished (Fields et al., 2001). For certain groups, like children and very old people equivalent databases are not yet available. The first dose–response data for children have been reported only recently (Lercher et al., 2000a). A major concern with this approach is that the dose–response data are valid only under steady-state conditions; however, most assessment questions (in Environmental Health Impact Assessment, Strategic Environmental Health Assessment and so forth) deal with changing environments. Often 'traffic calming' or other measures to reduce road traffic in residential areas have been discounted by mistakenly referring to the small benefit you could expect from dose–response curves. In this case powerful moderating variables such as safety concerns (of parents for their children) are neglected. The examples make the severe limitation of single-factor thinking in environmental health evident.

Job (1993) has raised the question whether the term 'annoyance' covers all the important negative reactions people experience from exposure to noise. In addition people may feel frustrated, helpless, fatigued, and so forth. Based on a review of research data he proposed to address noise problems in field surveys by the wider semantics of 'affectedness' instead of a single annoyance question only (Job et al., 2001).

The standard reply to Job's concern is that people account for all these effects when answering the general annoyance question (Langdon, 1987). Nevertheless, data to the contrary are available. Van Kamp (1990) found a stronger effect on health ratings in people exhibiting a coping style consisting of denial or avoidance ('noise is not a problem for me', 'it does not bother me'). In a community, where noise barriers have been installed, no correlation was found between noise level and annoyance, while a linear relationship between noise level and sleep disturbance still persisted (Lercher, 2001). In a large survey (Lercher and Kofler, 1996) noise-sensitive people were shown to exhibit lower average annoyance ratings (in the same noise categories) in spite of larger noise-associated health impairments (symptoms, medications) and less engagement in personal noise management (closing windows and so forth).

Recently, it has been recognized that the continuous monitoring of adverse effects other than annoyance should be a regular part of the assessment process (WHO, 2000). Hitherto, only one proposal for measuring sleep disturbance has been issued (Passchier-Vermeer, 1997). The EU Environmental Noise Directive (2002) mentions sleep disturbance in Annex 3 and promises an outline of assessment in future revisions. This is understandable because the current feasibility of monitoring other potential health effects of environmental noise has been questioned (Porter et al., 1998). Recent experience from the environmental health impact assessment around Schiphol airport has further indicated the limitations of available disease registers (Franssen et al., 2002). The health outcomes registered mostly cover severe pathologies (such as birth defects or hospital admissions) which are not suited to detect early signs of adverse health effects that surface first at the symptom level in the individual and at the general practitioners' level of health care. For instance, a longitudinal study found ambient noise exposure to be associated with a loss of physical function in older adults (Balfour and Kaplan, 2002). A standardized registry of such health outcome data is usually not available at the primary care level of health systems. This means that currently the appropriate monitoring of the health burden of environmental noise at the population level is rather limited.

## Environmental impact

We can distinguish direct and indirect effects of noise on the environment. An example of the direct impact of noise on the ambient environment is the reduced utility of balconies, gardens and common green spaces that should serve social and recreational purposes. It goes further, however: noise affects the way residents use their rooms (Morton-Williams et al., 1978; Lambert et al., 1984; Fields and Hall, 1986). While it is possible to move to rooms that are not affected by noise for some activities requiring quietness (reading, for example), this is more difficult for sleeping, TV viewing or conversations with visiting friends. Physical constraints in the design of flats often allow little choice and leave people with unsolved dilemmas (Figure 16.3). Another relationship of annoyance with house type is not yet fully understood (Bradley and Jonah, 1979; Sato et al., 1999, 2002). It could be that the design, insulation, density, social or other contextual factors associated with house type confound the relationship.

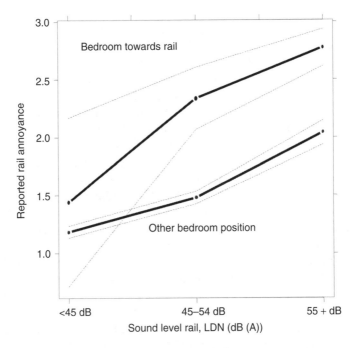

**Figure 16.3** Bedroom location and annoyance reporting.

Indirect effects mostly occur because road traffic noise is associated with traffic activities. The 'barrier' effect is such a complex example: the greater the traffic flow the fewer road crossings people make (Appleyard and Lintell, 1972). The difficulties in getting around on streets makes pedestrians (especially the elderly and children) feel unsafe (Hillman et al., 1991; TOI, 1991; Whitelegg, 1993). Paradoxically, this can increase the use of private cars and even affect health status: parents worried about their children's safety take them to school by car, resulting in poorer fitness (Armstrong, 1993). Further accompanying factors of vehicular traffic, such as air pollution and vibrations, substantially influence the noise annoyance ratings (Haider et al., 1990; Howarth and Griffin, 1991; Öhrström, 1997; Klæboe, 1998; Passchier-Vermeer, 1998; Zeichart, 1998, Lercher et al., 1999; Klæboe et al., 2000a, 2003).

### Noise is often clustered with other stressors, imperfect environments or lack of coping opportunities

The presence of multiple stressors reduces the effectiveness of coping efforts with noise. In cities, this situation makes it nearly impossible to detect noise effects against the background effects of other factors. In Alpine areas single houses are more vulnerable to the direct effects of transportation noise due to its exposure from more than one side (no quiet side).

The presence of multiple stressors reduces the effectiveness of coping efforts which depends on the expenditure of coping resources in the presence of other stressors (Lepore and Evans, 1996). A study in the Netherlands has found a high clustering of other environmental risks with noise exposure at local levels while risks due to radiation or chemical substances were more evenly distributed across the country (Pruppers et al., 1998).

The instance of the trans-Alpine traffic in the EU has shown that mountaineous areas are especially sensitive to negative environmental effects (Lercher et al., 1995; Lercher and Kofler, 1996; EEA, 2001; Knoflacher, 2001). Topography and meteorology unfavourably support the propagation of noise in such a way that the distant slopes of the valley often receive noise levels you hear in the second or third row along highways. Due to the low background levels in these distant areas the noise to background ratio increases and the noise impact on people is higher. For areas that have these characteristics that make them more vulnerable to the impact of environmental noise the term 'sensitive area' has been used, which is often applied in a more restrictive sense only (http://glossary.eea. eu.int/EEAGlossary/S/sensitive_area).

Finally, noise-impacted environments are generally judged as less attractive (Appleyard and Lintell, 1972; Fields and Hall, 1986; Kastka and Hangartner, 1986; Mace et al., 1999). Difficulties remain with the interpretation of these findings because noise is considered to be only one part of a cumulative negative effect of transportation activities on the quality of the environment. Road structures are typically associated with fewer green spaces or often in sharp contrast to residential gardens. In an early study, Langdon (1976) doubled the explained variance of individual annoyance ratings by including environmental ratings (visual, aesthetic) in the regression model. 'Incongruent' structures have been shown to reduce the liking for the neighbourhood (Wohlwill, 1979; Wohlwill and Harris, 1980; Tamura et al., 1992) and may further lead to less care being taken (Appleyard and Lintell, 1972). The visual appearance of the neighbourhood has been shown to influence auditory ratings (Sabadin et al., 1991; Maffiolo et al., 1999; Suzuki et al., 2000; Viollon et al., 2002). Kastka and Hangartner (1986) found that in visually attractive streets residents feel less annoyed. Japanese studies found the planting of tree belts reduces annoyance when the height of the tree belts is reasonable (Suzuki et al., 1989; Tamura et al., 1992; Hayashi et al., 1994; Kim and Fujimoto, 1994). Kim and Fujimoto (1994) concluded, from their analysis, that the tree arrangements brings back birds and insects and therefore more natural sounds can be heard in the area, which is judged more amenable by residents. In an Alpine valley, Lercher and Brauchle (2000b) found higher annoyance where the incongruence between ambient nature and the road was high and lower annoyance where the surroundings fitted more with the road structure. These results are compatible with both an attitudinal approach based on expectations and an environmental preference approach based on landscape assessment.

In summary, it seems rather difficult to single out the exact amount of the adverse impact of noise on the environment due to the multifaceted nature of the perceived quality of the environment. Moreover, the accounted variance depends strongly on the underlying theoretical model and whether constructive or reconstructive modelling approaches are applied (van Poll, 1997).

## Social impact

Predominantly experimental studies have been conducted on the potential impact of environmental noise on social behaviour. Evidence for a decrease in helping behaviour under loud noise conditions has consistently been found (Bell et al., 1996). Whether this finding is due to the masking, distracting or more narrow focusing effects of noise is still a matter of discussion. The early study by Appleyard and Lintell (1972) showed that residents in streets with lower traffic volume had three times as many friends and twice as many acquaintances as residents in streets with more traffic. They also found more casual social interactions among residents in the streets with lower traffic volume.

Furthermore, the average length of residence was highest for the low traffic area. The reported results could be confounded by selection factors though. Taking these results for further hypothesis generation it is imaginable that ambient noise also affects social support as it affects helping behaviour. One such finding has been reported (Lercher et al., 1999) and needs confirmation from other studies.

Wanting to move out of noisy areas is another well-known effect, indicating dissatisfaction with the existing situation. However, actual moving plans were not found to be associated with noise (Fields and Hall, 1986). Other reasons interfering with the wish to move were stronger. One important reason is the costs involved when moving. Linking this information with the consistent finding of an inverse association between indicators of social disadvantage (income, education, minority) and ambient noise levels (Glasauer, 1991; Forkenbrock and Schweitzer, 1999; Evans and Kantrowitz, 2002), it is not surprising that noise has been blamed for fostering social segregation. Following newer guidelines on the conceptualization of social impacts (Vanclay, 2002) we have to acknowledge the very limited database on this subject as far as the effects of environmental noise are concerned.

## Economic impact (individual and social)

Since the mid-1980s many economic studies have attempted to evaluate aimed at national cost estimates of noise pollution by various methods (Taylor et al., 1982; Weinberger et al., 1991; Soguel, 1996; Lambert et al., 1998; Sælensminde, 1999, 2000; Quinet, 2001). According to these studies, social costs range between 0.2% and 2.0% of the Gross National Product (Quinet, 1993; Maddison et al., 1996). A majority of these studies used hedonic price surveys by relating house prices and residential property values to noise levels or contingent valuation method surveys of willingness to pay (WTP). These studies usually report the decline in property values by means of the so-called noise depreciation index (NDI). The OECD recommends a noise depreciation index of 0.5% of property value per decibel increase if noise levels are above 50 dB (A) $L_{eq}$ (24 hours). Some research indicates that property value depreciation due to noise is non-linear and rises from 0.5% per dB (A) unit increase in the range 50–60 dB (A), to 0.8% per unit increase above 65 dB (A). These noise cost studies have been criticized on several grounds and are thought to underestimate total costs by a substantial amount (Verhoef, 1994, 1996). On the other hand, it was said the methodology is not able to separate clearly the effects of noise from other traffic impact ('focusing or interaction effects') and the studies did not consider contextual factors sufficiently (topography, double glazing, neighbourhood aspects, traffic flow, etc.). These concerns are supported by studies that indicate that residential property values along low-volume roads are quite sensitive to changes in traffic volume or to traffic on adjacent streets (Bagby, 1980; Hughes and Sirmans, 1992).

Other studies describe noise costs in cents per vehicle km/mile or cents per passenger km/mile for various sources (cars, buses, trucks) on different transportation routes (freeways, arterials, collectors). A summary of noise-cost estimates of European researchers by Quinet (1997) indicates an average estimate of approximately 0.7¢ per vehicle mile (US$). These estimates cannot be used for single sources such as heavy trucks, with costs five times higher per km/mile (Maddison et al., 1996).

Data from a tourist industry survey in the Alpine areas of Switzerland, Austria and Bavaria indicate a lower occupancy rate of rooms directed to the noise source. Furthermore, about 50% of guests in noisy rooms ask to be moved to quiet rooms and 16% of guests in noisy rooms leave early (Langer, 1996).

**Calculated economic impacts may be an underestimate**

Noise cost estimates for the society range between 0.2 and 2.0% of the GNP. The broad range of estimates is impressive, although, only hard facts (house depreciation) are typically considered, while more 'intangible' effects such as environmental, social and life quality issues are not yet sufficiently covered.

To sum up: noise impacts vary by source type and condition, location and time. Only rarely has a distinction been made between night- and daytime exposure. In general, noise costs are higher in urban areas due to the larger population impacted but a single vehicle in rural areas has a greater cost than an additional vehicle added to urban traffic. Several impacts have not been investigated (models do not account for non-residential impacts). Others, like health impacts, have never been addressed, probably due to the large uncertainties involved (Figure 16.4). Therefore, no attempt could be made to integrate the various impacts. All these are good reasons to assume that costs for some areas (sensitive areas) and for unfavourable combinations of source type, time and context are rather undervalued.

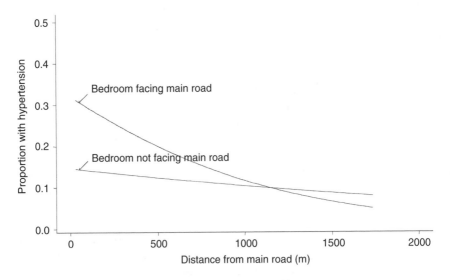

**Figure 16.4** Road distance, bedroom orientation and hypertension.

# Integrated management: policy perspectives

Environmental noise has been and still is a disliked subject with environmental health officers (EHOs), administrators and legislators. Noise has the label of the subjective (unwanted sound in standard definitions) and cannot be treated 'objectively' like radiation or particulate air pollution. However, policy approaches need objective data to build on. This has led to overemphasis on the dose–response database. These data hold quite well at the aggregated population level but they fail at the smaller neighbourhood level where the EHO should apply them (Grime, 2000). Only with the increasing need of governments and local administrations to deal with the notion of sustainability was it recognized that, despite its transitory nature, the effects of noise on the quality of life at the local level is cumulative and often mingled with other environmental and social problems.

To make the management of environmental noise compatible with the goal of a sustainable environment a clear *inter-* or *trans-sectoral* policy framework is required. As long as transport policies are not compatible with environmental or health policy (read the case study of the Alpine transit traffic, page 357) no progress is to be expected. To be successful reorientation is necessary (WHO, 2000). The core 'principles' of this reorientation are:

- *The precautionary principle.* In all cases, noise should be reduced to the lowest level achievable in a particular situation. Where there is a reasonable possibility that public health will be damaged, action should be taken to protect public health without awaiting full scientific proof.

- *The polluter pays principle.* The full costs associated with noise pollution (including monitoring, management, lowering levels and supervision) should be met by those responsible for the source of noise.

- *The prevention principle.* Action should be taken where possible to reduce noise at the source. Land-use planning should be guided by an environmental health impact assessment that considers noise as well as other pollutants.

At this point a cautious note is necessary. The pure reduction in intensity of environmental noise is not always necessary or sufficient. First, assessments need to consider and approach other determinants of impairment in the quality of life and the environment (TOI, 1991; Staples, 1997). The single pursuit of silence is an unnecessary and probably demotivating general goal (Job, 1999) – sounds are often meaningful. A variety of alternative approaches is available. Creative engineering allows noise to be overcome not only through silence but by masking sound (Zwicker and Fastl, 1999) and through the design of positive sound environments (Karlsson, 1999). Social and psychological approaches (Cederlöf et al., 1967; Sörensen, 1970; Job, 1991) have indicated the usefulness of changing people's attitudes and reactions to the sound – when appropriate – and through the timing and modification of the circumstances of exposure to sound (Job, 1999). As an overarching perspective, we have to modify the sound environment so that the meaningful information can come through to the receiver (soundscape approach). Nevertheless, there are some established 'principles' and tools that need to be considered when tackling environmental noise with this approach.

## Prevention

### Land-use planning

Land-use planning plays a central role in delivering sustainable development (Department for Transport, 1998; OECD, 2000; DEFRA, 2001; EEA, 2002). It works best by both providing incentives for sustainable plans and preventing harmful development by rigorous control. With foresight planning, some unnecessary noise exposure can be avoided. Classic noise zoning is an important tool and noise mapping can support this task. However, the traditional focus on zoning must be integrated with modern planning approaches that work against sprawling developments, support building layouts that provide a 'quiet side', and reduce the need for individual motorized travel by improving access to work, leisure activities and services (OECD, 2000; DEFRA, 2001). For instance, the Western Australian government is attempting to contain suburban sprawl through a new policy called Liveable Neighbourhoods (Jones, 2001). A slightly different concept from planning ahead is the new concept of 'environmental zoning'. This is an example of an active 'corrective' approach to ameliorate existing situations. It has been implemented in towns in North America, Sweden and recently Norway (Norway White Paper, 2002).

### Technical means

In general, noise can be combated most effectively at the source. Reliance on the control of noise emissions by setting standards for the individual sources is deceptive.

Sandberg (1995, 2001b) and the INCE working group have convincingly shown that the existing abatement policies for road traffic noise are inefficient. Sandberg (2001a) has blamed 13 common myths that seem to have been accepted among part of either the scientific or the administrative/ political community. The acceptance of these myths has delayed effective reduction of road noise in actual traffic. According to Sandberg, the most effective reduction would be delivered by speed limits, followed by road surfaces and tyre modifications. While speed limits would come at negligible costs, he and others (Nijland and Jabben, 2001) have shown the cost-effectiveness of low-noise tyres and road surface selection. Furthermore, Sandberg's (2000a, 2001b and Sandberg and Ejsmont, 2002) data support the view that a low-noise road surface may be competitive and even superior to building noise barriers in certain noise exposure situations. These data still show a potential to reduce noise at the source by a conventional engineering approach, however. As Nijland and Jabben (2001) pointed out: 'One of the major problems to overcome is the fact that, at present, costs are carried by other groups in society than those who would eventually be the beneficiaries. Solving this problem is far more a political than a scientific challenge.' This is probably the main reason why 'end of pipe' or 'downstream' technologies such as noise barriers and soundproof windows are still the most prevalent means of combating environmental noise. This is unfortunate because often – as case studies show – technical means close to the receiver *alone* are not sufficient to reduce health effects and to improve quality of life and more radical and expensive measures such as rerouting traffic by tunnels are eventually necessary to achieve this goal (Öhrström, 2000; Kolbenstvedt et al., 2005).

## Monitoring and assessment

Because reliance on 'source-oriented emission control' alone does not work, monitoring of both exposures (imissions) *and* adverse effects on humans and the environment is necessary to evaluate existing policies (WHO, 2000). Imission monitoring needs to contain simultaneous monitoring of other exposures from transportation as well. Within a sustainable perspective a much broader effect-based assessment needs to be implemented. The *surveillance of the adverse effects* in target populations should include:

---

**Preventive action through integrated assessment and management**

A clear **inter-** or **transsectoral** policy framework is required to combat noise at the various levels where it is generated by the 'driving' forces. Land–use planning, environmental zoning, sensitive areas, supportive sound environments are buzz words that have to be merged into a larger framwork. It should be guided by special needs in time and space and by the 'adaptive capacity' of the average individual.

---

- direct as well as cumulative adverse health effects from noise pollution (behavioural changes/aberrations, stress-related psycho-physiological effects, interference with communication, rest/relaxation and sleep);
- adverse effects on future generations (deterioration of residential, social and learning environments, impaired human development);
- sociocultural, aesthetic and economic effects (social isolation, run-down neighbourhoods, deterioration in the value of buildings).

Special attention in the evaluation should be directed towards vulnerable groups (children, the elderly and people with hearing deficits).

This means a 'cumulative assessment paradigm' is a necessary requirement; however, methodology and implementation seem to be difficult (Burris and Canter, 1997; Baxter et al., 1999; Fuller and Sadler, 1999; Cooper and Sheate, 2002).

Furthermore, existing tools, such as strategic environmental assessment (SEA) and environmental health impact assessment (EHIA) with citizen involvement, have to be applied at the earliest point, when major planning processes start. The orientation of these tools has to be more adapted to the sustainable policy orientation.

## Health promotion

Since the Ottawa charter of the WHO it has been recognized that the traditional 'hygiene approach' directed at prevention and protection does not suffice. The defensive character of such measures needs to be supplemented by approaches that provide direct control and support for citizens ('empowerment') and lead to general improvements of their environment in supporting the accomplishment of their daily tasks and challenges. Two scientifically supported approaches that can contribute to this process are concisely described below.

### Provision of control over the environment

Glass and Singer (1972) have directed our attention to the importance of control options in reducing adverse effects of sound on behaviour, cognition, motivation, emotion and well-being. Loss of control over one's environment is more likely to elicit feelings of helplessness in the long term (Hiroto, 1974; Seligman, 1975; Syme, 1991; Evans, 2001).

It is not surprising, therefore, that Taylor and Repetti (1997) mention 'the ability to predict and/or control aspects of the environment' as one of three main components of a 'healthy environment'. The underlying construct of perceived control (Wallston, 2001) is related to the concept of secondary appraisal in Lazarus and Folkman's theory of stress and coping, where a person is believed to judge the available sources to cope with the stressor. The greater the resources (or control options) the more likely it is that the individual will cope successfully.

Implementation of these ideas in practice is possible at different levels ranging from city planning, policy enforcement to health impact assessments (Lercher, 2001).

The quiet courtyards in many European cities are good examples of a highly effective and cost-efficient measure (Kihlman, 2001). The closed courtyards in blocks near busy roads provide an area for undisturbed communication (indoors and outdoors), recreation (recovery and sleep), optional social relations, and a place for small children to play safely. Both the Swedish Action Plan against Noise (Kihlman, 1993) and the EU Directive on Environmental Noise acknowledge the potential of this planning approach. A new Swedish research programme is investigating the potential of this approach with respect to health and well-being (Kihlman et al., 2001; Skånberg and Öhrström, 2002).

Silence is not the ultimate goal: the normalization of the soundscape is. No doubt – silence should be protected – most times, however, we need to modify the sound environment such that the meaningful information can come through to the receiver (soundscape approach). Noise can also be overcome through masking sound and through the timing and modification of the circumstances of exposure to sound. The goal should be 'person-environment-fit' and/or 'setting congruence'.

Active policy approaches such as community empowerment (McClendon, 1993; Rocha, 1997; Obermeyer, 1998; Ghose, 2001) have been proposed to increase perceived control. Recent research has actually shown the increase in personal efficacy and the feeling of control of the environment through capacity building and procedural involvement in neighbourhood improvement projects (Elwood, 2002).

Restrictions on noise pollution enforced for certain times in certain areas – although defensive in their nature – can also contribute to perceived control. Traffic calming has been shown to be effective not so much by its measured reduction in sound levels (which in terms of $L_{eq}$ is rather small) but more through its indirect effect on the reduction of impediments of (eg. easier crossings) and improved safety for children and the elderly on the streets. Such measures also indicate to the residents that those responsible for the environment are actually caring for their quality of life.

## Towards supportive environments: improving the environment

Sustainable development would mean that the acoustic environment *promotes* rather than endangers health and quality of life. The restoration perspective (Kaplan and Kaplan, 1989; Kaplan, 1995) complements the stress perspective. While stress research focuses on reducing demands, restoration research focuses on ensuring the necessary resources (Hartig, 2001).

A small body of this research is actually directed at the specific restorative effects of the environment, mainly natural scenery and parks (Bjork, 1986, 1995; Kaplan and Kaplan, 1989; Hartig et al., 1991, 1996; Ulrich et al., 1991; Korpela and Hartig, 1996; Hartig, 2001; Kaplan, 2001). This research gives some indication of positive effects on attention, mood and physiology when humans are exposed to natural and attractive surroundings. Furthermore, a questionnaire to measure the restorative quality of an environment has been developed (Hartig et al., 1997) and a monitoring tool for the provision of accessible urban green spaces is being published (Van Herzele and Wiedemann, 2002).

The notion of supportive environments is therefore clearly related to the concept of providing control and some overlap with general positive effects induced by attractive environments should happen in real life. There is, however, a difference. Providing supportive environments means more: it means to apply specific groups of actions that are directed at:

- special needs (working/studying, recreation and sleeping, conversation, opening windows, using balconies and gardens, protection of sensitive times);
- special sensitive areas (hospitals, school, kindergarten, playgrounds and common greens, parkland and recreational areas, residential and other areas with complex noise environments or other unfavourable conditions [terrain, meteorology, low-frequency components, lifestyle and time activity patterns] where a greater impact of noise is likely to be expected);
- special vulnerable groups (children, the elderly and people with hearing deficits).

Priority should be given in SEAs, EHIAs and other planning processes to these actions to support ongoing human activities by measures that improve the 'adaptive capacity' of the average individual. The measures may range from simple restrictions in time or space to the redesigning of roads and building blocks or an even larger redesigning of areas.

Not many such studies exist and few have directed their focus on noise impact. Studies of area redesign to move traffic away from residential areas in Gotenborg and Oslo are an example of such work in urban areas (Klæboe, 1998; Klæboe et al., 2000a; Öhrström and Skånberg, 2000; Kolbenstvedt et al., 2005). Redesigning a larger rural area to reduce the road traffic impact by building a new rail track mainly in tunnels was the subject of an EHIA in the Alpine area of Tyrol, Austria (Lercher et al., 1999).

## Conclusions

The road to solutions for the problem of environmental noise and its associated adverse effects relates to the measures that society takes to address the transportation problem. A sustainable perspective on traffic noise, environment and health requires integrative solutions that fit the specific local environment in its larger context. Only when the standardized assessment of climatic, architectural, geographical, sociocultural, psychological, health and ecological factors is an integrative part of the assessment process and added as another layer to the GIS is sufficient consideration of local and regional conditions possible. To guide the assessment process a contextually oriented environmental stress perspective is helpful for all activities – from scoping and planning of studies to the implementation of measures supporting a sustainable development.

## References

Alberola AJ, Mendoza LJ, Bullmore AJ, Flindell IH (2002) Noise mapping: uncertainties. In Forum Acusticum Sevilla 2002 CD–ROM Sociedad Espanola de Acustica.

Amphoux P (1993) L'identité sonore des villes européennes. Guide méthodologique. Grenoble: Travaux du Cresson.

Amphoux P (1995) Aux écoutes de la ville. La qualité sonore des espaces publics européens – Méthode d'analyse comparative – Enquête sur trois villes suisses. Rapport scientifique. Zürich: Nationales Forschungsprogramm 'Stadt und Verkehr'.

Ando Y (1998) Architectural Acoustics. Blending sound sources, sound fields and listeners. New York: AIP Press/Springer-Verlag.

Appleyard D, Lintell M (1972) The environmental quality of city stress: the resident viewpoint. Journal of the American Planning Association 38: 84–101.

Armstrong N (1993) Independent mobility and children's physical development. In M Hillman (ed.) Children Transport and the Quality of Life. London: Policy Studies Institute.

Augoyard J (1999) The Cricket Effect, which tools for the research on sonic urban Ambiences? In H Karlsson (ed.) (1999) From Awareness to Action. Proceedings 'Stockholm Hey Listen'. Conference on acoustic ecology. Stockholm: The Royal Swedish Academy of Music, pp. 1–7.

Augoyard J, Torgue H (1995) A L'Ecoute de L'Environement Sonore. Repertoire des effets sonores. Marseille: Parenthese.

Babisch W (2000) Traffic noise and cardiovascular disease: epidemiological review and synthesis. Noise and Health 8: 9–32.

Babisch W (2002) The noise/stress concept risk assessment and research needs. Noise and Health 4: 1–11.

Bagby G (1980) Effects of traffic flow on residential property values. Journal of the American Planning Association 46: 88–94.

Balfour JL, Kaplan GA (2002) Neighborhood environment and loss of physical function in older adults: evidence from the Alameda County Study. American Journal of Epidemiology 155: 507–15.

Baxter W, Ross W, Spaling H (1999) To what standard? A critical evaluation of cumulative effects assessments. Canada Environmental Assessment 7(2): 30–2.

Bell PA, Greene TC, Fisher JD, Baum A (1996) Environmental Psychology, 4th edn. Fort Worth: Harcourt Brace.

Berglund B, Nilsson ME (2001) Variation in perceived soundscape due to shielding building and façade. Proceedings of Internoise 2001. The Hague: INCE, pp. 1253–6.

Berglund B, Hassmen P, Job RF (1996) Sources and effects of low-frequency noise. The Journal of the Acoustical Society of America 99: 2985–3002.

Bjork EA (1986) Laboratory annoyance and skin conductance responses to some natural sounds. Journal of Sound and Vibration 109: 339–45.

Bjork EA (1995) Psychophysiological responses to some natural sounds. Acta Acustica 3: 83–8.

Blauert J, Jekosch U (1996) Sound-quality evaluation – a multi-layered problem. ACUSTICA United with Acta Acustica 83: 747–53.

Blumrich R, Heimann D (2002) A linearized eulerian sound propagation model for studies of complex meteorological effects. Journal of the Acoustical Society of America 112: 446–55.

Botteldooren D, Verkeyn A, Lercher P (2002) Noise annoyance modelling using fuzzy rule based systems. Noise and Health 4: 27–44.

Bradley JS, Jonah BA (1979) The effects of site selected variables on human responses to traffic noise Part I: type of housing by traffic noise level. Journal of Sound and Vibration 66: 589–604.

Burris RK, Canter LW (1997) Cumulative impacts are not properly addressed in environmental assessments. Environmental Impact Assessment Review 17: 5–18.

Campbell J (1983) Ambient stressors. Environment and Behavior 15: 355–80.

Carles J, Bernaldez F, De Lucio J (1992) Audio-visual interactions and soundscape preferences. Landscape Research 17: 52–6.

Carter NL (1996) Transportation noise sleep and possible after-effects. Environment International 22 : 105–16.

CEC (1996) Future Noise Policy European Commission Green Paper COM(96) 540. Luxembourg: Final Office for Official Publications of the European Communities.

Cederlöf R, Jonsson E, Sörensen S (1967) On the influence of attitudes to the source of annoyance reactions to noise. Nordistk Hygienisk Tidskrift 48: 16–59.

Cohen S, Evans GW, Stokols D, et al. Behavior, health and environmental stress. New York, London: Plenum Press, 1986.

Cooper LM, Sheate WR (2002) Cumulative effects assessment; a review of UK environmental impact statements. Environmental Impact Assessment Review 22: 415–39.

De Hollander AE, Melse JM, Lebret E, Kramers PG (1999) An aggregate public health indicator to represent the impact of multiple environmental exposures. Epidemiology 10: 606–17.

Department for Environment, Food and Rural Affairs (2001) Towards a National Ambient Noise Strategy. London: DEFRA .

Department for Environment, Food and Rural Affairs (2002) The UK National Noise Incidence Study 2000/01. London: DEFRA: wwwdefragovuk/ environment/noise/nis0001/.

Department for Transport (1998) White Paper: A New Deal for Transport. Better for Everyone. London: The Stationery Office.

Diaz J, Ekelund M, Gothe R, Huber M, Jordan A, Kalischnigg G, Kampet T, Kappus A, Lopez Santiago C, Mansfield T, Maschke C, Niemann H, Welkker D (2001) Traffic Noise Pollution. Similarities and Differences between European Regions. Berlin: Berliner Zentrum Public Health (BZPH).

Dougall AL, Baum A (2001) Stress health and illness. In A Baum, T Revenson, JE Singer (eds) Handbook of Health Psychology. Mahwah, NJ: Erlbaum, pp. 321–38.

Elwood SA (2002) GIS use in community planning: a multidimensional analysis of empowerment. Environment and Planning A 34: 905–22.

Embleton TFW (1996) Tutorial on sound propagation outdoors. Journal of the Acoustical Society of America 100: 31–48.

European Environment Agency (2000) Are We Moving in the Right Direction? Indicators on Transport and Environmental Integration in the EU. Environmental issue report No 12. Copenhagen: OPOCE.

European Environment Agency (2001) Road Freight Transport and the Environment in Mountainous Areas. Case Studies in the Alpine Region and the Pyrenees. Copenhagen: EEA.

European Environment Agency (2002) Towards an Urban Atlas: Assessment of Spatial Data on 25 European Cities and Urban Areas. Environmental issue report No 30. Copenhagen: EEA.

Evans GW (2001) Environmental stress and health. In A Baum, T Revenson, JE Singer (eds) Handbook of Health Psychology. Mahwah, NJ: Erlbaum, pp. 365–85.

Evans GW, Bullinger M, Hygge S (1998) Chronic noise exposure and physiological response: a prospective study of children living under environmental stress. Psychological Science 9: 75–7.

Evans GW, Hugge S, Bullinger M (1995) Chronic noise and phychological stress. Psychological Science 6: 333–8.

Evans GW, Kantrowitz E (2002) Socioeconomic status and health: the potential role of environmental risk exposure. Annual Review of Public Health 23: 303–31.

Evans GW, Lepore SJ (1997) Moderating and mediating processes in environment-behavior research In GT Moore, R Marans (eds) Advances in Environment Behavior and Design. New York: Plenum Press.

Fidell S, Barber DS, Schultz TJ (1991) Updating a dosage–effect relationship for the prevalence of annoyance due to general transportation noise. Journal of the Acoustical Society of America 89: 221–33.

Fields JM (1993) Effect of personal and situational variables on noise annoyance in residential areas. Journal of the Acoustical Society of America 93: 2753–63.

Fields JM, Hall FL (1986) Community effects of noise. In PM Nelson (ed.) Community Effects of Noise. London: Butterworth, Chapter 3.

Fields JM, De Jong RG, Gjestland T, Flindell IH, Job RFS, Kurra S et al. (2001) Standardized general-purpose noise reaction questions for community noise surveys: research and a recommendation. Journal of Sound and Vibration 242: 641–79.

Flindell I, Porter N (2000) The implications of context-based assessment for noise management. In D Cassereau (ed.) Proceedings of Internoise 2000, Vol 4. Nice: Société Française d'Acoustique, pp. 2297–301.

Folkman S, Moskowitz JT (2000) Positive affect and the other side of coping. American Psychologist 55: 647–54.

Folkman S, Lazarus RS, Gruen RJ, DeLongis A (1986) Appraisal coping health status and psychological symptoms. Journal of Personality and Social Psychology 50: 571–9.

Forkenbrock DJ, Schweitzer LA (1999) Environmental justice in transportation planning. Journal of the American Planning Association 65: 96–111.

Franssen EAM, Staatsen BAM, Lebret E (2002) Assessing health consequences in an environmental impact assessment. The case of Amsterdam airport Schiphol. Environmental Impact Assessment Review 22: 633–53.

Fuller K, Sadler B (1999) EC guidance on cumulative effects assessment. Environmental Assessment 7(2): 33–5.

Fyhri A, Klæboe R (1999) Exploring the impact of visual aesthetics on the soundscape. In J Cuschieri, S Glegg, Y Yong (eds) Proceedings of Internoise. Fort Lauderdale, FL: INCE pp. 1261–4.

Genuit K (2002) Psychoacoustics – importance and application in practice. In Forum Acusticum Sevilla, on CD-ROM. Sociedad Espanola de Acustica.

Ghose R (2001) Use of information technology for community empowerment: transforming geographic information systems into community information systems. Transactions in GIS 5(2): 141–63.

Glasauer H (1991) Städtische Verkehrsbelastung und die Betroffenheit der sozialen Schichten. Internationales Verkehrswesen 43: 37–42.

Glass DC, Singer JE (1972) Urban Stress Experiments on Noise and Social Stressors. New York: Academic Press.

Goldstein BD (1995) The need to restore the public health base for environmental control. American Journal of Public Health 85: 481–3.

Grime S (2000) All in the mind. Environmental Health Journal 108: wwwehjonlinecom/archive/2000/august/august03html.

Grosjean M, Thibaud JP (2001) L'Espace Urbain en Methodes. Marseille: Parenthese.

Haider M, Kundi M, Groll-Knapp E, Koller M (1990) Interactions between noise and air pollution. Environment International 16: 593–601.

Halpern D (1995) More Than Bricks and Mortar? Mental Health and the Built Environment. London: Taylor & Francis, pp. 37–69.

Hartig T (2001) Guest editor's introduction (special issue on restorative environments). Environment and Behavior 33: 475–9.

Hartig T, Mang M, Evans G (1991) Restorative effects of natural environment experiences. Environment and Behavior 23: 3–26.

Hartig T, Böök A, Garvill J, Olsson T, Gärling T (1996) Environmental influences on psychological restoration. Scandinavian Journal of Psychology 37: 378–93.

Hartig T, Korpela K, Evans GW, Gärling T (1997) A measure of restorative quality in environments. Scandinavian Housing and Planning Research 14: 175–94.

Hayashi M, Tamura A, Toyama N, Suzuki H, Kashima N (1994) Effects of planting on relief of annoyance – field survey at urban roadside. In S Kuwano (ed.) Proceedings Internoise 94. Yokohama, pp. 989–92.

Heimann D, Gross G (1999) Coupled simulation of meteorological parameters and sound level in a narrow valley. Applied Acoustics 56: 73–100.

Hempel T (2001) On the development of a model for the classification of auditory events. In DT Tsahalis (ed.) Proceedings of Euronoise 2001 on CD–ROM. Patras: LFME and EEA.

Hempel T, Blauert J (1999) Von der 'Sound Quality' zur 'Auditiven Systemqualität'. In B Feiten, F Hein, A Röbel, W Schaller (eds) Impulse und Antworten. Berlin: Wissenschaft und Technik Verlag, pp. 111–17.

Hillman M (1997) Health promotion: the potential of non-motorized transport. In T Fletcher, AJ McMichael (eds) Health at the Crossroads. Transport policy and urban health. Chichester: Wiley, pp. 177–86.

Hillman M, Adams J, Whitelegg J (1991) One False Move: A study of children's independent mobility. London: Policy Studies Institute.

Hinton J (2002) How to map noise. Noise and Health 4: 1–5.

Hiramatsu K (1999a) A method for comparing sonic environments. In J Cuschieri, S Glegg, Y Yong (eds) Proceedings of Internoise. Fort Lauderdale, FL: INCE, pp. 1305–8.

Hiramatsu K (1999b) Activities and impacts of Soundscape Association of Japan. In J Cuschieri, S Glegg, Y Yong (eds) Proceedings of Internoise. Fort Lauderdale, FL: INCE, pp. 1357–62.

Hiramatsu K (2001) Soundscapegraphy: the need method and utility. Proceedings of Internoise 2001, The Hague, pp. 1713–18.

Hiroto D (1974) Locus of control and learned helplessness. J Exp Psych 102: 187–193.

Howarth HVC, Griffin MJ (1991) The annoyance caused by simultaneous noise and vibration. Journal of Acoustical Society of America 89: 2317–23.

Hughes W, Sirmans CF (1992) Traffic externalities and single-family house prices. Journal of Regional Science 32: 487–500.

Ising H, Braun C (2000) Acute and chronic endocrine effects of noise: review of the research conducted at the Institute for Water Soil and Air Hygiene. Noise and Health 7: 7–24.

Iu KK, Li KM (2002) The propagation of sound in narrow street canyons. Journal of the Acoustical Society of America 112: 537–50.

Job R (1988) Community response to noise: a review of factors influencing the relationship between noise exposure and reaction. Journal of the Acoustical Society of America 83: 991–1001.

Job R (1991) Impact and potential use of attitude and other modifying variables in reducing community stress from noise. Transportation Research Record 1312: 109–15.

Job, R (1993) Psychological factors of community reaction to noise. In M. Vallet (ed) Noise as a Public Health Problem. Vol 3. Nice: Institute National de Recherche sur les Transports et leur Sécurité, pp 48–59.

Job R (1999) Internoise 98 – 'Sound and silence': setting the balance. Noise and Health 2: 78–9.

Job R, Hatfield J (2001) The impact of soundscape enviroscape and psychscape on reaction to noise: implications for evaluation and regulation of noise effects. Noise Control Engineering Journal 49(3): 120–4.

Job R, Hatfield J, Carter NL, Peploe P, Taylor R, Morrell S (2001) General scales of community reaction to noise (dissatisfaction and perceived affectedness) are more reliable than scales of annoyance. Journal of the Acoustical Society of America 110: 939–46.

Jones E (2001) Liveable neighbourhoods. World Transport Policy and Practice 7(2): 38–43.

Jonsson E, Kajland A, Paccagnella B, Sörensen S (1969) Annoyance reactions to traffic noise in Italy and Sweden. Archives of Environmental Health 19: 692–99.

Kaplan R (2001) The nature of the view from home. Environment and Behavior 33: 507–42.

Kaplan R, Kaplan S (1989) The Experience of Nature: A psychological perspective. New York: Cambridge University Press.

Kaplan S (1995) The restorative benefits of nature towards an integrative frameworks. Journal of Environmental Psychology 15: 169–182.

Karlsson H (ed.) (1999) From Awareness to Action. Proceedings 'Stockholm Hey Listen' Conference on acoustic ecology. Stockholm: Royal Swedish Academy of Music.

Kastka J, Hangartner M (1986) Machen hässliche Strassen den Verkehrslärm lästiger? Eine umweltpsychologische Analyse zum Einfluss architektonisch gestalterischer Elemente auf die Störwirkung von Verkehrslärm auf die Anwohner. Arcus 1: 23–9.

Kastka J, Noack R (1987) On the interaction of sensory experience causal attributive cognitions and visual context parameters in noise annoyance. In HS Koelega (ed.) Environmental Annoyance: Characterisation, measurement and control. Amsterdam: Elsevier, pp. 336–45.

Kihlman T (1993) Sweden's action plan against noise. Noise News International 1: 194–208.

Kihlman T (2001) Quiet side and high facade insulation – means to solve the city noise problem. Proceedings of Internoise 2001, The Hague, pp. 1227–36.

Kihlman T, Kropp W, Berglund B, Öhrström E (2001) Soundscape support to health. A cross-disciplinary research programme. Proceedings of Inter-Noise, The Hague, pp. 1237–46.

Kim B-C, Fujimoto K (1994) Amenity of environment in residential area on the basis of sound and green In S Kuwano (ed.) Proceedings Internoise 94. Yokohama, pp. 993–6.

Klæboe R (1998) The combined effects of road traffic – implications for environmental guidelines In NL Carter, R Job (eds) Noise as a Public Health Problem. Noise Effects 98. Vol. 2. Sydney: Pty Ltd. pp. 264–7.

Klæboe R (2001) The possible impact of the neighbourhood soundscape on exposure-effect relationships. Internoise 4, The Hague: INCE, pp. 1739–44.

Klæboe R, Kolbenstvedt M, Clench-Aas J, Bartonova A (2000a) Oslo traffic study – part 1: an integrated approach to assess the combined effects of noise and air pollution on annoyance. Atmospheric Environment 34: 4727–36.

Klæboe R, Kolbenstvedt M, Fyhri A (2000b) Changes in the sound – and urbscape following traffic changes in Oslo East: In DEGA (Hg) Fortschritte der Akustik. Oldenburg D: Deutsche Gesellschaft für Akustik e. v., pp 112–13.

Klaeboe R, Turunen-Rise IH, Harvik L, Madshus C (2003) Vibration in dwellings from road and rail traffic – Part II: exposure-effect relationships based on ordinal logit and logistic regression models. Applied Acoustics 64: 89–109.

Knauss D (2002) Noise mapping and annoyance. Noise and Health 4: 7–11.

Knoflacher H (2001) Problems caused by the motorway/railway freight traffic share in the Tyrol. Pl Mech Eng F-J Rai 215: 45–51.

Kolbenstvedt M, Klæboe R, Clench-Aas J, Bartonova A (2005) Environmental impacts of traffic diversion measures in Oslo. Study design and main results. Traffic and Air Pollution, in press.

Korpela K, Hartig T (1996) Restorative qualities of favorite places. Journal of Environmental Psychology 16: 221–33.

Kragh J (2001) News and needs in outdoor noise prediction. Proceedings of Inter-noise, The Hague, pp. 2573–82.

Lambert J, Simonnet F, Vallet M (1984) Patterns of behaviour in dwellings exposed to road traffic noise. Journal of Sound and Vibration 92: 159–72.

Lambert J, Kail JM, Quinet E (1998) Transportation noise annoyance: an economic issue. In NL Carter, R Job (eds) Noise as a Public Health Problem. Noise Effects '98, Vol. 2. Sydney: Pty Ltd., pp. 749–54.

Langdon FJ (1976) Noise nuisance caused by road traffic in residential areas: Parts I and II. Journal of Sound and Vibration 47: 243–82.

Langdon FJ (1987) Some residual problems in noise nuisance: a brief review In HS Koelega (ed.) Environmental Annoyance: Characterisation, measurement and control. Amsterdam: Elsevier, pp. 321–9.

Langer G (1996) Traffic noise and hotel profits – is there a relationship? Tourism Management 17: 295–305.

Lazarus RS (1991) Emotion and Adaptation. New York: Oxford University Press.

Lazarus RS (1993) Coping theory and research: past present and future. Psychosomatic Medicine 55: 234–47.

Lazarus RS (2000) Toward better research on stress and coping. The American Psychologist 55: 665–73.

Lazarus RS, Folkman S (1984) Stress Appraisal and Coping. New York: Springer.

Lepore JS, Evans GW (1996) Coping with multiple stressors in the environment. In M Zeidner, NS Endler (eds) Handbook of Coping Theory. Research Applications. New York: Wiley, pp. 350–77.

Lercher P (1996) Environmental noise and health: an integrated research perspective. Environment International 22: 117–29.

Lercher P (1998a) Deviant dose–response curves for traffic noise in 'sensitive areas'? In The New Zealand Acoustical Society Inc (ed.) Inter Noise 98 (Paper # 0242) Conference Proceedings on CD-ROM. Christchurch N.Z. Causal Productions.

Lercher P (1998b) Context and coping as moderators of potential health effects in noise-exposed persons. In D Prasher, L Luxon (eds) Advances in Noise Series, Vol. 1. Biological Effects of Noise. London: Whurr, pp. 328–35.

Lercher P (2001) Contextual and non-contextual perspectives in research and management of noise annoyance: an environmental health perspective. Proceedings Internoise 2001, The Hague (on CD-ROM).

Lercher P, Brauchle G (2000) Die wechselseitige Beeinflussung von externer akustischer und 'natürlicher' Umgebung in einem alpinen Tal: umweltpsychologische und gesundheitliche Perspektiven In DEGA (Hg) Fortschritte der Akustik. Oldenburg D, Deutsche Gesellschaft für Akustik eV pp. 118–20.

Lercher P, Kofler W (1993) Adaptive behavior to road traffic noise: blood pressure and cholesterol. In M Vallet (ed.) Noise as a Public Health Problem, Vol. 2. Nice: Institut National de Recherche sur les Transports et leur Sécurité, pp. 465–8.

Lercher P, Kofler WW (1996) Behavioral and health responses associated with road traffic noise along alpine through-traffic routes. Science of the Total Environment 189/190: 85–9.

Lercher P, Schmitzberger R, Kofler W (1995) Perceived traffic air pollution associated behavior and health in an alpine area. Science of the Total Environment 169: 71–4.

Lercher P, Stansfeld SA, Thompson SJ (1998) Non-auditory health effects of noise: review of the 1993–1998 period. In NL Carter, R Job (eds) Noise as a Public Health Problem. Noise Effects 98, Vol. 1. Sydney, Australia: pp. 213–20.

Lercher P, Brauchle G, Widmann U (1999) The interaction of landscape and sound-scape in the Alpine area of the Tyrol: an annoyance perspective. In J Cuschieri, S Glegg, Y Yong (eds) Proceedings of Internoise. Fort Lauderdale, FL: INCE, pp. 1347–50.

Lercher P, Brauchle G, Kofler W, Widmann U, Meis M (2000a) The assessment of noise annoyance in schoolchildren and their mothers. In D Cassereau (ed.) Proceedings of Internoise 2000, Vol. 4. Nice: Société Française d'Acoustique, pp. 2318–22.

Lercher P, Evans GW, Meis M, Kofler WW (2002) Ambient neighbourhood noise and children's mental health. Occup Environ Med 59: 380–386.

Leuner D (1992) Langfristige Entwicklung der Geräuschbelastung in Bayern. Nürnberg: Landesgewerbeanstalt Bayern.

McClendon B (1993) The paradigm of empowerment. Journal of the American Planning Association 59: 145–7.

Mace BL, Bell PA, Loomis RJ (1999) Aesthetic affective and cognitive effects of noise on natural landscape assessment. Society and Natural Resources 12: 225–42.

Maddison D, Pearce DW, Johansson O, Calthrop E, Littman T, Verhoef E (1996) The True Cost of Road Transport – Blueprint 5. London: CSERGE Earthscan.

Maffiolo V, Castellengo M, Dubois D, (1999) Qualitative judgments of urban sound-scapes. In J Cuschieri, S Glegg, Y Yong (eds) Proceedings of Internoise. Fort Lauderdale, FL: INCE, pp. 1251–4.

Miedema HM, Oudshoorn CG (2001) Annoyance from transportation noise: relation-ships with exposure metrics DNL and DENL and their confidence intervals. Environmental Health Perspectives 109: 409–16.

Miedema HM, Vos H (1998) Exposure-response relationships for transportation noise. Journal of the Acoustical Society of America 104: 3432–45.

Mirowska M (1998) An investigation and assessment of annoyance of low frequency noise in dwellings. Journal of Low Frequency Noise and Vibration 17: 119–26.

Morton-Williams J, Hedges B, Fernando E (1978) Road Traffic and the Environment. London: Social and Community Planning Research.

Namba S (1994) Noise – quantity and quality. Procceedings of the International Congress on Noise Control Engineering (Inter-Noise), Vol. 1, Yokohama, Japan, pp. 2–23.

NEHAP – Austria (1999) Austrian National Environmental Action Plan (NEHAP) Chapter 8, Traffic Vienna: Federal Ministry of Environment Youth and Family Affairs.

NEHAP – Switzerland (2000) Mobility and well-being. Nature and well-being. Housing and well-being. In Evaluation of the National Environmental Action Plan (NEHAP). Basel Institut für Sozial- und Präventivmedizin der Universität Basel, Basel (in German).

Neus H, Boikat U (2000) Evaluation of traffic noise-related cardiovascular risk. Noise and Health 7: 65–77.

Nijland H, Jabben J (2001) effects costs and benefits of noise measures in the Netherlands. Proceedings of Inter-noise 2001. The Hague, pp. 1831–4.

Norway White Paper (2002) Improving Urban Environment. Chapter 6. Oslo: Ministry of the Environment.

Obermeyer N (1998) The evolution of public participation. GIS Cartography and Geographic Information Systems 25(2): 65–6.

OECD (2000) Guidelines for Environmentally Sustainable Transport (EST). Vienna: OECD and Austrian Ministry of Agriculture Forestry Environment and Water Management.

Öhrstrom E (1997) Effects of exposure to railway noise – a comparison between areas with and without vibration. Journal of Sound and Vibration 205: 555–60.

Öhrström E (2000) Sleep disturbances caused by road traffic noise – studies in laboratories and field. Noise and Health 8: 71–8.

Öhrstrom E, Skånberg A-B (1996) A field survey on effects of exposure to noise and vibration from railway traffic part I: annoyance and activity disturbance effects. Journal of Sound and Vibration 193: 39–47.

Öhrström E, Skånberg A (2000) Adverse health effects in relation to noise mitigation – A longitudinal study in the city of Göteborg. In D Cassereau (ed.) Proceedings of Internoise 2000, Vol. 4. Nice: Société Française d'Acoustique, pp. 2112–15.

Passchier-Vermeer W (1997) Assessing noise exposure for public health purposes Rijswijk Health Council of the Netherlands Publication no. 1997/23E.

Passchier-Vermeer W (1998) Vibrations in the Living Environment. Factors related to vibration perception and annoyance. Leiden: TNO-PG.

Passchier W, Knottnerus A, Albering H, Walda I (2000) Public health impact of large airports. Reviews of Environmental Health 15: 83–96.

Paulsen R, Kastka J (1995) Effects of combined noise and vibration on annoyance. Journal of Sound and Vibration 181: 295–314.

Persson K, Rylander R (1988) Disturbance from low frequency noise in the environment – a survey among the local environment health authorities in Sweden. Journal of Sound and Vibration 121: 339–45.

Persson Waye K, Rylander R (2001) The extent of annoyance and long term effects among persons exposed to low frequency noise in the home environment. Journal of Sound and Vibration 240: 483–97.

Persson Waye K, Bengtsson J, Rylander R, Hucklebridge F, Evans P, Clow A (2002) Low frequency noise enhances cortisol among noise sensitive subjects during work performance. Life Sciences 70: 745–58.

Pesonen K (2000) On noise assessment and noise control engineering problems caused by seasonal variations of noise emission and excess attenuation. In D Cassereau (ed.) Proceedings of Internoise 2000, Vol. 3. Nice: Société Française d'Acoustique, pp. 1787–92.

Porter ND, Flindell IH, Berry FB (1993) An acoustic feature model for the assessment of environmental noise. Acoustics Bulletin November/December: 40–8.

Porter ND, Flindell IH, Berry BF (1998) Health effect-based noise assessment methods: a review and feasibility study. NPL Report CMAM 16. Teddington: National Physical Laboratory.

Pruppers MJM, Janssen MPM, Ale BMJ, Pennders, RMJ, van den Hout KD, Miedema HME (1998) Accumulation of environmental risks to human health: geographical differences in the Netherlands. Journal of Hazardous Materials 61: 187–96.

Pulles T, Biesiot W, Stewart R (1990) Adverse effects of environmental noise on health: an interdisciplinary approach. In B Berglund, T Lindvall (eds) Noise as a Public Health Problem, Vol. 4. Stockholm: Swedish Council for Building Research Stockholm, pp. 337–48.

Quinet, Emile: The Social costs of Transport: Evaluation and hunk with internalisation Policies, Working Document No 1 of a joint OECD/CEMT Seminar. Internalising the Social Costs of Transport 30.09.01.10.1993, Paris 1993.

Quinet E (1997) Full Social Cost of Transportation in Europe: The full costs and benefits of transportation. Berlin: Springer, pp. 69–111, Table A1.

Quinet E (2001) The cost in calculating transport noise disturbances in public decision making. Comptes Rendus de l'Academie Des Sciences, Serie III, Sciences de la Vie 324: 829–37.

Rocha E (1997) A ladder of empowerment. Journal of Planning Education and Research 17: 31–44.

Sabadin A, Suncic S, Hrasovec B, Verhovnik V (1991) Verkehrslärm und unterbewusste Wahrnehmung des Wohnumfeldes. Wissenschaft und Umwelt 3–4: 153–7.

Sælensminde K (1999) Stated choice valuation of urban traffic air pollution and noise. Transportation Research, Part D 4: 13–27.

Sælensminde K (2000) Valuation of nonmarket goods for use in cost-benefit analyses: methodological issues. TØI report 491/2000. Oslo: Institute of Transport Economics.

Sandberg U (1994) Noise emissions of road vehicles – effect of regulations. Report of an I–INCE working party. Osaka: INCE/J, and ASJ Proceedings of Internoise 94, Vol. 1, pp 67–76.

Sandberg U (ed.) (1995) The effects of regulations on road vehicle noise. Report by the International Institute of Noise Control Engineering Working Party. Noise News International 6: 85–113.

Sandberg U (2001a) Tyre/Road noise – myths and realities. Proceedings of Internoise 2001, The Hague, pp. 35–51.

Sandberg U (2001b) Noise emissions of road vehicles effect of regulations. Final Report 01–1 I-INCE. Working Party on Noise Emissions of Road Vehicles (WP-NERV): International Institute of Noise Control Engineering.

Sandberg U, Ejsmont J (2002) Tyre/road Noise – Reference Book. Harg, Sweden: Informex.

Sato T, Yano T, Björkman M, Rylander R (1999) Comparison of community responses to road traffic noise among residents of different types of housing. In J Cuschieri, S Glegg, Y Yong (eds) Proceedings of Internoise. Fort Lauderdale, FL: INCE, pp. 1321–6.

Sato T, Yano T, Bjorkman M (2002) Comparison of community response to road traffic noise in Japan and Sweden – Part I: Outline of surveys and dose-response relationships. Journal of Sound and Vibration 250: 161–7.

Schomer PD (2000) Loudness level weighting for environmental noise assessment. Acustica 86(1): 49–61.

Schomer PD, Suzuki Y, Saito F (2001) Evaluation of loudness-level weightings for assessing the annoyance of environmental noise. Journal of Acoustical Society of America 110: 2390–7.

Schulte-Fortkamp B (2002) Soundscapes and living spaces. Sociological and psychological aspects concerning acoustic environments. In Forum Acusticum Sevilla 2002 on CD–ROM. Sociedad Espanola de Acustica.

Schultz TJ (1978) Synthesis of social surveys on noise annoyance. Journal of the Acoustical Society of America 64: 377–405.

Seligman MEP (1975) Helplessness: On depression development and death. San Francisco: Freeman.

Skånberg A, Öhrström E (2002) Adverse health effects in relation to urban residential soundscapes. Journal of Sound and Vibration 250: 151–5.

Soguel N (1996) Contingent valuation of traffic noise reduction benefits. Swiss Journal of Economics and Statistics 132: 109–23.

Sörensen S (1970) On the possibilities of changing the annoyance reaction to noise by changing the attitudes to the source of annoyance. Nord Hyg Tidsk Suppl 1: 1–76.

Stallen PJM (1999) A theoretical framework for environmental noise annoyance. Noise and Health 3: 69–79.

Stanners D, Bordeau P (eds) (1995) Europe's Environment, the Dobris Assessment. Noise and Radiation. Copenhagen: European Environment Agency, pp. 359–74.

Stansfeld SA (1992) Noise, noise sensitivity and psychiatric disorder: Epidemiological and psychological studies. Psychological Medicine Monograph. Supplement 22, Cambridge, Cambridge University Press.

Stansfeld SA, Haines MM, Burr M, Berry B, Lercher P (2000) A review of environmental noise and mental health. Noise and Health 8: 55–8.

Staples SL (1996) Human response to environmental noise. Psychological research and public policy. American Psychologist 51: 143–50.

Staples SL (1997) Public policy and environmental noise: modeling exposure or understanding effects. American Journal of Public Health 87: 2063–7.

Stokols D (1987) Conceptual strategies of environmental psychology. In D Stokols, I Altman (eds) Handbook of Environmental Psychology. New York: Wiley.

Susini P, McAdams S, Winsberg S (1999) Multidimensional technique for sound quality assessment. Acta Acustica (Stuttgart) 85: 650–6.

Suter AH (1991) Noise and its Effects. Prepared for the Administrative Conference of the United States: wwwnonoiseorg/library/suter/suterhtm.

Sutherland LC (2000) Overview of outdoor sound propagation. In D Cassereau (ed.) Proceedings of Internoise 2000, Vol. 2. Nice: Société Française d'Acoustique, pp. 915–20.

Suzuki H, Tamura A, Kashima N (1989) Effects of planting on annoyance at urban roadside. Journal of Acoustical Society of Japan 45: 374–84 (in Japanese).

Suzuki Y, Abe K, Ozawa K, Sone T (2000) Factors for perceiving sound environments and the effects of visual and verbal information on these factors. In: A Schick, M Meis, C Reckhardt (eds) Contributions to Psychological Acoustics. Oldenburg: BIS, pp. 209–32.

Syme (1991) Control and health: a personal perspective. Journal of Mind-Body Health 16–27.

Tamura A (1997) Effects of landscaping on the feeling of annoyance of a space. In A Schick, M Klatte (eds) Contributions to Psychological Acoustics. Oldenburg: BIS, pp. 135–61.

Tamura A, Suzuki H, Kashima N (1992) Annoyance relief by planting belts. Journal of Acoustical Society of Japan 48: 776–85 (in Japanese).

Taylor SE, Repetti RL (1997) Health psychology: what is an unhealthy environment and how does it get under the skin? Annual Review of Psychol 48: 411–47.

Taylor SM, Breston BA, Hall FL (1982) The effect of road traffic noise on house prices. Journal of Sound and Vibration 80: 523–41.

Taylor SM, Wilkins PA (1986) Community effects of noise. In PM Nelson (ed.) Transportation Noise. London: Butterworth, Chapter 4.

TOI (1991) Traffic and the Environment: Summary Report. Oslo: Transport Economics Institute.

Torigoe K (1999) A strategy for environmental conservation developed through the concept of soundscape in Japan. In H Karlsson (ed.) From Awareness to Action. Proceedings 'Stockholm Hey Listen' Conference on Acoustic Ecology. Stockholm: Royal Swedish Academy of Music, pp. 103–9.

Truax B (1999) Models and strategies for acoustic design. In: Karlsson H (ed.) (1999) From Awareness to Action. Proceedings 'Stockholm Hey Listen' Conference on Acoustic Ecology Stockholm: Royal Swedish Academy of Music, pp. 8–16.

Ulrich RS, Simons R, Losito BD, Fiorito E, Miles MA, Zelson M (1991) Stress recovery during exposure to natural and urban environments. Journal of Environmental Psychology 11: 201–30.

Van den Berg GP (1998) Sound exposure measurements in cases of low frequency noise complaints. In: The New Zealand Acoustical Society Inc (ed.) Inter Noise 98 (Paper # 0454) Conference Proceedings on CD-ROM Causal Productions.

Van den Berg M, Gerretsen E (1996) Comparison of road traffic noise calculation models. Journal of Building Acoustics 3: 13–22.

Van Herzele A, Wiedemann T (2002) A monitoring tool for the provision of accessible and attractive urban green spaces. Landscape and Urban Planning 46: 1–18.

Van Kamp I (1990) Coping with noise and its consequences, dissertation, Groningen: Styx and PP Publications.

Van Kempen E, Kruize H, Boshuizen HC, Ameling CB, Staatsen BAM, De Hollander A (2002) The association between noise exposure and blood pressure and ischemic heart disease: a meta-analysis. Environmental Health Perspectives 110: 307–17.

Van Poll R (1997) The perceived quality of the urban residential environment. A multiattribute evaluation. Center for Energy and Environmental Studies (IVEM). Groningen: University of Groningen.

Vanclay F (2002) Conceptualising social impacts. Environmental Impact Assessment Review 22: 183–211.

Verhoef E (1994) External Effects and Social Costs of Road Transport Transportation Research 28A 273–87.

Verhoef ET (1996) The Economics of Regulating Road Transport. Cheltenham: Edward Elgar.

Viollon S, Lavandier C, Drake C (2002) Influence of visual setting on sound ratings in an urban environment. Applied Acoustics 63: 493–511.

Wallston KA (2001) Conceptualization and operationalization of perceived control. In: A Baum, T Revenson, JE Singer (eds) Handbook of Health Psychology. Mahwah, NJ: Erlbaum, pp. 49–58.

Weinberger M, Thomassen G, Willecke R (1991) Kosten des Lärms in der Bundesrepublik Deutschland. Zeitschrift für Lärmbekämpfung 39: 91–9.

Whitelegg J (1993) Transport for a Sustainable Future: The Case for Europe. London: Belhaven Press.

Wohlwill JF (1979) What belongs where? Research on the fittingness of man–made structures in natural settings. Landscape Research 3: 305–23.

Wohlwill JF, Harris G (1980) Response to congruity or contrast for man-made structures in natural recreation settings. Leisure Science 3: 349–65.

World Health Organization (2000) Guidelines for Community Noise. Geneva: WHO: www.who.int/peh/noise/noiseindex.html.

Wright P, Grimwood C (1999) Strategic management of noise: a UK Perspective. In J Cuschieri, S Glegg, Y Yong (eds) Proceedings of Internoise 99, pp. 1171–6.

Wrightson K (2000) An introduction to acoustic ecology. Soundscape 1: 10–13.

Yano T, Sato T, Björkman M, Rylander R (2002) Comparison of community response to road traffic noise in Japan and Sweden – Part II: path analysis. Journal of Sound and Vibration 250: 169–74.

Zeichart K (1998) Kombinatorische Wirkungen von Bahnlärm und Bahnerschütterungen. Zeitschrift für Lärmbekämpfung 45: 7–16.

Zwicker E (1982) Psychoakustik. Berlin: Springer.

Zwicker E, Fastl H (1999) Psychoacoustics – Facts and Models, 2nd edn. Berlin: Springer.

# CHAPTER 17

# Estimating the risk of hearing impairment due to impulse noise exposure

*Noise and Its Effects:* Edited by Linda Luxon and Deepak Prasher © 2007
John Wiley & Sons Ltd.

GUIDO F SMOORENBURG

## Introduction

Whereas the risk of hearing impairment due to exposure to continuous
and intermittent noise can be estimated to a satisfactory degree, estimating the risk for impulse noise still poses problems, in particular for
high-level impulses.

For continuous noise it has been possible, for example in weaving mills,
to identify retrospectively exposure conditions that did not change over
many years, so that noise-induced permanent shifts in hearing threshold
(permanent threshold shift or PTS) could be related with confidence to past
noise exposure. For intermittent noise and noises that lasted only part of the
day it has been difficult to derive reliable dose–effect relations because, retrospectively, these irregular exposures could not be assessed with sufficient
accuracy. Therefore, in the 1950s and 1960s, many experiments were started
in which one tried to assess the potential auditory damage risk of intermittent and short-duration noises by exposing human subjects to these noises
and measuring the temporary threshold shift (TTS) occurring shortly after
the exposure. Whether or not the results from these experiments are indicative of the permanent threshold shifts to be expected after years of exposure
to these noises remained a matter of conjecture. It led to different exposure
assessment rules. In the USA the TTS results were incorporated in the
Walsh–Healy Act, indicating that each reduction of the daily exposure duration by a factor of two allows for an increase of the exposure level by 5 dB.
In contrast, the US Environmental Protection Agency adopted the rule,
included in ISO 1999 (ISO, 1990), which states that the allowable exposure
level should be increased by no more than 3 dB.

The equal energy principle essentially reflects the view that risk of hearing
damage is determined by the total sound energy of the noise exposure.

Passchier Vermeer (1973) showed that the conclusions from TTS experiments depend considerably on the time interval between termination of the exposure and the threshold measurement. As one increases this time interval the results grow closer to the ISO rule. However, since one should avoid permanent damage in these experiments, increase of the time interval while not increasing exposure level implies smaller threshold shifts and, thus, less accurate data. At present, the standard ISO 1999 has received wide acceptance although it has been recognized that this standard may be overprotective in assessing the risk of short-duration and intermittent noise, but also underprotective for certain impact noises, in particular reverberating environments. Therefore ISO 1999 suggests a safety margin of 5 dB (see also Suvorov et al., 2001).

With respect to impulse noise, ISO 1999 indicates that 'Some users may wish to consider tonal noise and/or impulsive/impact noise about as harmful as a steady non-tonal noise that is approximately 5 dB higher in level'.

Thus, to some extent, the standard leaves it up to the user to estimate the harmfulness of impact and impulse noises. The problem of assessing the exposure retrospectively with a sufficient degree of accuracy, mentioned above for intermittent and short-duration noises, is even greater for impulse noises.

**Many variables are involved in impulse noise:**

- peak level;
- duration, rise and fall times;
- reverberation, impulse energy;
- inter-impulse time interval, impulse rate;
- the level of continuous background noise.

Moreover, subjects may also have been exposed to other types of noises. Records of these exposures, over years, are not available. Retrospective assessment of these exposures in relation to acquired hearing loss is impossible in view of the many variables involved. Therefore, estimating the risk of hearing impairment due to impulse noise exposure has to be based mainly on acute experiments measuring TTS.

In this chapter we shall summarize the series of TTS experiments conducted up to about 1980. This summary will show that risk of hearing damage from exposure to short-duration impulses (up to 1 ms in duration, for example from light-calibre weapons and fire crackers) can be approximated by the equal-energy principle. However, the result of this summary overestimates the risk for exposure to long-duration impulses, such as from blasts and large-calibre weapons. Analysis of new data, based on TTS but focusing on full recovery from TTS within 24 hours, provides new guidelines for risk assessment of these long-duration impulses.

# Summary of TTS studies until 1980

The TTS studies published in the open literature and in progress reports concerned impulse noises from light-calibre weapons (in free-field and in reverberating environments), wood and metal impacts, sparks, clicking toys (crickets) and synthetic impulses presented via loudspeakers. The exposure parameters specified and the TTS criteria applied differed from one experiment to the next. In order to be able to compile all data we defined a common impulse exposure measure and a common TTS criterion such that the data could be transformed to this common basis with a minimum of extrapolation. For full details the reader is referred to Smoorenburg (1982).

### Definition of impulse duration

Nearly always, the impulses were characterized in terms of peak sound level and some measure of impulse duration. The definitions of impulse duration most frequently used were A and B duration (Coles et al., 1967) and C duration (Pfander et al., 1975, 1980) (Figure 17.1). A duration applies to near-ideal Friedlander waves; the waves that occur with explosions in non-reverberating environments. B duration accommodates the impulses in a reverberating environment, including reflections. A duration is defined as the time interval between impulse onset and baseline crossing of the down-going slope of the wave form. B duration is defined as the time interval between impulse onset

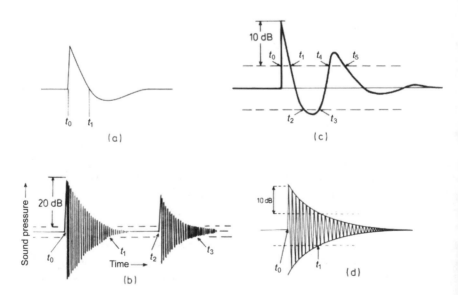

**Figure 17.1** (a–c) Three definitions of impulse duration from the literature and (d) the definition used in the present compilation of the data. Impulse duration is defined as the sum of the time intervals $t_1-t_0$, $t_3-t_2$, $t_5-t_4$, etc., if applicable. (From Smoorenburg, 1982.)

and the moment at which the down-going envelope of the waveform reaches a level 20 dB below peak level, including reflections. C duration is defined as the sum of all time intervals in the waveform microstructure, positive and negative, in which the absolute value of the instantaneous sound pressure exceeds a level 10 dB below the peak level. The common measure used in our compilation was coined the D duration, $\alpha_{-10}$. It is similar to the B duration, except for the $-10$ dB fall time. As mentioned before the introduction of the D duration was primarily based upon the need of a common denominator for impulse duration definitions used in the available studies, minimizing extrapolations.

However, the choice was also based on three additional considerations:

- In practice the ideal Friedlander wave will seldom occur; therefore a measure should be able to accommodate reverberating impulses.
- The definition of the C duration is physically less meaningful than that of the B duration.
- McRobert and Ward (1973) concluded that $-10$ dB fall time would be a better measure than $-20$ dB because reflections at 20 dB below peak level did not contribute to hearing loss.

Finally, in agreement with all studies, the number of impulses per exposure was incorporated in terms of a 'total duration' concept, the D duration of one impulse multiplied by the number of impulses.

### Definition of TTS criterion

Almost all investigators presented their data in terms of $TTS_2$, the temporary threshold shift measured 2 minutes after exposure. Thus, this measure was adopted in spite of its drawback quoted above (Passchier-Vermeer, 1973). The $TTS_2$ criterion was set at no more hearing loss than 15 dB, averaged across 1, 2 and 3 kHz. Compilation of the data required the application of this average measure, which would allow, in an extreme case, a loss of 45 dB at 3 kHz (and even higher above 3 kHz) if there was no loss at the other frequencies. The normative CHABA criterion (Committee on Hearing, Bioacoustics, and Biomechanics, 1968) set a limit of 30 dB to the losses at 3 kHz. Analysis of the data showed that, with the present 15 dB-average criterion, maximum TTS remained restricted to 30 dB. The percentage of cases in which hearing loss was allowed to exceed the 15 dB average, across 1, 2 and 3 kHz, varied in the respective studies from 25% to 5%. Statistical confidence of this compilation dictated that excess hearing loss could not be set lower than 10%.

### Angle of sound incidence

In free-field situations impulses that reach the ear with grazing incidence (from the front) are 2–6 dB less effective in inducing TTS than those that come from the side and, thus, face the ear (normal incidence). In this compilation all data have been transformed to normal incidence, applying an adjustment of –5 dB to the peak level if the original data concerned grazing incidence.

## Compilation of the data

The compilation is presented in Figure 17.2, plotting the peak level against total impulse duration at which 10% of the population exposed is expected to exceed the criterion $TTS_2$ of 15 dB on average, across 1, 2 and 3 kHz, with normal sound incidence. Table 17.1 shows essential aspects of the studies included. Figure 17.2 shows a near-linear relationship between peak level and total duration; linear regression yields a slope of –8 dB peak level per factor 10 increase of total duration. If one accepts that the data with total duration smaller than 0.01 s (indicated by L and E in Figure 17.2) may represent a critical maximum peak level of about 164 dB SPL then linear regression of the remaining data yields a slope of almost –10 dB per tenfold increase of total duration. This slope is in agreement with the equal energy principle. The regression line would represent $L_{eq}$ = 92 dB.

As the number of impulses increases, impulse noise gradually assumes the character of continuous noise. The duty cycle of the wood and metal impacts represented by C1 and W1 was about 10%. In order to examine

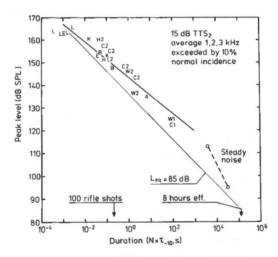

**Figure 17.2** Peak level in decibels and sound pressure level for a given total duration of N impulses multiplied by the duration of a single impulse, $\tau_{-10}$, at which the criterion of 15 dB temporary threshold shift (TTS), two minutes after exposure, averaged across the TTS at 1, 2 and 3 kHz, is exceeded by 10% of the population exposed. The peak level is given for normal incidence; the sound source facing the ear. The individual data are explained in Table 17.1. Results for steady noise, less than 8 hours in duration, are added to the figure, using the ordinate scale for effective level rather than peak level and adjusting duration such that a point in the figure represents a certain sound energy, irrespective of whether this point represents impulse or continuous noise. (From Smoorenburg, 1982).

**Table 17.1** Properties of the studies included in the compilation of Figure 17.2

| Symbol | Reference | Number of subjects | Sound source | Impulse duration (ms) | Number of impulses | Rate (impulses /s) |
|---|---|---|---|---|---|---|
| A | Acton and Forrest (1968) | 17 | Rifle | 70 | 100 | 0.06 |
| B | Bragg (1964) | 36 | Rifle | 2 | 25, 100 | – |
| C1 | Cohen et al. (1966) | 15 | Wood impact | 85 | 1170 | 1.3 |
| C2 | Rice & Coles (1965)* | 20 | Rifles | 2–4, 50 | 10–50 | 0.1–0.5 |
| E | Elwood et al. (1966) | 12, 110 | Rifle | 1, 2 | 1, 20 | – |
| H1 | Hodge et al. (1964)* | 12–16 | Rifle | 2 | 50 | 0.2–0.3 |
| H2 | Hodge and McCommons (1966)* | 28 | Rifle | 2 | 25, 50 | 0.2 |
| K | Kryter (1970) | 30, 9–16 | Rifle | 1 | 16, 100 | 0.2 |
| L | Loeb and Fletcher (1968) | 65–71 | Spark | 0.03–0.1 | 86–4 | 1 |
| W1 | Walker (1972) | 11 | Metal impact | 25 | 3, 840 | 3.2 |
| W2 | Ward et al. (1961) | 13 | Toy | 1.1 | 1, 800 | 1.25 |
| | | | Loudspeaker | 0.5 | 1, 800 | 1.25 |

*Also Coles et al. (1968).

how the results for impulse noises compare with those from short-duration continuous noise we have added some results from important TTS, short-duration experiments (Ward et al., 1959; Kylin, 1960). Since 1 s of total D duration at a certain peak level represents more sound energy than 1 s continuous noise at a certain effective decibel level the latter results have to be adjusted in order to be able to include them in Figure 17.2. This adjustment, based upon total sound energy, can be implemented in the duration dimension by multiplying duration by a factor of 4.6. As a result, 8 hours effectively becomes $1.3 \times 10^5$ rather than $8 \times 60 \times 60 = 2.9 \times 10^4$ s. Inclusion of the data for continuous noise shows that there is no discontinuity in the total set of data.

If one desires to apply a simple equal energy measure, irrespective of exact details of the noises, these data suggest that one can accept a maximum daily sound energy dose of $L_{eq} = 85$ dB.

This implies that one accepts overprotection, particularly in the total-duration range from 1 s to 100 s.

The above conclusion requires three comments:

1. One should be aware that with impulse noise TTS increases faster with an increase of sound level than with continuous noise (Smoorenburg, 1982). Thus, for example, when one has adopted an $L_{eq} = 90$ dB criterion for continuous noise, one should not apply the same criterion to impulse noise assuming the same risk of TTS. It will be higher for impulse noise. A similar warning concerns larger intersubject variability in susceptibility to impulse noise. When one considers the most

sensitive 5% (or less) of individuals in a population rather than the 10% used in this compilation, those 5% exposed to impulse noise may show more TTS than those exposed to continuous noise if TTS is comparable at the 10% bracket.

2. The above evaluation did not include frequency weighting whereas A weighting is applied when assessing continuous noise exposure. For most impulses included in this compilation A weighting implies a reduction of sound level by about 3 dB. However, in assessing exposure to continuous noise the angle of sound incidence does not play a role; random incidence is assumed. Assuming random incidence rather than normal incidence implies that the impulse exposure levels can be raised by about 3 dB. Thus, these minor corrections cancel out.

3. As stated before, the TTS data provide only an indication of auditory damage risk due to exposure to impulse noise. Application of these results should always be combined with a hearing conservation programme that includes regular audiometry.

# TTS from exposure to large-calibre weapons

The studies included in the previous section did not include large-calibre weapons. Once the results found for these weapons were compared with the conclusions drawn above it became rapidly apparent that the results from Figure 17.2 might well overestimate the risk of TTS from large-calibre weapons. The results, available up to about 1990, were collected and, as before, expressed in total duration, this being the product of the number of impulses and the D duration of a single impulse. TTS was compared with the damage risk criteria proposed by CHABA (1968), Pfander et al. (1975, 1980) and those derived above (Smoorenburg, 1982). The result is presented in Figure 17.3. A detailed description can be found in Smoorenburg (1992).

The maximum daily sound energy dose of $L_{eq}$ = 85 dB might overestimate the risk of hearing damage from large-calibre weapons.

### The different damage risk criteria

Figure 17.3 shows the CHABA criteria for 10 and 100 impulses (10 and 100 rounds in the figure since all data concerned weapon exposures), the Pfander criterion and the present criterion (Smoorenburg, 1992). The CHABA criterion, accepted in the UK and the USA, reflects the conclusion that the data can be described by a linear relation between peak level and total duration, the slope being about –8 dB (CHABA –7 dB) peak level per tenfold increase of total duration. Thus, CHABA stayed

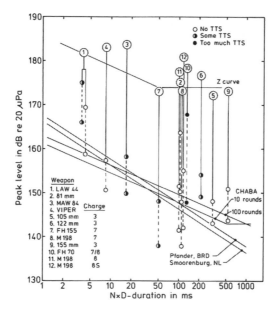

**Figure 17.3** Temporary threshold shift (TTS) produced by large-calibre weapons as a function of the peak level of the impulses and their total duration defined as the product of the number of impulses, $N$, and the D duration of a single impulse. TTS data are compared with the current damage risk criteria of CHABA (1968), Pfander et al. (1975, 1980) and Smoorenburg (1982). The Z curve represents the highest single exposure permitted, with hearing protection, in the USA. Too much TTS means that 5% of the subjects selected for highest TTS show more than 25 dB $TTS_2$ at any audiometric frequency; some TTS means more than 10 dB at any frequency. (From Smoorenburg, 1992.)

closer to the original data, not suggesting the equal energy simplification proposed above. Staying closer to the data also meant that separate curves were specified for different number of impulses. A tenfold increase in the number of impulses had to be compensated for by a 5-dB decrease in peak level. Pfander et al. proposed a criterion based on TTS experiments in which they focused on full recovery of TTS; 95% of the population exposed had to show no evidence of any change in their hearing ability 24 hours after exposure. They concluded that the damage risk criterion for impulse noise could simply be set at $L_{eq}$ = 90 dB. However, they took the C duration as the measure of duration without calculating the effective duration from their specific definition of impulse duration. A calculation based upon the assumption of an exponentially decaying impulse shows that the level specified by Pfander et al. has to be corrected by –3.6 dB, bringing their result down to $L_{eq}$ = 86.4 dB. This result is very close to the 85 dB derived in Figure 17.2 although the auditory damage risk criterion applied was considerably different.

## Comparison of TTS from large-calibre weapons to the current damage risk criteria

We have mentioned that A weighting of the sound energy distribution of short impulses would result in a small correction of about 3 dB. However, the impulses from large-calibre weapons are dominated by low-frequency energy. The effect of A weighting will be larger. In addition, all exposures to large-calibre weapons took place while the subjects wore hearing protection. The hearing protectors attenuate the low-frequency components of the sound less than the high-frequency components, which will increase the effect of A weighting. In this section we will compare experimental TTS with the current damage risk criteria, first without applying A weighting, then with A weighting.

The attenuation of the hearing protectors cannot be evaluated in terms of peak level and impulse duration. Therefore, we adopted the procedure used for continuous noise. Sound energy attenuation was calculated using the spectral energy distribution of the impulse and the frequency- dependent attenuation of the hearing protector, the latter as assessed for continuous noise. The resulting energy reduction was expressed as a corresponding reduction in peak level, keeping the impulse duration value measured without protection. The attenuation data used in this evaluation were experimenter-fit values, the values found when the hearing protector is placed under supervision of the experimenter. In practice, hearing protector placement might have been less well controlled, leading to less attenuation and, thus, higher effective exposures. In summary, it will be clear that the use of hearing protectors may have been a substantial source of error in the present evaluation.

In the present evaluation too much TTS means that only 5% of the subjects selected for highest TTS show more than 25 dB $TTS_2$ at one or more audiometric frequencies. Some TTS means 5% at more than 10 dB. This result is expected in a region 10–15 dB below the criterion levels shown in Figure 17.3.

The peak levels at the ear without protection are indicated by circles, including the weapon code. The Z curve indicates the free-field peak level of the highest single exposure, with hearing protection, permitted in the USA. Two data points are linked vertically to each circle with the weapon code. Each upper data point represents the unweighted exposure, including hearing protector attenuation. (The two pairs of data for weapon 1 represent attenuation while wearing glasses, left-hand pair, and without glasses, right-hand pair.) Figure 17.3 shows that there is only one upper data point with too much TTS (weapon 10), a data point well above the damage risk lines. Moreover, the upper data points representing some TTS are near or above the damage risk lines whereas they are expected at 10–15 dB below these lines. Thus, the experiments show much less TTS than expected.

The lower data point of each pair represents the exposures including A weighting of the impulse energy distribution under the hearing protector. These points are closer to the predictions although there still are a number of points near the damage risk lines with no TTS. This result suggests that including A weighting improves the estimation of TTS from large-calibre weapons but it also suggests that even this inclusion might not be sufficient. TTS may be less than predicted by all current damage risk criteria. Moreover, it may be less whereas some exposures may actually have been higher than calculated if hearing protection did not reach the experimenter-fit values assumed in this analysis.

### Improving TTS estimation applying alternative frequency-weighting schemes

Frequency weighting such that the low-frequency components of the impulse sounds contribute less to the exposure measure improve the risk estimate for impulses from large-calibre weapons.

The spectral energy distribution of Friedlander waves, generated by explosions in free-field, has two characteristic properties, illustrated in Figure 17.4: (1) the overall level of the high-frequency slope is uniquely determined by the peak level and (2) increasing impulse duration implies addition of low-frequency energy only (without affecting the overall level of the high-frequency slope). As A-weighting improves the relationship

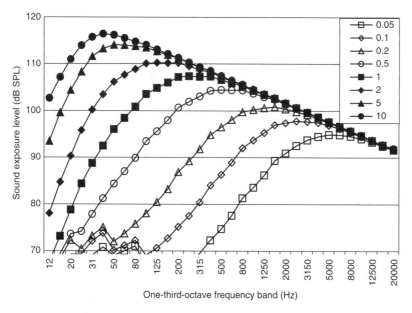

**Figure 17.4** Spectral energy distribution, expressed in sound exposure level being the effective sound pressure level of a 1 s sound burst with the same energy, of an ideal Friedlander wave with a peak level of 154 dB and A durations of 0.05–10 ms.

between TTS and sound exposure when short- and long-duration impulses are considered together, but does not yet provide full compliance, these results suggest that alternative frequency-weighting schemes, putting more emphasis on the high-frequency components, might yield better predictions.

Here we propose two alternative frequency weightings: (1) a weighting function corresponding to the threshold of hearing (T-weighting) and (2) a function representing the levels of bands of noise with limited bandwidth at which the same TTS is produced when the noise bands are presented with short durations (EqTTS-weighting). The first weighting is based on the consideration that the threshold-of-hearing curve closely matches the mechanical stimulus acting upon the receptor organ, the location where damage occurs. The curve is taken from the classic result of Sivian and White (1933). The choice of EqTTS-weighting seems trivial. However, it includes the assumption that TTS results found for short sound bursts presented non-simultaneously per frequency band are indicative of the simultaneous contributions from the spectral energy distribution of much shorter impulses. For the latter approach we adopted a result from Plomp et al. (1963), pertaining to 3-minute exposures. Figure 17.5 shows the two weighting functions in relation to A weighting. In agreement with the standardized weighting functions (such as A weighting) we fixed the attenuation of the new weighting functions at 0 dB for 1000 Hz. The effect of these functions on weighted sound energy is illustrated in Figure 17.6, using the Friedlander wave as a basic wave form in

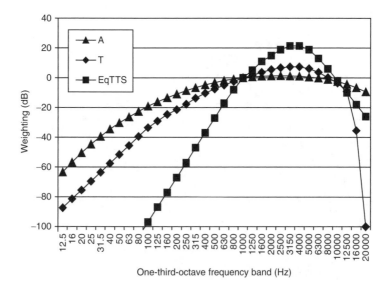

**Figure 17.5** Comparison of the three weighting contours used in the present analysis. A-weighting, T weighting corresponding to the threshold contour for random incidence sound in free-field (from Sivian and White, 1933) and EqTTS weighting corresponding to the level of noise bands producing about 5-dB TTS (from Plomp et al., 1963). The weighting has been fixed at 0 dB for 1000 Hz.

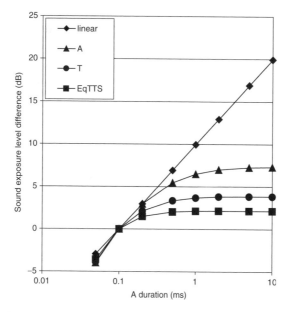

**Figure 17.6** Effective sound exposure level of Friedlander waves after applying frequency-dependent weighting as a function of impulse A duration. Linear: sound exposure level without weighting (the effective level increases proportionately with A duration), (A) the effect of A weighting, (T) effect of weighting corresponding to the threshold of hearing, (EqTTS) effect of weighting corresponding to bands of noise producing equal TTS. All sound exposure levels are presented relative to the level at A duration = 0.1 ms.

this calculation. Figure 17.6 shows that the effect of increasing impulse duration on impulse sound energy is reduced considerably by T weighting. Moreover, EqTTS-weighting implies that the weighted sound energy of a rifle (a fraction of a millisecond in the Friedlander, free-field condition) is about the same as the weighted sound energy of an impulse from a large-calibre weapon with a duration of 5 ms. Thus, these weightings might well be better candidates for damage risk criteria that should predict TTS equally well for short- and long-duration impulses. However, in terms of physical records of the exposures and detailed TTS measurements, the data used above are insufficient to allow for a systematic evaluation of the merits of these alternative weighting functions. Therefore, we will use new data collected within the so-called Blast Overpressure Project (BOP).

# Evaluation of the Blast Overpressure Project

In response to the lack of data on the effects of impulse noise and the urgent need to arrive at better auditory damage risk criteria it was decided, within a NATO research study group, chaired by the present author, that new TTS experiments had to be initiated.

The largest study was the BOP conducted at Kirtland Airforce Base, Albuquerque, New Mexico, USA under contract DAMD-17-88-C-8141 with EG&G Managements Systems, Albuquerque. The first preparatory report appeared in 1986 (Phillips et al., 1986). It was followed by a number of publications (Johnson, 1990, 1994, 1998; Johnson et al., 1990; Patterson et al., 1997; Chan et al., 1999, 2001). Here we present a recent analysis. A detailed description of this analysis can be found in Smoorenburg (2002).

## Impulse exposures

The blasts produced impulse sounds with peak levels depending on charge level and distance:

- At 1 m from 178.1 to about 196 dB SPL for charge levels from 1 to 7.
- At 3 m from 177.9 to 193.2 dB SPL for charge levels from 2 to 7.
- At 5 m from 172.9 to 189.4 dB for charge levels from 1 to 7.

The difference in peak level between two successive charge levels and two successive distances was about 3 dB. The number of impulses per exposure were 6, 12, 25, 50 and 100, in terms of energy also a 3-dB difference. The impulses were presented at a rate of about one per minute. Impulse duration varied between 0.9 and 3.0 ms. Subjects were exposed to conditions with increasing level and number until a certain $TTS_2$ criterion was reached. The right ear was always directed toward the sound source (normal incidence). It was covered by a standard US Army RACAL earmuff, which was placed under a standard infantry helmet. The left ear was also protected by the RACAL muff, but additionally by a foam earplug. The first series of experiments were conducted at the distance of 5 m. After this first series there was no TTS. Therefore, the muff of the right ear was modified by inserting eight plastic tubes (2.3 mm inside diameter) through the ear seal to produce a leak simulating a badly fitting muff. All subsequent series, at distances of 5, 3 and 1 m, were conducted with this modified muff. Waveforms were measured for at most three subjects per condition, at both the right and left ears, under the muffs near the ear canal, using miniature pressure transducers (low-pass cut-off frequency at 40 kHz). In addition, the free-field waveforms were measured at two locations representative of the locations of the right ears. The waveforms were sampled at a rate of 125 kHz. Each waveform consisted of $2^{15}$ samples (BOP, 1997).

## TTS criterion

All experiments were conducted with human volunteers. The results were primarily based on TTS measurements and secondarily on tinnitus complaints, and discomfort reported spontaneously. At any time volunteers were allowed to withdraw from the experiments. The TTS criterion was based on the target that there should be complete recovery within 24 hours. From the studies by Pfander et al. (1980) we concluded that this can be translated into $TTS_2 \leq 25$ dB (RSG.6, 1987). Subjects were exposed to conditions with increasing level and number until the target $TTS_2$ of 25 dB was reached. More specifically, as $TTS_2$ in excess of 25 dB had to be avoided, $TTS_2 > 15$ dB was considered to be a conditional failure in the sense that a one-step increase in exposure level or number was expected to produce $TTS_2 > 25$ dB. Thus, whenever $TTS_2 < 15$ dB the next step was considered to be a failure and it was not measured.

The study aimed at 95% protected with respect to the above $TTS_2$ criterion with 95% statistical confidence. This target implied 59 volunteers per condition; the actual number was 59–68.

## Optimal weighting of the spectral energy distribution

The results of the BOP experiments were analysed in terms of the percentage of the population exposed with $TTS_2 > 25$ dB versus the sound exposure level of the impulses subjected to the frequency-dependent weighting functions: A-weighting, T-weighting, EqTTS-weighting and, as a reference, linear (no) weighting. The percentage excess TTS was assumed to grow exponentially with sound exposure level.

In addition to the weighting function we included one more degree of freedom; the number factor. Rather than accepting the total duration measure we assumed that the effect of changing the number of impulses is unknown. The number of impulses, $N$, was included into the sound exposure level (SEL) by adding a term $\alpha^{10}\log(N)$ to the decibel value; $\alpha = 10$ corresponds to the total duration measure (and the equal energy principle), $\alpha = 5$ to the 5-dB adjustment included in the CHABA criterion. All combinations of frequency-dependent weighting and values of $\alpha$ from 0 to14 were tried.

Figure 17.7 presents the result. It gives the percentage of variance in the number of subjects with $TTS_2$ in excess of 25 dB explained using the four frequency-dependent weighting functions and the different number factors, assuming exponential growth of the number of subjects with excess TTS. The best prediction is found for T weighting and $\alpha = 5$. EqTTS weighting performs about equally well as T weighting if $\alpha = 7$ or greater. A weighting performs considerably worse, best at $\alpha = 3$. Linear weighting should not be considered. These results confirm the inference presented above: the high-frequency components of impulse noise are more important in predicting TTS than the generally accepted A weighting function would suggest. In addition, they suggest that the number of impulses is less important than implied in the total duration measure.

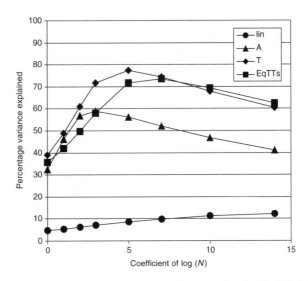

**Figure 17.7** Variance in percentage excess temporary threshold shift (TTS) explained by predicting TTS from sound exposure levels weighted as indicated in the legend and taking the number of impulses, $N$, into account by increasing the sound exposure level with the coefficient indicated on the abscissa multiplied by $\alpha^{10}\log(N)$. A coefficient of 10 corresponds to the equal energy principle.

## Exposure limits

When we focus on the sound exposure level at which we find 5% excess $TTS_2$, rather than the number of subjects in excess of the $TTS_2 < 25$ dB criterion, the number factor becomes even smaller. The results suggest that we may accept one critical sound exposure level for impulse numbers up to 100. The critical level would be 131 dB T-weighted SEL or 135 dB A-weighted SEL for the single impulse, irrespective of the number of impulses up to 100. (This value, and those to follow, concern the exposure level at the ear itself, under the hearing protector.) If one wishes to apply a total-energy-in-the-exposure measure then the energy limit would increase with the number of impulses given one critical level for the single impulse. Thus, proposing one total energy measure for all impulse numbers implies adoption of the energy found for the smallest number of impulses ($N = 6$ in this study), accepting overprotection for higher numbers (up to 100 in this study). With this approach the 8-hour energy equivalent becomes 96 dB, T-weighted, or 98 dB, A-weighted. These values are markedly higher than the value of 85 dB unweighted, proposed above when analysing the short-duration impulses. The difference is even greater than these numbers suggest because one has to take into account that the present TTS criterion is more stringent than the one proposed above and one has to apply a small adjustment of about –3 dB to that criterion in order to include A-weighting. (In both cases the angle of sound incidence was normal.)

# Optimized weighting of the spectral energy distribution function

Optimized weighting of the spectral energy distribution function does not provide a single impulse exposure measure suitable for estimating TTS from all types of impulses.

## Comparison of the results for short-duration impulses without hearing protection with those for long-duration, high-level impulses with hearing protection

Part of the data included in the second main section of this chapter concerning exposure to short-duration impulses without using hearing protection could be used for reanalysis, applying the TTS criterion used in the BOP project and A and T weighting. Again, this analysis suggests that there is a critical sound exposure level, irrespective of the number of impulses, this time for numbers up to 50. The critical SEL for the single impulse is 118 dB, T weighted, and 116 dB, A weighted. These values are much lower than those found in the previous section for long-duration, high-level impulses with hearing protection, which were 131 and 135 dB, respectively. Moreover, the equivalent 8-hour continuous-noise levels are quite different: 82 and 80 dB, T and A weighted respectively, compared with 96 and 98 dB for the long-duration impulses. Thus, A and T weighting (and also EqTTS weighting) do not provide an impulse exposure measure suitable for estimating TTS from all types of impulses. Yet, the present data suggest that the $L_{eq} = 80$ dB (A) limit, applied widely for continuous and intermittent noises, can be applied too when dealing with short-duration impulses reaching the unprotected ear.

## Low-frequency energy, contained in long-duration impulses, may reduce auditory damage risk from these impulses

The large difference between the findings for short- and long-duration impulses might be related to non-linear effects in sound conduction by the ear. Dancer et al. (1985) showed, in a well-controlled animal experiment, that increasing the A duration of Friedlander-type impulses, keeping the peak level constant at about 1.5 kPa (about 157.5 dB), produced systematically decreasing hearing loss, measured electro-physiologically one week after the exposure. As the energy will always increase with increasing impulse duration, whatever frequency-dependent weighting is applied, these results suggest that we have to assume non-linear interactions between the frequency components contained in the impulse.

Price and Kalb (1991) proposed a very promising method of evaluating damage risk for impulse noises assuming non-linear, compressive sound conduction in the ear. With such a compressive non-linearity, strong low-frequency components will suppress weaker high-frequency components.

Assuming that auditory damage risk is determined mainly by the high-frequency components of the impulse Price and Kalb showed how increase of low-frequency energy may reduce auditory damage risk. We have applied their model to the BOP data, using version 11-10-2000 supplied by DL Johnson, chairman of the S3-72 ANSI impulse noise working group (Smoorenburg, 2002). Although promising, the model has not yet produced the correct results. It appeared to be too compressive. The model requires further development. The number factor should be included in this further development. At present, the effect of impulse number is too large.

## Conclusions

Temporary threshold shift experiments suggest that risk of auditory hearing impairment due to impulse noise exposure can be estimated best by applying frequency-dependent weighting functions that emphasize the contribution from the high-frequency components in the spectral energy distribution. However, there is no single frequency-weighted sound exposure level that allows estimation of auditory damage risk for all types of impulses. For short-duration impulses, reaching the unprotected ear, the TTS data suggest that one may adopt the exposure limit of $L_{eq} = 80$ dB (A) (8-hour equivalent), using widely accepted A weighting. For long-duration, high-level impulses, reaching the protected ear, exposure of the ear itself (exposure level under the protector) can be higher. However, for these impulses adequate estimation of auditory damage risk requires further development of non-linear exposure assessment methods. The present results for these impulses pertain to the specific exposures included in this evaluation. Generalization of the present results to other sound sources should be conducted with extreme caution. It should always be accompanied by the installation of hearing conservation programmes including follow-up audiometry.

## References

Acton WI, Forrest MR (1968) Hearing hazard from small-bore weapons. Journal of Acoustical Society of America 44: 817–18.

BOP (1997) Blast Overpressure Measured under Earmuffs, Pressure-time Signatures and ACCESS Data Base. Review copy 4 of 6, 10 March 1997. Fort Rocker: US Army Aeromedical Research Laboratory. CDROM.

Bragg TS (1964) In Criteria for Assessing Hearing Damage Risk from Impulse-Noise Exposure, Technical Memorandum 13–67. Aberdeen Proving Ground: US Army Human Engineering Laboratories.

Chan P, Ho KH, Kan KK, Stuhmiller JH (1999) Evaluation of Impulse Noise Criteria using Human Volunteer Data. Jaycor Technical Report J299729-99–104. San Diego, CA: Jaycor.

Chan P, Ho KH, Kan KK, Stuhmiller JH, Mayorga MA (2001) Evaluation of impulse noise criteria using human volunteer data. Journal of Acoustical Society of America 110: 1967–75.

Cohen A, Kylin B, LaBenz PJ (1966) Temporary threshold shifts in hearing from exposure to combined impact/steady–state noise conditions. Journal Acoustical Society of America 40: 1371–80.

Coles RRA, Garinther GR, Hodge, DC, Rice CG (1967) Criteria for Assessing Hearing Damage Risk from Impulse-noise Exposure. Technical Memorandum 13–67. Aberdeen Proving Ground: Human Engineering Laboratories.

Coles RRA, Garinther GR, Hodge DC, Rice CG (1968) Hazardous exposure to impulse noise. Journal of Acoustical Society of America 43: 336–43.

Committee of Hearing, Bioacoustics and Biomechanics (1968) Proposed damage-risk criterion for impulse noise (gunfire). In W Dixon Ward (ed.) Report of the National Academy of Sciences – National Research Council, Committee on Hearing, Bioacoustics, and Biomechanics, Working Group 57. Washington, DC: CHABA.

Dancer A, Vassout P, Lenoir M (1985) Influence du niveau de crête et de la durée d'ondes de choc (bruits d'armes) sur l'audition du cobaye. Acustica 59: 21–9.

Elwood MA, Brasher PF, Croton LM (1966) A Preliminary Study of Sensitivity to Impulse Noise in Terms of Temporary Threshold Shifts. From: Criteria for Assessing Hearing Damage Risk from Impulse-Noise Exposure. Technical Memorandum 13–67. Aberdeen Proving Ground: US Army Human Engineering Laboratories.

Hodge DC, McCommons RB (1966) Reliability of TTS from impulse–noise exposure. Journal of Acoustical Society of America 40: 839–46.

Hodge DC, Gates HW, Helm CP, Soderholm RB, Blackmer RF (1964) Preliminary Studies of the Impulse-noise Effects on Human Hearing. Technical Memorandum 15–64. Aberdeen Proving Ground: US Army Human Engineering Laboratories.

International Organization for Standardization (1990) ISO 1999: Acoustics – Determination of occupational noise exposure and estimation of noise–induced hearing impairment. 2nd edition. Geneva: International Organisation for Standardisation.

Johnson DL (1990) Direct Determination of Occupational Exposure Limits for Freefield Impulse Noise. EG&G Report. Volumes I, II, and III.

Johnson DL (1994) Blast Overpressure Studies with Animals and Men: A Walk-up Study. USAARL Report No. 94-2. Fort Rucker: US Army Aeromedical Research Laboratory.

Johnson DL (1998) Blast Overpressure Studies. USAARL Contract Report No. CR–98–03. Fort Rucker: US Army Aeromedical Research Laboratory.

Johnson DL, Patterson JD, Nelson WR, Ripple G, Mundie TG, Christensen WI et al. (1990) Direct determination of occupational exposure limits for freefield impulse noise. Vol III of three appendices. Protocol for Study. Fort Detrick, Md.US Army Medical Research and Development Command.

Kryter KD (1970) The Effects of Noise on Man. New York: Academic Press.

Kylin B (1960) Temporary threshold shift and auditory trauma following exposures to steady-state noise. An experimental and field study. Acta Oto-Laryngol. Suppl. 152, 1–93.

Loeb M, Fletcher JL (1968) Impulse duration and temporary threshold shift. Journal of Acoustical Society of America 44: 1524–8.

McRobert and Ward, WD (1973) Damage - risk criteria: the trading relation between intensity and the number of nonreverberant impulses. Journal of the Acoustical Society of America 53: 1297–1300.

Passchier-Vermeer W (1973) Noise-induced hearing loss from exposure to intermittent and varying noise. Proc. Int. Congress on Noise as a Public Health Problem. Washington DC. US Environmental Protection Agency 169–200.

Patterson JH, Mozo BT, Gordon E, Canales JR, Johnson DL (1997) Pressure Measured under Earmuffs Worn by Human Volunteers during Exposure to Freefield Blast Overpressures. Report No. 98-01. Fort Rucker: US Army Aeromedical Research Laboratory.

Pfander F, in collaboration with Bongartz H, Brinkmann H (1975) Das Knalltrauma. Berlin: Springer Verlag.

Pfander F, Bongartz H, Brinkmann H, Kietz H (1980) Danger of auditory impairment from impulse noise: a comparative study of the CHABA damage-risk criteria and those of the Federal Republic of Germany. Journal of Acoustical Society of America 67: 628–33.

Phillips YY, Patterson J, Holland M, Steger J (1986) Direct Determination of Exposure Limits for Intense Freefield Impulse Noise. Fort Detrick, Md. US Army Medical Research and Development Command.

Plomp R, Gravendeel DW, Mimpen AM (1963) Relation of hearing loss to noise spectrum. J Acoust Soc Am 35: 1234–40.

Price R, Kalb, JT (1991) Insights into hazard from intense impulses from a mathematical model of the ear. J Acoust Soc Am 90: 219–27.

Rice CG, Coles RRA (1965) Impulsive noise studies and temporary threshold shift. In Proceedings of the Fifth International Congress Acoustics, paper B67, Liège, Belgium.

RSG.6 (1987) Effects of Impulse Noise. Report of NATO AC/243(Panel 8/ Research Study Group.6) D/9. G.F. Smoorenburg (Ed.) TNO-TM. Soesterberg, Netherlands.

Sivian LJ, White SD (1933) On minimum audible sound fields. Journal of Acoustical Society of America 4: 288–321.

Smoorenburg GF (1982) Damage risk criteria for impulse noise. In RP Hamernik, DH Henderson, R Salvi (eds) New Perspectives on Noise–Induced Hearing Loss. New York: Raven Press, pp. 471–90.

Smoorenburg GF (1992) Damage risk for low-frequency impulse noise: the spectral factor in noise-induced hearing loss. In AL Dancer, D Henderson, RJ Salvi, RP Hamernik (eds) Noise-Induced Hearing Loss. St Louis, MO: Mosby, pp. 313–24.

Smoorenburg GF (2002) Risk of hearing loss from exposure to impulse sounds. In: Reconsideration of the Effect of Impulse Noise. Report TM–02–I012. Soesterberg: TNO Human Factors. Also in: Reconsideration of the Effects of Impulse Noise, NATO RTO- TR-017 (HFM-022), ISBN 92-837-1105-X. Soesterberg, Netherlands.

Suvorov G, Denisov E, Antipin V, Kharitonov V, Starck J, Pyykko I et al. (2001) Effects of peak levels and number of impulses to hearing among forge hammering workers. Applied Occupational and Environmental Hygiene 16: 816–22.

Walker JG (1972) Temporary threshold shift caused by combined steady–state and impulse noises. Journal of Sound and Vibration 24: 493–504.

Ward WD, Glong A, Sklar DL (1959) Temporary threshold shift from Octave-band noise: applications to damage risk criteria. J. Acoust. Soc. Amer 31:522–528.

Ward WD, Selters W, Glorig A (1961) Exploratory studies on temporary threshold shift from impulses. Journal of Acoustical Society of America 33: 781–93.

# CHAPTER 18

# Occupational noise

*Noise and Its Effects:* Edited by Linda Luxon and Deepak Prasher © 2007
John Wiley & Sons Ltd.

WIESLAW J SULKOWSKI

## Introduction

Although the detrimental influence of work-related noise on health has
been known for centuries, it still remains a largely unsolved problem even
in highly mechanized and industrialized countries.

Noise-induced hearing loss (NIHL), a major byproduct of noisy machinery and/or technological processes in industrial settings, is considered as
one of the most common occupational health hazards, which carries not
only an enormous cost in workers' compensation and pensions but also
an even greater social cost due to loss of productivity and damage to quality of life.

Noise-induced hearing loss is the only indisputable permanent effect
of occupational noise; however, experimental research and epidemiological studies have shown that noise exposure may induce a
non-specific stress reaction, involving disturbances in communication,
task performance and sleep, as well as cardiovascular, biochemical, psychological and other changes (Passchier-Vermeer, 1994; Sulkowski,
1995), summarized in Table 18.1.

The impact of work-related noise on human health is manifold but due
to its largely slow and insidious nature the majority of people remain
unaware of the hazards of noise. The indisputable permanent effect of
occupational exposure is noise-induced hearing loss and there is a growing recognition of the threat to auditory function from high levels of
noise in work environments; they may also produce a non-specific stress
reaction, annoyance, disturbances in communication, task performance
and sleep, as well as to contribute in development of hypertension, psychiatric diseases, congenital defects, hormonal and immune disorders.

**Table 18.1** Possible long-term effects of exposure to occupational noise and the level below which no effects will be observable in an average population (Passchier-Vermeer, 1994)

| Effect | Effect observed[a] | No effect below | |
|---|---|---|---|
| | | *Unit* | *Value[b]* |
| Hearing loss | + | $L_{Aeq,8h}$ | 75 |
| Hypertension | + | $L_{Aeq,8h}$ | 80–85 |
| Ischaemic heart disease | + | $L_{Aeq,06-22h}$ | 65–70 |
| Hormonal effects | + | No data | ? |
| Immune effects | (+) | No data | ? |
| Birthweight | –? | No data | ? |
| Congenital effects | –? | No data | ? |
| Psychiatric disorders | + | No data | ? |
| Annoyance | + | $L_{Aeq,8h}$ | < 55 |
| Absentee rate | +? | $L_{Aeq,8h}$ | > 85? |
| Safety | +? | $L_{Aeq,8h}$ | > 85 |

[a]+, effect observed; –, no effect; +?, possibly an effect; –?, possibly no effect; (+), effect was observed in the laboratory only.
[b]?,unknown whether effect occurs.

With respect to hypertension, the question has arisen as to whether workers with severe high-frequency hearing loss are more sensitive to the acquisition of a noise-induced increase in blood pressure or hypertension than colleagues without or with only some high-frequency hearing loss. The question should be answered in the affirmative. The relative risk of hypertension for workers with high-frequency hearing loss is 1.6 compared with that of their colleagues; the mean systolic and diastolic blood pressure was 2.6 mmHg and 1.8 mmHg higher respectively (Passchier-Vermeer, 1994).

There is a growing recognition of the threat to auditory function from high levels of noise in occupational environments; according to the most recent estimations, more than 10 million US citizens are exposed in their jobs to noise of > 85 dB (A), and in Europe the number of employees put at risk of developing a significant NIHL is assessed as about 35 million. In the UK there are about 8 million people with bilateral hearing impairment of at least 25 dB HL, and noise exposure has a contribution to the prevalence (Davis, 1995, 1997).

The economic loss to society of this impairment has been estimated to range from 0.2% to 2% of gross domestic product in Europe, which at the lower figure of 0.2% equates to 12 billion euros.

The most reliable epidemiological data seem to be derived from the central state register of occupational diseases established in 1975 in Poland. The latest report of this unique register indicates that more than 650 000 workers (of a total 5 million employed in industry) are exposed to noise levels of 85 dB (A) or higher (Sulkowski, 2002; Sulkowski et al., 2004). The highest incidence of NIHL in the years 1999–2002 was found

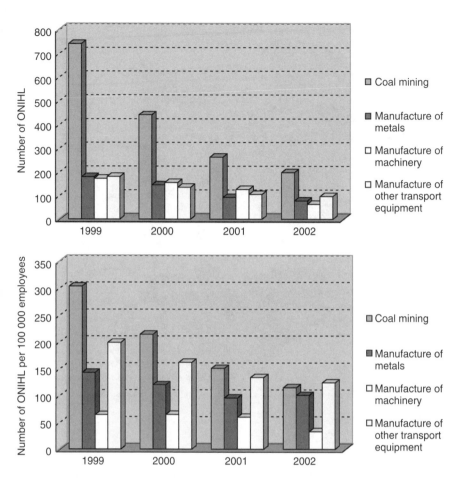

**Figure 18.1** Occupational noise-induced hearing loss in selected industrial branches in Poland according to the Statistical Classification of Economic Activities in the European Community.

in Polish coal mining (Figure 18.1); one may say that it differs little from the earliest extant reference which appears to be an observation recorded by Paracelsus in 1567 on hearing damage in miners (Sulkowski, 1980).

Other key industrial processes with a significant number of NIHL sufferers were – as shown in Figure 18.1 – iron and steel industries, as well as transport equipment production.

The majority of cases were recognized – as shown in Figure 18.2 – in the southern and western provinces of the country, mainly in the Silesian district, known for the high concentration of noisy enterprises. The most affected were workers aged 50–59 years (Figure 18.3) and exposed to noise over 20 years (Figure 18.4). This confirms that NIHL is an insidious, slow process of hearing deterioration that develops over a period of approximately 10–20 years, traditionally known as chronic acoustic trauma.

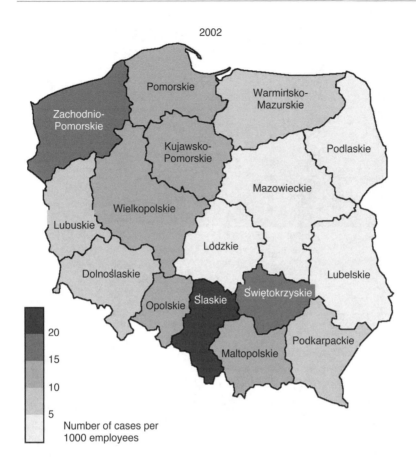

**Figure 18.2** Geographical distribution of occupational noise-induced hearing loss in Poland in 2002.

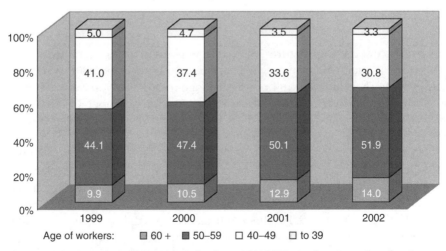

**Figure 18.3** Occupational NIHL in Poland in 1992–2002 as a function of workers' age.

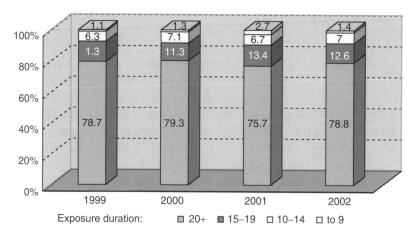

**Figure 18.4** Occupational NIHL in Poland in 1999–2002 as a function of exposures duration.

The only optimistic finding of the above data is a decreasing trend in the incidence of NIHL from 36 new cases in the years 1992–1998 annually per 100 000 employees to 20 cases per year since 1999 (Figure 18.5). One may presume that this results from the introduction in 1999 of the national programme of hearing conservation in industry, based on obligatory pre-employment and follow-up audiometric examinations, as well as the implementation of recommended noise regulations.

Undoubtedly, the adoption of noise standards is an important international step in averting NIHL in the workplace. However, in the light of some current research, there are many shortcomings and gaps. For instance,

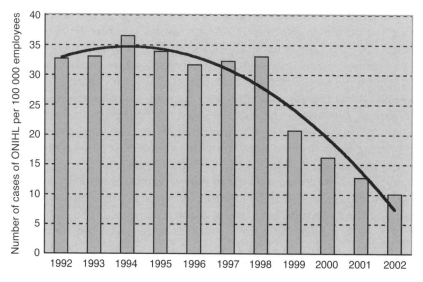

**Figure 18.5** Incidence of occupational noise-induced hearing loss in Poland in 1992–2002 with a line of trend.

none of the existing legislation, which concentrates on the legal thresholds for noise exposure (the most widespread is 85 dB (A) in the workplace), considers mixed exposures, which are very common in occupational environments, or exposure with a contribution of hand–arm or whole-body vibrations (Kowalska and Sulkowski, 1989; Pyykkö et al., 2003), toxic agents (Prasher et al., 2002) or temperature fluctuations (Parsons, 2003), which may interact to increase or modify the likelihood of adverse health effects. Another weakness of the noise standards is the general assumption that all noise exposures impair the inner ear in the same way and, therefore, can be evaluated by means of a common simple metric, namely the equal energy hypothesis or some variant thereof. Impulse noise in particular falls into this category as it cannot be covered by standards mainly designed for continuous noise exposures (Sulkowski, 1986; Kryter, 1994). Also individual differences in susceptibility to NIHL should not be ignored.

Thus, a reasonable objective for future planning is a new approach to identifying susceptible individuals, as well as an improvement in safety limits for noise exposures. This work should be based on animal models (although the question of extrapolation of such results to humans complicates the picture) and on longitudinal cross-sectional human data, which provide a better understanding of the relationship between temporary and permanent auditory threshold shift following noise exposure, and histopathological alterations in the ear.

# Types of hearing loss caused by noise

There are two main forms of hearing loss due to noise, traditionally termed acoustic trauma.

*Acute* acoustic trauma refers to a sudden hearing loss, which is the result of a short single exposure to a high sound pressure level usually exceeding the ear's pain threshold (for example, quarrymen too close to a blast or armed forces personnel near an explosion). Such cases are treated on medicolegal grounds as compensable accidents at work (Sulkowski, 1971) but clinically they may present as unilateral, more seldom binaural, rupture of the eardrum and/or damage of the ossicular chain with a conductive type of hearing loss, as well as sensorineural or mixed hearing impairment due to stretching of the elastic inner ear compartments beyond their limits by the impact of noise.

In contrast to this mechanical type of injury, *chronic* acoustic trauma is a product of metabolic cochlear damage through overstimulation of the inner ear resulting from repeated long-lasting multiannual exposure to moderate noise levels. It is manifest as a slow, gradually progressive and cumulative sensorineural hypoacusis, and the extent to which it develops depends on both the intensity and duration of noise exposure, as well as differences in individual susceptibility. In contemporary publications the term 'chronic acoustic trauma' has been replaced by 'noise-induced hearing loss' (NIHL) or 'noise-induced permanent threshold shift' (NIPTS). Such work-related

NIHL is treated in the legislation of many countries as a compensable prescribed occupational disease (Sulkowski, 1980; Dobie, 1993).

Hearing loss due to noise may have a form of the acute acoustic trauma i.e. sudden hearing loss caused by short single exposure to a high sound pressure level or – more common – the chronic acoustic trauma i.e. noise-induced hearing loss (NIHL) gradually progressive due to repeated long-lasting multiannual exposure.

NIHL is preceded by, and may be accompanied by a reversible temporary threshold shift (TTS). Application of rules relating the growth and recovery of TTS to the magnitude of the NIPTS is however equivocal.

Noise-induced hearing loss – the noise-induced permanent threshold shift (NIPTS) – is defined as the change of the hearing level in relation to a previously measured level (usually before starting the exposure) or, in the absence of such data concerning this hearing level, in relation to audiometric zero minus presbysocioacusis (auditory threshold changes caused by ageing and effects of non-occupational 'micronoise' traumas of everyday life) and nosoacusis (auditory threshold changes due to other external factors). So the term 'noise induced' should be applied only if it can be firmly established that no other reason for the threshold shift exists (Ward, 1976; Sulkowski, 1980; Kryter, 1994). An NIPTS is preceded by, and may at any time be accompanied by, a reversible temporary threshold shift (TTS).

Over the years, much information has been gathered about the TTS and its relationship to noise exposure. These relationships were earlier used as basic to defining the criteria of NIPTS risks. According to Ward (1973a) the terms 'auditory adaptation' and 'auditory fatigue' are synonyms of TTS and may be applied interchangeably. The magnitude of TTS is a function of many noise parameters, and the established relationship between them can be described by the following formulae (Ward, 1973a, 1976; Melnick, 1976; Meister, 1977; Dieroff, 1994; Kryter, 1994):

- A continuous, steady-state noise, depending upon the spectrum composition and the level, produces a TTS proportional to the logarithm of the exposure time, i.e. a doubling of TTS in decibels requires a tenfold increase of the exposure time. The recovery from a moderate magnitude of TTS has a similar exponential time course, recovering completely within 16 hours of exposure. In other words, both the growth and the recovery of TTS have a rapid development at the onset and then gradually slow down. Generally, threshold shift measured in decibels increases monotically during the first 8–16 hours (with individual variations) of exposure and, shortly thereafter, reaches a relatively stable plateau or asymptote (called the asymptotic threshold shift). However, when the TTS has reached 40 dB or more, the recovery may become linear in time, with the TTS requiring days or even weeks to disappear. This 40-dB or 50-dB TTS may represent some sort of critical TTS that should not be exceeded if the risk of permanent damage is to be avoided.

- Temporary threshold shift increases linearly with the moderate noise level, starting at about 70–75 dB SPL and ending at 130 dB (below 70 dB threshold shifts usually do not appear, or they are very short-term ones only, regardless of the exposure time); this means that the difference between TTS produced by 100 and 110 dB noises will be about the same as the difference between those produced by 110 and 120 dB.
- A noise with a maximum energy at low frequencies will produce less TTS than one in which the energy is at higher frequencies.
- The frequency range in which TTS occurs depends on the stimulus; in the case of broadband noise, the maximum TTS will be observed in the 3000- to 6000-Hz range; pure tones and narrow bands of noise produce a maximum TTS at a frequency higher than that of the TTS producing sound (from one-half to one octave higher); the most 'effective' producer of TTS is thus a stimulus of about 3000 Hz.
- An intermittent exposure is much less able to produce TTS than a steady one; this means that the ear can tolerate more total acoustic energy in the case of an intermittent stimulus. In such a case, the TTS is not only a function of the level but also of the ratio of noise duration to breaking time (effective quiet) and to the number of repeated cycles (noise 'on' and noise 'off'). Usually, an intermittent exposure for 8 hours has half of the value of an analogous TTS due to a continuous noise of the same level and duration, and it may be even lower if the breaks participate more in the total duration of the intermittent noise action.
- The characteristics of a TTS from impulse noise have not been explained completely. Usually, such a TTS is bigger in comparison with the TTS from the continuous noise, but, with simultaneous continuous and impulse noise, the final effect is less (Cohen, Klyin and LaBenz, 1966; Yamamura et al., 1974). The reason for this seems to be the increased efficiency of the protective reflex of the middle-ear muscles under the influence of the summing stimuli. The average maximum TTS (especially produced by gunfire) is often at 6000 Hz instead of at 4000 Hz, where the maximum usually occurs after broadband noise exposure. But the most striking difference between TTSs from steady noise and impulse noise is that the latter grows linearly with time instead of exponentially. This is reviewed in detail in Chapter 17 by Smoorenburg.

The development of NIPTS depends upon the same agents as TTS – level and noise duration, recurrence of exposure, other environmental features and individual susceptibility.

It has been assumed for years that permanent and temporary threshold shifts are very closely related, accepting certain assumptions, which may be summarized after Ward (1973b, 1976) as follows:

- Noises that produced equal average amounts of TTS would also produce equal amounts of NIPTS.

- If one noise produced twice as much TTS as another, it was also twice as dangerous in regard to NIPTS.
- If an exposed person showed half as much TTS as another he would suffer only half as much permanent hearing loss.

The observed relationships established the basis for the concept of predicting the size of NIPTS from $TTS_2$ measurements (TTS measured 2 minutes after the cessation of noise exposure) and specification of the hearing damage risk criteria. However, more recent data force one to be cautious in the application of these rules relating the growth and recovery of TTS to NIPTS and, although both are correlated, the relationship is not strong enough to use TTS to predict the magnitude of permanent hearing loss (NIH Consensus, 1990; Dieroff, 1994).

## Hearing damage risk criteria

Many attempts have been made to define the relationship between noise exposure and hearing loss, and to introduce protection for the ear through the use of engineering and/or administrative controls.

One of the approaches that can be used to encourage the limitation of noise exposure is to develop and enforce strict hearing damage risk criteria (DRCs). The term refers to specifications that define exposure limits – maximum acceptable noise exposure levels and durations and that relate the probability of inducing hearing loss to the properties of the noise environment. (Sulkowski, 1980; Kryter, 1994; Alberti, 1996).

Some of the DRCs have been incorporated, in one form or another, in legislation or regulations of particular countries, in documents of the International Organization for Standardization (ISO) and in the World Health Organization (WHO) recommendations that are concerned with hearing conservation. However, it was not easy to indicate permissible noise levels for particular durations that, if not exceeded, would result in no effect or an acceptably small effect on hearing over a working lifetime of exposure.

Unfortunately, no biological criterion represents an absolute borderline between safety and hazard, and the noise DRCs are no exception. Figure 18.6 (according to Mills, 1982) shows critical and safe levels of exposure demonstrating how difficult it is to define any one admissible noise intensity, bearing in mind that NIHL depends greatly on composite agents – level, duration, scheduling of exposure, and individal differences.

Thus, the 85 dB (A) limit for an 8-hour daily exposure, which is currently accepted internationally, expresses an economic and practical compromise, and a small proportion of any population exposed to this level for a working lifetime will suffer a hearing impairment. According to the international standard ISO 1999 (ISO, 1990) 'Determination of occupational noise exposure and estimation of noise-induced hearing impairment.', about 10% of workers after 40 years' exposure will experience, at this limit, an NIPTS of $\geq 25$ dB, judged by a pure-tone average of 500, 1000 and 2000 Hz (Lutman, 1996).

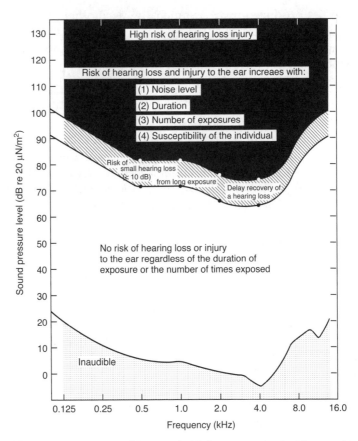

**Figure 18.6** Most of the range of human audibility categorized with respect to the risk of injury and hearing loss. (Reprinted with permission from Mills, 1982.)

Using the formula of 'material impairment' coined by the Occupational Safety and Health Administration (OSHA) in the USA, describing NIPTS as an average hearing threshold level of 25 dB across the frequencies 1000, 2000 and 3000 Hz, the risk would be somewhat larger.

Thus, the proportion of the population that should be protected (the acceptable level of risk in an exposed population) and the level of hearing loss that may be tolerated (the hearing loss formula that is used) are open to question, and there is no consensus (Suter, 1996).

At the present time, most countries use 85 dB (A) as the permissible occupational exposure limit, adopting the equal energy concept promulgated by Burns and Robinson (1970). It argues that the hazard to hearing is determined by the total energy (a product of sound level and duration) entering the ear during a typical work period, for example, one day or one week, and that equal quantities of the acoustic energy are equally injurious regardless of how they are distributed in time. This is true whether sound exposure is spread over a short or long period; in other words, *a given sound experienced for 8 hours does as much harm as twice that sound experienced for 4 hours or half that sound experienced for 16 hours*. Remembering that decibels are a logarithmic scale, doubling sound intensity is equivalent to increasing its intensity by 3 dB; thus a 93-dB sound is twice as intense as a 90-dB sound, and a 103-dB sound is twice as intense as a 100-dB sound. This concept allows a 3-dB increase in sound pressure level to indicate a halving of the duration (< 8 hours) of continuous daily steady-state exposure, in order to maintain an equal degree of hazard (Sulkowski, 1980; Kryter, 1994; Alberti, 1996).

The criteria (abbreviated DRC) refer to specifications defining exposure limits i.e. maximum permissible noise levels and durations which, if not exceeded, would result in no or acceptably small effect on hearing.

The 85 dB(A) limit for an 8-hour daily exposure is currently accepted internationally although a small proportion of any population exposed to this level for a working lifetime will suffer a hearing impairment.

The true 'no-adverse-effect' level for occupational noise exposure over the workday of 8 hours seems to be 75 dB(A).

The total received A-weighted energy[a] is a representative measure of noise exposure with respect to the hearing injury, expressed by the term 'equivalent sound level ($L_{eq}$) in dB (A)', which may be defined as equally dangerous for hearing and producing the same effect as the continuous noise of a constant level with the same value in dB (A).

However, the estimation of noise-induced hearing loss, which is most reliably determined from $L_{eq}$, requires considering the amount of permanent threshold shift that would occur 'normally' as an age-related phenomenon and, therefore, the international standard ISO 7029 (ISO, 1984) presents hearing threshold levels as a function of age – the data being identical to those of database A of ISO 1999, based on investigation from the 1960s. Figures 18.7 and 18.8 show the median age-related threshold shifts (presbycusis), which relate to otologically selected populations not exposed to noise during working hours; the median value at the age of 25 years was taken as zero. Both figures illustrate that presbycusis starts at the higher frequencies and, in general, women have somewhat better hearing acuity than males of the same age group.

The calculation of hearing threshold levels of populations occupationally exposed to noise allowed the second edition of ISO 1999. In these most comprehensive DRCs, the dose–effect relationships are characterized by the equivalent sound level normalized to an 8-hour working

---

[a]By convention, the occupational noises which include a wide band of frequencies are measured through the 'A' filter in the sound level meter and thus are designated in dB (A) units; the A-frequency weighting network approximates the ear's response characteristics and is a common measurement scale (see Chapter 2).

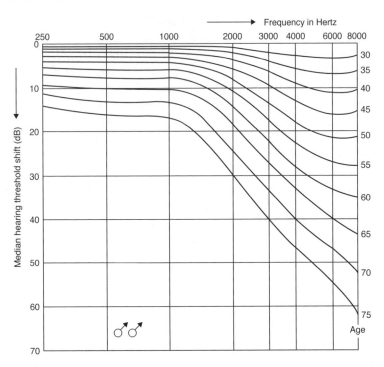

**Figure 18.7** Median values of the age-related threshold shifts of male otologically selected populations not exposed to occupational noise. (From ISO 7029 and database A of ISO 1999.)

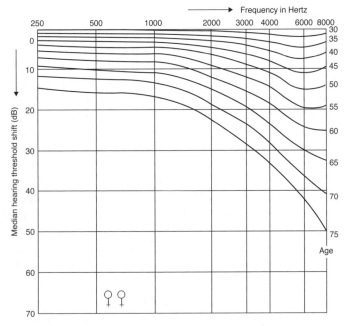

**Figure 18.8** Median values of the age-related threshold shifts of female otologically selected populations not exposed to occupational noise. (From ISO 7029 and database A of ISO 1999.)

day ($L_{EX,8h}$) and NIPTS for frequencies across the range 500–6000 Hz for exposure durations of 1–40 years.

Figure 18.9 gives percentile distribution of NIPTS at 4000 Hz (the most noise-vulnerable frequency) after noise exposure of 40 years' duration. It is worthy of note that NIPTS after 1 year's and 10 years' exposure is about 25% and 75% respectively of the NIPTS values given in Figure 18.9. It can be concluded from these relationships that the probability of NIHL is negligible below equivalent sound levels of 75 dB (A) over the workday of 8 hours. This level had previously been documented by the WHO (1997) as the 'no-adverse-effect' level for occupational noise exposure.

So, there appears to be reasonable agreement that sound levels below 75 dB (A) will not engender a permanent hearing loss, even at 4000 Hz. At higher levels of intensity, the hearing loss is directly related to sound level for comparable durations. Unfortunately, the mandatory DRC, $L_{eq,8h}$ of 85 dB (A), is unable to ensure the preservation of normal hearing

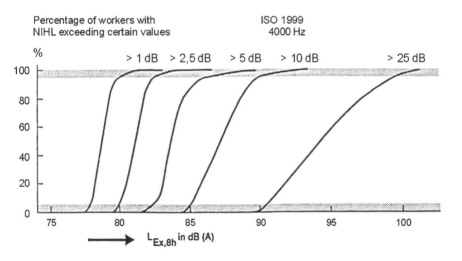

**Figure 18.9** Percentage of people with noise-induced permanent threshold shift at 4000 Hz exceeding certain values as a function of the equivalent sound level during the workday. Exposure time is equal to 40 years (ISO 1999).

(including 4000 Hz) in 100% of exposed individuals, but only in that part of the population with an average susceptibility. It is argued that acceptance of lower noise limits safe for all would be very costly, involving the necessity for further reduction of noise by engineering means, and instituting monitoring audiometry in greater numbers of employees (Sulkowski, 1986) as such a compromise between occupational health requirements aimed at maximal reduction of risk with optimal reduction of noise levels must be weighed against technical–economical possibilities of industry. This balance is impossible to maintain in the long term.

One should also remember – as emphasized by Passchier-Vermeer (1994) – that when evaluating the effects of noise, it is relevant to have some insight into the level of noise exposure not only in the working environment but also in the home/leisure activities, and to obtain information on total noise exposure during an average 24-hour period. However, there is usually a lack of such data.

A very crucial weakness of DRCs based on the $L_{eq}$ as a representative measure of noise exposure with respect to the hearing injury is the fact that they are based on data from continuous noise exposures and, therefore, cannot be used as DRCs for impulse noise, which damages the cochlea in a different way from a continuous noise (Dieroff, 1994; Sulkowski et al., 1999). Consequently, to evolve more comprehensive noise standards to cover both continuous and impulse noise there is a necessity for more data relating acoustic impulse noise parameters to NIHL. This is discussed in Chapter 17.

## Susceptibility to NIHL

Besides the acoustic parameters influencing the development of NIHL – noise level, spectral characteristics, dynamics of noise (steady-state or varying intensity), the duration of exposure and its distribution during the workday – there is another very important factor, noted by Fosbroke in 1830 over 140 years ago: individual susceptibility (Sulkowski, 1980) (see Chapter 7).

Although there is increasing effect with increasing levels and duration of exposure, what is perhaps more surprising is that people are not affected similarly. Both temporary threshold shift (TTS) and permanent threshold shift (PTS) in response to a given intense noise may differ by as much as 30–50 dB among individuals.

It is known that, apart from the basic group, which includes the majority of individuals, in which the hearing changes are proportional to the degree of exposure, two extreme groups are observed: one not showing any changes at all or minimal changes, and another with hearing impairment considerably surpassing the average for the whole population. Notwithstanding earlier presumptions that extreme groups amount to about 20% of an exposed population, it is to be expected that individual sensitivity in a given population would demonstrate a normal gaussian distribution; it means that the majority of people are characterized by the average, moderate sensitivity, and a small percentage display resistance, and a similar percentage high sensitivity to noise damage. Thus it makes it extremely difficult to predict hearing outcome resulting from a given noise exposure in any one individual (Dieroff, 1994; Sulkowski, 2002).

Several factors have been proposed to explain the differences in NIHL among individuals and over time in the same individual, although the biological bases of these differences are still unknown (Alberti, 1996; Kowalska and Sulkowski, 1997b).

Surprisingly, NIHL as well as TTS in response to a given intense noise may differ as much as 30 to 50 dB or even more among individuals. The reasons are still unexplained.

Among several factors which may influence an individual's susceptibility there are considered the resonant and transmission properties of the outer and middle ear, differences in the inner ear anatomy and physiology (e.g. poor blood circulation), auditory efferent system, genetic predisposition, gender and age, pigmentation, magnesium deficiency, ototoxic drugs and chemicals, human addictions. Ambiguity of opinions concerns also the role of a coexisting middle- and inner-ear pathology.

A number of extrinsic factors (for example, characteristics of the external ear canal and middle ear, drugs and prior exposure to noise) may influence an individual's susceptibility to NIHL. It is presumed that an unusually efficient acoustic transfer through the conductive ear system can be associated with increased risk of damage due to increased energy coupled to the inner ear; the effectiveness of sound transmission may indeed differ individually depending upon the mass and geometry of the auditory ossicles, and size of the tympanic membrane and oval window.

The strength of the protective contraction of the middle-ear muscles, reducing the transmission of at least the low-frequency tones, which is not the same in every individual, is probably of great importance.

Some animal studies suggest that individual differences in the inner-ear anatomy and physiology – such as density and spacing of the hair cells, rigidity of the cochlear partition, thickness of the tectorial membrane, blood supply to the cochlea, chemical characteristics of endolymph, rate of oxygen utilization, and density of afferent and efferent innervation – may also be significant (Dieroff, 1994; Kryter, 1994).

Considering that one of the possible mechanisms in the development of NIHL is the vascular pathology in the microcirculation of the cochlea as demonstrated by histological evidence of reduced cochlear blood flow following noise exposure, it is possible that localized ischaemia and microvascular alterations may occur during noise exposure. Thus poor blood circulation and/or oxygenation of the cochlea in individuals may render them more susceptible.

Ototoxic drugs and certain chemicals represent another cause of differences in susceptibility to noise exposure within individuals. In animal research, certain antibiotics (such as kanamycin), salicylates (such as aspirin) and cytotoxic chemotherapeutic agents (such as cisplatin) appear to exacerbate the damaging effects of noise exposure. Clinical evidence of corresponding effects in human patients has not been established, but precautions should be taken with regard to noise exposure in individual subjects treated with these medications (NIH

Consensus, 1990; Boettcher et al., 1992), particularly administered on a chronic basis. There is a growing list of industrial chemical substances that can – with the combination of noise – increase several-fold the risk to hearing (see Chapter 21). Recent studies have suggested that some chemicals, known as ototoxicants, such a toluene, styrene, xylene, trichloroethylene, carbon disulphide, and their mixtures, in addition to solvents, some heavy metals and asphyxiants (Sulkowski, 1990; Sulkowski et al., 2002), may have interactive synergistic effects with noise. Thus, although the individual noise exposure and chemicals may each be within exposure limits, in combination they may still pose a risk (Kowalska, Sulkowski and Sińczuk-Walczak, 2000; Morioka et al., 2000; Prasher et al., 2002).

The role of the auditory efferent system (the superior olivary complex in the brain stem with the crossed olivocochlear bundle to the contralateral cochlea) has recently been raised as particularly important (Henderson, Zheng and McFadden, 2001). Zheng et al. (1997), who completely sectioned the olivocochlear bundle fibres in chinchillas and exposed the animals to broadband noise of 105 dB SPL for 6 hours, found an increased susceptibility in de-efferented ears despite similar cytocochleograms in the efferent innervated and de-efferented ears. More recent studies (Śliwińska-Kowalska et al., 2000) have been able to confirm this effect using contralateral efferent suppression of auditory brain-stem response (ABR) and distortion product otoacoustic emissions (DPOAE) in guinea pigs.

There are currently some genetic speculations regarding susceptibility to NIHL (Erway and Willot, 1996). The first human genetic mutation responsible for development of deafness was identified in 1995 (Ahituv and Avraham, 2000). Now more than 70 genes are known to contribute to isolated hearing impairments (Van Lear and Van Camp, 2001). Therefore, a genetic predisposition for developing NIHL cannot be ignored. It is thought – in the light of molecular investigations – that mutations of mitochondrial DNA (mtDNA) may influence a generation of genetically related sensorineural hearing damage, also induced by noise. This is exemplified by the mutation *A3243G*, which causes hearing loss through dysfunction of the inner and outer hair cells (Ueda et al., 1998; Hutchin and Cortopassi, 2000; Griffiths et al., 2001; Usami et al., 2002).

Gender and age are other factors that are associated with variations in susceptibility. A slight difference in hearing thresholds between young boys and girls was observed to increase between ages 10 and 15 years, when boys begin to show reduced high-frequency auditory sensitivity relative to girls, who continue to demonstrate better hearing than men into advanced age (Lehnhardt, 1965, 1974; Sulkowski, 1980).

These gender differences are probably due to the greater exposure of males to noise (for example, during military service) and to the lower exposure of women (higher indices of absence at work due to pregnancy and maternity leave) rather than due to any inherent distinct susceptibility. Moreover, gender differences in hearing thresholds (better in females) exist in populations not exposed to noise (Corso, 1959; Hinchcliffe, 1959; ISO, 1990).

The relationship between NIHL and ageing is not completely explained. There is evidence that babies born to mothers working in noisy environments have an increased risk of high-frequency hearing loss (Szmeja, Slomko and Sikorski, 1979; Daniel and Laciak, 1982), and, in childhood, there may be a sensitive period related to the development of the efferent pathway. At the other extreme, increasing age has been hypothesized to be linked with decreasing susceptibility. This contention is based on the existence of presbycusis, hearing loss that increases with age and that is not known to be attributable to excessive noise exposure or other known aetiology. The traditional approach is to consider the effects of NIHL and age as additive (Corso, 1980); however, some data show that such an assumption cannot be used quantitatively for either groups or individuals (Mills et al., 1998; Hinchcliffe, 1999a). Nevertheless, retrospective studies (Sulkowski, 2002) indicated that subjects exposed for the first time to hazardous noise at a younger age showed a trend to develop smaller hearing loss than subjects who began their work at an older age.

Obviously, the relationships between advancing age and susceptibility to NIHL are confounded by presbycusis. Typical hearing levels at various ages have been incorporated in the ISO 7029 standard (see Figures 18.7 and 18.8), which may be used to estimate the portion of overall hearing loss that is attributable to exposure to excessive noise.

According to some investigations, pigmentation is considered to be a factor influencing the differences in susceptibility; melanin estimation with eye and skin colour in occupationally noise-exposed workers showed that black or dark-skinned individuals had fewer threshold shifts in comparison with white subjects with blue eyes (Carter, 1980). This was interpreted as demonstrating that melanin could protect the inner ear against acoustic trauma with a mechanism involving the generation and neutralization of free oxygen radicals (Barrenas, 1997; Tachibana, 1999).

Some animal and human studies have also demonstrated that magnesium deficiency may increase the risk of NIHL in a given noise exposure. Therefore, oral intake of magnesium supplement is recommended, as a method of reducing the magnitude of noise-induced TTS and PTS (Attias and Bresloff, 1999; Scheibe, Haupt and Ising, 2000). A contrary opinion results from the investigation of Walden, Henselman and Morris (2000), which has not confirmed any relationships between individual susceptibility to NIHL and level of magnesium in the blood serum.

Human addictions may also play a role in the development of NIHL; some data suggest that smoking is associated with an increased risk (Starck,

Topilla and Pykko, 1999), while a moderate alcohol consumption (140 g weekly) exerts a protective effect (Popelka et al., 2000).

Another phenomenon that should be taken into account is increasing resistance to hearing damage by pre-exposure sound conditioning. It has been found that prior exposure to a low level non-traumatic stimulus 'conditions' or 'toughens' the ear to subsequent damaging sound exposure (Henderson et al., 1996; Canlon, Fransson and Viberg, 1999; Niu and Canlon, 2001).

Is an ear that has already suffered NIHL more susceptible to further injury due to noise exposure than an undamaged ear? This difficult question is usually raised when a hearing-impaired worker attempts to move from one noisy industry to another, only to fail employment hearing screening. This is based on the belief that, because of previous damage to the ears, hearing is more likely to deteriorate more rapidly than normal. There are no data to suggest that such an ear will continue the degenerative process more quickly than a normal ear. Nevertheless, people already handicapped by hearing loss should be excluded from all further noise exposure because at this point over-conservatism is not only medically desirable but also economically justified as any further hearing deterioration will automatically be compensable (Alberti, 1996).

The outer- and middle-ear diseases resulting in conductive hearing losses are mostly considered to reduce the flow of acoustic energy to the cochlea and, therefore, diminish the amount of NIHL produced by a given noise (NIH Consensus, 1990). It is worth mentioning that the only proven case of a protective effect of a middle-ear pathology in relation to a cochlea exposed to noise is the observation (checked experimentally only on rats and guinea pigs) (Akoyoshi et al., 1966) that an explosion with a simultaneous rupture of the eardrum causes a considerably smaller NIPTS than in the situation where the tympanic membrane remains undamaged.

Burns and Robinson (1970) stated that there is no clear picture regarding development of NIHL complicated by pathologies of both the middle and/or the inner ear. However, in their examination of workers with such pathologies, exposed to noise, the hearing levels were more elevated than the anticipated levels in healthy ears. Similar findings were reported in our own study (Laciak and Sulkowski, 1973; Sulkowski and Laciak, 1973) on subjects employed in a textile industry who underwent radical or tympanoplastic surgery of the middle ear. Therefore, it remains unclear whether a middle-ear disorder provides protection against noise, like an earplug, or, on the other hand, exerts a worsening effect.

A particular ambiguity of opinions concerns otosclerosis. According to McShane et al. (1991) the disease partially protects from NIHL. Novotny and Pospisil (1960) report six cases, three of whom, after many years of work in noise, did not present any deterioration of hearing connected with the exposure, unlike three others with characteristic notches at 4000 Hz. Lehnhardt (1965, 1974) states that a pure 'stapedius' form of otosclerosis protects the cochlea against the traumatizing action of noise, while a mixed form with a considerable decrease of a cochlear reserve supports further hearing loss in exposure conditions. The four cases observed by Scevola (1967) suggest rather a decreased susceptibility to NIHL independent of the clinical form.

However, cutting middle-ear muscles during stapedectomy, which normally serves a protective function by contraction in response to intense sound, can result in increased susceptibility (Colletti and Sittoni, 1982; NIH Consensus, 1990).

In summary, scientific knowledge is currently inadequate to predict that any individual will be safe in noise that exceeds established damage risk criteria, or that specific individuals will show greater than average loss following a given exposure. Among the many proposed explanations, the hypothesis that the resonant and transmission properties of the outer and middle ear affect individual susceptibility deserves further attention. Empirical support for this hypothesis should not be difficult to obtain, but very few data have been collected on this question, for both TTS (experimentally) and PTS (retrospectively). Moreover, the effect of middle-ear problems (including otosclerosis) and conductive hearing loss, and whether they afford protection to the inner ear from damaging effects of noise exposure (rather like a built-in hearing defender) and, if so, to what degree, require clarification. Differences in susceptibility of the cochlear structures to NIHL may exist but no practical approach to predicting them is yet available. Identification of susceptible humans will almost certainly be delayed until a successful animal model is available (Henderson et al., 1996; Henderson, Zheng and McFadden, 2001).

# Clinical features and diagnosis of occupational NIHL – medicolegal assessment

The production of NIHL in healthy unprotected ears is a slow progressive and insidious process and years of exposure may elapse before any significantly noticeable loss of hearing occurs.

The mechanism of inner-ear damage is not completely known but it appears that overstimulation by noise for long periods of time produces metabolic changes in the organ of Corti, which in turn cause degenerative changes in the hair cells' structure. Experimentally, pathological changes can be observed in the mitochondria, subsurface cisternae, smooth endoplasmic reticulum and nucleus, and there are increases in lysosomes and Hensen bodies. Furthermore, membrane alterations lead to changes in ionic composition and herniation of cell contents. Vascular changes in the stria vascularis and the spiral ligament have also been reported. Thus, there are changes in cellular metabolism, damage to cellular architecture leading to alteration in function, although no direct relationship can be defined between pathology and function. Normal thresholds have been reported with considerable outer hair cell (OHC) and inner hair cell (IHC) loss. Accurate prediction of threshold is not possible on the basis of the extent of hair cell loss or conversely a prediction of pathology for a given threshold. However, noise characteristically causes a notch in the auditory sensitivity in the region of 2–8 kHz, leading to a reduction in the dynamic range of hearing and poorer frequency selectivity. There may be pitch distortion, reduced speech intelligibility and the troublesome symptom of tinnitus (Spoendlin, 1976; Saunders, Cohen and Szymko, 1991; Dieroff, 1994).

Unfortunately, there are no clear-cut clinical features that distinguish NIHL from several other causes of sensorineural hearing impairment. The diagnosis is based on history, physical examination and appropriate laboratory tests, including full hearing tests. Although there are audiometric configurations suggestive of the diagnosis, it may have many variations, and no one configuration fits all cases or excludes a case (Alberti, 1996; Luxon, 1998).

Clinically, the initial stage of NIHL is characterized in pure-tone audiometry by the presence of a bilateral, essentially symmetrical, high-tone notch at 4000 Hz, which may also occur at neighbouring frequencies – 3000 and 6000 Hz – not involving any subjective awareness of changes in hearing. The notch, as the years of exposure pass, grows deeper and broader, the high frequencies being more rapidly affected than the low frequencies; with incremental hearing loss at 2000 Hz, progressive deterioration of speech intelligibility appears, evincing complaints of hearing handicap.

Although 4000-Hz notches are characteristically associated with NIHL, it must be borne in mind that this particular shape of audiometric curves has been identified in a multiplicity of other otological pathology, including perilymph fistula, genetic hearing impairment, ototoxic drugs and idiopathic hearing loss, and has been specifically highlighted in cases of head trauma. Therefore, although the 4-kHz notch is the only characteristic sign of occupational noise damage to the inner ear, it is not specific for this condition (Luxon, 1997, 1998; Hinchcliffe, 2002).

Although 4000 Hz notches are characteristically associated with NIHL this particular shape of audiometric curves can be identified also in a multiplicity of other otological pathology.

So, the final diagnosis should be made by excluding other causes of sensorineural hearing losses, similar to those occuring in the population at large (e.g. Ménière's disease, acoustic neuroma).

In medicolegal evaluation of NIHL as prescribed occupational compensatable disease the objective audiometric measures (e.g. auditory evoked potentials) should be used to check up the accuracy of pure-tone audiometry or to detect an intentional exaggeration.

As time goes on, the notches disappear with hearing in the higher frequencies also worsening, so that the audiogram becomes indistinguishable from many other sensorineural hearing losses (Alberti, 1996).

Burns and Robinson (1970) stated that after 10 years of exposure to a given noise, the loss in the higher frequencies plateaus, but gradually the loss spreads into the lower frequencies (Figure 18.10). The rate of spread and the degree of loss are related to both the intensity of sound and the individual's susceptibility to noise. With significant hearing loss in the high frequencies, important speech information is often inaudible or unusable. Other interfering sounds, for example background noise, competing voices or room reverberation, may reduce even further the hearing-impaired listener's receptive communication ability. The presence of tinnitus may be an additional debilitating condition. Such impairment in hearing ability resulting from NIHL may vary from mild to severe.

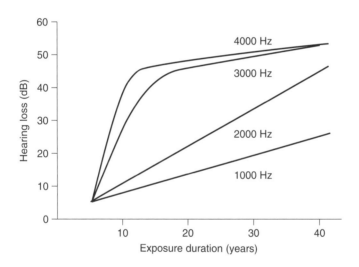

**Figure 18.10** Typical course of noise-induced hearing loss as a function of exposure duration (median hearing levels: simplified graphs). Hearing and Noise in Industry. London: HMSO. (Reproduced with permission from Burns and Robinson, 1970.)

A simplified, schematic development of occupational NIHL due to continuous steady-state industrial noise of $L_{eq}$ 90–100 dB (A) depending on exposure duration is shown in Figure 18.11. Individual audiograms should agree more or less with this typical idealized form (Dieroff, 1994; Sulkowski, 2002).

However, NIHL, like any other chronic disorder, may coexist with other diseases. Therefore, the final diagnosis should be made by exclusion – if

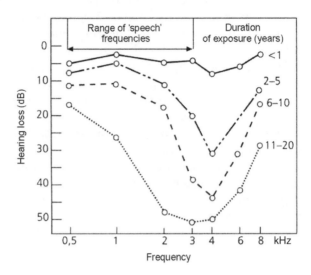

**Figure 18.11** Schematic development of occupational noise-induced hearing loss.

other causes of hearing loss have been excluded, noise exposure has been adequate and there is an appropriate hearing loss, it is customary to attribute the loss to that cause (Alberti, 1996; Luxon, 1998). The diagnosis must be made individually and one should avoid the error of believing that noise exposure and hearing loss are necessarily causally related. For instance, in our own series of 1805 medicolegal cases, in as many as 490 claims for NIHL (27%), other causes of hearing loss, similar to those occurring in the population at large, were recognized (Sulkowski and Śliwińska-Kowalska, 1995). In Table 18.2 many non-occupational ear diseases such as otosclerosis, Ménière's disease, otitis media, acoustic neuroma, ototoxicity as well as malingering are identified.

It is essential to take a full medical history to identify any known cause of sensorineural hearing loss other than noise exposure which may complicate the interpretation of hearing impairment. Important questions include those about familial hearing loss, length of symptoms, childhood illness, school screening (whether school hearing screening has ever been failed), ear discharge, other diseases related to hearing loss such as hypertension, diabetes or renal problems, use of ototoxic drugs and head injuries.

Where indicated, further investigation should be initiated, including haematologic, serological and imaging, including, if necessary, computed tomography (CT) or magnetic resonance imaging (MRI).

When noise exposure is believed to be the cause of the hearing loss, various causes of loss must be sought, for example recreational, military and occupational. Even within the realm of occupational hearing loss, it is often difficult to attribute the cause to a specific employer, and ultimately it may become a matter of clinical skill and exquisite judgment to establish both

**Table 18.2** Diagnosis of 490 patients from among 1805 referred with noise-induced hearing loss (NIHL) (Sulkowski and Śliwińska-Kowalska, 1995)

| Reasons for elimination of occupational aetiology of hearing loss | Number of cases | % |
|---|---|---|
| Malingering | 117 | 23.9 |
| Otosclerosis | 19 | 3.9 |
| Ménière's disease | 29 | 5.9 |
| Chronic purulent otitis media | 44 | 9.0 |
| Past surgery of the middle ear | 39 | 7.9 |
| Otitis media adhesiva | 78 | 16.0 |
| Congenital deafness | 3 | 0.6 |
| Post-traumatic lesions of the inner ear | 8 | 1.6 |
| Acoustic neuroma | 2 | 0.4 |
| Toxic injuries of the inner ear | 7 | 1.4 |
| Central hearing disorders | 3 | 0.6 |
| Average hearing loss <30 dB (low fence)[a] | 74 | 15.1 |
| Lack of essential noise exposure[b] | 67 | 13.7 |
| Total | 490 | 100 |

[a] Since 2002 Polish regulations define NIHL in terms of prescribed occupational compensable disease as bilateral cochlear hearing loss with the average pure-tone threshold of at least 45 dB at 1, 2 and 3 kHz in the better ear; before, the compensation scale has required at least 30 dB at 1, 2 and 4 kHz in the better ear but after subtracting the age corrections.

[b] Noise exposure records pointed out a short-lasting exposure ($\leq 5$ years) to the noise levels $\leq L_{eq}$ 70 dB(A).

the cause of the hearing loss and the proportion of it that should be attributed to any given employer (Alberti, 1996).

The basic diagnostic test is pure-tone audiometry, which quantifies the hearing loss; the pattern of audiogram may give a clue towards the diagnosis because it may help to distinguish among various sites of lesion: conductive, cochlear and retrocochlear. Habitual exposure to industrial noise cannot cause conductive hearing losses. Although, in a significant number of medicolegal cases referred to us (see Table 18.2) a conductive hearing loss that had not been discernible in the audiograms sent in with the patients was identified. The presence of an air–bone gap should lead to the suspicion of deliberate exaggeration or that there are either calibration errors or there is excess airborne radiation from the bone-conduction transducer. In cases with mixed hearing loss, the sensorineural element may be the result of, or be associated with, the middle-ear disorder.

The supplementary audiometric tests, namely tympanometry and stapedial reflex threshold measurements, are of importance both in excluding middle-ear pathology and in differentiating cochlear from retrocochlear dysfunction.

As mentioned earlier, the occupational NIHL typically presents a cochlear dysfunction with bilaterally symmetrical sensorineural hearing loss, worse in the higher frequencies.

Asymmetrical losses (>10 dB for pure-tone audiometry) are, however, fairly frequent in noise-exposed workers but it may be difficult to differentiate the precise causes. The most recent study, including a survey of the literature on the subject of asymmetry, confirmed left-ear inferiority irrespective of noise exposure (Luxon, 1997, 1998). Unilateral or asymmetrical sensorineural hearing loss has relatively serious connotations in otology, for it may be the first sign of a variety of cochlear – or, possibly more important, retrocochlear – disorders such as acoustic neuroma, posterior fossa meningioma and so forth (Alberti, Symons and Hyde, 1979, Alberti 1996). It should therefore be carefully investigated. Undoubtedly, the evaluation of NIHL is a complex and time-consuming exercise. The environmental and genetic factors predisposing an individual to the development of NIHL remain unclear and there is no single simple diagnostic test. An understanding of the current knowledge regarding the diagnostic pitfalls associated with NIHL is essential if accurate diagnoses are to be made, preventive and rehabilitative measures are to be set in place, and adequate but appropriate compensation is to be awarded to those who suffer injury leading to significant handicap and/or disability as a result of noise exposure.

The battery of tests employed includes hearing examinations such as conventional pure-tone air- and bone-conduction audiometry, tympanometry and stapedius reflex threshold estimation, speech reception threshold and speech discrimination tests and, if deemed necessary, otoacoustic emission measurement and evoked response audiometry. In cases of presumed asymmetrical hearing loss additional audiological tests such as reflex decay, tests for recruitment and so forth, should also be undertaken. Temporal bone tomograms (CT) to show the internal auditory meatus, vestibular tests and occasionally brain scans and MRI are recommended.

The clinician examining a patient suspected to have NIHL must establish or conversely exclude the existence of a hearing loss wholly attributable to noise. In the absence of a typical audiometric configuration and all too frequently the lack of serial audiograms and adequate noise exposure information, he must be alert to other causes of complaints for hypoacusis, as listed in Table 18.2, for example.

The next difficult task is to quantify the hearing loss due to noise exposure. The degree of accuracy required in the quantification for compensation purposes, when each additional decibel means an additional sum of money, is higher than is required for conventional diagnostic audiometry and more sophisticated methods are necessary (Alberti, 1996; Sulkowski, 2002).

It must be emphasized that pure-tone audiometric thresholds are a subjective measure, requiring the full cooperation of the subject if optimal thresholds are to be obtained. Objective audiometric measures should therefore routinely be obtained as a reliable means of assessing the accuracy of pure-tone audiometry and of detecting an intentional or unintentional exaggeration of the pure-tone thresholds.

In our medicolegal material the attempts of exaggeration of hearing loss manifested by feigned audiometric responses, also called non-organic hearing loss or malingering, were detected in 117 of 1805 patients claiming compensation for occupational NIHL (see Table 18.2). Many audiometric tests are designed to identify exaggerated hearing loss but few quantify it. Quantification for compensation purposes must be frequency-specific and parallel tonal audiometry. Objective verification of the audiogram has been sought for some time and evoked potential recordings offer several responses which may fulfil this role.

In the UK, cortical evoked potentials have been incorporated into practice for assessment of presence of a non-organic overlay of a loss (Prasher, Mula and Luxon, 1993), and the amplitude of the N1 component is considered as objectively determining the threshold of hearing at 1 kHz and 4 kHz. However, this procedure requires the active participation of the subject throughout the test to avoid any tendency to sleep, which adversely affects the response.

Our experience (Sulkowski et al., 1994; Sulkowski and Śliwińska-Kowalska, 1995; Sulkowski, 2002) suggests that ABR, particularly frequency-specific responses – measured according to a protocol (Table 18.3) – are more useful in the estimation of threshold and 'reconstruction' of pure-tone audiogram with a satisfactory precision within 5 dB nHL. Figure 18.12 illustrates the case of a malingerer subject; his true hearing thresholds have been determined by means of our frequency-specific ABR technique.

There are some important features in detecting malingering, which are well known to clinicians, and may be found during conventional testing (Sulkowski, 1980; Rossi et al., 1985). The most common pattern is a flattish audiogram at around 70–80 dB, lack of sharpness and repeatability of pure-tone thresholds, significantly less sensitive descending thresholds than ascending ones, and poor agreement of automatic Békésy audiometry with manual thresholds (Hinchcliffe, 1999b). A further guide is a discrepancy between speech reception thresholds and pure-tone thresholds; unfortunately, the weakness of the above is that a number of those who exaggerate pure-tone thresholds do not show this difference because they appear to be able to exaggerate their speech reception threshold as well as pure tones (Alberti, 1996; Dieroff, 1994). Also, the presence of a so-called type 5 Békésy audiogram, the configuration often seen in malingerers, in which the continuous tones are heard better than the interrupted ones,

**Table 18.3** Protocol of auditory brain-stem response(ABR) measurement procedure

| Stimuli | Tone pip, 1000 Hz (2-0-2 cycle) |
| | Tone pip, 2000 Hz (4-0-4 cycle) |
| | Tone pip, 3000 Hz (8-0-8 cycle) |
| | Click, 100 μs |
| Envelope | Gaussian |
| Polarity | Alternating |
| Repetition rate | 31/s |
| Band-pass filter | 200–2000 Hz |
| Time analysis | 20 ms for tone pips |
| | 10 ms for click |

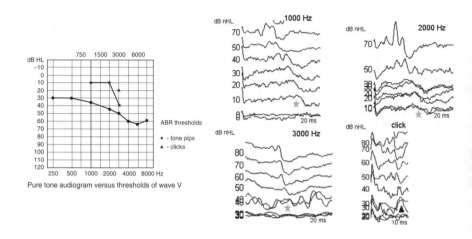

**Figure 18.12** Pure-tone audiogram versus auditory brain-stem response recordings (thresholds of wave V due to tone pips and clicks) in a malingerer.

can be misleading. There have been reports of both false negatives in malingering cases and false positives in genuine cases (Coles and Priede, 1971).

Acoustic reflex threshold (ART) measurements, which are easy to elicit in persons with normal middle-ear function, may provide predictive but not quantifiable evidence of exaggerated hearing loss. ARTs are always greater than pure-tone thresholds, and even in an ear with a severe cochlear loss are usually at least 20 dB higher than the pure-tone thresholds. Thus, if they are equal to or smaller than the latter, it constitutes convincing evidence of feigned hearing loss (Alberti, 1996; Sulkowski et al., 2002a).

Unlike the advantages of the frequency-specific ABR, otoacoustic emissions (OAEs) have rather limited applicability, when dealing with compensable occupational noise damage (Prasher and Sulkowski, 1999; Lucertini et al., 2001). The presence of click transient-evoked emissions (c-TEOAEs) merely reflects an audiometric threshold of less than 30 dB HL for the frequency range 1–4 kHz, or – as reported by Collet et al. (1993) (Kowalska and Sulkowski, 1997 by Collet et al. (1993) and Kowalska and Sulkowski (1997$^a/_b$))–corresponds to the best hearing frequency if the hearing loss in at least one frequency between 0.25 and 8 kHz is equal to or less than 40 dB HL. Distortion-product otoacoustic emissions (DPOAEs) provide a more promising objective measure of the configuration of the subjective audiogram (Prasher and Sulkowski, 1999). However, they can be measured only if behavioural hearing thresholds do not exceed about 50 dB HL (Kowalska and Sulkowski, 1998). Figure 18.13 shows the results of DPOAE measurements in the same malingering patient as illustrated earlier (see Figure 18.12) by use of the ABR.

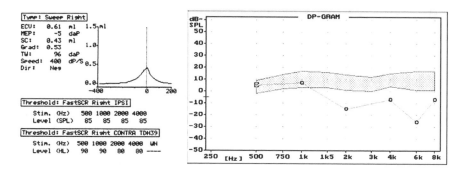

**Figure 18.13** Distortion product otoacoustic emissions and impedance audiometry results in a malingerer subject, the same tested earlier with auditory brain stem response (see Figure 18.12).

In summary, it may be concluded that a battery of tests including electrophysiological measurements is desirable to make the correct differential diagnosis and to quantify the hearing loss. Although evoked potentials or other physiological responses, considered to form the basis for 'objective audiometry', have some important limitations, their utility, for the prediction of the 'real' hearing thresholds in an uncooperative malingering claimant is undoubted.

For compensation purposes various formulae (scales) derived from pure-tone audiometric measures are used in different countries[b] (Sulkowski, 1980, 2002). The standard Polish formula (see comment on Table 18.2) approximates to the British approach (Hinchcliffe, 1997; Raglan, Sulkowski and Prasher, 1999). Both seem to combine a good correlation between auditory handicap, understood as a disadvantage in everyday life for a given individual resulting from a hearing disability that is compensable, and impairment that is measured in terms of decibel elevation of hearing threshold. In order to calculate an amount of indemnity and/or disability pension, the pure-tone average loss over a 45-dB fence is transformed into percentage of permanent loss of health (bodily impairment).

For tinnitus, which very often accompanies occupational NIHL and therefore increases the total handicap, an additional provision of 5% whole bodily impairment is awarded (Sulkowski and Śliwińska-Kowalska, 1995; Kowalska and Sulkowski, 2001; Guzek et al., 2002). It is estimated that tinnitus is present permanently in 50–60% of those with NIHL, its severity increases with increasing hearing loss, and the incidence seems to be higher in those exposed to impulse noise (Alberti, 1987; Sulkowski et al., 1999; Prasher et al., 2001).

---

[b]There is no consensus about the validity or utility of the scales, which scale should be used, whether measures of speech understanding should be included, or whether self-assessment ratings should be incorporated into either impairment rating scales of disability determinations (Coles and Sinclair, 1990; NIH Consensus, 1990; Dobie, 1993).

# Therapy, rehabilitation and prevention of occupational hearing loss

Acute acoustic trauma can be medically treated using carbogen, isobaric oxygen, hyperbaric oxygen and corticosteroid therapy. In the standardized animal study by d'Aldin et al. (1999) the most efficient treatment in terms of recovery of auditory function turned out to be the administration of corticosteroids combined with hyperbaric oxygen therapy. Clinical experience has shown that acute acoustic trauma in humans can be successfully treated with hyperbaric oxygen, conventionally supplemented with corticosteroid drugs (Lamm and Arnold, 1996, 1999; Kopke et al., 2001). Advances in inner-ear pharmacology and their clinical applications seem to be encouraging (Puel et al., 1999b) and in the future may also be applied to chronic acoustic trauma – NIHL. To date, NIHL is considered incurable, but preventable.

During the early 1980s several experiments demonstrated that the magnitude of hearing loss induced by noise could be modulated. It was apparent from these experiments that manipulations of cochlear metabolism directly altered the subsequent damage induced by noise. Increasing or decreasing body temperature during noise exposure resulted in an increased or decreased cochlear damage (Drescher, 1976; Henry and Chole, 1984). In addition, increasing the oxygen supply or removing the thyroid gland was also shown to protect the ear from NIHL (Berndt and Wagner, 1979).

Recently, it has been suggested that destruction of the primary auditory dendrites below the IHC, might be due to excessive release of neurotransmitter (probably glutamate) from the IHCs, which is toxic (excitotoxic) to the structure and function of spiral ganglion neurons (Puel et al., 1996). Consistent with this hypotensis is the high degree of protection against noise trama that is observed when the glutamate antagonist kynurenate is applied to the cochlea (Puel et al., 1999a).

Other protective agents include antioxidants. An important factor, associated with tissue destruction through metabolic stress, is the generation of reactive oxygen species (ROS) or free radicals. According to a major hypothesis, ROS formation results from increased mitochondrial activity, and may also follow changes in cochlear blood flow associated with intense sound exposure (Lamm and Arnold, 1996). These ROS can react with and damage cellular protein, DNA and unsaturated lipids. The body's normal antioxidant defences cannot counteract free radicals in excess. Several reports support the importance of ROS in NIHL (Ohlemiller, Wright and Dugan, 1999; Dehne et al., 2000; Ohinata et al., 2000).

Enhancing the antioxidant defence system with additional free radical scavengers could be useful in preventing/minimizing hearing loss caused by toxins and noise exposure. Promising therapeutic candidates with protective action against NIHL include caroverine (anti-glutaminergic agent) (Ehrenberger and Felix, 1995), sarthran (angiotensin receptor antagonist) (Goldwin et al., 1998), superoxide dismutase (Ohlemiller, Wright and Dugan, 1999) and allopurinol (Seidman, Shivapuja and Quirk 1993; Attanasio et al., 1999). Allopurinol and its major metabolite, oxy-purinol, are potent inhibitors of xanthine oxidase, one of the enzymes that produces ROS (Wippich et al., 2001). It has been shown that allopurinol not only blocks the formation of ROS, but can also scavenge ROS (Das et al., 1987; Moorhouse et al., 1987; Franze et al., 2003).

To date, NIHL is considered incurable although there are some promising results of treatment with hyperbaric oxygen, corticosteroids and antioxidants.

As far as rehabilitation is concerned the hearing aids are very useful for and well accepted by those with noise-induced impairment.

NIHL can be prevented or, at least, minimized by implementing the sound surveys to assess the degree of hazardous noise, engineering and administrative noise control to lower exposure, education of workers why and how to prevent hearing loss, usage of personal ear protectors and mandatory pre-employment and follow up audiometric tests.

Like presbycusis, NIHL cannot be reversed but unlike presbycusis it can be prevented or, at least, minimized. Therapeutic options are limited to rehabilitaion by use of hearing aids or implantable electronic protheses and they should not be withheld (Sulkowski, 2002).

It is hoped that implementing effective hearing-loss prevention programmes (also known as hearing conservation programmes) (see Chapter 31) will lead to a reduction in noise-induced impairments. Such programmes for occupational settings must include the following interactive components: sound surveys to assess the degree of hazardous noise exposure, engineering and administrative noise controls to lower exposures, education to inform at-risk individuals why and how to prevent hearing loss, hearing protection devices (earplugs, earmuffs and canal caps) to reduce the sound reaching the ear, and audiometric evaluations to detect hearing changes. Governmental regulations that currently apply to most noisy industries should be revised to encompass all industries and all employees, strengthened in certain requirements, and strictly enforced with more inspections and more severe penalties for violations (NIH Consensus, 1990; Sulkowski, 1998, 2002).

Carefully performed sound surveys measuring sound levels throughout the plant and throughout the working day indicate the absolute levels in a plant and help identify those for whom there is potentially hazardous noise. The exposure of individual workers, if the job is static, may be extrapolated from these measurements, but it is far better to undertake individual noise dosimetry studies (Alberti, 1996; Sulkowski and Olina, 1985; Sulkowski and Pawlaczyk-Luszczynska, 1994).

Personal hearing protectors should be used when noise levels remain hazardous even after appropriate engineering and administrative controls have been put in place. It is not, however, enough to provide protectors; there must be a programme to encourage their use and instruction in their proper fitting and maintenance. The plant/occupational physician has a major role to play in this area and should be familiar with the various types of protector, their advantages and disadvantages, and their application (Alberti, 1996; Kowalska and Sulkowski, 1997; Sulkowski, 1998, 2002).

Regular audiometric evaluation of workers' hearing is crucial to the success of any hearing conservation programme, because it is the only way to actually determine whether occupational hearing loss is being prevented. Because occupational hearing loss occurs gradually, affected employees often notice no change in hearing ability until a relatively large change in their hearing sensitivity has occurred. New employees must be subjected to routine pure-tone audiometry and the effectiveness of the programme monitored usually every year. Such follow-up testing has many functions; important among them is the opportunity that it provides to reinforce the hearing conservation programme and to monitor proper use of hearing protectors. It detects those with hearing loss, and identifies individuals' changes and whether a total programme is effective (Alberti, 1996). In some countries, including Poland, mobile audiological vehicles are employed for hearing screening (Sulkowski, Sward-Matyja and Matyja, 2001). By taking the vehicle to individual places and plants the testing is effected thoroughly and at lower cost than if workers (particularly those in small industrial enterprises without an in-huse health service) had to be examined at separate appointments in other locations.

With regard to most non-auditory effects, which usually occur at relatively high noise exposure levels, these might be prevented by enforcement of present regulatory limits in the occupational environment (Passchier-Vermeer, 1994).

# References

Ahituv N, Avraham KB (2000) Auditory and vestibular mouse mutants: models for human deafness. Journal of Basic and Clinical Physiology 11: 181–91.

Akoyashi M, Amemiya A, Sato K, Takeda T, Shoji T (1966) On the pathogenesis of acoustic trauma of the cochlea in rabbits and guinea pigs due to explosion. International Audiology 5: 270–6.

Alberti PW (1987) Tinnitus in occupational hearing loss: nosological aspects. Journal of Otolaryngology 16: 34–45.

Alberti PW (1996) Occupational hearing loss. In JJ Ballenger, JB Snow (eds) Otorhinolaryngology: Head and Neck Surgery. Baltimore: Williams and Wilkins, pp. 1087–101.

Alberti PW, Symons F, Hyde ML (1979) Occupational hearing loss: the significance of asymmetrical hearing thresholds. Acta Otolaryngologica 87: 255–63.

Attanasio G, Cassandro E, Sequino L, Mafera B, Mondola P (1999) Protective effect of allopurinol in the exposure to noise pulses. Acta Otorhinolaryngologica Italiana 19: 6–11.

Attias J, Bresloff I (1999) Oral magnesium reduces noise induced temporary and permanent hearing loss. In D Prasher, B Canlon (eds) Cochlear pharmacology and noise trauma. London: NRN Publishers, p. 43–52.

Barrenas ML (1997) Hair cells loss from acoustic trauma in chloroquine treated red, black and albino guinea pigs. Audiology 36: 187–201.

Berndt H, Wagner H (1979) Influence of thyroid state and improved hypoxia tolerance on noise induced cochlea damage. Archives of Otorhinolaryngology 224: 125–8.

Boettcher FA, Gratton MA, Bancroft BR, Spongr V (1992) Interaction of noise and other agents. In A Dancer, D Henderson, R Salvi, RP Hamernik (eds) Recent advances in noise-induced hearing loss. St. Louis: Mosby Year Book.

Burns W, Robinson DW (1970) Hearing and Noise in Industry. London: HMSO

Canlon B, Fransson A, Viberg A (1999) Medial olivocochlear efferent terminals are protected by sound conditioning. Brain Research 850: 253–60.

Carter NL (1980) Eye colour and susceptibility to noise-induced permanent threshold shift. Audiology 19: 86–93.

Cohen A, Klyin B, LaBenz PJ (1966) Temporary threshold shifts in hearing from exposure to combined impact/steady-state noise conditions. Journal of the Acoustical Society of America 40: 1371–9.

Coles RRA, Priede VM (1971) Nonorganic overlay in noise-induced hearing loss. Procedings of the Royal Society of Medicine 64: 194–9.

Coles RRA, Sinclair A (1990) Hearing. In FC Edwards, RI McCallum, PJ Taylor (eds) Fitness for Work. Oxford: OUP, pp. 70–98.

Collet L, Levy V, Veuillet E, Truy E, Morgon A (1993) Click-evoked otoacoustic emissions and hearing threshold in sensorineural hearing loss. Ear and Hearing 14: 141–3.

Colletti V, Sittoni W (1982) Noise history, audiometric profile and acoustic reflex responsivity. In RJ Salvi, D Henderson, RP Hamernik, V Colletti (eds) Basic and Applied Aspects of Noise Induced Hearing Loss. New York: Plenum Press, pp. 247–69.

Corso JF (1959) Age and sex differences in pure tone thresholds. Journal of the Acoustical Society of America 31: 498–503.

Corso JF (1980) Age correction factor in noise-induced hearing loss: a quantitative mode. Audiology 19: 221–32.

d'Aldin C, Cherny L, Dancer A (1999) Medical treatment for acoustic trauma. In D Prasher, B Canlon (eds) Cochlear pharmacology and noise trauma. London: NRN Publishers, pp. 54–72.

Daniel T, Laciak J (1982) Observations clinique et experiences concernant l'etat de l'appareil cochleo-vestibulaire des subjects exposes au bruit durant la vie foetable. Revue de Laryngologie, Otologie e Rhinologie 103: 313–18.

Das DK, Engelman RM, Clement R, Otani H, Prasad MR, Rao PS (1987) Role of xanthine oxidase inhibitor as free radical scavenger: a novel mechanism of action of allopurinol and oxypurinol in myocardial salvage. Biochemical and Biophysical Research Communications 148: 314–19.

Davis A (1995) Hearing in adults. London: Whurr Publishers.

Davis A (1997) The epidemiology of hearing impairment in the UK, with particular attention to the impact of noise. Proceedings of the British-Polish Workshop on Noise-induced Hearing Loss. Slok-Belchatow, Poland: The Nofer's Institute Editorial Office, pp. 4–7.

Dehne N, Lautermann J, den Cate WJ, Rauen U, de Groot H (2000) In vitro effects of hydrogen peroxide on the cochlear neurosensory epithelium of the guinea pig. Hearing Research 143: 162–70.

Dieroff HG (1994) Lärmschwerhörigkeit. Jena-Stuttgart: Gustav Fischer Verlag.

Dobie RA (1993) Medical-legal evaluation of hearing loss. New York: Van Nostrand Reinhold.

Drescher DG (1976) Effect of temperature on cochlear response during and after exposure to noise. Journal of the Acoustical Society of America 59: 401–7.

Ehrenberger K, Felix D (1995) Receptor pharmacological models for inner ear therapies with emphasis an glutamate receptors: a survey. Acta Otolaryngologica 115: 236–40.

Erway LC, Willot JF (1996) Genetic susceptibility to noise-induced hearing loss in mice. In A Axelsson, H Borchgrevink, RP Hamernik, P-A Hellstrom, D Henderson, RJ Salvi (eds) Scientific Basis of Noise-induced Hearing Loss. New York: Thieme, Stuttgart-New York: George Thieme Verlag, pp. 56–64.

Franze A, Sequino L, Saulino C, Attanasio G, Marciano E (2003) Effect over time of allopurinol on noise-induced hearing loss in guinea pigs. International Journal of Audiology 42: 227–34.

Goldwin B, Khan MJ, Shivapuja B, Seidman MD, Quirk WS (1998) Sarthran preserves cochlear microcirculation and reduces temporary threshold shifts after noise exposure. Otolaryngology, Head and Neck Surgery 118: 576–83.

Griffiths TD, Blakemore S, Elliot C, Moore BC, Chinnery PF (2001) Psychophysical evaluation of cochlear hair cell damage due to the A3243 G mitochondrial DNA mutation. Journal of the Association for Research in Otolaryngology 2: 172–9.

Guzek W, Sulkowski WJ, Kowalska S, Makowska Z (2002) Tinnitus Center at the Nofer Institute of Occupational Medicine- first experience. Medycyna Pracy 53: 461–4 (in Polish).

Henderson D, Subramaniam M, Henselman LW, Portalatini P, Spongr VP, Sallustio V (1996) Protection from continuous, impact or impulse noise provided by prior exoposure to low-level noise. In A Axelsson, H Borchgrevink, RP Hamernik, P-A Hellstrom, D Henderson, RJ Salvi (eds) Scientific Basis of Noise-induced Hearing loss. New York: Thieme, Stuttgart-New York: George Thieme Verlag, pp. 150–8.

Henderson D, Zheng X, McFadden SL (2001) Cochlear efferent system-a factor in susceptibility to noise? In D Henderson, D Prasher, R Kopke, R Salvi, R Hamernik (eds) Noise-induced Hearing Loss: Basic mechanisms, prevention and control. London: NRN Publishers, pp. 127–39.

Henry KR, Chole RA (1984). Hypothermia protects the cochlea from noise damage. Hearing Research 16: 225–30.

Hinchcliffe R (1959) The threshold of hearing as a function of age. Acustica 9: 303– 8.

Hinchcliffe R (1997) Editorial review: WHO and its role in the prevention of deafness and hearing impairment. Journal of Laryngology and Otology 111: 699–701.

Hinchcliffe R (1999a) Noise hazards to the general population: hearing surveys reassessed. Journal of Audiological Medicine 8: 113–21.

Hinchcliffe R (1999b) György Bekesy (1899-1972) Fifty years of Bekesy audiometry (1947-97). Journal of Audiological Medicine 8: 72–91.

Hinchcliffe R (2002) The clinical picture of occupational noise-induced hearing loss – the historical perspective. Journal of Audiological Medicine 11: 63–74.

Hutchin TP, Cortopassi GA (2000) Mitochondrial defects and hearing loss. Cellular and Molecular Life Sciences 57: 1927–37.

ISO 7029 (ISO, 1984) Acoustics - threshold of hearing by air conduction as a function of age and sex for otologically normal persons. Geneva: International Organization for Standardization.

ISO 1999 (ISO, 1990) Acoustics - determination of occupational noise exposure and estimation of noise-induced hearing impairment. Geneva: International Organization for Standardization.

Kopke RD, Hoffer ME, Wester D, O'Leary MJ, Jackson RJ (2001) Targeted topical steroid therapy in sudden sonsorineural hearing loss. Otology and Neurology 22: 475–9.

Kowalska S, Sulkowski WJ (1989) Inner ear impairment in the vibration syndrome caused by local vibrations. Medycyna Pracy 40: 169–76 (in Polish).

Kowalska S, Sulkowski WJ (1997a) Measurements of click-evoked otoacoustic emission in industrial workers with noise-induced hearing loss. International Journal of Occupational Medicine and Environmental Health 10: 441–59.

Kowalska S, Sulkowski WJ (1997b) Present and future activities concerning protection against noise in the European Union. Medycyna Pracy 48: 703–12 (in Polish).

Kowalska S, Sulkowski WJ (1998) Measurements of distortion product otoacoustic emissions in industrial workers with noise-induced hearing loss. In D Prasher, L Luxon (eds) Advances in Noise Research. London: Whurr Publishers, pp. 205–12.

Kowalska S, Sulkowski WJ (2001) Tinnitus in noise-induced hearing impairment. Medycyna Pracy 52: 305–13 (in Polish).

Kowalska S, Sulkowski WJ, Sińczuk-Walczak H (2000) Assessment of the hearing system in workers chronically exposed to carbon disulfide and noise. Medycyna Pracy 51: 123–38 (in Polish).

Kryter KD (1994) The Handbook of Hearing and the Effects of Noise: Physiology, psychology, and public health. San Diego, New York, Boston, London, Sydney, Tokyo, Toronto: Academic Press.

Laciak J, Sulkowski WJ (1973) The effect of industrial noise upon hearing organ after radical operations of the middle ear. Otolaryngologia Polska 27: 485–91 (in Polish).

Lamm K, Arnold W (1996) Noise-induced cochlear hypoxia is intensity dependent, correlates with hearing loss and precedes reduction of cochlear blood flow. Audiology and Neuro-Otology 1: 148–60.

Lamm K, Arnold W (1999) Therapeutic strategies for improving cochlear blood flow. In D Prasher, B Canlon (eds) Cochlear Pharmacology and Noise Trauma. London: NRN Publishers, pp. 150–65.

Lehnardt E (1965) Die Berufsschäden des Ohres. Archiv für Ohren- Nasen- und Kehlkopfheilkunde 185: 11–242.

Lehnardt E (1974) Zur Begutachtung der Lärmschwerhörigkeit. Medycyna Pracy 25: 59–68 (in Polish).

Lucertini M, Viaggi F, Pasquazzi F, Cianfrone G (2001) Medico-legal use of otoacoustic emissions in the audiological selection process for employment. Scandinavian Audiology 30, suppl 52: 146–51.

Lutman ME (1996) Estimation of noise-induced hearing impairment for compound noise exposures based on ISO 1999. Journal of Audiological Medicine 5: 1–7.

Luxon LM (1997) The clinical diagnosis of noise induced hearing loss. Proceedings of the British-Polish Workshop on Noise-induced Hearing Loss. Slok-Belachatow, Poland: The Nofer's Institute Editorial Office, pp. 1–3.

Luxon LM (1998) The clinical diagnosis of noise-induced hearing loss. In D Prasher, LM Luxon (eds) Advances in Noise Research. London: Whurr Publishers.

McShane DP, Hyde ML, Finkelstein DM, Alberti PW (1991) Unilateral otosclerosis and noise-induced hearing loss. Clinical Otolaryngology 16: 70–5.

Meister FI (1977) Dependence of the temporary threshold shift on the immediately preceding exposure to noise. Audiology 16: 260–4.

Melnick W (1976) Human asymptotic threshold shift. In D Henderson, RP Hamernik, DS Dosanjh, JH Mills (eds) Effects of Noise on Hearing. New York: Raven Press, pp. 277–89.

Mills JH (1982) Effects of noise on auditory sensitivity, psychophysical tunning curves, and suppression. In RP Hamernik, D Henderson, RJ Salvi (eds) New Perspectives on Noise-induced Hearing Loss. New York: Raven Press, pp. 249–63.

Mills JH, Dubno JR, Boettcher FA (1998) Interaction of noise-induced hearing loss and presbycusis. Scandinavian Audiology 27, supp. 48: 117–22.

Moorhouse PC, Grootveld M, Halliwell B, Quinlan JG, Gutteridge JM (1987) Allopurinol and oxypurinol are hydroxyl radical scavengers. FEBS Letters 213: 23–8.

Morioka I, Miyai N, Yamamoto H, Miyashita K (2000) Evaluation of combined effect of organic solvents and noise by the upper limit of hearing. Industrial Health 38: 252–7.

NIH Consensus Statement (1990) Noise and hearing loss. Vol. 8 Bethesda: National Institutes of Health, pp. 3–24.

Niu X, Canlon B (2001) Theories of sound conditioning. In D Henderson, D Prasher, R Kopke, R Salvi, R Hamernik (eds) Noise Induced Hearing Loss: Basic mechanisms, prevention and control. London: NRN Publishers, pp. 255–67.

Novotny Z, Pospisil A (1960) Vztach prevednich poruch sluchu k profesionalni nedoslychavosti z hluku. Ceskoslovenska Otolaryngologie 6: 339–43 (in Czech).

Ohinata Y, Miller JM, Altschuler RA, Schacht J (2000) Intense noise induces formation of vasoactive lipid peroxidation products in the cochlea. Brain Research 878: 163–73.

Ohlemiller KK, Wright JS, Dugan LL (1999) Early elevation of cochlear reactive oxygen species following noise exposure. Audiology and Neuro-Otology 4: 229–36.

Parsons K (2003) Noise and temperature. Proceedins of the WHO/NOPHER Meeting "Combined Environmental Pollutants and Health", Bonn: Regional WHO Office, pp. 35–9.

Passchier-Vermeer W (1994) Noise and health. Report of a Committee of the Health Council of the Netherlands, The Hague, publication no 1994/15E, pp. 7–101.

Popelka MM, Cruickshanks KJ, Wiley TL, Tweed TS, Klein BE, Klein R, Nondahl DM (2000) Moderate alcohol consumption and hearing loss: a protective effect. Journal of American Geriatric Society 48: 1273–8.

Prasher D, Sulkowski WJ (1999) The role of otoacoustic emissions in screening and evaluation of noise damage. International Journal of Occupational Medicine and Environmental Health 12: 183–92.

Prasher D, Mula M, Luxon L (1993) Cortical evoked potential criteria in the objective assessment of auditory threshold: a comparison of noise induced hearing loss with Meniere's disease. The Journal of Laryngology and Otology 107: 780–6.

Prasher D, Ceranic B, Sulkowski WJ, Guzek W (2001) Objective evidence for tinnitus from spontaneous emission variability. Noise and Health 3: 61–73.

Prasher D, Morata T, Campo P, Fechter L, Lund SP, Pawlas K, Starck J, Sulkowski WJ, Sliwinska-Kowalska M (2002) NoiseChem: A European Commission research project on the effects of exposure to noise and industrial chemicals on hearing and balance. International Journal of Occupational Medicine and Environmental Health 15: 5–11.

Puel J-L, d'Aldin C, Ruel J, Ladrech S, Pujol R (1999a) Perspectives in inner ear pharmacology and clinical applications. In D Prasher, B Canlon (eds) Cochlear Pharmacology and Noise Trauma. London: NRN Publishers, pp. 1–8.

Puel J-L, d'Aldin C, Ruel J, Pujol R (1999b) Protective effect of glutamate antagonist kynurenate in noise-induced hearing loss. In D Prasher, L Luxon (eds) Advances in Noise Research. London: Whurr Publishers, pp. 261–70.

Puel J-L, d'Aldin C, Saffiedine S, Eybalin M, Pujol R (1996) Excitoxicity and plasticity of IHC-auditory nerve contributes to both temporary and permanent threshold shift. In A Axelsson, H Borchgrevink, RP Hamernik, P-A Hellstrom, D Henderson, RJ Salvi (eds) Scientific basis of Noise-induced hearing loss. New York: Thieme, Stuttgart-New York: George Thieme Verlag, pp. 36–42.

Pykko I, Zou J, Starck J, Topilla E (2003) Interaction of noise and vibration in noise-induced hearing loss - a study on mechanisms. Proceedings of the WHO/NOPHER Meeting, Combined Environmental Pollutants and Health, Bonn: Regional WHO Office, pp. 40–3.

Raglan E, Sulkowski WJ, Prasher D (1999) A comparison of noise induced disability assessments in the UK and Poland. International Journal of Occupational Medicine and Environmental Health 12: 41–6.

Rossi G, Sulkowski WJ, Olina M, Avolio G, Giordano C (1985) Malingering and occupational hearing loss. Audiologia Italiana 2: 1–8.

Saunders JC, Cohen YE, Szymko YM (1991) The structural and functional consequences of acoustic injury in the cochlea and peripheral auditory system: a five year update. Journal of the Acoustical Society of America 90:136–46.

Scevola A (1967) Il trauma acoustico professionale negli otosclerotici. Archivio Italiano di Otologia 78: 474–8.

Scheibe F, Haupt H, Ising H (2000) Preventive effect of magnesium supplement on noise-induced hearing loss in the guinea pig. European Archives of Otorhinoloryngology 257: 10–16.

Seidman MD, Shivapuja B G, Quirk WS (1993) The protective effects of allopuriol and superoxide dismutase on noise-induced cochlear damage. Otolaryngology, Head and Neck Surgery 109: 1052–6.

Śliwinska-Kowalska M, Sulkowski WJ, Kotylo P, Pawlaczyk-Luszczyńska M (2000) Contralateral suppression of ABR and DPOAE and susceptibility to noise-induced hearing loss. In D Prasher, L Luxon (eds) Advances in Noise Research. London: Whurr Publishers, pp. 114–20.

Spoendlin H (1976) Anatomical changes following various noise exposure. In D Henderson, RP Hamernik, D Dosanjh, JH Mills (eds) Effects of Noise on Hearing. New York: Raven Press, pp. 69–89.

Starck J, Topilla E, Pykko I (1999) Smoking as a risk factor in sensory hearing loss among workers exposed to occupational noise. Acta Otolaryngologica (Stockh) 119: 302–5.

Sulkowski WJ (1971) Industrial sudden deafness. Proceedings of the XVIII Acoustical Seminar, Warsaw: Polish Acoustical Society, pp. 138–40 (in Polish).

Sulkowski WJ (1980) Industrial Noise Pollution and Hearing Impairment: Problems of prevention, diagnosis and certification criteria. Warsaw: Foreign Scientific Publications Department of the National Center for Scientific, Technical and Economic Information.

Sulkowski WJ (1986) Hearing damage risk criteria: present status and controversies. Audiologia Italiana 3: 53–60.

Sulkowski WJ (1990) Occupational exposure to carbon disulfide and dysfunction of the vestibular system: a clinical study. Cahiers de Notes Documentaire 139: 472–5 (in French).

Sulkowski WJ (1995) Environmental noise and future research programme. Proceedings of the International Advanced Research Workshop, Turin: Minerva Medica, pp. 245–53.

Sulkowski WJ (1998) Principles of health care of workers at risk for occupational noise-induced hearing loss in Poland. In N Carter, RFS Job (eds) Proceedings of 7th International Congress on Noise as a Public Health Problem. Sydney: PTY Ltd, pp. 122–6.

Sulkowski WJ (2002) Principles of Preventing Occupational Noise-induced Hearing Loss. Lodz: The Nofer's Institute Editorial Office (in Polish).

Sulkowski WJ, Laciak J (1973) The effect of industrial noise upon hearing organ after conservative operations of the middle ear. Otolaryngologia Polska 27: 617–27 (in Polish).

Sulkowski WJ, Olina M (1985) Orientamenti attuali nella mizurazione del rumore per la prevenzione della ipoacusia professionale. Audiologia Italiana 2: 113–20.

Sulkowski WJ, Pawlaczyk-Luszczyńska M (1994) Evaluation of occupational exposure to noise from the hearing conservation point of view. International Journal of Occupational Medicine and Environmental Health 7: 167–75.

Sulkowski WJ, Śliwinska-Kowalska M (1995) Compensable noise-induced hearing loss and medicolegal aspects of diagnosis. In R Schoonhoven, TS Kapteyn, JAMP de Laat (eds) Proceedings of European Conference on Audiology in Noordwijkerhout: Leiden: Nederlandse Voreniging voor Audiologie, pp. 364–71.

Sulkowski WJ, Śliwinska-Kowalska M, Kowalska S, Bazydlo-Golińska G (1994) Electric response audiometry and compensational noise-induced hearing loss. Otolaryngologia Polska 48: 370–4.

Sulkowski WJ, Kowalska S, Lipowczan A, Prasher D, Raglan E (1999) Tinnitus and impulse noise-induced hearing loss in drop-forge operators.

International Journal of Occupational Medicine and Environmental Health 12: 177–82.

Sulkowski WJ, Sward-Matyja M, Matyja W (2001) Audiobus - the first Polish audiological mobile unit. International Journal of Occupational Medicine and Environmental Health 14: 79–80.

Sulkowski WJ, Guzek W, Kowalska S, Matyja W, Sward-Matyja M (2002a) Occupational hearing loss: new diagnostic opportunities. Medycyna Pracy 53: 457–9 (in Polish).

Sulkowski WJ, Kowalska S, Matyja W, Guzek W, Wesolowski W, Szymczak W, Kostrzewski P (2002b) Effects of occupational exposure to a mixture of solvents on the inner ear: a field study. International Journal of Occupational Medicine and Environmental Health 15: 247–56.

Sulkowski WJ, Szymczak W, Kowalska S, Sward-Matyja M (2004) Epidemiology of occupational noise-induced hearing loss (ONIHL) in Poland. Otolarynglogia Polska 58: 233–6.

Szmeja Z, Slomko Z, Sikorski K (1979). The risk of hearing impairment in children from mother exposed to noise during pregnancy. International Journal of Pediatric Otorhinolaryngology 1: 221–9.

Suter AH (1996) Current standards for occupational exposure to noise. In A Axelsson, H Borchgrevink, RP Hamernik, PA Hellstrom, D Henderson, RJ Salvi (eds) Scientific Basis of Noise-induced Hearing Loss. New York: Thieme, Stuttgart-New York: George Thieme Verlag, pp. 430–6.

Tachibana M (1999) Sound needs melanocytes to be heard. Pigment Cell Research 12: 344–54.

Ueda N, Oshima T, Ikeda K, Abe K, Aoki M, Takasaka T (1998) Mitochondrial DNA deletion is predisposing cause for sensorineural hearing loss. Laryngoscope 108: 580–4.

Usami SI, Koda E, Tsukamoto K, Otsuka A, Yuge I, Asamura K (2002) Molecular diagnosis of deafness: impact of gene identification. Audiology and Neurootology 7: 185–90.

Van Lear L, Van Camp G (2001) Genes in the ear: what have we learned over the last years. Scandinavian Audiology 53: 44–53.

Walden BE, Henselman LW, Morris ER (2000) The role of magnesium in the susceptibility of soldiers to noise-induced hearing loss. Journal of the Acoustical Society of America 108: 453–6

Ward WD (1973a) Adaptation and fatigue. In J Jerger (ed) Modern developments in audiology. New York: Academic Press, pp. 301–44.

Ward WD (1973b) Noise-induced hearing damage. In MM Paparella DA Shumrick (eds) Otolaryngology. Philadelphia: Saunders, pp. 377–90.

Ward WD (1976) Noise-induced hearing loss. In J Northern (ed) Hearing Disorders. Boston: Little, Brown and Co; pp. 161–76.

WHO (1997) Conclusions and recommendations of first informal consultation on future programme development for the prevention of deafness and hearing impairment. Geneva: World Health Organization.

Wippich N, Peschke D, Peschke E, Holtz J, Bromme HJ (2001) Comparison between xanthine oxidases from buttermilk and microorganisms regarding their ability to generate reactive oxygen species. International Journal of Molecular Medicine 7: 211–16.

Yamamura K, Takashima H, Miyake H, Okada A (1974) Effect of combined impact and steady-state noise on temporary threshold shift (TTS). Medicina del Lavoro 65: 215–21.

Zheng XY, Henderson D, McFadden SL, Hu BH (1997) The role of the cochlear efferent system in acquired resistance to noise-induced hearing loss. Hearing Research 104: 191–203.

# CHAPTER 19

# Military noise-induced hearing loss

*Noise and Its Effects:* Edited by Linda Luxon and Deepak Prasher © 2007 John Wiley & Sons Ltd.

J Attias, AY Duvdevany, I Reshef-Haran, M Zilberberg, B Nageris

## Introduction

Active military service is necessarily accompanied by repeated exposure to high doses of noise, which potentially may damage hearing. While training to become a qualified soldier, the recruit passes through critical periods during which the risk of hearing loss is high. One of these periods is during basic training. For the first time, recruits are exposed to repeated high doses of impulsive noise. Thus, basic training is considered one of the most dangerous periods in military service (Gold et al., 1989). A variety of factors contributes to the high risk of hearing loss during military service.

**Factors contributing to NIHL in the military**

- high levels of noise
- impulse and continuous noise
- inappropriate hearing protections
- exercise

These include extremely high levels of noise, in terms not only of intensity but also of range of frequencies, combined exposure to both impulsive and continuous noise, inappropriate hearing protection, high intrinsic susceptibility to hearing damage and physical exercise that aggravates the hearing loss (Lindgern and Axelsson, 1988; Colletti et al., 1991).

The importance of perfect hearing in military environments is well recognized. During certain activities, especially those that threaten life, the soldier must have a perfect ability to localize and detect the source of danger. In addition, he must understand the orders he is receiving from his commander, particularly for safety reasons (Price et al., 1989; Price, 1995). Due to the background noise that results in a poor signal to noise ratio, the detection and discrimination of speech in a noisy environment are especially difficult. Moreover, as the soldier is acting in a demanding environment, auditory discrimination is even more difficult. All the above factors are aggravated when a high-frequency hearing loss occurs as a result of military NIHL.

As with all prevention, early detection of hearing loss, appropriate protection and treatment are essential. Thus, repeated quick screening to detect the highly susceptible individual is mandatory before and after noise exposure. Obviously, efficient ear protectors must always be used during the noise exposure, in addition to engineering and administrative interventions to reduce noise at its source.

In this chapter the prevalence of military noise-induced hearing loss (M-NIHL) is reported. Methods for early detection and diagnoses of M-NIHL as well as methods for prevention are discussed. In addition, the acoustic features of the military environment are described.

## Prevalence of M-NIHL

The prevalence of M-NIHL is significantly influenced by the exact physical characteristics of the noise (level, duration and frequency) and the total dosage reaching the ear. Individual susceptibility probably plays a significant role in the eventual severity of auditory damage.

Figure 19.1 depicts the prevalence of M-NIHL in a large sample of 4000 Israeli soldiers in the armour and infantry corps in four phases: before and after basic training, during professional training and during active operational service. In the professional training phase the soldier is studying a specific specialization such that during this period the exposure is reduced. In active operational service, the soldier is again exposed to high levels of noise.

Each soldier was tested in a mobile sound-attenuated room using calibrated earphones and audiometers. Skilled audiologists performed the audiological tests. To prevent temporary threshold shift (TTS) contamination, the auditory thresholds across 0.25–8 kHz were measured only after at least 48 hours of non-exposure to noise.

The M-NIHL was classified into two categories:

- more than 25 dBHL in the range 6–8 kHz (pre-acoustic trauma);
- more than 25 dBHL in the range 2–4 kHz (M-NIHL).

In both corps, the incidence of M-NIHL increased compared with the pre-basic training. In the armour division, the prevalence of hearing impairment pre-acoustic trauma increased from 11% before training to

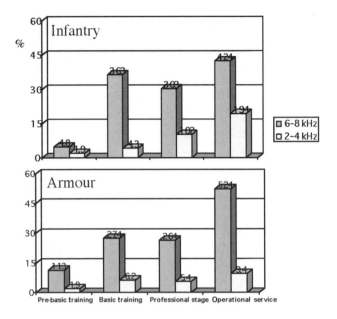

**Figure 19.1** Bar graphs to show prevalence of hearing loss in 4000 Israeli soldiers in two divisions (infantry and armour) at different career stages.

almost 52% (five times greater) at the end of active operational service. In contrast, the incidence of M-NIHL in the infantry increased 10 times compared with the pre-basic training. The significant differences reflect the extremely high doses of impulsive noises and inappropriate ear protection in the infantry when compared to the armour division. The armour soldier usually uses a helmet and is shielded by the tank cabin, both reducing the exposure to noise. In contrast the infantry soldier is less protected and more vulnerable.

The incidence of M-NIHL in Israeli troops is obviously high, most probably due to the intensive exposures to military noises. It is difficult to compare these figures with others worldwide because susceptibility of the variabilities in subjects, the methods of hearing evaluation and the training profiles are wide. Pelausa et al. (1995) reported that 11% of the infantry in the Canadian military had sustained mild-to-moderate hearing loss, greater than 25 dB HL across a frequency range of 3–6 kHz, associated with the use of small-calibre weapons. In the Swedish army, 29% were found to have hearing defects, predominantly in the high-frequency region. Following basic training, NIHL progression was found in 5%. In 0.5% this deterioration reached symptomatic level and 0.03% had significant NIHL (Klockhoff et al., 1986). In professional soldiers in the Finnish army, 26% had a hearing loss. In the French army, the prevalence of significant high-frequency hearing loss among 18- to 24-year-old soldiers was 9%. (Job et al., 2000).

## M-NIHL in various countries

| Country | Personnel | Frequency |
|---------|-----------|-----------|
| Israel | Full-time soldiers | 2 – 8% depending on age (Tinnitus: 22% of cases M-NIHL) |
| Canada | Infantry | 11% (mild-to-moderate HL) |
| Sweden | Army | 5% |
| Finland | Professional soldiers | 26% |
| France | Army | 9% |

(NB. Variability depending on age, susceptibility, military role, exposure, protection, criteria of hearing impairment, test technique etc.)

Figure 19.2 shows the incidence of M-NIHL in a sample of 2200 noise-exposed Israeli full-time soldiers. The incidence gradually increases as a function of age in an almost linear manner. In the age group 45 years and older the incidence can reach up to 70% of the soldiers. The increase of prevalence reflects the effects of total duration of exposure to noise.

Thus, the incidence of M-NIHL in both regular and full-time army personnel is high, due to the intensive training that necessarily includes repeated exposures to impulse and continuous noises.

Hearing loss is only one of the negative effects of noise exposure. Other auditory and extra-auditory adverse effects may occur following exposure to military noise. Tinnitus accompanies up to 22% of all NIHL depending on the age of the soldier (Figure 19.2). This symptom manifests as a neural dysfunction, which is difficult to treat and may lead to serious disruption in the daily life of certain sufferers (Attias et al., 1995, 2002).

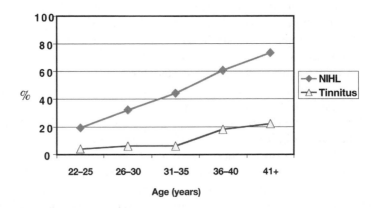

**Figure 19.2** The incidence of military noise-induced hearing loss (M-NIHL) and tinnitus in a sample of 2200 exposed Israeli full-time soldiers.

These figures of prevalence of M-NIHL in army personnel have not only social and medical implications but also significant economic ramifications. In 1996, 966 soldiers suffering from acute acoustic trauma were treated in French hospitals at a $US4 million cost. In the same year, France spent $US60 million on compensation for M-NIHL in veterans. Similarly in the USA in 1997, more than $US270 million were spent on M-NIHL compensation (Dancer et al., 1999).

# The acoustical features of military noise

### Blast noise

Blast noise is probably the main source of NIHL in armies. It is differentiated from the more 'common' industrial type noise by rapid changes of the pressure from the atmospheric level. The pressure pulse can reach a peak of 160–190 dB SPL in a very short time (less than 1 ms). This positive pressure wave is followed by a negative wave (relative to that of an atmospheric pressure) creating a shape of a 'freightliner wave'. This characterizes the blast or impulse noise (see Chapters 13 and 17).

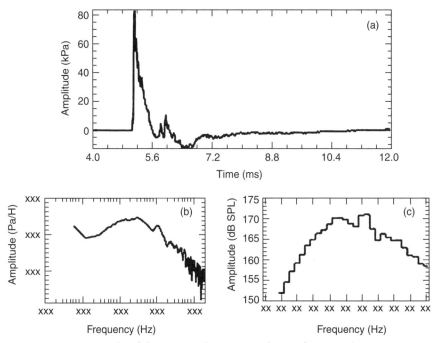

**Figure 19.3** An example of the time and spectrum shape of an impulse noise. This figure is reproduced by courtesy of Dr. Armand Dancer, French – German Research Institute, Saint – Louis, France.
(a) Signal time (ms) as function of amplitude (KPa)
(b) Signal spectrum – amplitude (Pa) as function of frequency (H$_z$)
(c) Signal frequency band amplitude

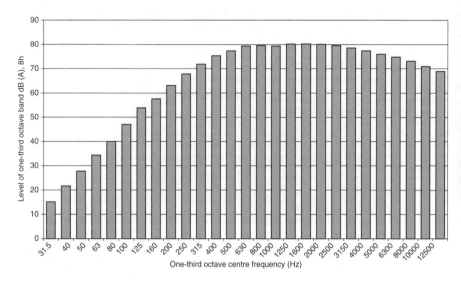

**Figure 19.4** An example of blast noise one-third octave spectrum (M16, 1 m from muzzle).

The spectrum of the blast noise is continuous, reaching a peak according to the duration of the pulse (the longer the pulse, the shorter the frequency peak).

Depending on certain standards the pulse duration can be defined. The US military standard MIL-STD-1474D uses the B duration, which is the time needed for a pulse to reduce from the pressure peak to 10% of its onset value.

Table 19.1 demonstrates characteristics of blast noise measured at 1 m distance or near the shooter's ears. The blast noise resulted from one shot. In addition examples of continuous noise characteristics are also detailed.

**Table 19.1** Characteristics of blast noise measured at 1 m or near the shooter's ears

| Type of weapon and vehicle | Peak level (dB SPL) | B duration (ms) | Peak spectrum level |
|---|---|---|---|
| M16, Uzi | 155–170 | 4–6 | 1–1.25 kHz $1/3$-octave band $L_{Aeq,8h}$ – 100–105 dB (A) |
| Cannons | (Next to muzzle) 185–19 | 30–50 | 50–100 Hz One-third octave band |
| Hand grenades | 175–185 | 3–6 | |
| Antitank missiles | 180–185 | about 10 | |
| Armoured vehicle | 95–115 dB (A) | | 50–150 Hz |

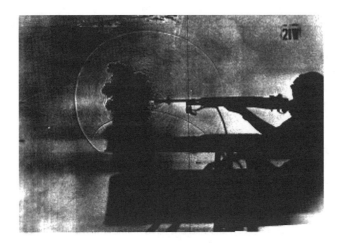

**Figure 19.5** An example of blast noise – shock wave produced by M14 muzzle.

# Protection against M-NIHL

As for all occupational or public health-related diseases, the primary approach to 'treat' NIHL is by prevention. The prevention of hearing loss is based simply upon the reduction of the sound energy entering the inner ear. To this end, hearing conservation programmes typically incorporate reduction of the noise at source, decreasing the noise exposure time, the use of ear defenders and regular audiometric monitoring.

**Hearing conservation includes:**

- Noise reduction at source
- Reduction of duration of exposure
- Use of ear defenders
- Regular audiometric monitoring

Without doubt, where hearing conservation programmes can be fully implemented, a significant reduction in NIHL is obtained (Henselman et al., 1995). Unfortunately, there are number of conditions that may result in only partial implementation, such as poor awareness, military restrictions, physical incompatibility and/or financial incapacity.

**Reasons for poor hearing protection in military**

- Poor awareness
- Military restrictions
- Physical incompatibility
- Financial constrictions

Reducing the intelligibility of commands, and difficulty in localizations and comfort reported by the soldier, may also be associated with the attenuation offered by the earplugs. Furthermore, for high levels of exposure (>120 dB (A)), a proportion of the sound energy may be bone conducted to the inner ear, resulting in cochlear damage despite of the use of ear protection.

# Ear protectors

Ear protectors' attenuation is a measure of their acoustic performances 'blocking' the hazardous noise. They are generally divided into groups: earplugs (foam – roll-down, formable – like wax plugs, premoulded, pod plugs and custom-fit plugs), earmuffs, semi-insert protectors and helmets. (see Chapter 30).

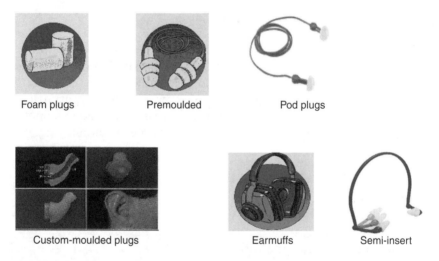

| Foam plugs | Premoulded | Pod plugs |

| Custom-moulded plugs | Earmuffs | Semi-insert |

**Figure 19.6** Different groups of ear protectors. This figure is reproduced by courtesy of AERO Company, Indianapolis IN 46268 USA.

The insertion loss (IL) is the common reference(Figure 19.7), and is quoted where attenuations are specified.

The attenuation of ear protectors is frequency dependent, and is usually better at high frequencies. This phenomenon is more pronounced with earmuffs. Hence, the attenuation of ear protectors is dependent upon noise spectrum and should be calculated and specified accordingly. The calculation is made by measuring the noise spectrum and then subtracting from the ear protector's attenuation provided by the manufacturer, or that measured separately. The real ear

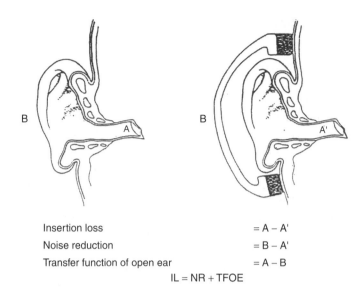

Insertion loss = A – A'

Noise reduction = B – A'

Transfer function of open ear = A – B

IL = NR + TFOE

**Figure 19.7** The acoustic attenuation of ear protectors can be specified as an insertion loss (IL) or a noise reduction (NR). TFOE, transfer function of open ear. This figure is reproduced by permission of Dr. Armand Dancer, French – German Research Institute, Saint – Louis, France.

protector's attenuation is the difference between the total level of attenuation with and without ear protectors. An alternative method of evaluation is using a single number, which describes the attenuation of 'flat' (uniform) spectrum noise, either by SNR (single number rating) or NRR (noise reduction rating).

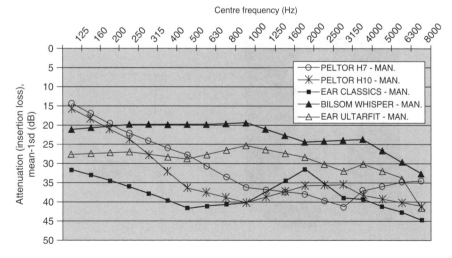

**Figure 19.8** The spectral attenuation of ear protectors according to manufacturers' data.

There are three different ways to measure the ear protector's attenuation at each frequency:

* REAT (real ear attenuation at threshold): with this method, audiometry is performed in subjects with and without earplugs. The difference in the auditory thresholds at each frequency represents the attenuation provided by the earplug. The advantages of this method include using real ears and having statistics for different ears. However, the disadvantages include subjective measures needing full cooperation from the subject, long procedures that require large samples (at least 30 subjects) and the response is strongly affected by the installation. Since measures are performed at threshold levels, this may not represent the real attenuation at high levels of exposures. Furthermore, the inner noise coming from the electronic ear protectors may disturb the auditory thresholds at certain frequencies.
* ATF (artificial test fixture – Figure 19.9): with this method an artificial head and simulation is used. By presenting a known noise to an ATF with ear protectors and measuring the pressure at the tympanic membrane, the noise reduction is calculated (subtracting the noise measured by an extra microphone). The advantages of this method include very fast and objective measurements, continuous frequency information and performance at real noise exposure even at very high stimulus levels. Disadvantages of this method may consist of great dependence upon simulation accuracy, no statistics (different ears) and the approach is highly expensive. There are only few comprehensive ATFs that are suitable for blast noise measurements.

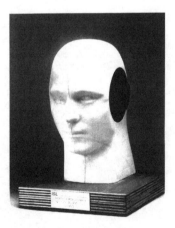 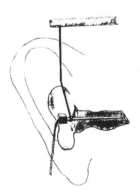

**Figure 19.9** Artificial test fixture.
This figure is reproduced by permission of Dr.Armand Dancer, French–German Research Institute, Saint–Louis, France.

- MIRE (microphone inside real ear): using microphones to measure the pressure behind EP on real subjects. A small tube is added to the microphone, and inserted into the ear canal (its end is a few millimetres from the tympanic membrane). The advantages of this method include having real ears and real noise exposure. It is an objective and short procedure, providing a continuous frequency measurement with strong statistics. However, the disadvantages may include the need to expose subjects to high levels of stimulations and to multi-exposure types. Thus, a serious restriction is the measurement of blast noises. It is difficult both to implement this method and to measure earplug attenuation at high frequencies because of the cut-off frequency of the tube (approximately 5 kHz).

**Attenuation of some common ear protectors is described below:**

1. SNR (REAT), [1]: foam plugs – approximately 20 dB, pre-moulded: 11–12 dB.
2. Small arms blast noise:
   (a) foam plugs (REAT), [1] – ~20dB.
   (b) foam plugs (ATF), [2]: $L_{Aeq}$ – approximately 40 dB, $L_{peak}$ – approximately40 dB.
   (c) pre-moulded plugs (REAT), [1] – 12–13 dB.
   (d) earmuffs (MIRE), [4]: $L_{Aeq}$ – 14–17 dB, $L_{Cpeak}$ – 22–27 dB.
   (e) earmuffs (ATF), [2]: $L_{Aeq}$ – approximately 25 dB, $L_{peak}$ – 26–27 dB.
3. Cannons:
   (a) foam plugs (MIRE), [5] $L_{peak}$ – 17.5 dB.
   (b) foam plugs (ATF), [2] – $L_{Aeq}$ – approximately 40 dB, $L_{peak}$ – approximately 40 dB.
   (c) earmuffs (MIRE), [5] $L_{peak}$ – 7.7–17.4 dB, according to volume size.
   (d) earmuffs (ATF), [2] $L_{peak}$ – 15–24 dB, $L_{Aeq}$ – 15–20 dB, according to volume size.
4. Armoured vehicle noise (ATF), [1]: earmuffs – approximately 15 dB.

# Biological protection

The novel biological strategies for preventing and treating NIHL offer a supplementary approach to mechanical ear protectors. Recent studies have shown that a small daily dose of 122 mg of magnesium (Mg) may reduce significantly the M-NIHL resulted from impulsive noise (Attias et al., 1994). Furthermore, similar doses resulted in smaller TTS in humans exposed to brief experimental noises (Attias et al., 2003). Moreover, Mg was found to be efficient in treating hearing loss in patients suffering from sudden deafness.

**Possible mechanisms of auditory protection by magnesium**

- Maintenance of selective membrane permeability.
- Effects on calcium.
- Effects on inner ear microcirculation.

The mechanism by which Mg provides protection is not well understood, but may involve basic molecular events; the involvement of Mg in maintaining selective membrane permeability (Horie et al., 1987), its effects on calcium (White and Hartzell, 1988) and on inner ear microcirculation (Guenther et al., 1989). No side effects of these levels of Mg ingestion were found in these studies.

These results strongly suggest the use of Mg supplements as an adjunct to existing mechanical protection regimes for several reasons. Active subject cooperation or motivation is not required and, therefore, Mg can be administrated to almost all populations especially in the military. Secondly, Mg has no side effects and has other beneficial effects, for example on the myocardial musculature. Thirdly, it can be easily and quickly administrated to very large populations (dissolved in juice, for example). Finally, in certain situations in which mechanical hearing protectors cannot be used, such as in specific military operations or activities, Mg may be the only alternative.

# Audiometric characteristics of M-NIHL

Most probably, the earliest and most common audiometric feature of M-NIHl is 6-to 8-kHz loss, which with continuation of exposure, affects the lower frequencies, particularly 3–4 kHz (see Figure 19.1). Most of the M-NIHL in the regular soldiers is of mild-to-moderate severity. The configuration of M-NIHL is usually bilateral, but more severe in the left ear (see below), without affecting the speech frequencies (0.25–2 kHz). With increased exposure, not only the severity increases but also other auditory complaints are reported such as tinnitus, hyperacusis and difficulties in understanding in noisy environments.

As the variability of noise exposures in the army is large, it is very difficult to predict the natural progression of NIHL. Hearing loss in military service appears to progress not at a steady rate but almost in a linear manner (see Figure 19.2). However, the progression rate of the lower frequencies is slower. Obviously individual susceptibility plays a significant role in the eventual NIHL (Gold et al., 1989).

In contrast to the log–time relationship between TTS and the intensity level of continuous noise, clinical experiences and studies have shown that this pattern does not necessarily occur with impulsive noise (Luz and Hodge, 1971; Hamernik et al., 1989). Delayed TTS (rebound recovery function – Luz and Hodge, 1971) ranging from 5 minutes up to 4 hours after the cessation of the impulsive exposure may occur. Furthermore, an increase of TTS at 1 or 4 hours after the exposure was also noted (Dancer et al., 1991).

# Otoacoustic emissions in the detection of NIHL

Currently, NIHL is established using a pure-tone audiogram performed in an attenuated room with calibrated earphones. Such testing needs the cooperation of the subject, is time-consuming and requires special equipment and skilled audiologists. Furthermore, pure-tone audiometry suffers from insensitivity to subtle noise-induced cochlear damage. These disadvantages limit the use of the pure-tone audiogram in active military personnel needing close audiological monitoring. To overcome these pitfalls partially, an alternative or supplementary approach has been introduced since the identification of otoacoustic emissions (OAE). This objective measure is a sensitive indication of the activity at the threshold level of the outer hair cell situated within the cochlea. With a miniature probe sealed in the outer ear and following brief click stimuli, the emissions can be recorded almost immediately. Using other types of pure-tone stimuli ($F_1$ and $F_2$) a distortion product ($2f_1 - f_2$) of OAEs is recorded reflecting the suprathreshold activity of the outer hair cells. Thus, the OAE has the necessary features to serve as an objective, sensitive and quick tool for screening and diagnosing NIHL.

In general, the presence of click evoked OAEs (CEOAEs) mostly indicates behavioural auditory thresholds better than 25 dB HL (Attias et al., 1996). However, the absence of CEOAEs is not necessarily accompanied with changes in the behavioural thresholds, as this may reflect the higher sensitivity of OAE over the audiogram in noting sub-clinical changes (Probst et al., 1987; Franklin et al., 1991; Attias and Bresloff 1996; Attias et al., 1996, 1998). In general, in military personnel with NIHL, the 'loss' noted using CEOAEs is bilateral, affecting primarily the high frequencies, the OAE response level is reduced and the frequency range of the emissions is narrowed (up to 2 kHz). Thus, recording emissions in the lower-frequency region with absence in the high frequency strongly indicates noise-induced emission loss and this is closely related to NIHL. If distortion product OAEs (DPOAEs) are used, information on the configuration of the behavioural audiogram can be also obtained (Attias and Bresloff, 1996).

The OAEs are efficient not only in helping the diagnosis of NIHL but also in screening between ears with and ears without NIHL.

Previous studies have shown that if the absence of CEOAEs at 2 kHz and 3 kHz was taken as an indication of NIHL, 92.1% sensitivity (correct discrimination of NIHL) and 79% specificity (correct identification of normal) would have been achieved. The simplicity and speed of the OAEs should encourage their use in military noise environments, where large samples of soldiers could be screened quickly and monitored by an objective and reliable tool.

# Laterality of M-NIHL

Although exposure to noise is expected to affect the two ears symmetrically, clinical observations and studies reporting on laterality document higher incidence and greater severity of NIHL on the left compared with

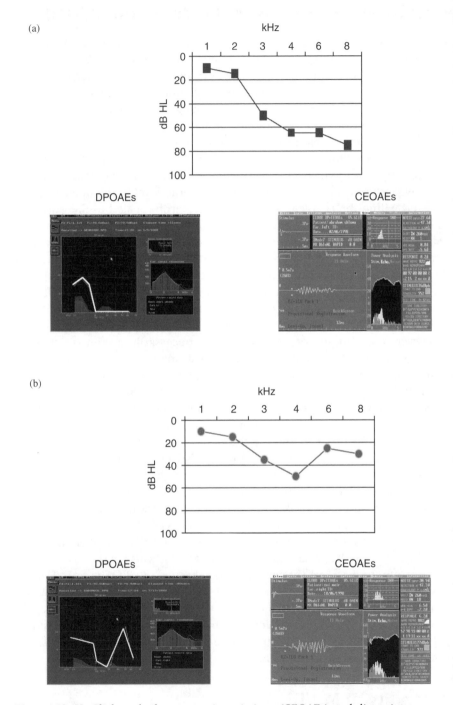

**Figure 19.10** Click-evoked otoacoustic emissions (CEOAEs) and distortion product otoemissions (DPOAEs) in a typical acoustic trauma for each ear separately. (a) A high-frequency hearing loss and (b) a 4-kHz notch.

the right ear (Rudin et al., 1988; May et al., 1990). This phenomenon is seen both in military (Cox and Ford, 1995) and in industrial exposures (Pirila et al., 1991a). The left-ear priority can be seen across the frequency range 2–6 kHz, and particularly at 4 kHz (Pirila et al., 1991b).

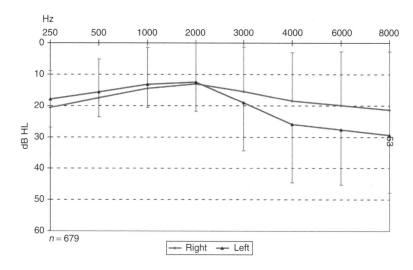

**Figure 19.11** Average audiometric thresholds in right and left ears across 4277 army personnel.

To explore further the association between M-NIHL and laterality, we analysed the audiograms of 4277 army personnel being exposed to military noises. Asymmetry was defined if the severity of NIHL in one ear was worse than that in the other ear by at least more than 15 dB HL at one frequency between 2 and 8 kHz.

**Table 19.2** Table showing symmetry/asymmetry of noise-induced hearing loss (NIHL), in 4277 army personnel

| Percentage | n | NIHL – side |
| --- | --- | --- |
| 34.2 | 1462 | Left |
| 16.3 | 699 | Right |
| 49.5 | 2116 | Symmetrical |
| 100 | 4277 | Total |

Figure 19.11 summarizes the average audiogram across all subjects and Table 19.2 shows the results. About 50% had a symmetrical NIHL, while more than 34% showed left ear dominance compared with 16% with more severe NIHL in the right ear. This phenomenon was found across all ages (Figure 19.12).

In order to explore the association between handedness and NIHL laterality, Table 19.3 details the prevalence of NIHL in military personnel

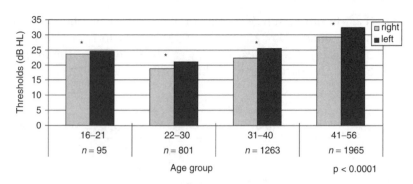

**Figure 19.12** Auditory thresholds 3–8 kHz in the different age groups in 4277 army personnel.

with right and left handedness. It was found that there is no association between handedness and NIHL laterality. Irrespective of the handedness, the left ear was more vulnerable. Subsequently, a detailed examination of the acoustic reflexes was carried out in order to test the possibilities that the NIHL laterality is due to differences in efficacy of the acoustical reflexes. Studying the acoustical reflexes measures in right- and left-handed normal subjects revealed no differences.

**Table 19.3** Tabulation of handedness and symmetry/asymmetry of noise-induced hearing loss (NIHL) in 119 military personnel

| Total | Symmetrical (%) | Right handed (%) | Left handed (%) | NIHL – side of most severe loss |
|-------|-----------------|------------------|-----------------|----------------------------------|
| 93 | 43.01 $n = 40$ | 13.98 $n = 13$ | 43.01 $n = 40$ | Right |
| 26 | 38.46 $n = 10$ | 19.23 $n = 5$ | 42.3 $n = 11$ | Left |
| 119 | 50 | 18 | 51 | Total |

Furthermore, analysis of the acoustic properties of right- and left-handed soldiers firing could not explain the NIHL laterality. According to the expansion of the pressure wave in the firing positions, the right handers shooting from the right shoulder bend their head to the right, and thus the right ear, which is in the shadow of the rifle barrel, is exposed to a lower level compared with the left ear, making the left ear more vulnerable. Inversely in left handers, the damage would be more in the right ear. However, the results of this study, as of another (Chung et al., 1983), show that this cannot fully explain the asymmetry in the left ear.

It seems that cortical and another retrocochlear factor may contribute to this asymmetry.

# Conclusion

Intensive military training is necessarily accompanied by repeated exposure to both impulse and continuous noise resulting in NIHL. The clinical course and properties of the M-NIHL is similar to industrial NIHL but seems to be much more accelerated. The NIHL laterality to the left is more pronounced in the army personnel. Handedness, acoustic reflex measures and firing position could not explain this phenomenon. Although ear protectors can reduce the damage, they cannot prevent it, partly because of the extremely high levels of noise reaching the inner ear by the bone-conduction acoustical pathway. Promising results using biological agents such as Mg are encouraging, suggesting that coupling both types of protection would be more beneficial for the army.

# References

Attias J, Bresloff I (1996) Noise-induced temporary otoacoustic emissions shifts. J Basic Clin Physiol Pharmacol 7: 221–3.

Attias J, Weisz J, Almog S, Shahar A, Wiener M, Joachims Z et al. (1994) Oral magnesium intake reduces permanent hearing loss induced by noise exposure. Am J Otolaryngol 15: 26–32.

Attias J, Shemesh Z, Bar-Or Z, Solomon A, Bleich A, Sohmer H (1995) Psychological profile of help and non-help seeking chronic tinnitus patients. Scand Audiol 24: 13–18.

Attias J, Bresloff I, Reshef I, Horowitz G, Furman V (1998) Evaluating noise induced hearing loss with distortion product otoacoustic emissions. Br J Audiol 32: 39–46.

Attias J, Sapir S, Bresloff I, Reshef-Haran I, Ising H (2004) Reduction in noise induced temporary threshold shift in humans following oral magnesium intake. Clin Otolaryngol 29(6): 635–41.

Chang H (1989) Application of the probe microphone method to measure attenuation of hearing protectors against high impulse pressure levels. Appl Acoust 27: 13–25.

Chung DY, Willson GN, Gannon RP (1983) Lateral differences in susceptibility to noise damage. Audiology 22: 199–205.

Colletti V, Fiorino FG, Verlato G, Montresor GZ (1991) Reduced active protection to the cochlea during physical exercise. Acta Otolaryngologica 111(2): 234–9.

Cox HJ, Ford GR (1995) Hearing loss associated with weapons noise exposure: when to investigate an asymmetrical loss. Journal of Laryngology and Otology 109: 291–5.

Dancer A, Grateau P, Cabanis A, Vaillant T, Lafont D (1991) Delayed temporary threshold shift induced by impulse noise (weapon noises) in men. Audiology 30: 345–56.

Dancer A, Buck K, Hamery P, Parmentier G (1999) Hearing protection in the military environment. Noise and Health 2(5): 1–16.

Franklin DJ, Lonsburry-Martin BL, Stanger BB, Martin GK (1991) Altered susceptibility of 2fl-f2 acoustic-distortion products to the effects of repeated noise exposure in rabbits. Ear and Hearing 53: 185–208.

Gold S, Attias J, Cahani M, Shahar A (1989) Incidence of hearing loss amongst conscripts before and following basic training in the IDF. Harefuah April 7, 377–9.

Guenther T (1981) Biochemistry and pathobiochemistry of magnesium. Magnes Bull 3: 91–101.

Hamernik RP, Ahroon WA, Patterson JA (1989) Threshold recovery functions following impulse noise trauma. J Acoust Soc Am 84: 941–50.

Henselman LW, Henderson D, Shadoan J, Subramaniam M, Saunde S, Ohlin D (1995) Effects of noise exposure, race, and years of service on hearing in the US Army soldiers. Ear Hear 16: 382–91.

Horie M, Irisawa H, Noma A (1987) Voltage dependent magnesium block of ATP – sensitive potassium channel in guinea pig ventricular cell. J Physiol (Lond) 387: 251–72.

Job A, Raynal M, Tricoir A, Signoret J, Rondet P (2000) Hearing status of French youth aged from 18–24 years in 1997 a cross-sectional epidemiological study in the selection center of the army in Vincennes and Lyon. Rev Epidemiol Sante Publique 48(3): 227–37.

Klockhoff I, Lyttkens L, Svedberg A (1986) Hearing damage in military service. A study on 38,294 conscripts. Scand Audiol 15: 217–22.

Lindgern F, Axelsson A (1988) The influence of physical exercise on sensibility to noise induced temporary threshold shift. Scand Audiol 17: 11–17.

Luz GA, Hodge DC (1971) Recovery from impulse-noise induced TTS in monkeys and men: a descriptive model. J Acoust Soc Am 49: 1770–7.

May JJ, Marvel M, Reagan M, Marvel LH, Pratt DS (1990) Noise induced hearing loss in randomly selected New York dairy farmers. Am J Ind Med 18: 333–7.

Paakkonen R, Lehtomaki K, Savolainen S (1998) Noise attenuation of communication hearing protectors against impulse from assault rifle. Milit Med 163: 40–3.

Pelausa EO, Abel SM, Simard J, Dempsey I (1995) Prevention of noise-induced hearing loss in the Canadian military. J Otolaryngol 24: 271–80.

Pirila T, Ervasti KJ, Sorri M (1991a) Hearing asymmetry among left-handed and right-handed persons in a random population. Scand Audiol 20: 223–6.

Pirila T, Sorri M, Ervasti KJ, Sipila P, Karjalainen H (1991b) Hearing asymmetry among occupationally noise exposed men and women under 60 years of age. Scand Audiol 20: 217–22.

Price G (1995) Weapon Noise and Performance. Bourges: Etablissement Technique de Bourges.

Price G, Kalb J, Garinther G (1989) Toward a measure of auditory handicap in the Army. Ann of Oto-Rhinol-Laryngol Supplement 140: 42–52.

Probst R, Lonsburry-Martin BL, Marin GK, Coats AC (1987) Otoacoustic emissions in ears with hearing loss. Am J Otolaryngol 8: 73–81.

Rudin R, Rosenhall U, Svarsudd K (1988) Hearing capacity in samples of men from the general population. Scand Audiol 17: 3–10.

White RE, Hartzell HC (1988) Effects of intracellular free magnesium on calcium current in isolated cardiac myocytes. Science 239: 778–80.

# CHAPTER 20

# The hazardous aspects of music

*Noise and Its Effects:* Edited by Linda Luxon and Deepak Prasher © 2007
John Wiley & Sons Ltd.

ROSALYN A DAVIES

For the large numbers of us for whom music is either a hobby or enjoyable relaxation, the possibility that music itself might cause noise damage in the form of a hearing disorder is disconcerting. On further study, however, some interesting insights emerge. It would appear that music sound levels that would be regarded as hazardous in an industrial context do not cause the same degree of hearing loss in the musician, that auditory 'training' might contribute to this advantage, that violinists and violists have a left-ear deficit, and that by the age of 79 there is no longer a difference between those who have been exposed to noise and those who have not – eventually presbycusis becomes a much more dominant factor.

There are many aspects to determining whether exposure to music will result in hearing loss. These include factors relating to the spectral profile of the noise pressure wave, factors relating to the instrument played and the concert venue, and factors affecting the susceptibility of individuals, whether they are the musicians or the music lovers. This chapter will look at each of these aspects and the evidence to link music to a hearing disorder.

## The music

It has been well established that symphony orchestras, popular orchestras, rock bands and personal stereo headphones produce music with sound pressure levels intense enough to cause permanent hearing loss (Sataloff and Sataloff, 1998). Such hearing loss may be accompanied by tinnitus, hyperacusis or diplacusis, and be severe enough to interfere with performance (Reid, 2001).

The units decibels (A) (or dB (A)) refers to a weighting protocol used to measure broadband noise. A weighted noise measurement integrates the various component frequencies of a broadband acoustic signal and quantifies the noise in a similar way to the healthy human ear that is most sensitive for the mid-frequencies (approximately 500–4000 Hz). A-weighting is the most commonly used weighting scheme in industrial noise measurement. The Occupational Safety and Health Administration (OSHA) of the USA (Kryter et al., 1966) put forward a hearing conservation regulation to protect the hearing of industrial workers. The 85 dB (A) 8-hour time-weighted average action level is used as a standard for determining potentially damaging noise. At this level, implementation of a hearing conservation programme is required in the USA, and is the 'first action level' in the UK and European Union (Noise at Work Regulations, 1989).

However, studies summarized by Johnson (1991) indicate that the threshold of noise (determined using the International Organization for Standardization's ISO 1999 (ISO, 1990)) that induces a hearing loss is frequency dependent (Table 20.1). He advocates that further longitudinal studies of the effects of long-term exposure should focus on frequencies of 3, 4 and 6 kHz for which critical sound levels can be exceeded even within the noise protection programme.

**Table 20.1** A-weighted levels that will cause no hearing loss from exposure to 8 hours of broadband noise, re: R-1999

| Frequency (Hz) | Level (dB) |
| --- | --- |
| 500 | 93 |
| 1000 | 89 |
| 2000 | 80 |
| 3000 | 77 |
| 4000 | 75 |
| 6000 | 77 |

(Reproduced from Johnson et al., 1991).

### Orchestral music

Sound levels within many orchestras have been shown to exceed allowable OSHA criteria. Jansson and Karlsson (1983), calculated that players received a maximum allowable noise dose in 10–25 hours' working time. They used tripod-mounted microphones and measured $L_{eq}$ values of 93.1 dB (A) for heavy exposure positions and 88.9 dB (A) for light exposure positions during performance. Royster et al. (1991), in detailed studies using Larson Davis 700 integrating sound level meters (dosimeters) clipped onto the musician's collar, measured sound exposures in orchestral musicians. These were evaluated in terms of their potential to cause noise-induced permanent threshold shift, according to the model presented in ISO 1999 (ISO, 1990). These personal dosimeters, measured the musicians' $L_{eq}$ values, allowing a complete time history of sound levels during the measurement period to be recorded and statistically analysed. Sample durations were usually 2–3 hours. These $L_{eq}$ values were then converted to equivalent daily 8-hour exposures to use the ISO 1999 model. The mean noise exposure thus measured was 85.5 dB (A) (maximum 94.7 dB (A); minimum 74.7 dB (A)); mean peak sound pressure level (SPL) was 124.9 dB (A) with maximum of 143.5 dB (A). The authors concluded, nevertheless, that the chance of acoustic trauma occurring during orchestral music was quite small.

Other studies have measured the noise exposure of different pieces in the classical repertoire. Kingston (1998), in his article identified music that might exceed the UK recommended 'mandatory action level' of 90 dB (Noise at Work Regulations, 1989) (Table 20.2). Prior to this, Camp and Horstman (1992) had identified noise levels of more than 110 dB(A) in some parts of the orchestra during playing of *Götterdämmerung* from Wagner's *Ring Cycle*.

**Table 20.2** Who is the loudest of them all?

* *Poem of Ecstasy*, Scriabin
* *Rite of Spring*, Stravinsky
* *1812 Overture*, Tchaikovsky
* *Also Sprach Zarathustra*, Richard Strauss
* *Symphony of a Thousand*, Mahler
* *Symphony No. 3*, Prokofiev
* *Earth Dances*, Birtwhistle
* *Symphony No. 2*, Shostakovich

(Reproduced with permission from Kingston, 1998).

## Rock-and-roll/popular music

Common to rock-and-roll and popular music is the uniform intensity range achieved by the sound engineer. In the late 1960s and early 1970s, levels of 120 dB (A) were routinely measured (Rintelman and Borus, 1968; Lebo et al., 1970). Lebo and Oliphant (1968) measured maximum outputs of 120 dB at 500 Hz through 300-W amplifiers, noting that only small speakers face the musician. Thus the musicians could hear the other instruments and keep time, but most of the high sound level, low-frequency component was produced in front of the musicians.

With the advent of lower distortion amplifiers, the volume can be increased further without audible distortion. The loud noise not only provides atmosphere but also masks out discrepancies between the high technology of the recording studios and the low fidelity of the concert venues. Thus modern pop concerts often produce much higher sound levels of over 135 dB (A) (Drake-Lee, 1992), with peaks even exceeding 150 dB (C) (Kähäri et al., 2003). By comparison, jazz, blues, and country and western are generally quieter with levels of 80–101 dB (A) measured on stage.

### Personal cassette players with earphones

Personal cassette players are capable of producing potentially damaging noise levels of up to 136 dB (A) in artificial ears (Wood and Lipscombe, 1972).

However, higher averaged thresholds have not been demonstrated in vivo, in young people who listen to pop music through headphones. Rice et al. (1987) have studied the sound levels at which young people listen to personal stereos and although their results tend to be reassuring they were correlated to subjective reports of hearing disability rather than by measurement of audiometric thresholds. They estimated the risk of hearing loss consequent upon a 10-year listening period, to be 1 in 1500.

## The instrument

There are now many studies that indicate that the SPLs of selected orchestral instruments are loud enough to cause noise damage (Teie, 1998).

**Four different instrument groups according to their measured $L_{eq}$ values, Royster et al. (1991):**

- Group 1: violin and viola.
- Group 2: horn, trumpet and trombone.
- Group 3: clarinet, flute, bassoon and percussion.
- Group 4: bass, cello, harp and piano.

Frequency histograms of sampling-period $L_{eq}$ values measured for the four different groups are shown in Figure 20.1. The values for the brass and percussion tend to be in the upper portion of the overall range. The $L_{eq}$ values for violins and violas are spread throughout the entire range whereas the values for group four (bass, cello harp and piano) fall in the lower half of the range.

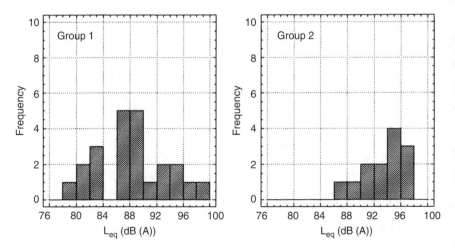

**Figure 20.1** Frequency histograms of sampling $L_{eq}$ values measured for four different groups. (Reproduced with permission from Royster et al., 1991.)

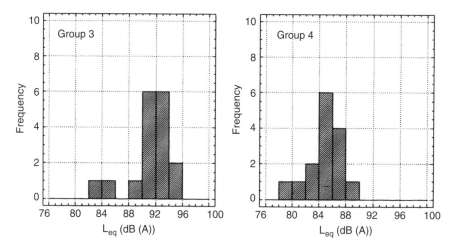

**Figure 20.1** continued.

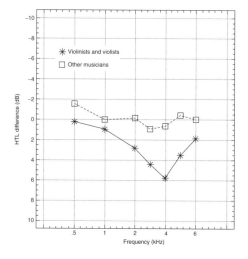

**Figure 20.2** Mean interaural threshold difference (left ear hearing threshold level (HTL) minus right ear HTL) for violinists and violists and for other musicians. (Reproduced with permission from Royster et al., 1991.)

The mean hearing threshold levels (HTLs) for the four different groups from Royster et al. (1991) were grossly similar to each other when analysed by decade. However ear-specific deficits have been demonstrated in violinists and violists, the left ear showing a greater hearing loss than the right (Ostri et al., 1989; Royster et al., 1991) (Figure 20.2). This is presumably because the left ear has a greater noise exposure as it is closer to the sound board, the right ear being protected by the head shadow effect.

**Table 20.3** Sound levels of various instruments

| Instrument | Sound level (dB (A)) |
|------------|:--------------------:|
| Violin | 84–103 |
| Cello | 84–92 |
| Bass | 75–83 |
| Piccolo | 95–102 |
| Flute | 85–11 |
| Clarinet | 92–103 |
| French horn | 90–106 |
| Oboe | 80–94 |
| Trombone | 85–114 |
| Xylophone | 90–92 |

(From Folprechtova and Miksovska, 1978.)

# Factors affecting hearing loss

In the investigation of the hazardous effects of music, studies have included both large-scale field studies and experiments with animal models (Johnson, 1991).

## Temporary threshold shift and permanent threshold shift

Measurements used to determine the effects of different factors in causing hearing loss include the temporary threshold shift (TTS) and the permanent threshold shift (PTS), as determined by pure-tone audiometry. The TTS is the temporary elevation of threshold at one or more test frequencies and is often associated with a numbness or dullness in the ears, with or without tinnitus, and typically lasts 16–18 hours. It is considered to be an early warning sign for a potentially PTS, and, if the noise does not cause a TTS, then it will not cause a PTS. The TTS tends to occur half an octave above the stimulus frequency, and is at 3000–6000 Hz for most noise sounds and for music. For very-low-frequency sound, < 500 Hz, the TTS is 300–750 Hz (Mills et al., 1983). Recovery from the TTS depends on the duration and intensity of the noise exposure (Melnick, 1991).

Attempts to standardize measurements of noise exposure date back to 1966 with the formation of the Committee on Hearing and Bioacoustics (CHABA – Kryter et al., 1966). A model of 'damage risk contours' was developed but did not take account of the less damaging effects of intermittent noise with regular quiet periods (Speaks et al., 1990; Ward, 1991). Since that time, further models have been developed such as ISO 1999 (ISO, 1990) which are sufficiently accurate to support the needs of most regulators, administrators and others who need guidance in setting acceptable limits for noise exposure.

It is generally considered that it is the intermittent nature of hazardous peak sound levels that contributes significantly to the reduced noise damage identified in musicians, when compared with those exposed to apparently equivalent noise levels. A study of impulse noise allows further insight into the hazards imposed (Price and Kalb, 1991). For example, although the peak SPLs of some percussionists – wooden blocks in popular music or orchestral cymbals – may be up to 150 dB SPL, it is the shape of the pressure wave and its spectral intensity that determine noise damage.

## Spectral shape and spectral intensity

The individual components of music that relate to noise damage include both the spectral shape and the spectral intensity of the music. Lebo and Oliphant (1969) showed that the spectral shape of orchestral noise was from 500 to 4000 Hz, whereas for rock-and-roll music most of the sound energy was at 250–500 Hz. They concluded that the spectral intensity varied depending on:

- the piece of music being performed;
- the performance hall in which the piece was being played;
- the acoustic conditions;
- the preferences of the conductor;
- the technique of the individual musician.

The concept of 'effective quiet' has evolved whereby estimates have been made of the upper sound level limit that would produce no TTS. For example, rock bands might never achieve an effective quiet level whereas the noise exposure of a quartet player might never exceed this value. The estimate would depend on the musical piece, the size of the band/orchestra and the exact location of the musician within the group.

## Exchange rates

Further sophistication has been achieved in measuring the dose of hazardous noise levels by the introduction of the term 'exchange rate'. Following on from the CHABA document (Kryter et al., 1966), the contours of equal risk of permanent hearing loss can be determined by the specified intensity and the specified duration of exposure. A 3-dB exchange rate means an identical risk if the sound level is increased by 3 dB but for only half the time of exposure – damage of a 95 dB (A) noise level for 8 hours is the equivalent of a 98 dB (A) noise level for 4 hours. The same logic is applied for a 5-dB exchange rate and implicit in this is that a 5-dB exchange rate identifies a lower risk than a 3-dB exchange rate. The report on the results from the International Institute of Noise Control Engineering Working Party considered that the 3-dB rule was probably a more reasonable exchange rate for daily noise exposure (Embleton, 1995).

# The musician/the listener

For the purpose of studying the hazardous effects of music, the term 'musician' has been used to include all those who actively work with music, that is songwriters, musicians of different genres, singers, disc jockeys and sound technicians. For all, whether they are rock-and-roll artists, orchestral players or the next Pavarotti, their chosen profession may confer a risk to their hearing. The vocational hearing requirements of musicians are greater and more specific than in most professions. Raised auditory thresholds in a violinist may incline the player to over-bowing to create the perceived sound intensity. Noise-induced tinnitus may interfere with hearing crucial to a good performance or a right entry. The songwriter/musician may have difficulties mixing recorded music in the studio to achieve the right balance.

## Symptoms

In response to confirmation of noise damage in some orchestral musicians, the Association of British Orchestras (ABO) commissioned a report attempting to deal with the issues confronting the musicians with regard to their hearing (Reid, 2001). A questionnaire was sent to 500 players in the UK. The auditory symptoms reported by players included tinnitus, hearing loss, hyperacusis, recruitment, 'cocktail party' effect and diplacusis. Frequent or occasional tinnitus was reported by 35–40% of the players, often triggered by noise, with woodwind players most likely to report this symptom. Of those reporting tinnitus, 30% found it bothersome and 6% were 'very bothered'. A fifth of players had perfect pitch at the outset of their musical careers, and a third of these felt that it had drifted. A quarter of woodwind players reported hyperacusis.

A similar questionnaire study was reported by Kähäri et al. (2003) from the responses of 139 Swedish rock/jazz musicians. Hearing loss or other hearing disorder was reported in 74%, with women being more likely to report hyperacusis, or hyperacusis plus tinnitus, than men. However, women showed bilateral, significantly better hearing thresholds at 3–6 kHz than men. They stressed the importance of evaluating all kinds of hearing problems in musicians because of their occupational dependence on optimally functioning hearing.

## Pure-tone audiometry

Musicians do develop noise-induced hearing loss (NIHL): 52% and 30% of classical and rock/pop musicians, respectively, were found to have a permanent hearing loss (as reviewed by Chasin, 1999) measured by pure-tone audiometry. Some studies have found that their notches centred on 6 kHz, probably because music has a greater high-frequency content than industrial noise, but the use of TDH39 headphones raises the possibility of the 6-kHz notch being artefactual. Musicians also often show more damage in the ear closer to the output of their instrument.

The effect of hearing loss at 3000–6000 Hz is to make it difficult for the musicians to hear some tones and some harmonics. Inability to hear these sounds can affect perception of timbre and balance. All tones are associated with overtones (harmonics) that occur at the same time. It is these overtones and the way in which they cluster into areas of strong harmonics that characterize the timbre of the instrument. Thus loss of some of the harmonics will affect music perception and recognition, and carries the risk of interfering with performance.

## PTS in orchestral musicians

Studies on orchestral musicians (Axelsson and Lindgren, 1981; Johnson et al., 1985; Ostri et al., 1989; Royster et al., 1991) have been relatively consistent as to the impact of orchestral music noise on HTLs when age-related reference data, that is ISO 7029 (ISO, 1984) has been used (Table 20.4).

**Table 20.4** Showing the main conclusions of 4 studies of the hearing loss in orchestral musicians

| Reference | Musicians | Conclusions |
| --- | --- | --- |
| Axelsson and Lindgren (1981) Götebotg | 139 musicians (some with previous military noise exposure) | • Notches seen<br>• Poorest HTL at 6 kHz<br>• Degree of loss small<br>• Greatest loss in bassoon, brass and left ears of violin and viola players |
| Johnson et al. (1985) Minnesota | 60 orchestral members from the Minnesota Orchestra | • Differences between actual HTLs and age-related thresholds < 10 dB<br>• Notches identified at 6 kHz |
| Ostri et al. (1989) Denmark | 95 orchestral musicians from the Royal Danish Theatre (presbyacusis reference material: ISO 7029) | • Median hearing thresholds (0.5, 1, 2, 4, 8kHz) increased for all age groups<br>• Notched configuration in 50% male and 13% female musicians<br>• Left ear deficit among violinists |
| Royster et al. (1991) North Carolina | 59 musicians from the Chicago Symphony Orchestra (reference material: ISO 7029) | • 53% musicians showed notched audiograms consistent with NIHL<br>• Violinists and violists showed poorer HTLs at 3–6 kHz in the left ear<br>• Bass, cello, harp and piano players, and right ears of violinists had better HTLs in both ears than other musicians |

HTLs, hearing threshold levels; NIHL, noise-induced hearing loss.

It is worth noting that ISO 7029 age-related reference data from 'oto-logically normal' persons, are considered by some audiologists to be a 'supernormal' data set. When compared with an unscreened, age-related normal population (Robinson, 1988; Davis, 1994), these musicians would be found to have a smaller degree of hearing loss.

### Permanent threshold shift in popular music and rock-and-roll

Rintelman and Borus (1968) assessed 42 college rock musicians and found no evidence of threshold shift in 95% of the musicians, suggest-ing that the risks are generally overrated. Axelsson et al. (1995) followed up 53 out of the 83 pop/rock musicians, whom they had studied in 1975, for evidence of progression of hearing loss. In their first study 13% of the musicians had a hearing loss of more than 20 dB HL at a high-frequency pure-tone average (3, 4, 6 and 8 kHz). Interestingly the median pure-tone audiogram recorded 20 years later was within 20 dB HL at all test frequencies. These musicians had been performing for 26 years and had been exposed to more or less continuous sound levels of more than 85 dB HL while playing. The range of HTL distribu-tion had increased and the median HTLs for the eight musicians who played percussion – those most exposed to impulsive sounds – showed the poorest hearing (Figure 20.3).

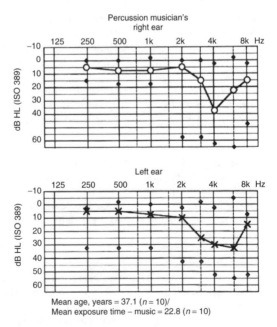

Figure 20.3 Pure-tone thresholds for musicians playing percussion instruments, median, 10th and 90th percentiles. (Reproduced with permission from Axelsson et al., 1995.)

The Swedish study from Kähäri et al. (2003) showed that female musicians had bilaterally better hearing thresholds at 3, 4 and 6 kHz when compared with men, who showed a broader distribution within the 10th to 90th percentiles than a reference population. The men also showed a left-ear deficit. They concluded, however, that studying hearing loss in musicians only, without consideration of other hearing disorders, minimizes the hazardous effects of music faced by rock and jazz musicians.

Both Axelsson and Lindgrendate and Kähäri et al., proposed a protective effect from a continuous contraction of the stapedius muscle at sound levels at and above 85 dB, and the 'training effect' (see below) to explain the very moderate influence on hearing sensitivity after performing pop/rock music for many years.

## TTS and popular music

Drake-Lee (1992) studied three of the four members (ages 25–37) of a heavy metal band, Man O War, with pre- and post-concert audiograms. He found that the pre-concert audiograms from the three out of the four players without a history of ear problems all had a 6-kHz dip suggestive of early noise damage (Figure 20.4). The chief sound engineer regularly

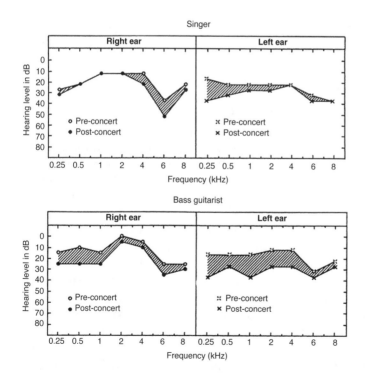

**Figure 20.4** Temporary threshold shifts, post-concert, in two musicians in a heavy metal band (the singer wore protection to the right ear during the concert). (Reproduced with permission from Drake-Lee, 1992.)

recorded levels of more than 135 dB (SPL-A) both on the stage and in the auditorium. The frequency of output rarely measured more than 8000 Hz and the peak was 500–1000 Hz. Interestingly, the post-concert audiogram showed a shift at all frequencies except for that of the singer who wore ear protection in the right ear. Audiograms for the singer and one of the other performers are shown in Figure 20.4.

Although the pop music venue delivers music loudly, the earphones of the personal hi-fi are capable of delivering levels of over 115 dB, and transient threshold shifts have been documented after 3 hours' exposure, although returning to normal within 24 hours (Katz et al., 1982). Bradley et al. (1987) reported on the exposure of schoolchildren to amplified music and reported that 37% of the children studied owned a personal cassette player. Hearing difficulties and tinnitus were reported more frequently by those children who owned a personal cassette player than by those who did not.

# Further assessment of the musician

Diagnostic measures for the early identification and prevention of NIHL include standard pure-tone and Békésy audiometry; otoacoustic emissions (OAEs) (transient emission OAEs or TEOAEs and distortion product OAEs or DPOAEs) and psychophysical measurements. The role of measurement of OAEs and psychophysical parameters is discussed below.

### Otoacoustic emissions

The outer hair cells (OHCs) of the cochlea are the first to show damage with hazardous noise levels. OAEs allow the objective, non-invasive quantification of OHC function and have an important role in the assessment of musicians before a PTS develops. Exposure to intense levels of music may induce mechanical and/or metabolic dysfunction of the OHCs. It is known that damage occurs to the OHC without variability at 130 dB (Spoendlin, 1975).

Noise exposure has been used as a tool to examine the relationship between OAE level and hearing threshold, as noise affects emissions and thresholds at specific frequencies (Attias et al., 1995). In their study comparing new recruits with noise-exposed military personnel, the noise-exposed but normal hearing subjects – those with normal hearing thresholds – had reduced overall click-evoked OAE power with a narrower frequency range compared with the new recruits with normal hearing. Further groups of military personnel with different degrees of hearing loss, as assessed by audiometry, were also studied (groups C, D, E, F and G) and the spectral analysis of their click-evoked OAEs, and the median audiograms are shown in Figure 20.5.

Lack of emissions did not necessarily indicate hearing thresholds worse than 20 dB HL, suggesting that emission loss should always be considered a more sensitive and therefore earlier indicator of cochlear damage.

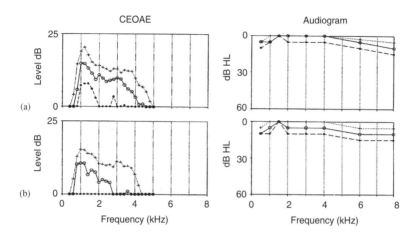

**Figure 20.5** Spectral analysis of the median click-evoked otoacoustic emissions (CEOAEs) and the median audiograms of (a) the normal, non-exposed to noise group, and (b) the normal-hearing, noise-exposed group. o, the median power of the emission response; •, low quartile; +, high quartile. (Reproduced with permission from Attias et al., 1995.)

## The effects of loss of OHC function

- Reduction of *cochlear amplification* leading to loss of hearing sensitivity to soft to moderate sounds (40–60 dB).
- Reduction of *frequency selectivity* and *spectral resolution* leading to diplacusis, i.e. an abnormal perception of pitch.
- Lack of *cochlear compression* leading to recruitment, an abnormal perception of loudness.

All these conditions are serious for the musician, the first driving the musician to play harder, causing strain and more hearing loss, the second causing difficulties with judgment of pitch, and the third effectively spoiling the musician's judgment of loudness.

### Distortion product otoacoustic emissions

Distortion product otoacoustic emissions are considered to be the OAEs the most specific for frequency. Two tones are presented simultaneously and a third tone (the distortion product) is created. DPOAEs were studied by Guthrie (2001) on 16 male musicians and 16 male non-musicians with normal hearing thresholds of 0–20 dB, as measured by pure-tone audiometry; 63% of the musicians displayed impaired OHC function at 4000 Hz on the right (56% on the left) and 25% of the non-musicians showed impaired function at the same frequency in the same ear (25% on the left). These statistically significant results support the concept that DPOAEs might be able to identify music-induced hearing loss with a 4-kHz noise notch before it is detectable by audiometry.

### Efferent suppression of OAEs

Further understanding of auditory physiology suggests that the OHCs of the cochlea are more susceptible to noise trauma than the inner ear cells (IHCs) (Saunders et al., 1985). OHCs are known to have an important role in the frequency selectivity of the cochlea and have energy-dependent motile properties. OHCs may act to attain adaptation to high sound pressure and to control the damping characteristics of the basilar membrane.

The medial efferents carried in the olivocochlear bundle are thought to be involved with the specific motile properties of the OHCs and may modulate the calcium-induced slow motility, which in turn alters the active mechanisms dependent on the fast OHC electromotility. The functional significance of medial efferents on cochlear micromechanics is thought to be a protective effect on the OHCs, mediated by acetylcholine, reducing the OHC active mechanism.

The suppression of OAEs mediated by the efferent system can be assessed using contralateral noise. Micheyl (1997) showed a significant difference in suppression figures between musicians and non-musicians, with musicians showing a greater TEOAE amplitude reduction upon contralateral noise stimulation than non-musicians. The medial olivocochlear bundle is the final link in the descending pathway from the auditory cortex to the OHCs and Micheyl provided anatomical and functional data to support the hypothesis that increased olivocochlear bundle activity is the result of increased activity in higher centres.

Thus, on the basis that the efferent system has a protective role on the health of the OHCs, those musicians with better contralateral suppression will be better protected against the damaging effects of noise. The findings of Micheyl argue for the possibility that the finding of enhanced contralateral suppression reflects a state of auditory training achieved in musicians (see below).

### Psychophysical tests

In 1990, West and Evans studied 60 subjects (non-musicians) aged 15–23 years (from the University of Keele) looking for hearing loss caused by amplified music. They used 'high resolution' (4 minutes per octave) sweep frequency Békésy tracking audiometry and measurement of auditory frequency resolution at 4 kHz using the psychophysical, comb-filtered, noise-masking technique. They noted that the earliest sign of hearing loss was a decrease in frequency resolution, and that pitch discrimination was reduced in subjects who had experienced TTS or tinnitus following exposure to amplified music. There was a significantly increased occurrence of audiometric notches in the 3.5- to 6-kHz frequency range in the 'older exposed' group than in the 'younger exposed' and control groups. Few of these notches were centred at 4 or 6 kHz and the majority would not have been detected by fixed frequency audiometry at conventional audiometric frequencies. Equivalent rectangular auditory bandwidths were significantly wider in subjects who reported TTS and/or post-exposure tinnitus (lasting more than 5 minutes following exposure) compared with those who did not. The finding of widened auditory bandwidth has been correlated with poor speech recognition – difficulties of a 'cocktail party' nature – and implies some damage to the cochlear filtering mechanism.

# Individual susceptibility

It had always been considered that individual susceptibility to NIHL related to genetic factors such as pigmentation (melanoderms having superior survival of hearing when compared with leucoderms), sex (females having superior survival of hearing) and age (Robinson, 1988). It has become apparent following controlled studies that the influence of these intrinsic variables is relatively small and cannot explain the wide range of hearing loss in demographic studies (Henderson and Hamernik, 1988). Increasingly, biological factors are thought to contribute to susceptibility to NIHL – acoustic reflex effectiveness, cochlear efferent activity and interactions of environmental factors (such as drugs) with noise (Henderson et al., 1993).

Cardiovascular function and overall fitness reduce the probability of hearing loss following noise trauma. Sanders and Axelsson (1981) showed a reduction in the TTS in shipyard workers exposed to industrial noise after an 8-month training programme. The interplay of low $O_2$ levels with noise in increasing the TTS to noise is postulated to occur as a result of metabolic exhaustion. It is also thought possible that smoking increases the risk of noise damage by increasing carbon monoxide levels.

# Auditory toughening/training

It has emerged that the auditory system is able to modify its susceptibility to damage from noise, depending on previous exposure. Miller et al. (1963) first showed the 'toughening effect' of prior exposure to spectrally similar noise by demonstrating a reduction in hearing loss when a damaging level of that same noise was then administered. Subramaniam et al. (1991) exposed chinchillas to octave-band noise at 0.5 kHz for 6 hours/day for 10 days at 95 dB and then after 5 days exposed them to the same noise at 106 dB for 48 hours. By comparison with a control group, the previously exposed group was rendered less susceptible to damage from traumatic exposure. In a group of 12 teenage volunteers, Miyakita et al. (1992) demonstrated that the TTS induced by a 105 dB SPL noise at 2000 Hz for 10 minutes, was reduced by prior exposure to music at 70 dB (A) for 6 hours/day during the 9-day training period. To date the exact timing of a possible maximum training effect is unknown and probably will depend on a variety of experimental conditions, not all controlled for by existing studies. The exact physiological mechanisms underlying this type of training effect still remain unclear.

## Emotional factors

Clearly an important distinction between occupational noise as experienced by industrial workers and music experienced by the musician/or concert lover relates to the pleasure given. One explanation for the apparent reduction in PTS experienced by the musician in comparison to the industrial worker for the same noise exposure level is the activity of the higher central pathways which feed onto the olivocochlear bundle, affecting the activity of the OHCs. Axelsson et al. (1995) have suggested that the emotional responses to the music played, including boredom, can affect the NIHL. Earlier studies from Lindgren and Axelsson (1983) indicate that there is a significant reduction in TTS if the sound is non-informative noise, but of equal intensity and duration. Swanson et al. (1987) showed that the TTS was less in a group of 10 who liked a particular type of popular music than in 10 who disliked that pop music, following exposure for 10 minutes. This supports the view that sounds perceived as offensive produce greater TTS than sounds perceived as enjoyable.

On the assumption that 'nice music results in less damage', the musicians in the ABO study (Reid et al., 2001) were asked if they were happy and relaxed: 5% of brass players felt that they spent all their time playing music that they strongly disliked; 18% of woodwind players spent half their time making a 'loathsome' noise; and 10% of the orchestra spent more than half their time playing music that they strongly disliked.

This possible stress-mediated emotional effect is to some degree supported by animal models where prednisolone was associated with a partial restoration of the cochlear microphonic and full restoration of the auditory brain-stem responses in guinea-pig ears exposed to noise (Lamm and Arnold, 1997).

# Room acoustics

Musical venues may vary from recording studio to clubs, churches and dedicated concert halls. It is well established that four features are essential for a good performance venue: an adequately intense sound level; an early first sound reflection; evenly distributed sound; and appropriate reverberation time (Chasin, 1996).

The use of baffles in concert halls helps to fulfil at least three of these criteria. Baffles are large, rigid, reflective surfaces, sometime known as 'clouds', which enhance sound levels and are angled in such a way (as calculated by ray acoustics) to give an early first sound reflection. The distance between the lateral walls determines the 'intimacy' of the music, which is heightened if the first sound reflection is less than 20 ms. Subsequent reflections merge into a reverberation pattern that characterizes the hall. Baffles can also stop 'flutter echo', the effect that occurs when the incident and reflected waves interact constructively and destructively. When the lateral walls of the concert venue are parallel, standing waves can be set up, again preventing even distribution of sound.

The Boston Symphony Hall, built in 1900, was designed according to the principles of Walter Sabine's studies on reverberation time (RT). The RT is the time, in seconds, for a sound to decay by 60 dB and is directly proportional to the volume of the hall and indirectly proportional to the total sound absorption. Various styles of music are flattered differentially according to the RT of a particular concert venue. Low RTs tend to deaden the sound but high RTs degrade speech clarity. For example, baroque music is best performed in venues with an RT of 1.6–2.0 ms (matching the RT of the palace music rooms of that era), and the romantic music of the nineteenth and twentieth centuries is best played within halls with longer RTs of 2.0 ms or more.

Rehearsal rooms can potentially pose a risk to hearing because of hazardous sound levels produced by the practising musician. To minimize this risk, a minimum volume of at least 17 m$^3$ is required, and ideally, the room is irregularly shaped and fitted with well-selected acoustic finishes (Chasin, 1996).

# Recommendations for noise protection

Knowing that hearing disorders are a possible consequence of an occupation associated with music, it becomes paramount to provide effective hearing protection for musicians. The approaches that are recommended are similar to those offered to workers at risk from industrial noise damage and include environmental modification as well as customized ear protection for the individual.

The simplest of strategies to minimize the hazardous effects of music is humming. Humming elicits the stapedial reflex causing the ossicular chain to tighten and slightly attenuating the sound transmitted to the cochlea. If humming is started just prior to a loud external noise and continued throughout, the humming will afford some protection to hazardous noise levels. Clearly this is not always an appropriate measure for sound protection!

One rationale for the reduced susceptibility of certain musicians to the hazardous noise levels of music is that appertaining to woodwind and brass players. These musicians constantly blow against resistance resulting in the Valsalva effect. This creates a mild middle-ear dysfunction resulting in an 'earplug' effect.

## Four ear protection alternatives

The following ear protection approaches have been found to be of most use in the Musicians Clinic at the Centre for Human Performance and Health Promotion in Hamilton, Canada (Chasin and Chong, 1991):

- ER-15: this device uses an acoustic amplifier embedded in the earplug. Higher frequencies, normally lost by placement of an obstruction in the ear canal, are pre-emphasized and a uniform attenuation of about 15 dB is achieved.
- ER-15 SP: a more recent version of the of the ER-15, which is physically smaller and with less high-frequency attenuation.
- ER-20/HI-FI: an acoustic amplifier is used, but with different characteristics to the ER-15. This device allows for about 20-dB attenuation but with a high-frequency roll-off. (Note that the ER series is predicated to the relative attenuation of both the fundamental and the harmonic structure of music.)
- Vented/tuned: this is a custom-made swimmer's earplug with a tunable vent drilled through the centre. With a 3-mm diameter vent, the earplug is acoustically transparent up to 2000 Hz, but has 30 dB of high-frequency attenuation.

Musicians are counselled that an earplug in both ears is better than an earplug in just one.

Chasin and Chong (1991) have developed a protocol to assess spectral levels at the musician's eardrum with and without ear protection, while playing their instruments. This provides the tester with the range of intensities and frequencies that can be produced by the musician, and therefore the requirements made of ear protection.

Knowledge of the individual musicians' strategies for intensity monitoring and definition of quality help to refine the choice of ear protection (Chasin, 2003). For example, reeded woodwinds are likely to use a high-frequency cue for intensity monitoring and therefore an ER-15 is the attenuator of choice. For the violinist, it is crucial to have significant harmonic audibility, and again a low, broadband attenuation earplug such as the ER-15 is likely to be appropriate. Other woodwinds and larger string instruments possess little fundamental and harmonic energy in the higher frequencies, and the ideal ear protection would let through the low-frequency sounds but attenuate the high-frequency sounds from the brass section sitting nearby. A vented/tuned ear plug is useful for these musicians (Chasin, 2000). For the percussionist, the high hat cymbal, typically on the left side of the drummer, provides the most damaging element, resulting in a left ear hearing deficit for these players. An ER-20/HI-FI will provide a level of attenuation of the high frequencies without interfering with the player's monitoring ability. The solo vocalist is also at risk of self-induced hearing loss and can benefit from vented/tuned earplugs, but can use ER-15 earplugs if singing with other instruments.

To verify the performance of the chosen earplugs, a probe-microphone system is used to measure the real-ear occluded gain. After measuring the unaided response, the response with the earplug in place is measured with the probe tube just extending beyond the end of the earplug bore in the ear canal (Chasin and Chong, 1991). The frequency-specific protection provided by a range of earplugs is shown in Figure 20.6

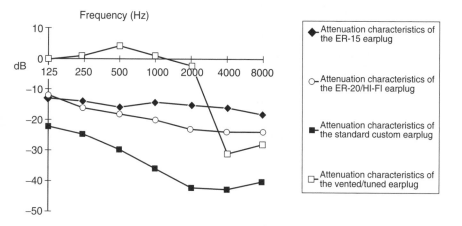

**Figure 20.6** The real-ear attenuation characteristics of the three types of musicians' earplugs and of a standard custom earplug for reference. (Reproduced with permission from Chasin and Chong, 1991.)

## Moderation

Alternation of noisy days with quiet days for musicians is a principle of noise protection with a good theoretical basis. Studies show a resolution of the TTS caused by noise or music after 16–18 hours, and regulations regarding exposure require an upper limit of 'off-time' to minimize the noise-exposure rating. Violinists and violists can use mutes while playing reducing overall daily noise exposure.

## Environmental strategies

Shielding the noise source or increasing the distance between the noise source and the listener can minimize noise exposure. Elevation of the trumpet players on stage ensures that much of the damaging mid-and high-frequency energy goes over the heads of the players in front. Plexiglas baffles can be erected between the cymbals and jazz/blues woodwind players but should not extend higher than a drummer's ear. This ensures that drummers are not subject to their own high-frequency reflections.

Violins and violas should always be played away from overhangs such as those commonly found in orchestral pits. The loudness of high-frequency harmonic components is reduced by the acoustic proofing of these overhangs and induces the violin and viola players to play harder to compensate for this lost energy, producing an unnecessary increased sound level with consequent arm strain.

**The ABO (Reid, 2001) have made the following recommendations:**

- playing of quieter pieces;
- balancing of concert programme to include quieter pieces;
- use of quieter instruments;
- placing of brass on risers of at least 50 cm and preferably 1 m high;
- avoiding putting one row of brass in front of another;
- allowing 2 metres of clear space in front of the orchestra;
- use of baffles at 45° to the floor, behind the horns;
- not putting violins under overhangs that come within 1 m of their heads;
- using Perspex/polycarbonate screens to shield players from noisy sections;
- creation of an in-house expert team;
- auditory training of players.

**Table 20.5** Strategies and devices for reducing hearing loss in musicians

| Instrument | Problems | Solutions |
| --- | --- | --- |
| Small strings | Overhang | Move away from overhang |
| | Own music | ER-15 earplugs |
| | Practising | Practise with mute in place |
| Large strings | Brass section | Vented/tuned earplugs |
| | | Brass on risers |
| | Monitoring | Acoustic monitor tube (cello) |
| Brass | Other musician complaints | Brass on risers |
| | Practice | Acoustic/electronic practice mute |
| | Other brass | Baffles |

**Table 20.5** continued

| Instrument | Problems | Solutions |
|---|---|---|
| Woodwinds | Instruments to rear | Brass on risers |
| | | Earplugs |
| | Amplified instruments | Move parallel to speakers |
| Percussion | High hats | Practice pads |
| | | Closed high hats |
| | Monitoring | Shakers |
| | | Custom earphones |
| | Wrist strain | ER-25 |
| Amplified instruments | Speakers | Move parallel to the speaker |
| | | Elevate speakers |
| | | ER-15 earplugs |
| | Monitoring | Shakers |
| | | Custom earphones |
| Vocalists | Speakers | ER-15 or vented/ tuned earplugs |
| | Monitoring | Custom earphones |

(From Chasin (1996) with permission.)

Chasin (1996) includes a table in his appendices that summarizes the strategies and devices for reducing hearing loss in musicians (Table 20.5).

# Conclusion

Some preliminary conclusions can be drawn. First, the net evidence indicates that NIHL loss occurs in a small proportion of both pop and classical musicians and is causally related to hazardous noise levels. Secondly, the hearing loss is not severe enough to interfere with speech perception, but the effects of mild high-frequency hearing loss have not been well established. Thirdly, if hearing disorders other than hearing loss alone are taken into account – tinnitus, hyperacusis, diplacusis – the chance of a musician experiencing a hazardous effect of music increases.

Detailed studies are required to explore further the factors causing the reduced noise damage in musicians when compared with industrial workers exposed to apparently equivalent noise levels. These factors include the effects of intermittence of noise, the effects of higher centres on olivocochlear bundle function and the resulting dampening of the OHC effects on the basilar membrane.

Finally, there are good reasons to expect that attempts at hearing conservation should not interfere with performance.

# References

Attias J, Furst M, Furman V, Reshaf (Havau) I, Horowitz G, Bresloff I (1995) Noise induced otoacoustic emission loss with or without hearing loss. Ear and Hearing 16: 612–18.

Axelsson A, Lindgren F (1977) Does pop music cause hearing damage? Audiology 16: 432–7.

Axelsson A, Lindgren F (1981) Hearing in classical musicians. Acta Otolaryngologica Supplementum 377: 3–74

Axelsson A, Eliasson A, Israelsson B (1995) Hearing in pop/rock musicians: a follow up study. Ear and Hearing 16: 245–53.

Bradley R, Fortnum H, Coles R (1987) Research note: patterns of exposure of schoolchildren to amplified noise. British Journal of Audiology 21: 119–25.

Camp JE, Horstman SW (1992) Musicians sound exposure during performance of Wagner's Ring Cycle. Medical Problems of Performing Artists 7(2): 37–9.

Chasin M (1996) Musicians and the Prevention of Hearing Loss. San Diego, CA: Singular Publishing Group Inc.

Chasin M (1999) Musicians and the prevention of heaing loss: the A, B, C#. Hearing Review 6(2): 10–16.

Chasin M (2000) Music Appreciation 101: Woodwinds, large stringed instruments, violins and violas. Hearing Review 7(1): 46.

Chasin M (2003) Playing it safe: How to minimize the effects of loud noise and music on hearing. Hearing Professional 52(1): 57.

Chasin M, Chong J (1991) In situ hearing protection program for musicians. Hearing Instruments 42(12): 26–8.

Davis A (ed.) (1994) Hearing in Adults: MRC Institute of Hearing Research. London: Whurr, pp. 327–74.

Drake-Lee AB (1992) Beyond music: auditory temporary threshold shift in rock musicians after a heavy metal concert. Journal of the Royal Society of Medicine 85: 617–19.

Embleton T (1995) Upper limits on noise in the workplace. International Institute of Noise Control Engineering Working Party. Canadian Acoustics 23(2): 11–20.

Folprechtova A, Miksovska O (1978) The acoustic conditions in a symphony orchestra. Pracov Lek 28: 1–2.

Guthrie OW (2001) DPOAEs among normal hearing musicians and non-musicians. The Hearing Review 6(May): 26–8.

Hellstrom PA (1991) The effects on hearing from portable cassette players. A follow–up study. Journal of Sound Vibration 51: 461–9.

Henderson D, Hamernik RP (1988) Impulse noise: a critical review. Journal of Acoustical Society of America 1086, 80(2): 569–84.

Henderson D, Subramaniam M, Boettcher FA (1993) Individual susceptibility to noise induced hearing loss: an old topic revisited. Ear and Hearing 14(3): 152–68.

International Organization for Standardization (1984) ISO 7029: Hearing threshold level assocaited with age for an otologically normal population. Geneva: ISO.

International Organization for Standardization (1990) ISO 1999, 2nd edn: Acoustics – Determination of noise exposure and estimation of noise-induced hearing impairment. Geneva: ISO.

Internationals Organization for Standardization (1991) ISO 389: Acoustics–Standard reference zero for the calibration of pure–tone audiometers 3rd edn. Geneva: ISO.

Jansson E, Karlsson K (1983) Sound levels recorded within the symphony orchestra and risk criteria for hearing loss. Scandanavian Audiology 14: 215–21.

Johnson DL (1991) Field studies: industrial exposures. Journal of the Acoustical Society of America 90(1): 170–4.

Johnson DW, Sherman RE, Aldridge J, Lorraine A (1985) Effects of instrument type and orchestral position on hearing sensitivity for 0.25–20 kHz in the orchestral musician. Scandanavian Audiology 14: 215–21.

Kähäri K, Zachau G, Eklöf M, Sandsjö L, Möller C (2003) Assessment of hearing and hearing disorders in rock/jazz musicians. International Journal of Audiology 42: 279–88.

Katz A, Gerstman H, Sanderson R, Buchanan R (1982) Stereo ear phones and hearing loss. New England Journal of Medicine 307: 1460–1.

Kingston P (1998) Why these people must be protected from themselves. Guardian 20 January: 9.

Kryter KD, Ward WD, Miller JD, Eldredge DH (1966) Hazardous exposures to intermittent and steady-state noise. Journal of the Acoustical Society of America 39: 451–64.

Lamm K, Arnold W (1997) The effect of prednisolone and non-steroidal anti–inflammatory agents on the normal and noise-damaged guinea pig inner ear. Hearing Research 115: 149–68.

Lebo CP, Oliphant KP (1969) Music as a source of acoustic trauma. Laryngoscope 72: 1211–18.

Lebo CP, Oliphant KP, Garrett J (1970) Acoustic trauma from rock and roll music. California Medicine 107: 378–80.

Lindgren F, Axelsson A (1983) Temporary threshold shift after exposure to noise and music of equal energy. Ear and Hearing 4: 197–201.

Melnick W (1991) Human temporary threshold shifts (TTS) and damage risk. Journal of the Acoustical Society of America 90: 147–54.

Micheyl C (1997) Differences in cochlear efferent activity between musicians and non–musicians. NeuroReport 8: 1047–58.

Miller JD, Watson CS, Covell WP (1963) Deafening effects of noise on the cat. Acta Otolaryngologica Supplementum 176: 1–91.

Mills JH, Osguthorpe JD, Burdick CK, Patterson JH, Moza B (1983) Temporary threshold shifts produced by exposure to low-frequency noises. Journal of the Acoustical Society of America 73: 918–23.

Miyakita T, Hellstrom PA, Frimansson E, Atelisson A (1992) Effect of low level acoustic stimulation on temporary threshold shift in young humans. Hearing Research 60: 145–55.

Ostri B, Eller N, Dahlin E, Skylv G (1989) Hearing impairment in orchestral musicians. Scandanavian Audiology 18(4): 243–9.

Price GR, Kalb JT (1991) Insights into hazard from intense impulses from a mathematical model of the ear. Journal of the Acoustical Society of America 90(1): 219–27.

Reid AW (2001) A sound ear: exploring the issues of noise damage in orchestras. London: Association of British Orchestras.

Rice CG, Breslin M, Roper RG (1987) Sound levels from personal cassette players. British Journal of Audiology 21: 273–8.

Rintelman WF, Borus JF (1968) Noise–induced hearing loss in rock and roll musicians. Archives of Otolaryngology 88: 377–85.

Robinson DW (1988) Threshold of hearing as a function of age and sex for the typical unscreened population. British Journal of Audiology 22: 5–20.

Royster JD, Royster L, Killion M (1991) Sound exposures and hearing thresholds of symphony orchestra musicians. Journal of the Acoustical Society of America 89: 2783–803.

Sanders A, Axelsson A (1981) Comparison of cardiovascular responses in noise-resistant and noise-sensitive workers. Acta Otolaryngologica 76 (suppl 377): 75–100.

Sataloff RT, Sataloff J (1998) Hearing loss in musicians. In RT Sataloff, AG Brandfonbrenner, RJ Lederman (eds) Performing Arts Medicine. London: Singular Publications Inc., pp. 85–98.

Speaks C, Nelson D, Ward W (1970) Hearing loss in rock and roll musicians. Journal of Occupational Medicine 12: 216–19.

Spoendlin HH (1975) Anatomical changes following various noise exposures. In D Henderson, RP Hamernick, DS Dosanjh, JH Mills (eds) Effects of Noise on Hearing. New York: Raven Press, pp. 69–87.

Subramaniam M, Henderson D, Spongr V (1991) Frequency differences in the development of protection against NIHL by low level 'toughening' exposures. Journal of the Acoustical Society of America 89: 1865–74.

Swanson SJ, Dengerink HA, Kondrick P, Miller CL (1987) The influence of subjective factors on temporary threshold shifts after exposure to music and noise of equal energy. Ear and Hearing 8: 288–91.

Teie PU (1998) Noise-induced hearing loss and symphony orchestra musicians: risk factors, effects, and management. Maryland Medical Journal 47(1): 13–18.

Ward WD (1991) The role of intermittence in PTS. Journal of the Acoustical Society of America 90: 164–9.

West PDB, Evans EF (1990) Early detection of hearing damage in young listeners resulting from exposure to amplified music. British Journal of Audiology 24: 89–103.

Wood WS, Lipscombe DM (1972) Maximum available sound pressure levels from stereo components. Journal of the Acoustical Society of America 52: 484–7.

CHAPTER 21

# Organic solvent exposures and occupational hearing loss

*Noise and Its Effects:* Edited by Linda Luxon and Deepak Prasher © 2007 John Wiley & Sons Ltd.

MARIOLA ŚLIWIŃSKA-KOWALSKA, EWA ZAMYSLOWSKA-SZMYTKE

Organic solvents are frequent contaminants of the atmosphere in industry, and are used in paint and lacquer factories, dockyards and plants manufacturing ships/boats, furniture, plastic, fibres, rubber tyres and many other products. Many types of solvents, such as paints and lacquers, are also used in non-occupational activities – mostly household procedures. A number of these substances, including xylene, toluene, styrene, ethyl benzene, trichloroethylene and *n*-hexane have been shown to impair hearing in animals, when applied at high concentration (Table 21.1).

Some of them (toluene and styrene) display a synergistic effect with noise exposure on hearing and cochlear hair cell damage (Lataye and Campo, 1997; Lataye et al., 2000).

**Table 21.1** Evidence on the effects of exposure to organic solvents alone and in combination with noise on hearing

| Substance | Animal studies | | Human studies | |
|---|---|---|---|---|
| | *Without noise* | *With noise* | *Without noise* | *With noise* |
| Xylene | + | No data available | + | + probable additive effect |
| Toluene | + | + synergism | + | + probable additive effect |
| Styrene | + | + synergism | + | + probable additive effect |
| Ethyl benzene | + | + synergism | No data available | No data available |
| Trichloroethylene (TCE) | + | + synergism | + | No data available |
| *N*-Hexane | + | + | Under evaluation | Under evaluation |
| Carbon disulphide | + | + synergism | + | + probable synergism |

477

Otoxicity of organic solvents in occupationally exposed humans is more difficult to elucidate. The concentration of chemicals is much lower than that used in animal studies, and workers are usually exposed to a mixture of solvents at widely varying compositions and concentrations, making assessment of the effect of a single substance difficult to establish. Furthermore, in industrial settings, exposure to chemicals often coexists with an increased level of noise, which is the most common occupational and environmental factor damaging the inner ear. It is thus hard to distinguish the solvent effect from noise-induced hearing loss.

This chapter summarizes current knowledge on the influence on the auditory organ of occupational exposures to organic solvents, alone or in combination with noise, and its contribution to hearing conservation programmes for workers at risk.

## Literature overview

The main human study results dealing with the ototoxicity of organic solvents are presented in Table 21.2.

**Table 21.2** Human studies on the effects of organic solvents (alone and in combination with noise) on auditory organ

| Reference | Population | Exposure | Results |
| --- | --- | --- | --- |
| Biscaldi et al. (1981) | Six accidentally poisoned workers of electromechanical industry | Toluene | EEG abnormalities and vestibular hyporeflexia after the accident. Hearing loss recorded in three subjects (reversible in one) |
| Barregård and Axelsson (1984) | Four painters of a shipyard | Noise and solvent mixture | Workers exposed to noise and solvents had much more pronounced sensorineural hearing loss than would be expected from their noise exposure only |
| Bergström and Nyström (1986) | 319 subjects working in sawmills, paper pulp production and chemicals division | Noise-only (95–100 dB (A)) ($n = 164$) Noise (80–90 dB (A)) and solvent mixture ($n = 47$) | The prevalence of hearing loss at 4 kHz was more frequent in noise- and solvent-exposed group than in noise-only exposed subjects |
| Chang (1987) | 34 workers of printing factories (22 with polyneuropathy) | $n$-Hexane | Prolongation of the wave I–V interpeak latencies in the ABR, corresponding with the severity of the polyneuropathy |

**Table 21.2** (continued)

| Reference | Population | Exposure | Results |
|---|---|---|---|
| Ödkvist et al. (1987) | 31 workers exposed to solvents and jet fuel | Mixtures of aliphatic and aromatic solvents | Abnormal results of interrupted speech and evoked cortical potential audiometry. Pathology in central vestibular tests (visual suppression test, saccades test) |
| Muijser et al. (1988) | 59 workers of a company maufacturing glass-fibre-reinforced plastic products | Styrene, mean concentration: directly exposed – 138 mg/m$^3$ indirectly exposed – 61 mg/m$^3$ | No differences in hearing thresholds between exposed group and controls. Significantly higher hearing threshold at 8 kHz in directly exposed workers compared with indirectly exposed group |
| Möller et al. (1990) | 18 workers of a plastics boat plant | Long-term exposure to styrene < 110 mg/m$^3$ | PTA$^2$ did not indicate hearing loss due to causes other than age. Abnormal results in central auditory pathways in seven subjects (distorted speech, cortical response audiometry). Abnormal central vestibular function in 16 subjects (posturography and rotatory visual supression test) |
| Morata et al. (1993) | Workers of rotogravure printing and paint manufacturing divisions | Noise-only (88–97 dB (A)) ($n = 50$) | Prevalence of hearing loss – 26% Adjusted RR – 4.1 (95%CI: 1.4–12.2) |
| | | Organic solvent mixture (toluene, xylene, benzene and others) ($n = 39$) | Prevalence of hearing loss – 18% Adjusted RR – 5.0 (95%CI: 1.4–17.5) |
| | | Noise (88–98 dB (A)) and toluene at high concentrations (100–370 p.p.m.) | Prevalence of hearing loss – 53% Adjusted RR – 10.9 (95%CI: 4.1–28.9) Higher prevalence of ears with acoustic reflex decay as compared to noise-only and solvent mixture-only groups |

**Table 21.2** (continued)

| Reference | Population | Exposure | Results |
|---|---|---|---|
| Jacobsen et al. (1993) | Self-assessed questionaire study on 3284 subjects | Organic solvent mixture, more than 5 years of employment | Adjusted RR 1.4 (95%CI: 1.1–1.9) |
| | | Noise only | Adjusted RR 1.9 (95%CI: 1.7–2.1) |
| | | Noise and organic solvent | Adjusted RR 1.8 (95%CI: 1.6–2.1), the effect of the noise dominated and no additional effect from solvent was found |
| Laukli and Hansen (1995) | 33 men reffered to otorhino-laryngology department from neurology and occupational medicine departments | A variety of organic solvents and lead-containing fumes | Mild-to-moderate sen-sorineural hearing loss in some subjects; varying degrees of abnormality in the central tests (filtered speech and cognitive responses – MMN, P300, P400) |
| Sass-Kortsak et al. (1995) | 299 subjects of the fibre-rein-forced plastics manufacturing industry | Styrene (mean 73.5 mg/m³) and noise (87.2 ± 6.5 dB (A)) | Age and noise exposure positively correlated with hearing loss. No evidence for a chronic styrene-induced effect on hearing acuity in noise and styrene exposed. A high correla-tion between noise and styrene exposures |
| Vrca et al. (1996) | 49 workers of printing press | Low concentra-tions of toluene | A significant prolongation of P1 wave latency and increased interval of interpeak latency P3–P5 in the ABR |
| Morata et al. (1997a) | 124 rotogravure printing workers | Noise (71–93 dB (A)) and organic solvent mixture (toluene, ethyl acetate, ethanol) at low concentrations | The prevalence of bilateral high-frequency hearing loss – 49.2%. The OR estimates for hearing loss were 1.07 times significantly greater for each increment of 1 year of age and 1.76 times significantly greater for each gram of hippuric acid per gram of creatinine |

**Table 21.2** (continued)

| Reference | Population | Exposure | Results |
|---|---|---|---|
| Morata et al. (1997b) | 438 petroleum refinery workers | Organic solvent mixture (benzene, toluene, xylene, ethyl benzene and cyclohexane) at concentrations within exposure limits; with and without noise | The prevalence of hearing loss in exposed to solvents groups – 42–50%, in non-exposed groups – 15–30%. Adjusted OR estimates for hearing loss: 2.4 (95%CI: 1.0–5.7) for solvents-only group; 1.8 (0.6–4.9) for noise-only group and 3.0 (1.3–6.9) for noise and solvents group. Acoustic reflex decay test suggested a retrocochlear or central pathway involvement in certain job categories |
| Niklasson et al. (1998) | 60 workers with suspected solvent-induced chronic toxic encephalopathy | Organic solvent mixture (white spirits, thinner, toluene, xylene) | No difference between study groups and controls in PTA; abnormality in the central auditory tests (distorted speech and cortical response audiometry) in solvent-exposed. No correlation between clinical neurological and neuro-physiological investigation and audiological test results |
| Morioka et al. (2000) | 48 male workers of a factory producing plastic buttons | Noise (58–92 dB (A)) and styrene (most exposures within the OELs; in Japan OEL = 210 g/m³) | No significant differences between exposed and control grups in PTA. The prevalence rate of upper limit of hearing below 75th percentile curve higher in noise- and solvent-exposed group than noise-only and control groups |
| Śliwińska-Kowalska et al. (2001a) | Workers of paint and lacquer factory and metal industry | Organic solvent mixture at low concentrations ($n = 207$). Noise (up to 88 dB (A)) and organic solvent mixture at low concentrations ($n = 96$). Unexposed control group ($n = 214$) | Adjusted RR for hearing loss in the solvent-only exposed group significantly increased (2.8; 95%CI: 1.8–4.3); no additional risk in the solvent- and noise-exposed group. Mean hearing thresholds (at 2–4 kHz) higher in workers exposed to noise and solvents than solvent-only group |

**Table 21.2** (continued)

| Reference | Population | Exposure | Results |
|---|---|---|---|
| Morata et al. (2002) | 313 workers of fibreglass and metal products manufacturing plants | Noise (85–108 dB (A)) and styrene (below recommended values) | Adjusted ORs for hearing loss were 1.19 for each increment of 1 year of age (95%CI: 1.11–1.28), 1.18 for every decibel > 85 dB (A) of noise exposure (95%CI: 1.01–1.34) and 2.44 for each millimole of mandelic acid per gram of creatinine in urine (95%CI: 1.01–5.89). Hearing thresholds (2, 3, 4 and 6 kHz) in noise- and styrene-exposed workers significantly worse than in noise-only exposed group and controls |
| Śliwińska-Kowalska et al. (2003) | 290 yacht yard and plastic factory workers | Styrene (61.8 mg/m³) with and without noise Noise ($L_{eq}$ 89.2 dB (A)) | Adjusted OR fourfold higher in the styrene-exposed group compared with controls, and twofold higher for combined exposure to noise and styrene than sole exposure to styrene. A positive linear relationship between averaged lifetime styrene concentration and hearing threolds at the frequencies 6 and 8 kHz |
| Chang et al. (2003) | 66 metal factory workers 131 viscose rayon plant workers exposed to noise and carbon disulphide ($CS_2$) 105 workers of electronic industries | $CS_2$ (average 1.6–20.1 p.p.m.), noise (80–91 dB (A)) Noise-only (83–90 dB (A)) | Higher prevalence of hearing loss in workers co-exposed to noise and $CS_2$ (67.9%) than noise-only group (32.4%) and controls (23.6%). Adjusted ORs of hearing loss increasing with the exposure to $CS_2$ from 3.8 (95%CI: 1.5–9.4) for exposures of 37–214 year-p.p.m. to 70.3 (95%CI: 8.7–569.7) for exposures above 453 year-p.p.m. |
| Śliwińska-Kowalska et al. (2004) | 701 dockyard workers (517 exposed to noise and solvents and 184 to noise only) | Noise (85–102 dB (A)) and mixture of organic solvents containing mainly xylenes (mean concentration 245 mg/m³) | Adjusted OR of hearing loss significantly (threefold) higher in noise-only exposed group, and almost fivefold higher in noise- and solvent-exposed group compared with controls Adjusted ORs for hearing loss 1.12 for each increment of 1 year of age, 1.07 for every decibel of lifetime noise exposure (dB (A)), and 1.004 for each increment of the index of lifetime exposure to solvents in the air At 8 kHz a moderate effect of solvent on hearing thresholds additional to noise-induced hearing loss |

95%CI, 95% confidence interval; ABR, auditory brain-stem responses; OEL, occupational exposure limit; OR, odds ratio; p.p.m., parts per million; PTA, pure-tone audiometry; RR, relative risk;

## Solvent mixtures

In 1984, Barregård and Axelsson were the first to describe hearing loss in four people with a history of occupational exposure to noise and a mixture of organic solvents. The hearing loss due to this combined exposure was more profound than that found after exposure to noise alone (Barregård and Axelsson, 1984). Two years later, Bergstöm and Nyström (1986) studied the occurrence of hearing loss in 319 workers in the paper industry, who were exposed solely to noise, or to both noise and organic solvents. At a frequency of 4 kHz, hearing loss was more common in people exposed to noise and solvents than in those who were exposed only to noise. Morata et al. (1993) demonstrated an increased relative risk of hearing loss in lacquer and paint industry workers exposed to a mixture of organic solvents containing toluene, xylene and methyl ethyl ketone (MEK) as the main components. An increased (2.4-fold) risk of hearing loss was also demonstrated in employees of petroleum refineries, who were exposed to a mixture of toluene, xylene, ethyl benzene and cyclohexane at relatively low concentrations, not exceeding currently admissible exposure limits (Morata et al., 1997b). Similarly, we demonstrated that low concentration exposure to a mixture of organic solvents with xylene as the main compound resulted in almost threefold higher probability of developing hearing loss in paint and lacquer factory workers (Śliwińska-Kowalska et al., 2001).

| Industries affected by hazardous organic solvents include: | | | |
|---|---|---|---|
| Paper | Fibres | Paint | Furniture |
| Lacquer | Dockyards | Plastics | Boatbuilders |
| Tyres | Dry cleaning | Printing | Herbicides |
| Viscose/rayon | Explosives | Shoe making | Leather |
| Optic goods | | | |

A questionnaire cohort study by Jacobsen et al. (1993), performed on 3284 subjects with a history of occupational exposure to different organic solvents confirms the field study findings cited above.

The results of studies on the combined exposure to noise and a mixture of organic solvents in humans are equivocal. An additive effect of organic solvents to noise might be seen from the data of Morata et al. (1993). The authors reported that occupational exposure was associated with fourfold, fivefold and elevenfold increases in the risk of hearing loss in cases of noise-only, solvent-only and combined noise/toluene exposures, respectively. In another report, the same authors showed that the exposure of petroleum refinery workers to a mixture of solvents only (toluene, xylene, ethyl benzene, cyclohexane) was associated with an adjusted odds ratio (OR) of hearing loss of 2.4 (95%CI 1.0–5.7), while in the solvents and noise group this value was slightly higher (relative risk or RR 3.0; 95%CI 1.3–6.9) (Morata et al., 1997b). On the other hand, the cohort study by Jacobsen et al. (1993) showed a dominant effect of noise and no additional hearing risk due to solvents in cases of combined exposure. The adjusted RR values in that survey were 1.4 for the solvent-only group, 1.9 for the noise-only group and 1.8 for the noise and solvent group. However, in the last study, the evaluation of hearing acuity was based on a self-assessment questionnaire, which could lead to the underestimation of hearing loss, particularly at high frequencies. Similarly, in our study on paint and lacquer factory workers (Śliwińska-Kowalska et al., 2001a), we were not able to show any additional hearing loss risk upon combined exposure to noise and organic solvent mixture when compared with isolated exposure to solvents. Since the levels of workplace noise were only slightly elevated above the threshold limit value (up to 88 dB (A)), the negative results of that investigation might have been due to poor dichotomy between the populations exposed (85–88 dB (A)) and not exposed to noise (below 85 dB (A)). Our recent study in dockyard workers exposed to noise and a mixture of organic solvents containing mainly xylene indicate an additive risk effect of co-exposure on hearing impairment (see below) (Śliwińska-Kowalska et al., 2004).

Hearing threshold shift due to exposure to organic solvents seems to be mild or moderate, and the most sensitive frequencies are 4–8 kHz. Our epidemiological field study performed in paint and lacquer factory workers and shipyard workers showed that a mean hearing threshold shift due to solvent mixture ototoxicity was from 6 dB at 4 kHz to 8 dB at 6 kHz and 10 db at 8kH(Śliwińska-Kowalska et al., 2005). A previous clinical study performed by Laukli and Hansen (1995) also showed only a mild-to-moderate hearing loss in the majority of 33 subjects exposed to different organic solvents at the workplace, and referred to the otorhinolaryngology department from neurology and occupational medicine departments. Niklasson et al. (1997) did not find any difference in pure-tone audiometry and a monosyllabic speech recognition test between the unexposed group and workers exposed to the mixture of solvents containing white spirits, thinner, toluene and xylene. However, in both of these studies, central auditory abnormalities were reported: Laukli and Hansen identified abnormal cognitive responses in approximately one-third of patients, while Niklasson et al. observed that the distorted speech-recognition scores were significantly lower, and cortical response audiometry latencies were significantly longer, in the solvent group than in the control group.

### Site of pathology

| | |
|---|---|
| Noise | Predominantly cochlear |
| Organic solvents | Cochlear/metrocochlear/central auditory and vestibular |

Similar results were found earlier by Ödkvist and co-workers in subjects exposed to a mixture of aliphatic and aromatic solvents. These results would suggest that organic solvents, apart from possible cochlear ototoxicity shown in animals, might significantly damage the central auditory pathway. Also, central vestibular abnormalities were often found in solvent-mixture exposed workers (Ödkvist et al., 1983, 1987, 1992; Niklasson et al., 1997, 1998).

## Xylene

Xylene used technically is a combination of three isomers (o-, m- and p-xylene) and ethyl benzene. It is commonly used as a solvent in paints and lacquers, and during the synthesis of several chemicals. It is inhaled via the airways, although some amounts of xylene can also be absorbed through the skin. It is metabolized to methylhippuric acid, which is determined in urine and serves as an exposure index. Xylene is irritant to the respiratory tract and displays neurotoxic activity similar to that of toluene. In general, xylene forms a part of solvent mixtures (see above).

In our study in the paint and lacquer factory, workers exposed to a solvent mixture with xylene as the main component (moderate concentrations from 1 to 110 mg/m$^3$, mean 28 mg/m$^3$) showed an increased relative risk of hearing loss that could be attributed to solvent exposure (Śliwińska-Kowalska et al., 2001a). Co-exposure to noise and solvents containing predominantly xylene could exacerbate noise-induced hearing loss. An additive effect of such co-exposure with adjusted OR measures around 3 and almost 5 in noise-only and noise- and solvent-exposed group, respectively, were observed in dockyard workers (Śliwińska-Kowalska et al., 2004). The same authors also reported a hearing threshold at 8 kHz as being significantly poorer in workers co-exposed to noise and solvents. This was positively correlated with the concentration of solvents in the workplace air during the time of employment.

## Toluene

Toluene is a colourless, transparent liquid with a very characteristic odour. It is used mostly in the production of paints, lacquers, rubber and glue, dyes and degreasing agents, and in some (for example, rotogravure) printing processes and in the leather tanning industry. It is absorbed through the airways, digestive tract and skin. Toluene is metabolized to hippuric acid. The rate of urinary benzoic acid excretion at the end of the day is used as the biological exposure index. Toluene is known to exert a damaging effect on the central nervous system and liver. It may also irritate the respiratory tract.

The first study suggesting ototoxicity of toluene was published in 1981 (Biscaldi et al., 1981). Three out of six workers acutely overexposed to this solvent developed hearing loss. In only one subject were the changes reversible. Several years later, a cross-sectional field study in paint and lac-quer factory workers (Morata et al., 1993) showed that exposure to a mixture of solvents, of which the main component was toluene, was asso-ciated with as high as a fivefold increased probability of developing hearing loss compared with that found in non-exposed controls. More recently, it has been shown that the adjusted OR of hearing impairment is increased in printing industry workers, even though the concentrations of toluene are within currently admissible occupational exposure limits (Morata et al., 1997b).

A combined exposure to noise and toluene seems to be more haz-ardous than exposure to noise alone. In the rotogravure printing industry, workers exposed to noise (at 88–97 dB (A)) and 98% pure toluene at con-centrations exceeding the admissible levels (from 100 to 370 p.p.m., with admissible limit in the USA of 100 p.p.m. = 375 mg/m$^3$), the risk of hear-ing loss was 11 times higher than in non-exposed controls, while in noise-only exposed population the corresponding value was only 4 (Morata et al., 1993).

Although clear cochlear damage due to toluene exposure has been shown in rats, currently available data in humans indicate that the expo-sure to toluene is related to retrocochlear or central auditory rather than cochlear damage. Abnormalities of stapedial reflex decay (Morata et al., 1993) and auditory brain-stem responses (Vrca et al., 1996) have been shown in the toluene-exposed population.

| Type of solvent exposure | | | |
| --- | --- | --- | --- |
| Risk | Mixture (main Xylene) | Toluene | Styrene |
| Solvent only | 2.8 | 5.0 | 5.2 |
| Solvent + noise | 4.9 | 10.9 | 10.9 |

## Styrene

Pure styrene is a colourless, volatile liquid with a characteristic sweetish odour, sparingly soluble in water. However, it usually contains some addi-tional chemicals responsible for its sharp, disagreeable odour. It occurs mainly in the production of polyester laminates and plastics, plastic products, synthetic rubber and insulating materials (such as polyurethane foam), and in the glass fibre-reinforced plastic products industry (such as yachts, lavatory pans and wash basins). Styrene is absorbed through the airways and skin and is metabolized primarily to mandelic acid (MA) and phenylglyoxal acid (PGA). Styrene affects the functions of various human organs and systems, the most significant being the mucosa, liver and cen-tral nervous system. In animal studies, styrene and its metabolite – styrene oxide – have been found to be more ototoxic than toluene.

The effect of styrene on hearing was first assessed by Muijser et al. (1988) in 59 employees of a company producing glass fibre-reinforced plastic products. Compared with the non-exposed control group, and after adjustment for presbycusis, these employees did not reveal increased hearing thresholds when assessed by pure-tone audiometry, either at standard or at extended high frequencies. A statistically significant difference in hearing thresholds was found, however, between the workers directly exposed to styrene (at the mean concentration of 138 mg/m$^3$) and those indirectly exposed to styrene (at 61 mg/m$^3$). Two years later Möller et al. (1990), who examined the employees exposed to styrene at concentrations remarkably below the Swedish occupational exposure limit (OEL 119 mg/m$^3$ in 1990), did not note any significant hearing loss in the solvent-exposed group compared with the non-exposed controls. However, 17 of 18 examined workers revealed abnormal results of central auditory and vestibular tests.

Although the first studies failed to indicate a significant effect of styrene on the audiometric threshold, recent papers document that occupational exposure to that solvent may increase the OR of hearing loss. In the workers of a plant manufacturing yachts, and in employees of the plastics industry, we have shown that exposure to styrene at mean concentration of 61.8 mg/m$^3$ (Polish OEL for styrene is 50 mg/m$^3$) was associated with an almost 4-fold increased OR of hearing loss (value adjusted to the age, gender, current occupational exposure to noise and noise exposure in the past) (Śliwińska-Kowalska et al., 2003). Mean hearing thresholds adjusted for age, gender and noise exposures were significantly higher in the styrene-exposed group than in non-exposed controls at all standard frequencies tested (1–8 kHz).

Two other studies also showed poorer hearing thresholds in a population of workers exposed to styrene, even though the concentration of this solvent did not exceed the threshold limit value. Hearing impairment related to the extended high frequencies only, and was seen in workers exposed to styrene for more than 5 years. This effect was associated with styrene concentrations in air and mandelic acid concentrations in urine (Morioka et al., 1999, 2000).

The results of the studies performed in populations exposed to both noise and styrene are equivocal. An early study did not provide evidence of chronic styrene-induced hearing acuity impairment in 299 employees exposed to styrene and noise at fibre-reinforced plastics manufacturing enterprises (Sass-Kortsak et al., 1995). In that study, noise (L$_{eq}$ 87.2 ± 6.5 dB (A)) and styrene (concentration 73.5 ± 88.6 mg/m$^3$) exposures were highly correlated, and the effect of noise was shown to be predominant. On the other hand, our latest study assessing the OR of hearing loss in styrene-only, noise-only, and styrene- and noise-exposed population suggests an additive effect of co-exposure (Śliwińska-Kowalska et al., 2003). The chance of developing hearing loss increased 3.3-fold in noise-only exposed workers, 5.2-fold in styrene-only exposed workers, 10.9-fold in noise and styrene co-exposed subjects and over 21.5-fold in noise, styrene and toluene co-exposed individuals. Moreover, after adjustment for age and noise a linear correlation between styrene concentration in the air and hearing threshold at 6 and 8 kHz was found.

As for toluene, although animal studies show cochlear damage due to styrene exposure, human data point to a central rather than a peripheral auditory effect. In styrene-exposed workers, pathological results of distorted speech audiometry and central auditory potentials, in addition to abnormalities in central vestibular function were recorded by Möller and co-workers (1990). However, this study involved a limited number (18) of patients visiting an outpatient clinic and was compared with a control group. Thus, the results should be interpreted with caution. In our recent clinical investigation on over 100 styrene-exposed workers, we were able to show clear signs of cochlear damage (distortion product otoacoustic emission or DPOAE impairment) that were significantly greater in this group than in control subjects without a history of occupational exposure to chemicals (Sliwinska-Kowalska, submitted).

### n-Hexane

Pure n-hexane is a colourless volatile liquid, with an unpleasant odour; it is relatively immiscible with water. It is used mainly in laboratories as a component of solvent mixtures (textile, furniture, shoe manufacturing and printing industry). n-Hexane is inhaled, absorbed in the respiratory tract and metabolized in the liver. Its predominant toxic effects are related to the central nervous system and comprise peripheral neuropathy (sensory or sensorineural) and muscle wasting. A prolonged neural transmission time, with accompanying nerve fibre demyelination, was shown in electromyography (Kuwabara et al., 1999).

The evidence of n-hexane-induced toxicity to the auditory organ is based mainly on animal studies (Rebert and Sorensen, 1983; Nylén and Hagman, 1994; Nylén at al., 1994). Longer inter-wave I–V latencies in the auditory brain-stem responses of patients with n-hexane neuropathies were reported as early as 1987 (Chang, 1987). Our recent study in workers of a shoe factory exposed to moderate concentrations of n-hexane and toluene showed an eightfold increased OR of hearing loss when compared with non-exposed controls and this value increased to 20.2 with combined exposure to solvents and noise (Śliwińska-Kowalska, 2005). In contrast to previously described solvents (toluene, styrene), n-hexane does not influence hearing threshold in animals when acting alone. However, it may cause hearing impairment in combined exposures with toluene or xylene (Pryor and Rebert, 1992; Nylén and Hagman, 1994; Nylén et al., 1994).

### Trichloroethylene

Trichloroethylene is a colourless liquid with an aromatic odour. It is used as a solvent for various types of fat, grease, wax and resin. It was extensively used to clean clothes (dry cleaning). It is absorbed through airways, alimentary tract and skin. In industrial exposures, this substance is present as a minor constituent of the mixtures of solvents. It has been shown in animal studies that trichloroethylene damages spiral ganglion cells, and not cochlear hair cells (Fechter et al., 1998).

### Carbon disulphide

Carbon disulphide ($CS_2$) is a colourless volatile (46°C boiling point) liquid with a sweetish odour. It is used in the manufacturing processes of viscose, rayon and paper, to degrease leather, optic glass, and in the manufacture of herbicides, paints, varnishes or explosives. Current examples of carbon disulphide exposure include workers of laboratories assessing carbon disulfide environmental pollution by gas chromatography. Carbon disulphide is toxic primarily to the nervous, circulatory, haematopoietic systems and the skin. It is metabolized to thiocarbamide, 2-thioazolidinone-5 and thiothiazolidine-4-carboxylic acid (TTCA).

Most of the data on carbon disulphide toxicity have been obtained from studies on exposed workers, who show increased frequency of sensorineural hearing loss. Most cases involve retrocochlear damage with changes typically located in the auditory nerve and brain stem (longer latency of waves I, III and V) (Hirata et al., 1992).

A recent study performed in viscose rayon plant workers exposed to noise ($L_{eq}$ 80–91 dB (A)) and $CS_2$ (concentration 1.6–20.1 p.p.m.) shows a substantially higher prevalence of hearing loss in the group exposed to $CS_2$ than in the noise-exposed and non-exposed populations (67.9% in $CS_2$ group versus 32.4% in the noise-only group and 23.6% in the control group) (Chang et al., 2003). Hearing loss occurred mainly for speech frequencies (0.5, 1 and 2 kHz). The adjusted OR of hearing loss increased with the exposure level and years of employment (from 3.8 for $CS_2$ exposure of 37–214 year-p.p.m. to 70.3 for $CS_2$ exposure more than 453 year-p.p.m.).

# Hearing outcomes

Summarizing the data from the literature, several hearing outcomes were taken into account to assess the influence of sole exposure to solvents and combined exposure to solvents and noise on the auditory organ. The first one is RR, or OR, of hearing impairment. This outcome is usually defined as a chance of developing hearing loss exceeding 25 dB HL in at least one frequency in the range 125–8000 Hz, as assessed by pure-tone audiometry. All research studies showed a significantly (1.4–5.2 times) increased adjusted OR measures for hearing loss in solvent-only exposed populations, that is within a similar range as the risk of hearing loss in noise-only exposed population (1.8–4.1) (Figure 21.1). A combined exposure to noise and solvents seems to have an additive effect on the risk of hearing loss. All papers, except one, showed that the probability of developing hearing impairment was higher in the populations co-exposed to noise and solvents, and in that case adjusted odds ratio values ranged from 2.8 to 21.5 (Figure 21.1). One study contradicting this conclusion was based on self-assessed questionnaire data not confirmed by audiometric or exposure measurements (Jacobsen et al., 1993).

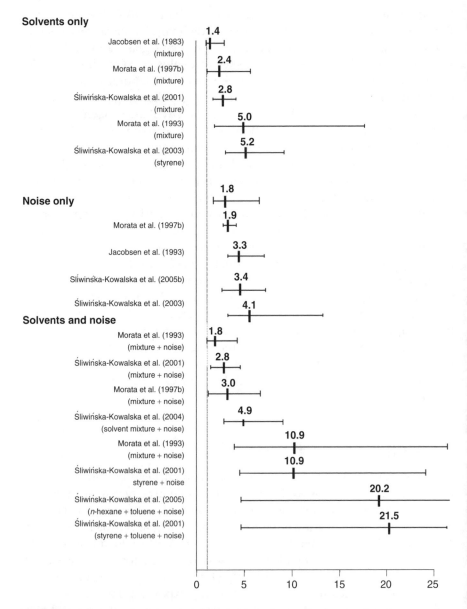

**Figure 21.1** Adjusted odds ratio/relative risk measures for hearing loss by type of exposure.

An assessment of the odds of developing hearing loss does not provide information about the severity of hearing impairment. Thus, the second hearing outcome used in human research studies was permanent hearing threshold shift. Sole exposure to organic solvents seems to exert only mild-to-moderate impairment of hearing. Hearing loss concerns predominantly the region of high frequencies (4, 6 and 8 kHz) in case of solvent mixture exposure (Śliwińska-Kowalska et al., 2005) and the entire range of frequencies in case of styrene exposure (Śliwińska-Kowalska et al., 2003).

**Configuration of hearing loss**

| | |
|---|---|
| Organic solvents alone | Mild-to-moderate hearing loss |
| + noise | Noise component predominates |
| Solvent mixture | High-frequency hearing loss |
| Styrene | All frequencies affected |

Some studies have shown hearing loss also in extended high frequencies in styrene-exposed workers (Morioka et al., 1999, 2000). In the case of combined exposure to noise and organic solvents, the noise effect is predominant. In some studies no additional effect of solvents was seen (Sass-Kortsak et al., 1995); in others, published by our group, an additive effect was observed at 8 kHz (Śliwińska-Kowalska et al., 2003, 2004, 2005).

Since organic solvents are well-known neurotoxic substances, central auditory pathology must be considered as an auditory outcome measure. Damage of the auditory cortex may influence speech understanding even though hearing thresholds are normal. Indeed, some previous clinical studies suggested that organic solvents primarily damage the central auditory pathway, and extensive auditory tests assessing these sites should be considered in the population exposed to those substances. This is particularly important in the case of combined exposure to noise and organic solvent. The different sites of damage caused by noise (purely cochlear – some evidence of central involvement) and organic solvents (central, retrocochlear and cochlear) may contribute to the exacerbation of noise-induced hearing loss by solvents in exposed populations.

# Relationship between exposure level and hearing outcome

Based on the biological monitoring, it has been shown that, in the population of printing industry workers exposed to noise and a mixture of organic solvents, the OR estimates were 1.76 times higher for each increment of hippuric acid (metabolite of toluene) per gram of creatinine in urine (95%CI 1.00–2.98) (Morata et al., 1997a) (Table 21.3). Recently, it has been shown by the same authors that, in noise- and styrene-exposed workers, the adjusted OR for hearing loss was 2.44 for each millimole of mandelic acid (metabolite of styrene) per gram of creatinine in urine (95%CI: 1.01–5.89) (Morata et al., 2002). In both these studies, biological measurements were performed only once at the time of audiometric data collection, which makes it impossible to

**Table 21.3** Odds ratio (OR) measures for hearing loss by age, noise and organic solvent exposure

| Reference | Parameters | OR | 95% CI[a] |
|---|---|---|---|
| Morata et al. (1997a) | Age (years) | 1.07 | 1.03–1.11 |
| | Hippuric acid[b] in urine (in millimole per gram of creatinine) | 1.76 | 1.00–2.98 |
| Morata et al. (2002) | Age (years) | 1.19 | 1.11–1.28 |
| | noise > 85 (in dB (A)) | 1.18 | 1.01–1.34 |
| | mandelic acid[c] in urine (in millimole per gram of creatinine) | 2.44 | 1.01–5.89 |
| Śliwińska-Kowalska et al. (2004) | Age (years) | 1.12 | 1.10–1.14 |
| | Lifetime noise (in dB (A)) | 1.07 | 1.04–1.09 |
| | Lifetime exposure index for solvents in the air (in numerical values) | 1.004 | 1.00–1.01 |

[a]95%CI, 95% confidence interval; [b]Biomarker for toluene; [c]Biomarker for styrene.

**Table 21.4** Biomarkers of organic solvents

| Toxic agent | Biomarkers of exposure | Admissible values in urine |
|---|---|---|
| Xylene | Methylhippuric acid | 1.4 g/l, for urine of density 1.024 mg/m³ |
| Toluene | Benzoic acid | 80 mg/h |
| Styrene | Mandelic acid | 16 mg/h |
| | Mandelic acid + phenylglyoxylic acid (MPA) | 25 mg/h |
| n-Hexane | 2,5-Hexanedione | 2.5 mg/l, for urine of density 1.016 mg/m³ |
| Trichloroethylene | Trichloroacetic acid | 20 mg/l |
| Ethyl benzene | Mandelic acid | 20 mg/h |
| Carbon disulphide | 2-Thiothiazolidine-4-carboxylic acid | 3 mg/g creatinine |

extrapolate those data to the cumulative exposure to a given solvent over each employee's working lifetime. On the other hand, positive results of these investigations showing a dose–response relationship would suggest that biological monitoring of solvent exposure might be important. Organic solvent metabolites to be measured are presented in Table 21.4.

Our recent study in a population of dockyard workers exposed to noise and a mixture of organic solvents shows that the OR for hearing loss adjusted for age and noise effect was 1.004 for each increment of the index of lifetime exposure to solvents (Śliwińska-Kowalska et al., 2004). Also, a relationship between solvent exposure and hearing threshold shift at 8 kHz was confirmed in that population. According to our knowledge, this is the first paper showing a dose–response effect between cumulative measure of exposure to solvents and hearing outcomes.

# Contribution of current knowledge on organic solvent ototoxicity to hearing conservation programmes

## Medical prevention

In view of current knowledge on organic-solvent ototoxicity it should be concluded that appropriate preventive measures must be taken in all workers exposed to organic solvents with special regard to those co-exposed to noise and solvents.

As the hearing effect of organic solvents may be small, and located only at high and very high frequencies or masked by noise-induced hearing loss, a high index of clinical suspicion and special regard must be paid to patient complaints regarding problems with understanding speech, as well as vertigo and dizziness (Śliwińska-Kowalska et al., 2001b). Occupational exposure to noise does not cause vestibular organ pathology, while in cases of exposure to organic solvents, vestibulacerebellar balance disorders could be a first symptom of neurotoxicity (Ödkvist et al., 1983, 1987, 1992; Yokoyama et al., 2002). Pure-tone audiometry, which is the gold standard test for noise-exposed population, is probably not the 'best' test for solvent-exposed workers. In view of our latest study (Sliwinska-Kowalska, submitted) on the styrene-exposed population, otoacoustic emission might be more helpful. Bearing in mind a possible central auditory effect of the exposure to solvents, central auditory tests or electrophysiology measures (for example, P300) may be more appropriate in some cases. In n-hexane-exposed subjects, the auditory brain-stem response should be considered for assessing exposure-related neuropathy of the auditory nerve.

In the everyday practice of occupational medicine it might be important to distinguish between the hearing effect of noise-only exposure and
co-exposure to noise and solvents. In medical prevention for noise- and
solvent-exposed subjects, hearing loss at 8 kHz higher than predicted
could indicate an additional effect of solvent ototoxicity (Figure 21.2).

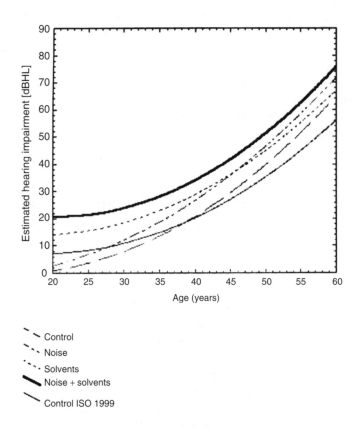

**Figure 21.2** Effects of solvent ototoxicity.

## Action levels

The protection of workers is commonly based on the so-called admissible
OELs or threshold limit values (TLVs) assessed separately for a given physical or chemical hazardous agent. The currently recommended OELs for
organic solvents, including xylene, toluene and styrene, are based on
their neurotoxic and hepatotoxic activities, and vary among different
countries. In view of the latest data, it seems that currently applied action
levels may be insufficient to protect human populations from solvent-
induced auditory damage (Morata et al., 1997b; Morioka et al., 2000;
Śliwińska-Kowalska et al., 2001a), and more reliable procedures should
be implemented in the future.

# Conclusion

In conclusion, the epidemiological data currently available indicate that the population of workers exposed to organic solvents is at high risk of developing hearing loss. The implementation of audiometric screening for those workers, in addition to environmental and biological monitoring, seems to be urgently needed, especially as hearing loss might be the early symptom of chronic toxic encephalopathy (Ödkvist et al., 1987).

# Acknowledgments

Supported by the 6th European Framework Project under the Marie Curie Host Fellowship for the Transfer of Knowledge (Project "NoiseHear" - Contract No MTKD-CT-2004-003137/UE), and by the project of the Polish Ministry of Education and Science No 0911/P05/2004/26.

# References

Barregård L, Axelsson A (1984) Is there an ototraumatic interaction between noise and solvents? Scandinavian Audiology 13(3): 151–5.

Bergström B, Nyström B (1986) Development of hearing loss during long-term exposure to occupational noise. A 20-year follow-up study. Scandinavian Audiology 15(4): 227–34.

Biscaldi GP, Mingardi M, Pollini G, Moglia A, Bossi MC (1981) Acute toluene poisoning. Electroneurophysiological and vestibular investigations. Toxicological European Research 3: 271–3.

Chang SJ, Shih TS, Chou TC, Chen CJ, Chang HY, Sung FC (2003) Hearing loss in workers exposed to carbon disulfide and noise. Environmental Health Perspectives 111(13): 1620–24.

Chang YC (1987) Neurotoxic effects of *n*-hexane on the human central nervous system: evoked potential abnormalites in *n*-hexane polyneuropathy. Journal of Neurology, Neurosurgery, and Psychiatry 50(3): 269–74.

Fechter LD, Liu Y, Herr DW, Crofton KM (1998) Trichloroethylene ototoxicity: evidence for a cochlear origin. Toxicological Sciences: An Official Journal of the Society of Toxicology 42(1): 28–35.

Hirata M, Ogawa Y, Okayama A, Goto S (1992) A cross-sectional study on the brainstem auditory evoked potential among workers exposed to carbon disulfide. International Archives of Occupational and Environmental Health 64(5): 321–4.

International Organization for Standardization (1990) ISO 1999. Acoustics–Determination of Occupational Noise Exposure and Estimation of Noise Induced Hearing Impairment. Geneva: ISO.

Jacobsen P, Hein HO, Suadicani P, Parving A, Glytelberg F (1993) Mixed solvent exposure and hearing impairment: an epidemiological study of 3284 men. The Copenhagen male study. Occupational Medicine 43: 180–4.

Kuwabara S, Kai MR, Nagase H, Hattori T (1999) *n*-Hexane neuropathy caused by addictive inhalation: clinical and electrophysiological features. European Neurology 41(3): 163–7.

Lataye R, Campo P (1997) Combined effects of a simultaneous exposure to noise and toluene on hearing function. Neurotoxicology and Teratology 19: 373–82.

Lataye R, Campo P, Loquet G (2000) Combined effects of noise and styrene exposure on hearing function in the rat. Hearing Research 139(1-2): 86–96.

Laukli E, Hansen PW (1995) An audiometric test battery for the evaluation of occupational exposure to industrial solvents. Acta Oto-Laryngologica 115(2): 162–4.

Möller C, Ödkvist L, Larsby B, Tham R, Ledin T, Bergholtz L (1990) Otoneurological findings in workers exposed to styrene. Scandinavian Journal of Work Environment and Health 16: 189–94.

Morata T, Dunn D, Kretschmer L, Lemasters G, Keith R (1993) Effects of occupational exposure to organic solvents and noise on hearing. Scandinavian Journal of Work Environment & Health 19(4) 245–54.

Morata TC, Fiorini AC, Fischer FM, Colacioppo S, Wallingford KM, Krieg EF, Dunn DE, Gozzoli L, Padrão MA, Cesar CL (1997a) Toluene-induced hearing loss among rotogravure printing workers. Scandinavian Journal of Work Environment & Health; 23: 289–98.

Morata TC, Engel T, Durão A, Costa TR, Krieg EF, Dunn DE, Lozano MA (1997b) Hearing loss from combined exposures among petroleum refinery workers. Scandinavian Audiology 26(3): 141–9.

Morata TC, Johnson AC, Nylén P, Svensson EB, Cheng J, Krieg EF, Lindblad AC, Ernstgård L, Franks J (2002) Audiometric findings in workers exposed to low levels of styrene and noise. Journal of Occupational Environmental Medicine 44(9): 806–14.

Morioka I, Kuroda M, Miyashita K, Takeda S (2000) Evaluation of organic solvent ototoxicity by the upper limit of hearing. Archives of Environmental Health 38(2): 252–7.

Morioka I, Miyai N, Yamamoto H, Miyashita K. Evaluatiou of combined effect of organic solvents and noise by the upper limit of hearing. Ind Health 1999; 54(5): 341-46

Muijser H, Hoogendijk E, Hooisma J (1988) The effects of occupational exposure to styrene on high-frequency hearing thresholds. Toxicology 49: 331–40.

Niklasson M, Möller C, Ödkvist LM, Ekberg K, Flodin U, Dige N, Skoldestig A (1997) Are deficits in the equilibrium system relevant to the clinical investigation of solvent-induced neurotoxicity? Scandinavian Journal of Work Environment and Health 23(3): 206–13.

Niklasson M, Arlinger S, Ledin T, Möller C, Ödkvist L, Flodin U, Tham R (1998) Audiological disturbances caused by long-term exposure to industrial solvents. Relation to the diagnosis of toxic encephalopathy. Scandinavian Audiology 27(3): 131–6.

Nylén P, Hagman M (1994) Function of the auditory and visual systems, and of peripheral nerve, in rats after long-term combined exposure to *n*-hexane and methylated benzene derivates. II. Xylene. Pharmacology and Toxicology 74: 124–9.

Nylén P, Hagman M, Johnson AC (1994) Function of the auditory and visual systems, and of peripheral nerve, in rats after long-term combined exposure to *n*-hexane and methylated benzene derivates. I. Toluene. Pharmacology and Toxicology 74: 116–23.

Ödkvist L, Larsby B, Tham R, Hyden D (1983) Vestibulo-oculomotor disturbances caused by industrial solvents. Otolaryngology-Head and Neck Surgery 91(5): 537–9.

Ödkvist LM, Arlinger SD, Edling C, Larsby B, Bergholtz LM (1987) Audiological and vestibulo-oculomotor findings in workers exposed to solvents and jet fuel. Scandinavian Audiology 16(2): 75–81.

Ödkvist L, Möller C, Thuomas KA (1992) Otoneurologic disturbances caused by solvent pollution. Otolaryngology-Head and Neck Surgery 106(6): 687–92.

Pryor GT, Rebert CS(1992) Interactive effects of toluene and hexane on behavior and neurophysiologic responses in Fischer-344 rats. Neurotoxicology 13(1) 225–34.

Rebert CS, Sorenson SS (1983) Concentration-related effects of hexane on evoked responses from brain and peripheral nerve of the rat. Neurobehavioral Toxicology and Teratology 5(1): 69–76.

Sass-Kortsak AM, Corey PN, Robertson JM (1995) An investigation of the association between exposure to styrene and hearing loss. Annals of Epidemiology 5(1): 15–24.

Śliwińska-Kowalska M, Zamyslowska-Szmytke E, Szymczak W, Kotylo P, Fiszer M, Dudarewicz A, Wesolowski W, Pawlaczyk-Luszczynska M, Stolarek R (2001a) Occupational solvent exposure at moderate concentration increases the risk of hearing loss. Scandinavian Journal of Work Environment and Health 27(5): 335–42.

Śliwińska-Kowalska M, Zamyslowska-Szmytke E, Pawlaczyk-Luszczynska M, Kotylo P, Dudarewicz A, Wesolowski W (2001b) Ototoxic effects of organic solvents: Prophylactic guidelines (in Polish). M Sliwinska-Kowalska (Ed.) Editorial Office of Nofer Institute of Occupational Medicine: 1–48.

Śliwińska-Kowalska M, Zamyslowska-Szmytke E, Szymczak W, Kotylo P, Fiszer M, Wesolowski W, Pawlaczyk-Luszczynska M (2003) Ototoxic effects of occupational exposure to styrene and co-exposure to styrene and noise. Journal of Occupational and Environmental Medicine 45(1): 15–24.

Śliwińska-Kowalska M, Zamyslowska-Szmytke E, Szymczak W, Kotylo P, Fiszer M, Wesolowski W, Pawlaczyk-Luszczynska M Bak M, Gajda-Szadkowska A (2004) Effects of co-exposure to noise and mixture of organic solvents on hearing loss in dockyard workers. Journal of Occupational and Environmental Medicine Jan 46(1): 30–8 [b].

Śliwińska-Kowalska M, Zamyslowska-Szmytke E, Szymczak W, Szymczak W, Kotylo P, Fiszer M, Wesolowski W, Pawlaczyk-Luszczynska M (2005) Exacerbation of noise-induced hearing loss by co-exposure to workplace chemicals. Environmental Toxicology and Pharmacology 19: 547–53 [a].

Yokoyama K, Araki S, Nishikitani M, Sato H (2002) Computerized posturography with sway frequency analysis: application in occupational and environmental health. Industrial Health 40(1): 14–22.

Vrca A, Karacic V, Bozicevic D, Bozikov V, Malinar M (1996) Brainstem auditory evoked potentials in individuals exposed to long-term low concentrations of toluene. American Journal of Industrial Medicine 30: 62–6.

CHAPTER 22

# Noise hazards in the medical environment

*Noise and Its Effects:* Edited by Linda Luxon and Deepak Prasher © 2007 John Wiley & Sons Ltd.

MOSHE CHAIMOFF, LINDA M LUXON

Noise has become a major environmental problem and a public health concern in most industrialized countries (Bowling and Edelman, 1987). Occupational hearing impairment is usually associated with factories and airports, healthcare institutions being traditionally regarded as safe and quiet workplaces. Conventional images of the hospital create two misconceptions in the minds of people who have sporadic or casual contact with it. First, that it is not really a workplace, in comparison with a factory, and second, that since the function of the hospital is to promote health and well-being, it is a healthy and safe place for those within it, both patients and medical staff. Both assumptions are far from the truth as each hospital employs hundreds to thousands of workers treating hundreds to thousands of patients and an even greater number of visitors who every day enter the hospital's doors, walk its corridors and are exposed to a variety of environmental conditions and noises. It is obvious that patients require favourable environments to assist their recovery, and staff need appropriate working conditions. In this chapter, the physiological as well as the psychological hazards of noise to patients and medical staff are reviewed and the noise levels and dangers of these modern hospitals discussed.

## Physiological and psychological hazards of noise

Most sounds can be described as a means of communication, which may be used to draw attention, to give warning, to entertain or to communicate. The term 'noise' is commonly used to designate an annoying or unwanted sound. In the hearing field, it means any excessively loud sound that can potentially harm hearing. The patterns of environmental noise are typically described as: continuous; relatively constant noise, fluctuating; noise rises and falls in level over time, and intermittent or impulsive; and sounds interrupted for varying time periods. Impulsive or impact noises caused by explosive or metal-on-metal mechanical events are intense and short lasting.

Sounds evoke different physiological and psychological responses depending on the amplitude, frequency and duration of sound (Clark, 1991).

**Physiological and psychological response to sound:**

- hearing loss;
- tinnitus;
- dysacusis;
- changes in heart rate;
- changes in blood pressure;
- changes in skin resistance;
- behavioural changes;
- cognitive changes;
- sleep disturbances.

**Hearing loss**

Exposure to excessive sound impairs hearing and may damage the cochlea. If the sound is moderately intense it may produce a temporary threshold shift (TTS). After exposure, if the TTS does not recover before the ear is re-exposed to excessive sounds, or sound pressure levels are greater than those creating the TTS, it may produce a much more severe TTS, or may give rise to a permanent threshold shift (PTS). The precise relationship between the TTS and the PTS in hearing loss resulting from noise exposure remains ill-defined (Clark, 1991; Gao et al., 1999). However, one common view is that the magnitude of the initial reversible threshold shift produced by a specific exposure sets the upper limit for growth of the PTS under the continual influence of the hazardous sound producing the TTS. Traditionally, the PTS can be caused by acoustic trauma – a single short exposure to a very intense sound such as an explosion that results in sudden loss of hearing – while noise-induced hearing loss (NIHL) results from chronic exposure to less intense but more prolonged levels of sound. The minimal intensity of sound that may result in a TTS is between 78 and 85 dB (A) and long-term exposure to noise levels exceeding 85 dB (A) for 8 hours per day is sufficient to cause a PTS (Clark, 1991). The frequency spectrum of the sound and the length of exposure are critical factors in inducing the PTS. The threshold for long-term TTS marks the upper limit of safe working conditions. The US Occupation Safety and Health Administration (OSHA) has established guidelines for permissible noise exposure levels and duration (Table 22.1).

**Table 22.1** OSHA permissible noise exposures

| Duration (hours/day) | Sound pressure level (on dB (A) scale slow response) |
| --- | --- |
| 8 | 90 |
| 6 | 92 |
| 4 | 95 |
| 2 | 100 |
| 1 | 105 |
| 0.5 | 110 |
| ≤ 0.25 | 115 |

From: Occupational Safety and Health Administration (1988) Chapters XVII 1910-176, Code of Federal Regulations. Washington DC: US Govt Printing Office.

## Psychological, physiological changes and disturbances of sleep

*Behavioural changes* such as annoyance are typical findings in studies of noise and the percentage of people annoyed increases by about 10% for each 5-dB (A) increase in the sound level in frequencies of 500–5000 Hz (Kryter, 1985; Kjellberg, 1990). The most obvious effect of noise is that it may mask speech and other sounds that one wants to hear. Several studies have shown that noise is especially annoying when this is the case (Williams et al., 1969; Moran and Loeb, 1977).

The *physiological responses* to noise are of three types, which may be distinguished by duration of the response and the relationship to the noise exposure.

### Physiological responses to noise

- Immediate short-lasting phasic response
- Persistent tonic response
- Long-term health hazards

First there is an immediate, short-lasting, phasic physiological response to noise changes. Any change in noise may lead to a subconscious response generally called an 'orienting reflex'. This response involves a redirection of sense organs towards the noise source and a series of physiological responses lasting no more than a few seconds, including lowered heart rate, blood pressure and peripheral blood flow, together with increased apocrine gland activity. Provided that the noise is perceived to be of no importance for the individual, the response habituates. If the noise has a very sudden onset it may evoke a startle reflex, which includes blinking and muscular jerks that may cause momentary disruption in the performance of manipulatory tasks (May and Rice, 1971).

Second, noise can give rise to a more persistent, tonic response during and for a short period after exposure. This type of response is still controversial, because inconsistent experimental results have been obtained as the studies by Frankenhaeuser and Lundberg show (Frankenhaeuser and Lundberg, 1974; Lundberg and Frankenhaeuser, 1978). In one study, subjects undertook mental arithmetic during exposure to low-level or high-level noise. There was no effect of noise on performance but an increased secretion of adrenaline and an increased effort was recorded qualitatively. Thus, the performance level was upheld at the price of increased physiological stress. In a second study, a lower performance standard was demanded and the opposite result was obtained: performance was impaired whereas the adrenaline level was unaffected by noise.

Third, long-term health hazards secondary to chronic noise exposure are reported. An increased incidence of hypertension and other cardiovascular problems have been suggested in several epidemiological studies of groups occupationally exposed to noise (Borg, 1981; Tarnopolsky and Clark, 1984). Moreover, as noise may cause annoyance and stress it is reasonable to hypothesize that it also contributes to the development of mental illness (Tarnopolsky and Clark, 1984). Although many studies have been conducted in this area, no definite conclusion has emerged although a higher incidence of admission to mental healthcare units and use of psychotropic drugs has been reported. Nevertheless, evidence argues against noise being a major causal factor (Tarnopolsky and Clark, 1984).

### Disturbances of sleep

Disturbances of sleep are another noise hazard. Sleep has been considered therapeutic throughout time but the scientific relationship between sleep and health is largely unknown (Krueger and Majde, 1990; Schwab, 1994). In rabbits there appeared to be a relationship between sleep pattern and recovery from infectious disease, with a correlation between increased mortality and morbidity and sleep disturbances in rabbits infected with *Staphylococcus aureus* (Krueger and Majde, 1990). Cytokines and bacterial cell wall products also have been shown to alter sleep patterns in animals (Krueger and Johannsen, 1989), data that suggest that sleep may play a role in aiding the host's defence against infectious diseases, as well as a wide spectrum of other pathological conditions.

# Noise in the medical environment

There are many possible noise hazards in the medical environment. A patient may be transferred by helicopter and/or ambulance to hospital, admitted to a medical ward, submitted to procedures in the imaging unit and operating theatre, before being transferred to the intensive care unit (ICU). Each situation may pose a noise hazard. Moreover, noise hazards are found in the laboratories and maintenance facilities of a modern hospital such as the kitchen, housekeeping or laundry.

## Sources of medical/rescue transport noise

* Aeroplane
* Helicopter
* Ambulance – siren, apparatus
* Fire engine – cutting equipment, siren

### The hospital-based helicopter

Use of hospital-based helicopters for emergency medical transport has increased over the last decade, leading to increased noise exposure of helicopter pilots, aircrew and transported patients. In their study, Pasic and Poulton (1985) studied the Bell 206L helicopter and found that the sound intensities to be between 85 and 90 dB (A), for the crew's average duration of 2.3 hours/day. Mean respiratory rate, an estimate of noise-induced stress, was found to be significantly increased in pilots without ear protection when compared with pilots with ear protection (Wichnan et al., 1979; Pasic and Poulton, 1985). Moreover, although pilots subjected to aircraft noise at 100 dB (A) for 8 hours showed no decrement in perceptive ability, the second 4 hours of exposure revealed a significant decrease in intellectual judgment (Pierson, 1971). However, the use of communication headsets with noise attenuation values of 30–40 dB (A) is standard in most current hospital-based helicopter programmes (Pasic and Poulton, 1985).

Considering patient care, noise makes it impossible to use a standard stethoscope to auscultate breath sounds and heart sounds, which are especially important in cardiac, pulmonary and trauma patients who are most likely to be transported by helicopter.

Moreover, in a study by Shenai (1977), sound levels were measured in a neonatal incubator during transport in a rotatory aircraft and fixed wing aircraft (Convair C131B and Cessna 421). Sound levels varied from 58 dB (A) to 68 dB (A) inside the transport incubator before air transport, but exceeded 90 dB (A) during transport. Young infants, particularly immature neonates, may be particularly susceptible to hazardous noise, as suggested by the fact that young animals show a greater susceptibility to noise-induced physiological and pathological alterations (Falk et al., 1974).

In conclusion, aside from the transport incubator, noise levels are not excessive and the duration is short. However, if the crews' mean daily duration of noise exposure were to be increased, or prolonged flight duration were expected for a patient, a hearing conservation programme would be required. Moreover, in regard to neonate transport by air, special attention should be paid to sound levels and hearing protection.

## Ambulance transport

Emergency medical service providers routinely travel to and from the scene of a medical emergency using a vehicle with flashing lights and siren. The aim is to ensure the attention of fellow drivers and pedestrians as a safety precaution and thus prevent accidents. A loud auditory signal may exert an immediate arousal effect (De Lorenzo and Eilers, 1991). Recommended attributes of a warning signal include sufficient power and wide frequency spectrum to overcome masking noise (Patterson, 1990). The recommended frequency range is between 1 kHz and 4 kHz, which is consistent with the peak sensitivity of human hearing (Fidell et al., 1974). A US Department of Transportation study (Skeiber et al., 1977) noted that the sound of sirens results in community annoyance and sleep disturbance, but concluded that the risk of hearing damage to the general population was insignificant. However a US Federal study (Skeiber et al., 1978) has demonstrated sound levels for an ambulance driver exceeding occupational standards. Other studies (Johnson et al., 1980; Pepe et al., 1985; Flesch et al., 1986) have linked hearing loss to siren-exposed emergency medical staff. Simple measures to reduce the risk of exposure include mounting the siren speakers on the front grill of the vehicle, rather than on the cabin roof, and closing the vehicle windows (Skeiber et al., 1978). Patients and crew members in the rear compartment of the ambulance were considered to be at minimal risk of hearing loss (Rasmussen et al., 1983). In a more recent study, the noise levels in the ambulance ranged from 58 dB (A) in the patient compartment to 84 dB (A) in the forward cab with the windows open and the siren in use (Price and Goldsmith, 1998). However, there appears to be no excessive loss of hearing acuity in ambulance personnel (Price and Goldsmith, 1998).

In conclusion, it seems that both the patient and the crew are at no risk of hearing loss as a consequence of the high-amplitude noise of the emergency siren. However, if the mean daily duration of noise exposure of emergency staff, mainly in the front cab, was to be increased a hearing conservation programme would be required.

# Noise in hospital

Many treatment and diagnostic areas are noisy.

## The sources of noise

- medical wards;
- imaging units;
- intensive care wards;
- other areas.

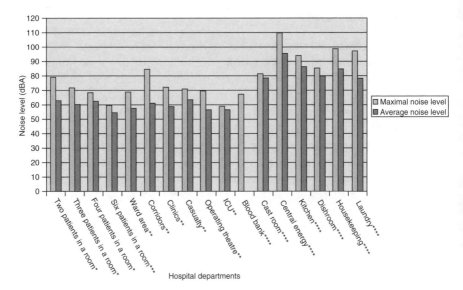

**Figure 22.1.** Maximal and average noise levels (dBA) recorded in different hospital departments as obtained from several references (\*=36,\*\*=34,\*\*\*=35,\*\*\*\*=57).

## Medical wards

The patients, staff, visitors and equipment contribute to the level of noise in medical and surgical wards. In a study performed by Tope (1983), the average noise level in surgical wards with two, three and four patients was measured. In a room with two patients, the peak noise was 79.3 dB (A) and the average noise level over 24 hours was 55.43 dB (A). In a room with three patients, the peak noise was 72 dB (A) and the average noise level was 54.45 dB (A). In the room with four patients, the peak noise was 68.8 dB (A) and the average noise level was 52.63 dB (A). The average noise in all the rooms, over 24 hours, was 54.17 dB (A). Other studies (Aitken, 1982; Bayo et al., 1995) showed similar sound levels of 58 dB (A) in ward areas. These noise levels are not loud enough to cause hearing loss, but may be of sufficient intensity to interfere with rest and sleep needed for the recovery of the patient (Minckley, 1968; Shapiro and Berland, 1972; Falk and Wood, 1973).

## Imaging units

Apart from noise contributors similar to those in any other department in the hospital, imaging units have one additional and significant source of noise: magnetic resonance imaging (MRI). The introduction of MRI has resulted in tremendous advances in medical diagnosis. However, one potentially adverse effect is that the equipment is extremely noisy (Liener et al., 2005). Sound pressure levels (SPLs) of MRI noise were measured at the position of the human head in the isocentre of five MRI systems, using ten different pulse sequences routinely acquired in clinical MRI, and were between 113 dB SPL and 117 dB SPL (Counter et al., 1997). The T1-weighted images generated more intense acoustic noise than the proton-dense T2-weighted measures. When patients' auditory thresholds were measured before and after an average of 39 minutes of MRI, a TTS of at least 15 dB HL was detected in one half of the patients compared with 10% of patients undergoing the same procedure but with ear plugs (Brummett et al., 1988). All TTSs returned to normal within 15 minutes and, thus, it seems that some people are at risk of TTSs but not PTSs. However, because patients with particular susceptibility to intense sound cannot be defined, it is advisable to offer hearing protection (Liener et al., 2005).

In addition to patients, the effect of noise on medical staff and their performance should be considered. In a study assessing the effect of noise on the efficiency of residents identifying radiological pathology, it was found that inaccuracies were greater in those clinicians who were upset or irritated by the high noise levels (Park et al., 1994). Similar results have been found in other studies looking at task performances in a noisy environment (Cohen, 1980; Fisher, 1983).

## Operating theatre

The dangers of air and water pollution in surgery were identified about a century ago and, as a result, aseptic and antipollution techniques are routinely practised. However, in the current pollution-aware age, surgery has fallen behind in its recognition of what has been called 'the third pollution'. This is noise that is defined as unwanted sound and an everyday nuisance that may have an effect on the well-being and work performance of those exposed to it. Operating theatres are as susceptible to noise pollution as other working environments. Shapiro and Berland (1972) linked the noise levels in an operating theatre to those encountered on a motorway. Staff and patients in the operating theatre are exposed to a barrage of sounds, produced by monitoring devices, alarms, suckers, diathermy machines, scavenging systems for anaesthetic gases, mechanical and pneumatic tools, heaters, pumps, paging devices and 'intercoms', telephones, by the clanging of metal bowls, instruments and trolleys, and, in some operating theatres, background music requested by the operating team. This cacophony (Love, 2003) is often exacerbated by noise from adjacent scrub-up areas, instrument rooms and sterilizers. For theatre staff, this noise can lead to impaired concentration and performance, interference with communication and increased levels of stress.

### Noise in the operating theatre

- Monitoring devices
- Paging devices
- Alarms
- 'Intercoms'

- Telephones
- Suckers
- Diathermy machines
- Scavenging systems
- Mechanical and pneumatic tools
- Heaters
- Pumps
- Clanging metal instruments

Patients who are conscious for part or all of the time in the operating theatre may develop a level of anxiety because of the noise (Mori and Murata, 1979; Davis et al., 1989; Hodge and Thompson, 1990). The sound level in an operating theatre has been measured to be between 52 and 108 dB (A), although the higher sound levels were only of a short duration (Fisher, 1983). The background noise levels in these studies were within the recommended levels for a satisfactory working environment in an operating theatre (Hodge and Thompson, 1990). However, the effect of noise on performance depends not only on its level and the stress tolerance of the individual but also on the complexity of the task being undertaken and the type of noise (Fisher et al., 1984).

Two features of the type of noise are important, namely whether it is predictable and whether it is controllable. Even high- level continuous noises (90–120 dB (A)) mainly have no effect on the performance of simple motor or mental tasks (Baum et al., 1985). However, noises of lesser intensity, especially when they are unpredictable, uncontrollable or both, can interfere with the performance of complex tasks (Baum et al., 1985). Moreover, members of a surgical team may be easily distracted by conversations between other members of the team, leading to suboptimal communication for mutual understanding and good performance of the necessary surgical procedures.

Noise can become an especially serious problem for a conscious patient during local or regional anaesthesia. An operation is stressful for most patients and added stress and anxiety should be avoided by keeping noise to a minimum. Sudden loud noises not only raise the stress level for the patient, but may also cause a startle response with movement of that part of the body upon which the surgery is being performed.

Recommendations to ensure a more pleasant and quiet environment in the operating theatre include: earplugs or headphones for the conscious patient, background music played in the theatre at low volume, which may mask other sounds without impairing communication or psychomotor performance (Hawksworth, Sivalingam and Asbury, 1998) and redesigning and reducing the noise levels of alarms, so that the surgeon and the anaesthetist will be alerted without extreme noises.

Noise pollution should be considered in the design of new operating theatres (for example, installation of sound insulation between scrub-up and sterilization areas and the theatre itself by avoiding the use of hard, sound-reflecting ceilings and floors) (Fisher et al., 1984). The need for paging devices, intercoms and telephones in operating theatres must be carefully assessed because of their potential to distract staff and disturb the conscious patients. In order to avoid exposure to sudden loud noises with consequent higher levels of anxiety, the patient should not be in the operating theatre during preparation for the procedure.

Noise hazard during operations on the skull, teeth or even the ear should be considered. The noise from drilling and shaving the bone is transmitted directly through the skull to the cochlea. It is known that the surgical drill in ear surgery generates bone-conducted noise levels of about 100 dB (A) around the cochlea. This type of noise has its main energy in the 2- and 4-kHz octave bands (Kylen and Arlinger, 1976; Arlinger and Kylen, 1977). Drilling during ear surgery is often maintained for about 1 hour and a 2.4- to 4.8-kHz noise band of intensity 100 dB (A) for 1 hour may produce a TTS of about 40 dB HL at 4 kHz (Miller, 1974). Soudijn et al. (1976), studying surface preparations of cochlea from drill-noise-exposed guinea pigs, found distinctive lesions in the organ of Corti. To begin with, there was a large circumscribed lesion, which involved total destruction of the organ of Corti over several tenths of millimetres. Second, there was a combination of lesions of a row of inner cells with lesions of first-row outer hair cells. Finally, there was a scattered loss of hair cells, solitary or in small groups, which involved the outer hair cells of the second and third rows more than those of the first row, leaving the inner hair cells entirely intact. Kylen et al. (1977a) measured pure-tone thresholds before and after otological surgery and found TTSs of up to 40 dB HL for a duration of up to 1 month with a direct correlation between the threshold shift and the duration of drilling. It was found that exposure to 100 dB (A) for 5 minutes gave an average TTS of 15 dB HL, for 40 minutes gave approximately 35 dB HL and for 60 minutes gave about 40 dB HL in the 4-kHz band.

The type of drill and the shape and size of the burr are also important (Soudijn et al., 1976; Kylen et al., 1977b). The low-speed drill (12 000 r.p.m.) produces more noise (up to 10 dB (A) higher) than the high-speed (20 000 r.p.m.) or the very-high-speed drill (100 000 r.p.m.). This is due not so much as to the difference in revolutions per minute as to the difference in torque. The higher torque of the low-speed drill permits greater pressure of the burr on the bone, thus involving an increased intensity of noise. Conical burrs were found to be noisier than spherical burrs of the same diameter. All burrs of larger diameter were noisier than burrs of smaller diameter (Soudjin et al., 1976). However a study of high-powered ENT instruments did not demonstrate a noise hazard (Prasad and Reddy, 2003).

**Noise in the ICU**

Intensive care units are especially designed for severely ill patients and only those who need highly specialized care and attention are transferred to the ICU. However, several studies have demonstrated that, with regard to noise, the ICU environment is potentially hazardous. In Falk and Wood (1973), Hrgest (1979), Soutar and Wilson (1986) and Yassi et al. (1991), sound monitoring in an acute care unit revealed an average sound level of 66 dB (A). This demonstrates that noise pollution in the ICU setting is not a rare problem in a small number of specialised hospitals, but a more general problem. Other studies (Aaron et al., 1996; Carley et al., 1997; Kahn et al., 1998) demonstrated a significant association with sound peaks (80 dB (A)) and arousal from sleep and sleep fragmentation, detected as transient EEG arousals. This sleep deprivation has been demonstrated to affect task performance, general mood and level of alertness, and increase daytime fatigue. Observation studies (Helton et al., 1980; Hansell, 1984) have shown that at least one-third of sleep-deprived subjects have symptoms consistent with 'ICU psychosis' syndrome and that patients identify staff noises as the most disturbing. It is also possible that sleep deprivation may adversely affect respiratory muscle function (Chen and Tang, 1989) and ventilatory control (White et al., 1983), and potentially hinder weaning from mechanical ventilation. Noise has also been implicated in causing hearing loss, especially in patients concomitantly receiving ototoxic drugs such as aminoglycosides (Dayal et al., 1971; Falk, 1972). Additionally, from a staff perspective noise has been reported to contribute to critical care nurse burnout (Topf and Dillon, 1988).

In a study undertaken by Robertson and Cooper-Peel (Robertson et al., 1998), the measured peak noise distribution in a neonatal intensive care nursery (NICU) exceeded 90 dB (A) in 31.3% of minute measurements. Background sound levels in the NICU ranged from 45 to 135 dB (A) and may have lasted for prolonged periods at 80 dB (A) (Zahr and Traversay, 1995). Some common sounds, such as closing the incubator porthole, can reach 120–135 dB (A). These noise levels are in excess of the recommendations of the American Academy of Paediatrics that noise levels in the NICU should not exceed 58 dB (American Academy of Pediatrics Committee on Environmental Health, 1994).

The frequent and high-intensity noise in the NICU is considered a factor in altering the behavioural and physiological responses of infants, and may be responsible for hearing loss seen in premature infants (Gottfried, 1985; Ostfield et al., 1990). This is because premature infants have less developed neuronal organization and are thus more sensitive to, yet less competent in handling, environmental stimuli (Gottfried, 1985; Gorski and Huntingdon, 1988; Ostfield et al., 1990). They usually react to NICU stimuli with physiological rather than interactive responses. Physiological responses to noise are manifested by heart rate accelerations, colour changes and decreased oxygen saturation levels, while behavioural responses are manifested by disturbed sleep and excitement (Gorski and Huntingdon, 1988; Krawciw et al., 1990).

**Neonatal responses to noise**

- Heart rate acceleration
- Increase in blood pressure
- Colour changes
- Decreased oxygen saturation levels
- Disturbed sleep
- Excitability

Sudden loud noises, such as telephones ringing and alarms, are associated with a decrease in oxygen saturation levels, an increase in blood pressure and possibly intraventricular haemorrhage (Blennow et al., 1974; Long et al., 1980; Beckham and Mishoe, 1982). Auditory stimulation can also interfere with sleep and heart rate in infants (Gorski et al., 1988; Ostfeld et al., 1990). Furthermore, it has been argued that the increased energy infants expend on responding to noise may impair their growth (Thomas, 1989).

### Other departments

Noise levels in other hospital departments are reported in several studies (Minckley, 1968; Aitken, 1982; Bayo et al., 1995) to average 68 dB (A) in the blood bank, 79 dB (A) in the cast room, 96 dB (A) in generator, pumps, compressors and boiler rooms, 82 dB (A) in the kitchen and 75 dB (A) in the laundry. In these departments, staff members are exposed to high levels of noise, which can cause constant irritation and fatigue. Long-duration exposure may lead to noise-induced hearing loss.

In modern society it is the employer's responsibility to identify all workers who are or are likely to be exposed to sound levels of sufficient intensity and duration to cause hearing impairment. In the USA, the OSHA requires a hearing conservation programme at 85 dB (A) using an 8-hour time-weighted average (see Table 22.1). Thus, for areas with noise exposure of 80–85 dB (A), a hearing conservation programme (including audiometry and education) must be implemented; the employer must provide hearing protection for workers exposed to noise levels above 85 dB (A).

# Conclusion

Environmental noise in hospitals has received scant attention in the medical literature. The US Environmental Protection Agency (EPA) recommends that noise levels in the hospital setting do not exceed 45 dB (A) during the day and 35 dB (A) at night (EPA, 1974).

In the hospital-based helicopter, the use of headsets for crew and short transmitting time reduce the danger of noise-induced hearing loss (Pasic and Poulton, 1985), but it can raise the level of anxiety and discomfort for the patient and interfere with simple medical tasks such as auscultation. Therefore, all diagnostic examination should be performed before or after transport, while, during flight, monitoring should use electronic devices with on-screen information. In the case of long transport time, the patient should be provided with hearing protection devices.

Ambulance staff are not at risk of siren noise damage in the case of short transport time (Rasmussen et al., 1983; Price and Goldsmith, 1998). However, when they are repeatedly called upon, the siren should be used more cautiously, and only with the vehicle windows closed. If the siren is required for a long duration, hearing protection devices should be used. Monitoring the patient required the same considerations in the ambulance as in the helicopter.

Noise levels in the medical wards and ICU are not loud enough to cause a PTS but they are of sufficient intensity to interfere with rest and sleep needed for the recovery of the patient (Minckley, 1968; Haslam, 1970; Shapiro and Berland, 1972; Falk and Wood, 1973). The main problem in the intensive care setting is sleep deprivation, which has been demonstrated to affect the well-being of the patient and interfere with recovery (Falk and Wood, 1973; Hrgest, 1979; Soutar and Wilson, 1986; Yassi et al., 1991). 'ICU psychosis' syndrome (Helton et al., 1980; Hansell, 1984) can affect a third of patients and it is also possible that sleep deprivation may hinder weaning from mechanical ventilation. Patients concomitantly receiving ototoxic drugs are more susceptible to noise-induced hearing loss (Dayal et al., 1971; Falk, 1972) and, from the staff perspective, noise has been implicated in contributing to critical care nurse burnout (Topf and Dillon, 1988).

In the imaging department the main noise hazard is MRI. It seems that due to the short duration of exposure some patients are at risk of TTS but not PTS. However, because patients with particular susceptibility to intense sound cannot be defined, it is advisable to offer hearing protection to all those who undergo the test.

In the operating theatre matters are even more complicated. Staff and patients are exposed to a barrage of sounds that can lead to impaired concentration and performance, interference with communication and increased levels of stress. Recommendations to ensure a more pleasant and quiet environment in the operating theatre include earplugs or headphones for the conscious patient and background music played in the theatre at low volume, which may mask other sounds without impairing communication. Operating theatres should be updated with particular attention to redesigning and reducing the noise levels of alarms, paging devices, intercoms and telephones.

As for the procedure itself, any skull surgery, especially ear surgery, entails a risk of development or exacerbation of sensorineural hearing loss, and individual sensitivity certainly plays a role in this respect. In ear operations involving the use of an otological drill, one takes an additional acoustic risk by exposing the diseased ear to sound intensities that can have a traumatic effect on the organ of Corti. This risk increases if the bone involved is more sclerotic, for this requires longer drilling and an increased pressure of the burr against the bone, by which duration and intensity of the drill noise increase.

Special care should be taken in neonates. Noise levels in NICUs have a negative effect on the infants' physiological and behavioural responses. When noise intensities are decreased, infants have higher saturated oxygen values, less fluctuation in physiological responses, sleep better, and have more quiet alert states and fewer state changes (Zahr and Traversay, 1995). Studies (Thomas et al., 1981; Linn et al., 1985; Tynan, 1986) have found that infants with frequent state changes or those with state instabilities have higher rates of developmental delays, behavioural deficit and subsequent medical problems. Therefore by reducing the noise levels in NICUs the long-term outcome of premature infants may be improved.

It can be understood from this chapter that both patients and staff are affected by noise in the medical environment. In most cases, when compared with the OSHA criteria (see Table 22.1), the noise levels are not high enough to cause noise-induced hearing loss. However, it does cause irritability, chronic fatigue, lack of concentration and disturbance of sleep pattern, and excite a negative influence on the recovery of patients. Noise-induced hearing loss is most likely in NICUs, in ICUs when combined with ototoxic drug administration, and during scalp or ear surgery.

Acoustic modifications in the structure of hospitals have been suggested (Minckley, 1968), and should be extended to hospital equipment and furniture. Furthermore, patients might be offered some control over noise through relaxation techniques or through listening to their preferred stimuli supplied by headphones. Distress and interpersonal conflict might be reduced if patients with dissimilar reactions to noise were not placed in the same room. Finally, hospital staff should attempt to lower noises that are under their control such as socioacusis of visitors, telephones, television, radios, beepers and general conversation. Monitors, alarms, respirators, incubators and other equipment should be designed to produce only low-intensity noise. It is possible that reorganization of the day's schedule is needed, combined with re-education of staff about the negative consequences of noise and its prevention.

# Acknowledgement

We would like to thank Ms Hannah Derry, MSc, for her assistance in producing this chapter.

# References

Aaron JN, Carlisle CC, Carskadon MA et al. (1996) Environmental noise as a cause of sleep distruption in an intermediate respiratory care unit. Sleep 19: 707–10.

Aitken RJ (1982) Quantitative noise analysis in a modern hospital. Archives of Environmental Health 37: 361–4.

American Academy of Pediatrics Committee on Environmental Health (1994) Noise pollution: neonatal aspects. Pediatrics 54: 476–9.

Arlinger SD, Kylen P (1977) Bone-conducted stimulation in electrocochleography. Acta Otolaryngologica 84: 377–84.

Baum A, Fosher J, Singer J (1985) Social Psychology. New York: Random House.

Bayo MV, Garcia AM, Garcia A (1995) Noise levels in urban hospital and workers' subjective responses. Archives of Environmental Health 50: 247–51.

Beckham RW, Mishoe SG (1982) Sound levels inside incubators and oxygen hoods used with nebulizers and humidifiers. Respiratory Care 35: 1272–9.

Blennow G, Svenningsen N, Almquist B (1974) Noise levels in infant incubators. Pediatrics 53: 29–32.

Borg E (1981) Physiological and pathogenic effects of sound. Acta Otolaryngologica Supplement 381: 1–68.

Bowling A, Edelman R (1987) Noise in society: a public health problem? Health Promotion 2: 75–83.

Brummett RE, Talbot JM, Charuhas P (1988) Potential hearing loss resulting from MR imaging. Radiology 169: 539–40.

Carley DW, Applebaum R, Banser RC et al. (1997) Respiratory and arousal responses to acoustic stimulation. Chest 112: 1567–71.

Chen H, Tang R (1989) Sleep loss impairs respiratory muscle endurance. American Review of Respiratory Disease 140: 907–9.

Clark WW (1991) Noise exposure for leisure activities: a review. Journal of the Acoustical Society of America 90: 175–81.

Cohen S (1980) After effects of stress on human performance and social behaviour: a review of research and theory. Psychological Bulletin 88: 82–108.

Counter SA, Olofsson A, Grahn HF, Borg E (1997) MRI acoustic noise: sound pressure and frequency analysis. Journal of Magnetic Resonance Imaging 7: 606–11.

Davis JM, Ewen A, Cuppage A, Gilbert D, Winkelaar R (1989) Noise levels in the operating rooms - a comparison of Canada and England. Anaesthesia and Intensive Care 17: 98–9.

Dayal VS, Kokshanian A, Mitchell DP (1971) Combined effects of noise and kanamycin. Annals of Otology 80: 897–902.

De Lorenzo RA, Eilers MA (1991) Lights and siren: a review of emergency vehicle warning system. Annals of Emergency Medicine 20: 1331–5.

Environmental Protection Agency (1974) Information on Levels of Environmental Noise Requisite to Protect Public Health and Welfare with an Adequate Margin of Safety. Washington DC: Government Printing Office.

Falk SA (1972) Combined effects of noise and ototoxic drugs. Environmental Health Perspectives 2: 5–22.

Falk SA, Wood NF (1973) Hospital noise-levels and potential health hazards. New England Journal of Medicine 289: 774–81.

Falk SA, Cook RO, Hoseman JK, Sanders GH (1974) Noise-induced inner ear damage in new born and adult guinea pigs. Laryngoscope 84: 444–53.

Fidell S, Pearson KS, Bennet R (1974) Prediction of aural detectability of noise signals. Human Factors 16: 373–83.

Fisher JD, Bell PA, Baum A (1984) Environmental Psychology, 2nd edn. New York: Holt, Reinhart & Winston.

Fisher S (1983) Memory and search in laud noises. Can J Psychol 37: 439–49.

Flesch I, Tubbs R, Carpenter J (1986) Siren noise. Emergency 18: 42.

Frankenhaeuser M, Lundberg U (1974) Immediate and delayed effect of noise on performance and arousal. Biological Psychology 2: 127–33.

Gao WW, King DL, Zheng XY, Ruan FM, Liu YJ (1999) Comparison in the changes in the steriocilia between temporary and permanent threshold shift. Hearing Reserch 62: 27–41.

Gorski PA, Huntington L (1988) Physiological measures to tactile stimulation in hospitalised preterm infants. Pediatric Research 23: 210a.

Gottfried AW (1985) Environments of newborn infants in special care units. In AW Gottfried, IL Gaiter (eds) Infant Stress under Intensive Care. Baltimore, ML: University Park Press, pp. 23–54.

Hansell HN (1984) The behavioural effect of noise on man: the patient with intensive care unit psychosis. Heart Lung 13:59–65.

Haslam P (1970) Noise in hospitals: its effect on the patient. Nursing Clinics of North America 5: 715–24.

Hawksworth CR, Sivalingam P, Asbury AJ (1998) The effect of music on anaesthetists' psychomotor performance. Anaesthesia 53(2): 195–7.

Helton MC, Gordon SH, Nunnery SL (1980) The correlation between sleep deprivation and the intensive care unit syndrome. Heart Lung 9: 464–8.

Hodge B, Thompson JF (1990) Noise pollution in the operating theatre. Lancet 335: 891–4.

Hrgest TS (1979) Clinical engineering practices: noise – the new hospital contaminant. Clinical Engineering 7: 38–40.

Jerger J, Jerger S, Pepe P et al. (1986) Race difference in susceptibility to noise-induced hearing loss. American Journal of Otology 7: 425–9.

Johnson DW, Hammond RJ, Sherman RE (1980) Hearing in the ambulance paramedic population. Annals of Emergency Medicine 9: 557–61.

Kahn DM, Cook TE, Carlisle CC et al. (1998) Identification and modification of environmental noise in an ICU setting. Chest 114(2): 535–40.

Kjellberg A (1990) Subjective, behavioural and psychophysiological effects of noise. Scandanavian Journal of Work and Environmental Health 16(1): 29–38.

Krawciw N, Ostfeld B, Burke S, Hiatt M, Hegyi T (1990) Computer based system for the assessment of environmental impact on the neonate. Pediatric Research 27: 1257 (212a).

Krueger JM, Johannsen L (1989) Bacterial products, cytokines and sleep. Journal of Rheumatology 19 (suppl): 52–7.

Krueger JM, Majde JA (1990) Sleep as host defence: Its regulation by microbial products and cytokines. Clinical Immunology and Immunopathology 57: 188–99.

Kryter KD (1985) The Effects of Noise on Man. New York: Academic Press.

Kylen P, Arlinger SD (1976) Drill-generated noise levels in ear surgery. Acta Otolaryngologica 82: 402.

Kylen P, Arlinger SD, Berholtz LM (1977a) Peroperative temporary threshold shift in ear surgery. Acta Otolaryngologica 84: 393–401.

Kylen P, Stjernvall JE, Arlinger SD (1977b) Variables affecting the drill-generated noise levels in ear surgery. Acta Otolaryngologica 84: 252.

Liener K, Wunderlich A, Ehret G, Bachor E (2005) Measurement of noise protection in functional magnetic resonance imaging. Laryngorhinootologie 84(2): 108–12.

Linn P, Horowitz FD, Fox H (1985) Stimulation in the NICU: is more necessarily better? Clinical Perinatology 12: 407–23.

Long J, Lucy J, Philip A (1980) Noise and hypoxemia in the intensive care nursery. Pediatrics 65: 143–5.

Love, H (2003) Noise exposure in the opthopaedic operating theatre: a significant health hazard. Australia and New Zealand Journal of Surgery 73(10): 836–8.

Lundberg U, Frankenhaeuser M (1978) Psychophysiological reactions to noise as modified by personal control over noise intensity. Biological Psychology 6: 51–9.

May DN, Rice CG (1971) Effects of startle due to pistol shots on control precision performance. Journal of Sound and Vibration 15: 197–202.

Miller JD (1974) Effect of noise on people. Journal of Acoustical Society of America 56: 729.

Minckley BB (1968) A study of noise and its relationship to patient discomfort in the recovery room. Nursing Research 17: 247–50.

Moran SLV, Loeb M (1977) Annoyance and behavioural after-effects following interfering and non–interfering aircraft noise. Journal of Applied Psychology 62: 719–26.

Mori H, Murata H (1979) A study of noise in the operating room. Japanese Journal of Anaesthesiology 10: 1102–6.

Ostfeld B, Krawciw N, Burk S, Hiatt M, Hegyi T (1990) Impact of environment on the high–risk infant: the effect of monitoring alarms. Pediatric Research 27: 1295: 218A.

Park SH, Song HH, Han JH, Park JM et al. (1994) Effect of noise on the detection of rib fractures by residents. Investigational Radiology 29(1): 54–8.

Pasic TB, Poulton TJ (1985) The hospital-based helicopter, a threat to hearing? Arch Otolaryngologica 111: 507–8.

Patterson RD (1990) Auditory warning sound in the work environment. Philosophical Transactions of the Royal Society of London 327: 485–92.

Pepe PE, Jerger J, Miller RH et al. (1985) Accelerated hearing loss in urban emergency medical services firefighters. Annals of Emergency Medicine 14: 438–42.

Pierson WR (1971) Noise and aircrew effectiveness. Aerospace Medicine 42: 861–4.

Prasad KR, Reddy KT (2003) Live recordings of sound levels during the use of powered instruments in ENT surgery. Journal of Laryngology and Otology 117(7): 532–5.

Price TG, Goldsmith LJ (1998) Changes in hearing acuity in ambulance personnel. Prehospital Emergency Care 2: 308–11.

Rasmussen JA, Mclean JM, Stasiak RS (1983) Sound levels in emergency medical service. Journal of Environmental Health 45: 176–8.

Robertson A, Cooper-Peel C, Vos P (1998) Peak noise distribution in the neonatal intensive care nursery. Journal of Perinatology 18: 361–4.

Sanders AF (1975) The foreperiod effect revisited. Quarterly Journal of Experimental Psychology 27: 591–8.

Schwab RJ (1994) Disturbances of sleep in the intensive care unit. Critical Care Clinics 10: 681–94.

Shapiro RA, Berland T (1972) Noise in the operating room. New England Journal of Medicine 287: 1236–8.

Shenai JP (1977) Sound levels for neonates in transit. Journal of Pediatrics 90: 811–12.

Skeiber SC, Mason RL, Potter RC (1977) Effectiveness of Audible Warning Devices on Emergency Vehicles. Washington, DC: US Department of Transportation, National Highway Traffic Safety Administration. Publication No. DOT-TSC-OST-77–38.

Skeiber SC, Mason RL, Potter RC (1978) Effectiveness of audible warning devices on emergency vehicle. Sound and Vibration 1(2): 14–17, 20–2.

Soudijn ER, Bleeker JD, Hoeksema PE et al. (1976) Scanning electron microscopic study of the organ of Corti in normal and sound-damaged guinea pigs. Annals of Otology, Rhinology and Laryngology 85 (supplement 29): 1–58.

Soutar RL, Wilson JA (1986) Does hospital noise disturb patients? BMJ 292: 305.

Tarnopolsky A, Clark C (1984) Environmental noise and mental health. In H Freeman (ed.) Mental Health and the Environment. London: Churchill Livingstone, pp. 250–70.

Thomas EB, Denenberg VH, Sievel J, Zeidner LP, Becker PT (1981) State organisation in neonates: developmental inconsistency indicates risk for developmental dysfunction. Neuropediatrics 12: 45–54.

Thomas K (1989) How the NICU environment sounds to the preterm infant. Maternal Child Nursing Journal 14: 249–51.

Tope M (1983) Noise pollution in the hospital. New England Journal of Medicine 309: 43–4.

Topf M, Dillon E (1988) Noise-induced stress as a predictor of burnout in critical care nurses. Heart Lung 17: 567–73.

Tynan WD (1986) Behavioural stability predicts morbidity and mortality in infants from a neonatal intensive care unit. Infant Behaviour and Development 9: 71–9.

White DP, Douglas NJ, Pickett CK et al. (1983) Sleep deprivation and the control of ventilation. American Review of Respiratory Disease 128: 984–6.

Wichnan H, McIntyre M, Accomazzo E (1979) In-flight measures of stress reduction due to wearing expandable earplugs. Aviation Space and Environmental Medicine 50: 898–900.

Williams CE, Stevens KN, Klatt M (1969) Judgements of the acceptability of aircraft noise in the presence of speech. Journal of Sound and Vibration 9: 263–75.

Yassi A, Gaborrieau D, Gillespie I et al. (1991) The noise hazard in a large health care facility. Journal of Occupational Medicine 33: 1067–70.

Zahr LK, Traversay JD (1995) Premature infant responses to noise reduction by earmuffs: effects on behavioural and physiological measures. Journal of Perinatology 15: 448–55.

# CHAPTER 23

# Stress effects of noise

*Noise and Its Effects:* Edited by Linda Luxon and Deepak Prasher © 2007
John Wiley & Sons Ltd.

HARTMUT ISING, BARBARA KRUPPA

## Sound and noise

Sound creates numerous effects in humans. An essential and vital aspect is that of communication with fellow humans. Sound that is appraised as unwanted once it interferes with communication is regarded as *noise.* Accordingly, unwanted or hazardous sound effects are called *noise effects.* In principle, any perceptible sound may be experienced as disturbing and rated as causing annoyance (Interdisziplinärer Arbeitskreis, 1990).

To perceive a sound, the sound level must in the first place be above the hearing threshold of the listener and, secondly, should not be masked by another sound.

To give an example: in a quiet hotel room a guest is peacefully preparing for bed after a strenuous day at work. Just then, another guest enters the room next to his, promptly turning up his favourite music at a volume far above normal room level. The bass rhythms from the room next door are clearly recognizable. The guest's annoyance about such inconsiderate behaviour makes falling asleep all the more difficult for him. The following night, a heavy thunderstorm is going on. While the rain is drumming against the window panes, the guest feels comfortable in his warm, dry room. This time, the noise of the rain gusts masks the bass beats from his neighbour's room, leaving him undisturbed and making it easy for him to go to sleep. This example may demonstrate that the effect of the information transferred by sound is often more disturbing than the noise level.

## Disturbed communication

When concentrating on mental tasks, the most disturbing noises are those of the intermittent and impulsive type. As Arthur Schopenhauer once remarked: 'Hammer blows, barking dogs and screaming children are dreadful, but the true murderer of all thoughts is the crack of a whip.' Not only high-intensity impulse sounds such as those produced by whip cracking, but also impulsive sounds with peak levels lower to some degree can cause significant impairments of short-term memory, and consequently of mental efficiency (Klatte et al., 1995). In this case, the effects of irregular noise bursts with rapid sound pressure rises distinctly dominate the effect of the sound level.

In other types of communication disturbed by noise, the relevant aspect might be the relationship between steady noise disturbances and the necessity of perceiving a particular sound for practical reasons (Lazarus et al., 1985). The type of communication also plays a part in the degree of the disturbance. When listening to the news, a single overflight noise may render the one decisive sentence of the information incomprehensible. As the sentence will not be repeated, the loud noise event has in this case an extremely annoying effect. In noise-disturbed face-to-face conversations, however, it is to some degree possible to continue by repeating sentences, raising one's voice and intensely concentrating on the issue in order to compensate for the acoustic lack of information. But then, in a number of persons involved, such increased efforts produce stress reactions that may trigger an increased release of stress hormones (Ising, 1983b).

**Biological and adverse responses to 'noise'**

- Stimulation of the middle-ear protective reflex
- Stimulation of the autonomic nervous system
- Stress responses
- Acute auditory pain at high-intensity noise
- Inner-ear damage – mechanical and/or metabolic

Immediate physiological noise effects on the autonomic nervous system consist in activated vegetative functions, which begin at maximum noise levels of about 60 dB (A) in waking persons (Interdisziplinärer Arbeitskreis, 1990; Jansen, 1991). In sleeping persons, the threshold of central activation, vegetative reagibility and the release of stress hormones is no less than 10 dB lower than in waking persons. To provide undisturbed sleep, traffic noise immissions should therefore not exceed continuous noise levels of 30 dB (A) or maximum noise levels of 40 dB (A) at the ear of a sleeping person (Interdisziplinärer Arbeitskreis, 1982).

The auditory protective reflex of the middle ear is initiated at sound levels around 70 dB above hearing threshold (Moeller, 1983). Noise levels exceeding 80 dB (A) potentially induce reversible hearing impairments (temporary threshold shifts or TTSs), which increase in degree depending upon noise intensity and duration of exposure (Ward, 1963).

Long-term exposure to continuous noise with levels above 80 dB (A) (related to a 40-hour week) poses an increased risk of inner-ear damage – permanent threshold shifts (PTSs) or chronic tinnitus (Dieroff, 1994).

The pathomechanism of continuous noise-induced threshold shifts is primarily determined by excessive metabolic effects on the hair cells of the inner ear. Isolated impacts of impulse noises with peak levels above 150 dB (A), however, cause immediate permanent hearing loss through shock waves mechanically destroying outer and inner-ear hair cells (Pilgramm, 1994).

The onset threshold of auditory pain is established at around 120 dB (A). An exposure to pure tones in the frequency range 2–4 kHz at sound levels of 120 dB (A) and a minimum duration of 100 ms was in a self-inflicted experiment followed by a severe, piercing, inner-ear pain (Pfander, 1975). Dieroff (1991) sees such auditory pains as an effect of acoustical over-excitation analogous with the ophthalmological blinding effect. Excessive noise immissions connected with inner-ear pain lead to alterations in inner-ear structures. In the environment area, however, noise exposures to such an extent do not occur as a rule. Exposures to extremely high sound intensities, as were in the past caused by direct overflights of military fighter jets at low altitudes (MLAFs) (Spreng, 1994), have in a number of cases caused acute ear pain correlated with permanent auditory threshold shifts (Ising et al., 1991; Ising and Rebentisch, 1993).

# Noise effects on neuroendocrine regulation

Sudden, unexpected noise events set off a series of stress reactions with an initial startle reflex, followed by an orienting reaction directed towards locating and validating the sensory stimulus. This reaction habituates relatively fast. If, however, maximum levels of singular noise events exceed a certain limit value, which in adults is about 90 dB (A), then according to the stress concept a defence reaction sets in (Turpin and Siddle, 1980; Turpin, 1986). Depending upon individual behavioural patterns, the defence reaction leads to either a fight–flight or a defeat reaction. The defence reaction is equivalent to the fight–flight reaction variant of the stress model developed by Henry (1992). The sequence of the stress reactions under concern is genetically programmed. They provide biologically vital protection strategies without adverse effects on health as long as they seldom occur.

Henry and Stephens (1977) developed a psychophysiological stress model – then further developed by Henry (1992) – from which they derived two different physiological reaction types with regard to the mental capacity of coping with stress situations. If a stress situation is controlled with success the primary stress hormone to be released is noradrenaline. If, however, constant efforts are needed to gain or keep control, the predominant stress hormone is adrenaline. A loss of control may lead to a defeat reaction, which is characterized by an increase in ACTH and cortisol concentrations (Figure 23.1):

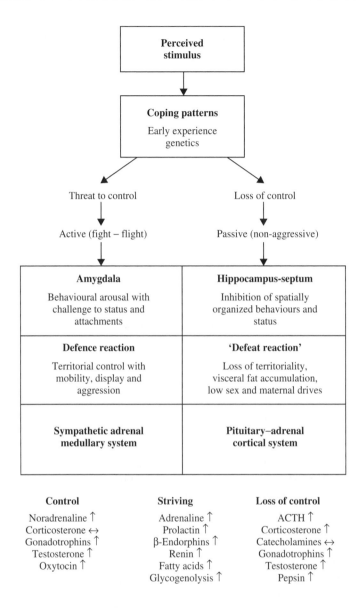

**Figure 23.1** Psychophysiological stress model according to Henry (1992).

A defence reaction is activated when an organism is challenged but remains in control. With loss of control there is activation of the hypothalamo-pituitary-adrenal axis, and the gonadotropic species preservative system shuts down. Visceral fat accumulates with a Cushingoid distribution, and there is a shift from active defence to a passive non-aggressive coping style. (Henry, 1992)

In analogy to this concept, three different types of psychophysiological stress responses can be observed in waking persons with regard to different intensities, duration and dynamic nature of the noise (Figure 23.2):

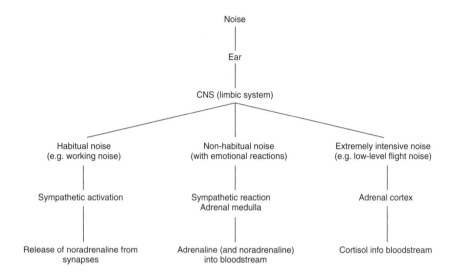

**Figure 23.2** Noise stress model (Ising et al., 1990).

- *Exposure to familiar noise* such as occupational noise, but with levels above 90 dB (A), predominantly induces a release of noradrenaline from synapses of the sympathetic nervous system and into the blood circulation from the adrenal medulla. A noradrenaline release is not connected with an increased central activation.
- *Exposures to unfamiliar noise,* and more so if signalling a threat or danger, the primary response is an orienting reaction. If a noise is subjectively associated with fear or anxiety, sympathetic activation evokes a reaction pattern which is directed towards elimination of the source of threat – the fight–flight reaction. The primary hormone in this case is adrenaline, released from the adrenal medulla, and it has a stimulating effect on the central nervous system (CNS). There are indications of an increased adrenaline effect of continued neural ß-stimulation for hours after plasma concentration has subsided to normal (Majewski et al., 1981; Blankenstijn et al., 1988).
- *Exposures to extremely high-intensity noise,* especially to unexpected noise with fast level rises and peak levels above 120 dB (A), are usually followed by a defeat reaction as a result of subjective lack of control of such stress situations. The primary hormone in this case is cortisol, released from the adrenal cortex. The *physiological* effect of increased releases of cortisol consists in balancing long-term effects of *exceeding*

activation processes. Glucocorticoids have a positive inotropic cardial effect, enhance the effect of catecholamines in the peripheral vascular system and exert an activating effect on the CNS.

Table 23.1 summarizes the results of our own investigations, illustrating the types of the noise-induced stress reactions given in Figure 23.2. In the majority of the studies, noise exposures were experimentally modified under real life conditions, and respective acute stress hormone reactions assessed. In a work noise study (Ising et al., 1980b), an additional cross-sectional comparison was performed among persons with long-term noise exposures of different duration, and a similar one was carried out for military low-altitude flight (MLAF) noise study (Ising et al., 1991). In these studies, manifest alterations in stress hormone excretion were observed. In the experimental studies all test persons were tested between two and ten times for results across time.

**Table 23.1** Investigations of the Institute for Water, Soil and Air Hygiene for testing stress hormone increases.

| Reference | Type of noise (duration) | Acute/ chronic | $L_{eq}$(dB (A)) ($L_{max}$) | Test persons ($n$) | Measure- ments ($n$) | Adrena- line | Noradrena- line | Free cortisol |
|---|---|---|---|---|---|---|---|---|
| Ising et al. (1990) | MLAF noise (5 s) | Acute | ($L_{max}$: 105/125) | 12 | 120 | = | = | + |
| Ising et al. (1991) | MLAF noise (years) | Chronic | **60–70** (125)[a] | 35 | 35 | (+) | (+) | + |
| Ising et al. (1980a) | Motorcycle racing (8 h) | Acute | **85** (100) | 57 | 114 | + | = | ø |
| Ising (1983a) | Low-frequency noise (8 h) | Acute | **50–60** | 18 | 54 | + | = | ø |
| Ising et al. (1980a | Occupational noise (8 h/years) | Acute & chronic | **71–102** | 47 | 77 | = | + | ø |
| Ising et al. (1982) | Road traffic noise (8 h) | Acute | **75** (90) | 18 | 54 | = | + | ø |
| Ising (1983b) | Road traffic noise (8 h) | Acute | **60** (75) | 43 | 82 | = | + | ø |

[a]Outside level; +, significant increase; (+), significant metanephrine increase; =, no alteration; ø, not tested; MLAF, military low-altitude flight.

Exposures to experimental MLAF noise of $L_{max}$ = 125 dB (A) resulted in significant increases in cortisol serum concentrations compared with noise exposures with levels of 20 dB less (Ising et al., 1990). Following exposures to MLAF noise at maximum outdoor levels up to 125 dB (A) lasting for years, a group of people involved showed significantly increased 24-hour excretions of cortisol and metanephrine (a catecholamine metabolite) compared with persons exposed to modest or no MLAF noise (Ising et al., 1991).

# Types of disturbing environmental noise

Exposures to unfamiliar noises, such as those that occur at motorcycle races (Ising et al., 1980a) with mean levels $L_m$ = 85 dB (A) and maximum levels $L_{max}$ = 100 dB (A), as well as exposure to low-frequency white noise (Ising et al., 1982; Ising, 1983a) at $L_m$ = 50–60 dB (A), induced significant increases in serum adrenaline.

In brewery workers exposed to noise of different intensities under plain work conditions (Ising et al., 1980b), an increase in noradrenaline excretion was assessed after experimentally increasing the noise exposure levels by not using ear protection. Comparing noradrenaline excretion values in three groups of long-term, differently noise-exposed persons (Ising and Braun, 2000) showed persistent noradrenaline increases in the case of work noise exposures above 95 dB (A) lasting for years.

Activities like concentrated work or verbal communication disturbed by noise of relatively low sound levels may still lead to stress reactions. Sophisticated manual tasks, carried out under play-back exposure to road traffic noise of 75 dB (A), induced significant increases in noradrenaline (Ising et al., 1982). During verbal communications disturbed by road traffic noise, a mean level of 60 dB (A) was sufficient for effecting a significant increase in noradrenaline (Ising, 1983b; Ising and Braun, 2000). During sleep, acute and chronic stress hormone increases are already detected at considerably lower noise levels (Table 23.2).

Earlier research has indicated that serum adrenaline will exceed standard values preferably if noise stress is associated with unknown, unpredictable and subjectively threatening situations (Frankenhaeuser and Patkai, 1965; Graham et al., 1967; Konzett et al., 1971). Konzett and co-workers (1971) found increased adrenaline excretion values in experimental tests using unpredictable auditory stimuli.

---

**Stress hormone responses**

Noradrenaline increases as a response to:
- increase in intensity of familiar noise
- noise situation under control
- long-term occupational noise above 95 dB (A)
- complex work tasks disturbed by low-level noise.

Adrenaline increases as a response to:
- noise stress associated with unknown, unpredictable and threatening situations
- time – correlated with subjective annoyance
- lack of control of noise situation.

Cortisol increases as a response to:
- exposure to high-intensity noise
- noise events causing substantial disturbance or stress
- noise events that signal a danger.

**Table 23.2** Overview of studies on the relationship of noise exposure and stress hormone increases

| First author | Year | Type of noise (duration) | Acute/ chronic | $L_{eq}$(dB (A)) ($L_{max}$) | Test persons | Measure- ments | Adrena- line | Noradren- aline | Free cortisol |
|---|---|---|---|---|---|---|---|---|---|
| Cavatorta | 1987 | Occupational noise (years) | Chronic | > 85 | 130 | 130 | + | + | ø |
| Sudo | 1996 | Occupational noise (years) | Chronic | 71–100 | 75 | 125 | + | + | + |
| Melamed | 1996 | Occupational noise (days/yrs) | Acute & chronic | > 55/> 85 | 35 | 350 | ø | ø | + |
| Maschke | 1992 | Flight noise (8 nights) | Acute | 29–55 (55–75) | 8 | 64 | + | = | ø |
| Maschke | 1995 | Flight noise (8 nights) | Acute | 29–45 (55–65) | 28 | 224 | + | = | + |
| Evans | 1998 | Flight noise (1.5 years) | Chronic | 53/62[a] | 217 | 217 | + | + | ø[c] |
| Harder | 1999 | Flight noise (40 nights) | Acute & chronic | 42 (65) | 15 | 600 | = | = | + |
| Ising | 1999 | Flight noise (1–3 × 10s) | Acute | (90–100)[a] | 68 | 272 | = | = | = |
| Carter | 1994 | Road traffic noise (2 nights) | Acute | 32 (65–72) | 9 | 18 | = | = | ø |
| Babisch | 1996 | Road traffic noise (years) | Chronic | 45–75[a] | 200 | 200 | = | + | ø |
| Braun | 1999 | Road traffic noise (yrs/2n.) | Acute & chronic | 45/ 53–69[a] | 26 | 152 | = | + | + |
| Evans | 2001 | Road traffic noise (years) | Chronic | 47/ 62[a] (day) | 115 | 115 | = | = | + |
| Ising | 2002 | Road traffic noise (years) | Chronic | $L_{max}$ = 20–53 (night) | 56 | 56 | ø | ø | +[b] |

[a]Outside level; [b]First half of night; [c]Total cortisol assessed; +, significant increase; =, no change; ø, not measured.

Adrenaline concentrations measured across time of noise exposure agreed well with the corresponding time-related subjective annoyances (which in cases eased off). Therefore, adrenaline concentrations measured across time seem to reflect a person's subjective annoyance better than the respective noise levels (Cesana et al., 1982; Fruhstorfer et al., 1990). However, adrenaline concentrations are probably not only connected with aspects of individual experience, but with the entirety of impressions conveyed both by direct effects on the structures of the CNS and by indirect psychological effects.

Cortisol increases were found for intermittent noises (Follenius et al., 1980; Yamamura et al., 1982) under the condition of unexpectedness or inability to cope with a noise event (Mason, 1968; Hansen et al., 1976), especially in cases of noise events that have to be considered as causing substantial disturbance and stress. Several authors have tested

ACTH (corticotrophin) instead of cortisol. Following a single simulated MLAF noise event at a maximum level of 105 dB (A) and a duration of 3 seconds, ACTH concentration was significantly increased, and in 48% of the test persons the values amounted to two times the standard concentration (Marth et al., 1988). Following noise exposures of 85 dB (A) with a duration of several days, only minor rises in ACTH concentration were observed.

When assessing cortisol excretion, a method ought to be used that guarantees the specific assessment of free cortisol – the biologically effective component of total cortisol.

## Stress effects of exposure to work noise, flight and road traffic noise

Table 23.2 gives a survey of recent research on noise-induced stress hormone increases. In two work noise studies, permanent rises in adrenaline, noradrenaline and cortisol were found (Cavatorta et al., 1987; Sudo et al., 1996). Melamed and Bruhis (1996) succeeded in normalizing the chronically disturbed circadian rhythm of cortisol in noise-exposed workers by introducing the use of ear protection.

Only one out of five flight-noise studies (Ising et al., 1999) found no significant noise-induced stress hormone increase. In this case, exposures were too short in duration and the number of exposures was rare – single overflights of military aircraft in the late evening hours. In contrast to that, two studies by Maschke (Maschke, 1992; Maschke et al., 1995) comprised laboratory and field investigations employing simulated electro-acoustical flight noise for four nights, and four control nights without exposure. In the laboratory study, only catecholamines were assessed, yielding an increase in adrenaline. In the field study, increased adrenaline excretion was found for the first two test nights, but increased cortisol for the third and fourth test nights.

In a prospective intervention study with children by Evans (Evans et al., 1998), significant increases in adrenaline and noradrenaline excretion were found after a new airport had been opened. There was also a tendency for total cortisol to increase, but free cortisol was not assessed. Harder et al. (1999) determined free cortisol excretion after 3 test nights without noise and 37 nights with simulated flight noise by means of loudspeakers in the test persons' bedrooms. Only for the second and third night with flight noise exposure, an acute increase of mean group values in cortisol excretion was found. The mean cortisol values then returned to standard, except for a 7-day fluctuation overlapping the circadian cortisol rhythm. The key results were increases in cortisol concentrations which significantly exceeded standard values during the final 2 weeks of nocturnal flight noise exposure (Maschke et al., 2002).

This study (Maschke et al., 2002) shows that long-term nocturnal noise exposures may in vulnerable individuals lead to persistent cortisol values that even exceed the normal range.

Three out of four road-traffic noise studies showed significant relationships between long-term noise exposure and stress hormone increases. The negative finding of Carter et al. (1994) resulted from an incorrect method, as stress hormone concentrations were given but no reference values.

In the framework of the project 'Traffic and health in densely populated Berlin areas' measurements of overnight catecholamine excretion were carried out, with 200 women exposed to traffic noise of different intensities in their homes (Babisch et al., 1996). Women with their bedrooms oriented towards streets with high traffic noise (mean sound level/night-time/outside $L_m$ > 57 dB (A)) showed significantly increased excretions of noradrenaline compared with women living on streets with relatively low traffic noise ($L_m$ < 52 dB (A)). Results remained stable after adjustment for smoking habits, alcohol consumption and social parameters.

In the same study, stress hormones were assessed in test persons living on noisy streets who were asked to leave their bedroom windows open to further increase the indoor noise level (Braun, 1999). These test persons had been exposed to night-time traffic noise for several years. Opening the windows produced noise level increases of 9–18 dB. Mean indoor noise levels with windows closed were between 30 and 50 dB (A).

Acute noise level increases induced mean increases in free cortisol excretion rates by one-third. A follow-up comparison with a control group living in a quiet area has shown that noradrenaline and cortisol excretions in test persons exposed to substantial traffic noise were significantly increased also with closed windows, while adrenaline concentrations remained unaltered.

Evans et al. (2001) compared children exposed to moderate road-traffic noise of daytime outside levels $L_m$ >60 dB (A) with children living in quiet areas with $L_m$ <50 dB (A) and found increases in free cortisol and cortisol metabolites. Catecholamines remained unaltered.

In a study on children exposed to day and night lorry noise with low-frequency characteristics (Ising and Ising, 2001), distinct increases in free cortisol and cortisol metabolites were assessed from urinary excretion in the first half of the night, but not in the second half. In the traffic noise-exposed children, clear evidence was found for a disturbed circadian cortisol rhythm compared with children living in quiet areas.

### Noise situations causing elevation of hormone levels

- Noisy occupational environment
- Aircraft noise
- Proximity of airport
- Home on a noisy street

Only 2 out of the 13 presented studies do not report stress hormone increases associated with noise exposure. It is emphasized, however, that apart from predominantly increased stress hormone concentrations, there are also reports of the odd case of noise-associated decreases in stress hormone concentrations (Harder et al., 1999; Ising and Braun, 2000). From the presented research it can be concluded that long-term environmental noise exposure lasting for years may in a number of exposed people lead to chronic dysregulations in their endocrine systems.

# Noise-induced stress effects during sleep

The following focuses on why the human organism responds to low noise levels with considerable cortisol increases. Our ears are on the alert day and night, serving as our most important sensory warning system. This is why environmental sounds are perceived and processed whether a person is awake or asleep. In sound processing, specific subcortical areas of the CNS play an essential part in increases of cortisol concentration during sleep at low sound levels. In explanation of these processes Spreng (2001) gives the following details:

> With regard to sensory activation processes of the CNS one has to differentiate between two systems which are primarily controlled by subcortical centres, but differ in their major functions. These are the ascending reticular activating system (ARAS) and the vegetative nervous system (VNS).
>
> The ascending reticular activating system (ARAS) activates the cerebral cortex, thereby regulating among others the central rhythm of the sleep-phases and in addition controlling arousal. The leading element in this system is the subcortical formatio reticularis, a network of neurons reaching from the brainstem to the midbrain, containing neurons essential for circulatory regulation. The reticular formation is instigated by sensory stimuli on the one hand, and by the limbic system or 'emotional brain' on the other. Therefore, internal as well as external stimuli can influence the waking and the sleeping organism.
>
> The lateral core region of the amygdaloid body constitutes a regulatory component of the auditory system. Numerous findings of recent research suggest that the amygdala is a cerebral structure which plays an important role in emotional learning processes especially with regard to coping with anxiety. This central anxiety-related system is of a remarkable plasticity, or learning capacity in judging adverse noise events as negative noise stimuli.
>
> The amygdaloid body closes the causal chain between over-excitations of the central auditory system with ensuing over-activations of the hypothalamic–pituitary–adrenal axis and the effects of extra-hypothalamic hormone excretion. This might explain why quite often noise stimuli below the critical noise limit values of auditory damage, i.e. noise-induced hearing loss, and those below waking level may both have adverse effects on health.

During undisturbed sleep the cortisol concentration declines to a minimum, then rises to maximum values at around wake-up time in the morning. The cortisol nadir coincides with the onset of slow-wave sleep phases. During the early hours of the night, slow-wave sleep phases are associated with a minimum cortisol release. This circadian neuroendocrine regulation pattern is characteristic of undisturbed sleep (Born and Fehm, 2000). If this specific pattern loses balance through nocturnal noise disturbances, there will be a decline in the recovery function of sleep, which is achieved only at minimum cortisol levels.

# Time dependency of stress responses

A relevant aspect in health outcomes connected with noise-stress reactions is the response time. Acute noise effects that do not directly cause permanent health impairments are considered irrelevant for health. This holds for all reactions to noise, which completely habituate after repeated stress events. The problem with certain effects of noise-induced stress responses consists, however, in an apparently accomplished habituation, but is in fact maintained only under constant efforts on the part of the organism.

**According to Selye (Selye, 1953), the so-called *adaptation syndrome* develops in three stages:**

1. *The alarm phase,* characterized by an immediate response to a stressor.
2. *The resistance phase,* which includes habituation to a large extent, but involves: 'costs' – constant efforts of the organism to adapt to an altered equilibrium following persistent stress situations can lead to collapse of the organism, and eventually, according to Selye, to the third stage.
3. *Exhaustion.*

In persons with long-term noise exposure, and consequently with chronically increased stress hormone concentrations or permanent dysregulations of the stress hormone balance, such symptoms must, in view of their chronic process, be considered a potential cause of organic damage, and as indicating a risk to health.

# Neuroimmune responses to traffic noise

Previous studies that have assessed the concentrations of neurohormones such as the interleukins (especially of IL-2) and of cellular immune resistance in connection with either refreshing sleep or sleep deprivation. Born and Fehm (2000) have given the first indications of a supportive effect of a stress-free, refreshing sleep on the immune memory. Correspondingly, it was assumed that repeated long-term, nocturnal, noise-induced stress may contribute to the promotion of allergic diseases.

The pathogenesis of allergies can be stimulated by adjuvant effects caused by both air pollutants such as $NO_2$ and exhaust particles from diesel engines, as well as by traffic-related nocturnal noise (Ising et al., 2002, 2003, 2004). During sleep, noise signals that are known to be associated with danger, as for instance from lorry noise, have the potential to trigger stress reactions even if the noise level is low (Spreng, 2001). Associated increases of cortisol in the first half of the night seem to play an important role (Ising and Ising, 2002).

# Studies on children exposed to traffic-induced noise and air pollution

The hypothesis of an association between road-traffic immissions and allergic diseases has been put to the test in a three-phase study on health effects on children.

In a study on sleep disturbance in relation to stress hormone regulation during the night (Ising and Ising, 2002), correlations were found by assessing children's free cortisol excretions in their night urine collected at 1am and in the morning at wake-up time. Prior to this, all participating 56 children, aged 7–10 years, had a medical check-up and were interviewed, while their mothers completed corresponding questionnaires. The children lived either at a busy road with 24-hour lorry traffic, or in quiet areas, each half in number of the total group. During five consecutive nights the noise level was registered at the side of the road. In the children's bedrooms, representative measurements of the short-term maximal sound level ($L_{Amax}$ and $L_{Cmax}$) and of the frequency spectrum were taken.

Regarding the higher noise-exposed children, lorries with $L_{max} >$ 80 dB (A) passed by their houses at 2-minute intervals all night. The indoor levels were $L_{max} = 33$–52 dB (A) and 55–78dB (C) respectively with the maximum of frequency spectrum below 100 Hz.

## The following were found:

- The results gave strong indications of circadian rhythm dysfunction of nocturnal cortisol excretion in children who were living on streets with day and night lorry noise compared with less exposed children.
- The endocrine dysfunctions were correlated with substantial sleep disturbances and elevated prevalence of bronchial asthma and dermatological allergies.
- Children diagnosed with bronchial asthma or an allergy were found to have significantly higher excretion rates of cortisol metabolites – but not of free cortisol – in the first half of the night compared with the second half (Ising and Ising, 2002).

With specific reference to nocturnal lorry noise, that causing indoor noise levels rated up to now as not interfering with a healthy sleep (Interdisciplinärer Arbeitskreis, 1982) may according to the presented results be considered as detrimental to health, if the C-weighted indoor level exceeds $L_{max} = 60$ dB (C).

In a practice-based study using a blind interview design (Ising et al., 2002, 2003), the combined effects of chronic exposure to traffic-related air pollution and noise upon the risk of skin and respiratory diseases in children were investigated. The study sample comprised 401 children aged 5–12 years seeing their paediatricians in their clinics. The diagnoses for each child or the respective treatments in an observation period of one month were analysed, together with the parents' interview answers concerning the density of road traffic on their street, and several confounding factors. Multiple regression analyses resulted in significant increases of the relative risks of bronchial asthma, chronic bronchitis and neurodermitis in children living on heavy traffic streets. A comparison of the results with the literature on health effects caused by air pollution alone showed that traffic noise at night seems to have an additional, adjuvant effect on the pathogenesis of the quoted diseases.

In a current study, traffic-related air pollution and noise were measured outside the bedroom windows of approximately 10% of the same patients. Based on these measurements, immission charts were prepared to assess an objective categorization of air pollution and noise for the total group ($n$ = 401). In addition, the contact rates of the children with their physician during the previous 5 years for bronchitis and neurodermatitis were determined. The final step will be an analysis of the correlation between the traffic-related immissions and the annual contact frequencies with the physician for the quoted allergic diseases. For bronchitis the results were in agreement with our previous results (Ising et al., 2002, 2003, 2004).

# Conclusion

An overview is given on the results of earlier and recent investigations of the complexity of noise disturbances and the diversity of ensuing responses of the stress hormones noradrenaline, adrenaline and cortisol. The presented studies include acute and chronic occupational, flight and road traffic noise at day and night as well as environmental noise effects on adults and children. The results are gained from serum and urine measurements in experimental and field studies and evaluated in correlation with different subjective situations, intensities and duration of noise exposures. Taken into consideration are noise stress effects on verbal communication, manual or mental tasks and influences on sleep with regard to endocrine and neuro-immune health effects. As a general rule, increased serum *noradrenaline* values are predominant in long-term elevated, mentally controlled noise stress situations. *Adrenaline* is the primary stress hormone if longer efforts are needed to keep control. Thus, increased adrenaline agreed well with time-related subjective annoyances. A defeat reaction with loss of mental control is characterised by increases in serum *free cortisol* induced by unexpected high-intensity or intermittent noise events. Long-term disturbances of the circadian rhythm of cortisol release have proved to interfere with the normal sleep stages, causing poorer achievements during the day. In children living on streets with heavy traffic, increased cortisol values were correlated with substantial sleep disturbances and elevated prevalences of bronchial asthma and allergies.

# References

Babisch W, Fromme H, Beyer A, Ising H (1996) Katecholaminausscheidung im Nachturin bei Frauen aus unterschiedlich verkehrsbelasteten Wohngebieten. WaBoLu Hefte 9/96. Berlin: Institut für Wasser-, Boden- und Lufthygiene, Umweltbundesamt.

Blankenstijn PJ, Tulen J, Boomsma F, Eck HJRV, Mulder P, Schalekamp MADH, Man Int Veld AJ, Mairacker AHVD, Derkx FHM, Lamberts SJ (1988) Support for adrenaline-hypertension hypothesis: 18 hour pressor effect after 6 hours adrenaline infusion. The Lancet 17:1386–9.

Born J, Fehm H (2000) The euroendocrine recovery function of sleep. Noise & Health 2000, 7: 25–37.

Braun C (1999) Nächtlicher Straßenverkehrslärm und Stresshormonausscheidung beim Menschen. Dissertation, Berlin.

Carter NL, Hunyor SN, Crawford G, Kelly D, Smith AJM (1994) Environmental noise and sleep – a study of arousals, cardiac arrhythmia and urinary catecholamines. Sleep 17: 298–307: I–33.

Cavatorta A, Falzoi M, Romanelli A, Cigala F, Ricco M, Bruschi G, Franchini I, Borghetti A (1987) Adrenal response in the pathogenesis of arterial hypertension in workers exposed to high noise levels. Journal of Hypertension 5 (Suppl. 5): 463–6.

Cesana GC, Ferrario M, Curti R, Zanettini R, Grieco A, Sega R, Palermo A, Mara G Lebretti A, Algeri S (1982) Work-stress and urinary catecholamines excretion in shift workers exposed to noise, I: Epinephrine (E) and norepinephrine (NE). Medicina del Lavoro 73: 99–109: I–18.

Dieroff H-G (1991) Expertise zum Problemkomplex des akustischen Traumas sowie zur audiologischen Bewertung der das Gehör betreffenden Resultate der Hauptstudie zu gesundheitlichen Auswirkungen des militärischen Tieffluglärms. In Gesundheitliche Wirkungen des Tieffluglärms. H Ising, I Curio, H Otten, E Rebentisch, W Schulte (eds.) Forschungsbericht 91-105 01 116 des Umweltbundesamtes, Anhang pp 86–103.

Dieroff H-G (1994) Ohrgeräusche. In H-G Dieroff (ed.) Lärmschwerhörigkeit Gustav Fischer Verlag Jena Stuttgart. Chapter 4.7, pp 228–31

Evans GW, Bullinger M, Hygge S (1998) Chronic noise exposure and physiological response: a prospective study of children living under environmental stress. American Psychological Society, Vol.9: 75–7

Evans G, Lercher P, Meis M, Ising H, Kofler W (2001) Typical community noise exposure and stress in children. Journal of the American Society of Audiology.

Follenius M, Brandenberger G, Lecornu C, Simeoni M, Reinhardt B (1980) Plasma catecholamines and pituitary adrenal hormones in response to noise exposure. European Journal of Applied Physiology 43: 253–61.

Frankenhaeuser M, Patkai P (1965) Interindividual differences in catecholamine excretion during stress. Scandinavian Journal of Pyschology 6:117–23.

Fruhstorfer B, Pritsch MG, Fruhstorfer H, Sturm G, Wesemann W (1990) Effects and after-effects of daytime noise load. In B Berglund, T Lindvall (eds.) New Advances in Noise Research, part II. Proceedings of the 5th international congress on Noise as a Public Health Problem in Stockholm 1988. Swedish Council for Building Research, Stockholm, pp 81–91.

Graham LA et al. (1967) Some methodological approaches to the psycho-physiological correlates of behavior. In L Levi (ed.) Emotional Stress Karger, Basel New York, pp 178–91.

Hansen JD, Larson ME, Snowdon LT (1976) Effects of control over high intensity noise on plasma cortisol levels in rhesus monkeys. Behavioral Biology 16:333.

Harder J, Maschke C, Ising H (1999) Längsschnittstudie zum Verlauf von Stressreaktionen unter Einflußss; von nächtlichem Fluglärm. WaBoLu-Hefte, Institut für Wasser-, Boden- und Lufthygiene, Umweltbundesamt, Berlin.

Henry JP (1992) Biological basis of the stress response. Integrative Physiological and Behavioral Science 27: 66–83.

Henry JP, Stephens PM (1977) Stress, Health and Social Environment. Springer Verlag. Berlin.

Idzior-Walus B (1987) Coronary risk factors in man occupationally exposed to vibration and noise. European Heart Journal 8: 1040–6.

Interdisziplinärer Arbeitskreis für Lärmwirkungsfragen beim Umweltbundesamt (1982) Wirkungen von Lärm auf die Arbeitseffektivität. Zeitschrift für Lärmbekämpfung 30: 1–3.

Interdisziplinärer Arbeitskreis für Lärmwirkungsfragen beim Umweltbundesamt (1990) Belästigung durch Lärm: Psychische und körperliche Reaktionen. Zeitschrift für Lärmbekämpfung 37: 1–6.

Ising H (1983a) Effects of 8-hour exposure to infrasound in man. Proceedings of the Fourth International Congress on Noise as a Public Health Problem. Centro Ricerche e Studi Amplifon, Milano.

Ising H (1983b) Streßreaktionen und Gesundheitsrisiko bei Verkehrslärmbelastung. Dietrich Reimer, Berlin.

Ising H, Braun C (2000) Acute and chronic endocrine effects of noise: review of the research conducted at the Institute for Water, Soil and Air Hygiene. Noise & Health 7: 7–24.

Ising H, Ising M (2001) Stressreaktionen von Kindern durch Lkw-Lärm. Umweltmedizinischer Informationsdienst 1: 12–14.

Ising H, Ising M (2002) Chronic cortisol increases in the first half of the night caused by road traffic noise. Noise & Health 4 16: 13–21.

Ising H, Rebentisch E (1993) Ergebnisse einer Tieffluglärmstudie in der Bundesrepublik Deutschland: Aurale Wirkungen. In H Ising, B Kruppa (eds.) Lärm und Krankheit. Gustav Fischer, Stuttgart, pp 339–58.

Ising H, Dienel D, Günther T, Markert B (1980a) Health effects of traffic noise. International Archives of Occupational and Environmental Health 47: 179–90.

Ising H, Günther T, Melchert HU (1980b) Nachweis und Wirkungsmechanismen der blutdrucksteigernden Wirkung von Arbeitslärm. Zentralblatt für Arbeitsmedizin 30: 194–203.

Ising H, Markert B, Schenoda F, Schwarze C (1982) Infraschallwirkungen auf den Menschen. VDI Verlag, Düsseldorf.

Ising H, Rebentisch E, Babisch W, Curio I, Sharp D, Baumgärtner H (1990) Medically relevant effects of noise from military low-altitude flights – results of an interdisciplinary pilot study. Environment International 16: 411–23.

Ising H, Curio I, Otten H, Rebentisch E, Schulte W, Babisch W et al. (1991) Gesundheitliche Wirkungen des Tieffluglärms - Hauptstudie. Umweltbundesamt Berlin.

Ising H, Pleines F, Meis M (1999) Beeinflussung der Lebensqualität von Kindern durch militärischen Fluglärm. Umweltbundesamt, Berlin.

Ising H, Lange-Asschenfeldt H, Lieber G-F, Weinhold H, Eilts M (2002) Auswirkungen langfristiger Expositionen gegen ber Straßenverkehrsimmissionen auf die Entwicklung von Haut- und Atemwegserkrankungen bei Kindern. Bundesgesundheitsblatt 2: 807–13.

Ising H, Lange-Asschenfeldt H, Lieber G-F, Weinhold H, Eilts M (2003) Respiratory and dematalogical diseases in children with long-term exposure to road traffic immissions. Noise & Health 5(19) 41–50.

Ising H, Lange-Asschenfeldt H, Lieber G-F, Moriske H-J, Weinhold H (2004) Exposure to Traffic-Related Air Pollution and Noise and the Development of Respiratory Diseases in Childeren. Journal of Children's Health: Vol 2, No.2 145–147.

Jansen G (1991) Physiological effects of noise. In 2nd Edition. CM Harris (ed.) Handbook of Noise Control McGraw-Hill, New York, Chapter 25.

Klatte M, Kilcher H, Hellbrück J (1995) Wirkungen der zeitlichen Struktur von Hintergrundschall auf das Arbeitsgedächtnis und ihre theoretischen und praktischen Implikationen. Zeitschrift für Experimentelle Psychologie XLII (4): 517–44.

Konzett H et al. (1971) On the urinary output of vasopressin, epinephrine and norepinephrine during different stress situations. Psychopharmalogia, Berlin 21: 247–56.

Lazarus H, Lazarus-Mainka G, Schubeius M (1985) Sprachliche Kommunikation unter Lärm Kiehl; Ludwigshafen

Majewski H, Rand MJ, Tung LH (1981) Activation of prejunctional ß-adrenoceptors in rat atria by adrenaline applied exogenously or released as a co-transmitter. British Journal of Pharmacology 73: 669–79.

Marth E, Gallasch E, Fueger GF, Möse JR (1988) Fluglärm: Veränderungen biochemischer Parameter. Zentralblatt Bakterielle Hygiene B 185: 489–509.

Maschke C (1992) Der Einflußss; von Nachtfluglärm auf den Schlafverlauf und die Katecholaminausscheidung. Dissertation TU Berlin 1992.

Maschke C, Arndt D, Ising H (1995) Nächtlicher Fluglärm und Gesundheit: Ergebnisse von Labor- und Feldstudien. Bundesgesundheitsblatt 38, 4: 130–7.

Maschke C, Harder J, Ising H, Hecht K, Thierfelder W (2002) Stress hormone changes in persons exposed to simulated night noise. Noise & Health, 5: 17 35–45.

Mason JW (1968) A review of psychoendocrine research on the pituitary adrenal cortical system. Psychosomatic Medicine 30: 576–607.

Melamed S, Bruhis S (1996) The effects of chronic industrial noise exposure on urinary cortisol, fatigue and irritability. Journal of Occupational and Environmental Medicine 38: 252–6.

Moeller AR (1983) Auditory Physiology. Academic Press, New York.

Pfander F (1975) Das Knalltrauma: Analyse, Vorbeugung, Diagnose, Behandlung, Prognose und Begutachtung. Springer Verlag, Berlin.

Pilgramm M (1994) Akutes akustisches Trauma durch Schußbelastung. In H-G Dieroff (ed.) Lärmschwerhörigkeit. Gustav Fischer Verlag Jena Stuttgart, pp 142–58.

Selye H (1953) The Stress Of Life. Mcgraw-Hill, New York.

Spreng M (1994) Gehörschädigungsmöglichkeiten durch Tiefflugschallereignisse. In H-G Dieroff (ed.) Lärmschwerhörigkeit. Gustav Fischer Verlag Jena Stuttgart, pp 202–2.

Spreng M (2001) Periphere und zentrale Aktivierungsprozesse. In HE Wichmann, H-W Schlipköter, G Fülgraff (eds.) Handbuch der Umweltmedizin. VII-1 Lärm. Ecomed Verlag Landsberg. Chapter 4.4.1 pp 9–12.

Sudo A, Luong NA, Jonai H, Matsuda S, Villanueva MBG, Sotoyama M, Cong NT, Trinh LV, Hien HM, Trong ND, Sy N (1996) Effects of earplugs on catecholamine and cortisol excretion in noise-exposed textile workers. Industrial Health 34: 279–86.

Turpin G (1986) Effects of stimulus intensity on autonomic responding: the problem of differentiating orienting and defense reflex. Psychophysiology 23:1–14.

Turpin G, Siddle D (1980) Autonomic response to high intensity auditory stimulation (abstract). Psychophysiology 18:150.

Ward WD (1963) Auditory Fatigue and Masking. Modern Development in Audiology. Academic Press, New York

Yamamura K, Maehara N, Sadamoto T, Harabuchi I (1982) Effect of intermittent (traffic) noise on man - temporary threshold shift, and change in urinary 17-OHCS and saliva cortisol levels. European Journal of Applied Physiology 48: 303–14.

# CHAPTER 24

# Stress and noise – the psychological/physiological perspective and current limitations

*Noise and Its Effects:* Edited by Linda Luxon and Deepak Prasher © 2007
John Wiley & Sons Ltd.

CHRISTIAN MASCHKE, KARL HECHT

## Introduction

The term 'stress' is differently interpreted among experts. To avoid misunderstandings we therefore consider it advisable to give some preliminary explanation. Selye's theory (1953) of the general adaptation syndrome was based primarily on the functions of the hypophyseal–adrenocortical axis. Modifying this concept, Lazarus et al. (1957) developed a 'cognition stress' concept to adjust the rather mechanistic concept of a linear stimulus–reaction relationship. Levi (1967, 1974) later proposed a psychosocial stress concept, followed by other authors, such as Nitsch (1981), Balzer and Hecht (1989) and Hecht (2001), who with respect to regulatory theorems developed a concept of emotional stress based on earlier publications by Cannon (1929) and Lindsley (1951). The emotional stress concept includes interacting pathways of the feedback control system: cerebral cortex, limbic system, hypothalamo-vegetative hormonal immunological system, hypothalamo-limbic system, cerebral cortex.

Following this tradition, we define stress as a temporary or permanent disturbance of the individual psychophysiological homoeostasis.

> Stress represents a state of the organism in which all feedback processes are to be considered as influencing factors on all levels from molecular, cellular to organic, as well as viewed as a whole.
>
> Hecht et al. (1999)

Positive stress, called eustress, enhances efficiency and health, whereas distress is a deviation that features pathological systems. Stress stands for a reaction, whereas stressor is a factor that induces stress.

Eustress is usually a temporary condition, meaning that an individual successfully copes with his task and then relaxes. Distress, however, describes an unsuccessful process in which coping with a stress situation is not possible, or in which coping strategies are not applied appropriately.

Studies on biological behaviourism and neurobiology have demonstrated that distress leads to degenerated neural interactions and eventually causes disintegration of ineffective behavioural patterns (see, among others, Heine, 1997). Such processes do, in principle, offer an opportunity to part with habitual behavioural patterns and to develop new and more effective patterns instead. By employing new coping strategies, when coping with a stressor is unsuccessful, the system can regain its normal behaviour, often with a delay of the weekly (circaseptanian) rhythm (Perger, 1990; Hildebrandt et al., 1998).

Therefore one has clearly to differentiate acute from chronic stress.

An acute stress reaction is a short-term reaction that is usually characterized by an orienting or an adapting reaction (Sokolow, 1967). Chronic, long-term stress reactions are reactions indicating that the individual is making continued efforts to develop and employ compensating coping mechanisms.

Prolonged adaptation efforts do, however, constitute a health risk. Evidence of permanently outmanoeuvred biological rhythms (overstress) and the exhaustion stage of the general adaptation syndrome are objective criteria of such processes.

Reactions to physical strain are primarily determined by metabolic demands and therefore interindividually comparable. Identical stress loads, which are associated with only minor metabolic demands when coping with stress situations, are, on the other hand, interindividually followed by extremely differing reaction patterns.

Furthermore, daytime stress must be differentiated from nocturnal stress. During the day an individual has the option of voluntarily modifying a stress process once stress is perceived as such. During sleep, which is the usual state for the greatest part of the night, the conscious mind is set aside and the noise effect is dominated by uncontrolled autonomous and acquired patterns.

# Noise – activation – stress

A noise effect as the source of a stress reaction is best explained with regard to the relationship between noise perception and activational responses. Perception includes the psychological processing of information, which again allows an individual to perceive, analyse and evaluate information received from the environment (Sokolow, 1967).

Perception is, however, not confined to receiving particular environmental stimulations but includes cognitive awareness of sensory stimuli in all their facets. For humans, perception is an act that comprises mental and emotional processes, memory, attentiveness, imagination, fantasy, motivation and moods, as well as vegetative–endocrine and immune processes.

Perception of objects, persons or a noise is not bound to the existence of the item itself, but depends also upon the experience connected with it, the personal approach and emotional relationship, and upon the actual state of mind.

In the merry mood of a festive occasion, the level of a noise will be perceived differently from when one is in a depressed mood. In the perception process, the role played by a person's subjective attitude also becomes apparent in his evaluation of situations, outcomes, people, phenomena, etc. As a consequence, identical noise sources will evoke different points of view in the same person if perceived in different reactive situations. The perception of sound is associated with a number of characteristics. The hearing sense serves as a warning system. It is designed never to be out of function, and perceives acoustic information at any time and from all directions. The perception of a sound event is mainly conveyed by its sound pattern, sound level and time structure. A sound event that has entered the conscious mind through perception allows orientation in space and time (distances, movements, velocities), gives warnings of danger and provides information.

Through sound perception, activation processes are instigated in order to maintain adequate reactions in the individual. In early research, Cannon (1929) and Lindsley (1951) have seen emotional activation as a process that includes more or less all functional systems of the organism, foremost the vegetative–endocrine and neuroimmune systems, although of varying intensities. The functional structure of the psycho-neuro-vegetative regulatory systems is given in Figure 24.1.

In psychobiological studies on the evidence of vegetative reactions to noise, functions controlled by the autonomic nervous system have been taken into special consideration, as are heart rate, blood pressure, electrodermal reactions, pupillary width and vasomotor parameters (vasoconstriction). Stress-induced functional changes are known to have the effects illustrated in Table 24.1.

Hormones released by the autonomic nervous system in feedback control with the central nervous system (CNS) regulate the endocrine homoeostasis of the organism. Some of these hormones (such as noradrenaline) are also stored as neurotransmitters in synaptic structures of the sympathetic nervous system.

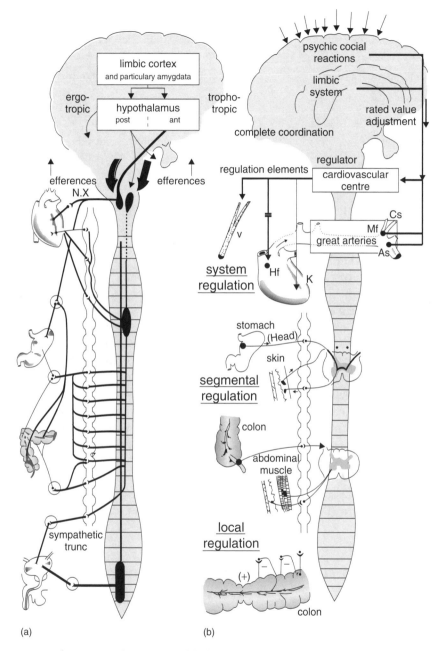

**Figure 24.1** Funtional structure of the psycho-neuro-vegetative regulatory systems.
a= vertically accentuated funtional structure
b= horizontally accentuated funtional structure
This figure is modified by Hecht and Maschke and the origin figure was published in Zwiener, and Langhorst, 1993

**Table 24.1** Functional changes caused by stress

| Questionnaire (interviews) | Emotional strain, elevated vigilance, increased attentiveness and concentration |
| --- | --- |
| Central nervous system | Electroencephalographic parameters |
| Cardiovascular system | Heart rate, blood pressure |
| Metabolism | Blood lipids |
| Motor system | Electromyographic parameters |
| Endocrine system | Hormones |

The pathogenic concept according to which psycho-physiological noise-induced effects are associated with health hazards is based upon the general stress concept. The activating hormones of the adrenal gland, catecholamines and cortisol, known as stress hormones (Croiset et al., 1987; Breznith et al., 1998; Sapolsky, 1998), are considered to be the main effectors. Stress hormones make it possible to survive in extreme situations.

*'They mobilize energy from storage tissue such as fat and liver in order to supply exercising muscle, and increase cardiovascular tone to accelerate the delivery of energy substrates. In addition, they inhibit long-term anabolic processes such as growth, tissue repair, bone recalcification, digestion and reproduction' (Sapolsky, 1998).*

Glucocorticoids play an essential part in these processes. The release of glucocorticoids from the adrenal cortex is the 'final step in a neuroendocrine cascade that begins with the perception of a stressor in the brain and the triggering of hypothalamic release of CRF (cortico-releasing factor)' (Sapolsky et al., 1986). In primates and humans, cortisol is the predominant glucocorticoid. Accordingly, immune parameters are equally subjected to the effects of stress reactions and also controlled by the CNS and the endocrine system (Benschop et al., 1994; Bonneau et al., 1997; Linthorst et al., 1997).

# Acute stress reactions to daytime noise

Acute noise-induced stress reactions in humans have been investigated in numerous experimental studies. In earlier research, Arguelles and colleagues (Arguelles et al., 1962; Arguelles and Disisto, 1970) have already determined increased serum cortisol in test subjects exposed to noise levels of 63 and 93 dB. Bondarev et al. (1970), on the other hand, observed decreased cortisol secretions with noise exposure to low-frequency sound pressure levels of 85 dB. Fruhstorfer et al. (1988a, 1988b) assessed the influence of daytime noise on hormone serum levels. The results show that exposure to high-intensity noise activates prolonged hypophyseal (pituitary gland) responses, but that they display a considerable variety of secretion patterns. Levi (1961) examined differences in noise susceptibility in groups of test subjects exposed to various combinations of stressors. Noise exposure combined with physiological and psychological activities resulted in larger increases of adrenaline than of noradrenaline, while cortisol secretion values remained at almost normal level.

Miki et al. (1998) found significant differences in cortisol excretion values when testing mental performance in relation to simultaneous noise exposure. Adrenaline secretion was, in contrast, increased during mental occupations independent of noise exposure or recreational periods.

Slob et al. (1973) submitted test subjects to a noise level of 80 dB and measured their endocrine reactions at different times of the day. In the mornings, an elevated release of adrenaline was determined and compared with that of a control group. In the afternoons, no excessive values were found in either group. It should be pointed out here that the test results may have been biased by overlapping circadian endocrine rhythms. A synopsis of serum levels over 24-hour periods for several hormones can already be found in a collective volume of aspects by Aschoff et al. (1974).

It can generally be concluded from the results that the secretion of glucocorticoids, triggered by the pituitary (hypophyseal) adrenocorticotropic hormone ACTH, and of catecholamines, shows distinct interindividual differences, and in parts is even controversial. Apart from influences of internal secretion processes associated with circadian rhythms, exogenous (mental or physical) effectors may additionally be involved in the development of stress situations.

# Acute stress reactions to night noise

Changes in nightly excretion values of stress hormones connected with acute road traffic noise exposure have been examined frequently in recent years following investigations by Maschke and colleagues (Maschke, 1992; Maschke, 1995) who verified increased urinary excretion rates in correlation to traffic noise during the night. Table 24.2 depicts a selection of relevant studies.

In studies of the effects of traffic noise, primarily catecholamine and cortisol concentrations were determined from cumulative total parameters in collective urinary secretion and analysed with regard to immission categories, or compared with controls (Ising and Braun, 2000). A striking result of a 40-day longitudinal study by Harder et al. (1998, 1999) was a second distinct increase after 3 weeks of night flight noise immission. The results were controversial in that they showed three reaction types of increasing, declining and unchanged cortisol levels. For the increased cortisol group, values exceeding the normal reference range were found in the sixth week (Maschke et al., 2003), indicating a permanently

**Table 24.2** Studies on the release of catecholamines (adrenaline and noradrenaline) and cortisol connected with acute exposure to traffic noise at night

| First author | year | Type of noise (observation period) | reaction type | $L_{eq}$(dB(A)) ($L_{max}$) | Test subjects ($n$) | Measurements | Adrenaline | Noradrenaline | Free cortisol |
|---|---|---|---|---|---|---|---|---|---|
| Maschke | 1992 | Flight noise (8 nights) | Acute | 36–56 (55–75) | 8 | 64 | + | = | |
| Maschke | 1995 | Flight noise (8 nights) | Acute | 29–45 (55–65) | 28 | 224 | + | | |
| Harder | 1999 | Flight noise (40 nights) | Acute | 42 (65) | 15 | 600 | = | = | + – |
| Carter | 1994 | Road traffic noise (2 nights) | Acute | 32 (65–72) | 9 | 18 | = | = | |
| Ising & Ising | 2001 | Road traffic acute noise (night-time) | (Chronic) | (20–53) | 56 | 56 | | | +ª |
| Basner | 2001 | Flight noise (13 night) | Acute | 28–53 (50–80) | 64 | 832 | = | = | = |

ªfirst half of night; +, increased; –, decreased; =, unchanged values

increased cortisol release in individuals sensitive to noise. Further, in a study of children living in streets with heavy truck traffic noise, Ising and Ising (2001) found an increase in free cortisol and metabolites for the first half of the night only and an additionally disturbed circadian cortisol rhythm. Basner et al. (2001) for their part observed no alterations of stress hormone excretions in adults, even when exposed to frequent loudspeaker playback overflight noises (8–24 times) with maximum levels between 50 dB (A) and 80 dB (A) during the night, nor did Carter et al. (1994) with an observation period of only two nights in which distinct effects were not to be expected. There seems to be no consistency in the diverse study results.

There is evidence that, during sleep, noise disturbances lead to imbalances in the physiological circadian rhythm of the primarily involved hormones that stimulate stress reactions dependent upon the mental and physical condition of the individual.

# Chronic noise-induced stress reactions

Stress hormone characteristics under long-term noise exposure have been studied throughout the 1980s in connection with occupational noise. However, it has only been since the mid-1990s that research on the endocrine effects of traffic noise has been carried out. As can be seen from Table 24.3, the results gained from occupational or traffic noise studies were also inconsistent with regard to stress hormone releases as indicators of chronic stress reactions.

**Table 24.3** Studies on catecholamines and cortisol releases associated with chronic noise exposure

| First author | Year | Type of noise (observation period) | reaction type | $L_{eq}$(dB(A)) ($L_{max}$) | Test subjects (*n*) | Measure-ments | Adren-aline | Noradren-aline | Free cortisol |
|---|---|---|---|---|---|---|---|---|---|
| Cavatorta | 1987 | Occupational noise (years) | Chronic | >85 | 130 | 130 | + | + | |
| Sudo | 1996 | Occupational noise (years) | Chronic | 71–100 | 75 | 125 | + | + | + |
| Babisch | 1996 | Road traffic (years) | Chronic | 45–75[a] | 200 | 200 | = | + | |
| Melamed | 1997 | Occupational noise (years/days) | Chronic | 0.55/>85 | 35 | 350 | | | + |
| Evans | 1998 | Flight noise (1.5 years) | Chronic | 53–62[a] | 217 | 217 | + | + | |
| Braun | 1999 | Road traffic (years) | Chronic | 53–69[a] | 26 | 152 | = | = | = |
| Evans | 2001 | Road traffic (years) | Chronic | >60/<50[a] (daytime) | 115 | 115 | = | = | + |
| Haines | 2001 | Road traffic (years) | Chronic | >63/<57[a] (school) | 451 | 451 | = | = | = |

[a]outside levels; +, increased; –, decreased; =, unchanged values.

Three of the studies were carried out in the framework of the project 'Traffic and health in densely populated Berlin areas'. Babisch et al. (1996) found significantly increased excretions of noradrenaline in women with their bedrooms oriented towards streets with relatively low traffic noise (mean value $L_m$ > 57 dB (A) measured outside) compared with women living on streets with relatively low traffic noise ($L_m$ > 52 dB (A)). Results remained stable after adjusting for age, social parameters and other factors. Braun (1999) assessed and analysed urinary stress hormone excretion, specifically of free cortisol, in women who had lived in noisy streets for years (30 to 50 dB (A) indoors). To examine stress hormone behaviour at further increased night noise levels, cortisol behaviour was measured when bedroom windows were left open, resulting in noise level differences of an additional 9–18 dB. Mean cortisol excretion values increased by one-third above the standard range. A follow-up comparison of the results in a control group living in a quiet area (Ising and Kruppa, 2001) showed significantly higher noradrenaline and cortisol excretions in the highly noise-exposed group even with windows closed, while adrenaline remained unchanged. In a study by Evans et al. (2001), increased cortisol and metabolite values but unchanged catecholamines were observed in children living in streets with a heavy traffic load of $L_m$ > 60 dB (A) compared with children exposed to $L_m$ < 50 dB (A). In contrast, Haines (2001) found no changes of cortisol excretion in primary schoolchildren exposed to high aircraft noise at school ($L_m$ > 63 dB (A) measured outside), in comparison with schoolchildren exposed to less strong aircraft noise (< 57 dB (A) measured outside).

A summary evaluation of the quoted studies on chronic noise-induced stress reactions is rather difficult because of their differing methodologies. However, it may be concluded that long-term noise exposure can, in a number of subjects, induce chronic regulatory imbalances in the endocrine system which are further influenced by strong intra- and interindividual varieties.

# Open questions, sources of error and problem areas

The measured results of free cortisol may be considered an indisputable indicator of acute stress reactions if the exposure situation and the functional state of the test subject preceding the exposure, as well as the circadian rhythm of cortisol releases, are taken into account. Reliable data are, however, obtainable only by blood sampling, which is in itself a stressor along with other invasive methods used in field studies, and which cannot, therefore, be employed as a matter of course (Maschke et al., 1998). For this reason, in many cases, night urine is gathered from the subjects and analysed. Collecting nightly urine, however, provides only cumulative total parameters of the test items, and no information on time-related processes. This is, according to Born and Fehm (2000), particularly the case with an increased cortisol nadir, which must be considered an essential indicator of chronic stress. In a sleeping subject with an undisturbed circadian rhythm, the cortisol nadir occurs in the first half of the night. Plasma cortisol releases in the morning are higher than nadir values by a factor of 10 (Born and Fehm, 2000). As cortisol release in the first half of the night is low, an increased cortisol nadir can be estimated by splitting urine collection. Under the condition of undisturbed sleep, the cortisol level in the first half of the night, divided by the cortisol level in the second half, has a fairly stable value of about 0.2. In addition, this scheme also allows interindividual differentiations with regard to minimized circaseptanian rhythms. The procedure of split analyses has been successfully carried out by Ising and Ising (2001). In contrast to children, split urine collection in adults usually entails full awakening by an alarm clock or full bladder (test subjects have the option of drinking a lot of liquid before bedtime instead of using an alarm clock). However, intentional awakenings can distinctly disturb sleep, particularly if the subject is unable to go back to sleep, and of itself induce stress. Furthermore, according to the general adaptation theory, one has to take into account an exhaustion stage as a reaction to chronic stress. In this case, the adrenocortical system is unable to function, and consequently a reduced stress hormone release reaction occurs to further stimuli (Hellhammer, 2001).

In addition to these problems, the measurement of free cortisol in urine samples strongly depends upon analysis methods. Competitive binding assays and radioimmune asssays, as the most frequently used tests in routine measurement, overestimate free cortisol levels due to other competitive cortisol-immunoreactive substances in the urine (Schöneshöfer et al., 1986). The specificity of these methods of analysis is too low to allow precise differentiation of free cortisol from its metabolites. Follow-up measurements of urine samples of the longitudinal study by Harder et al. (1998, 1999) using high-performance liquid chromatography (HPLC) analysis suggest that immune assays provide questionable results for free cortisol with regard to urine samples. There are distinct differences in analyses if free cortisol and cortisol metabolites show diverse reactions (Maschke et al., 2003).

The observed differences due to analysis techniques are of special significance. Various publications indicate that acute noise exposures specifically induce free cortisol changes but chronic noise exposures elevate values of cortisol metabolites. Schöneshöfer et al. pointed out in 1986 that an additional assessment of cortisol metabolites may assist in differentiating chronic hypercortisolism from acute stress reactions. From today's viewpoint it is mandatory, therefore, to determine free cortisol as well as specific metabolites from urine samples using HPLC analyses in order to reach comparable results. On the other hand, there is an urgent need to understand the rather complex endocrine reactions to chronic noise exposure in a better way than is the case at present. To reach this goal, further interdisciplinary studies are necessary.

Independent of the chosen analysis techniques, there is a remarkable weekly (circaseptanian) rhythm in the release of cortisol (Haus et al., 1998). In the longitudinal study by Harder et al. (1998, 1999), the fluctuation of 35–50% in the weekly rhythm of cortisol mean levels must not be neglected. To compensate for the weekly rhythm fluctuations, urine collections ought to be gathered over a period of at least 7 consecutive days, or corresponding weekdays should be compared.

Cross-sectional studies in which the weekly rhythms have not been taken into account are of little significance unless the nightly urine samples are split as described above. The weekly rhythm can also be compensated by calculating cortisol ratios (Ising and Ising, 2001).

## Prospective issues/outlook

The present arguments strongly suggest that in noise research it will be necessary to define uniform data collection methods as well as comparable cortisol analyses from urine samples. However, noise is not only a physical stimulus but also an individual experience. Adaptational and sensory processes therefore have to be taken into consideration when analysing cortisol values. For reasonably reliable comparisons of cortisol excretion values presented in various studies, a standardization of data collection procedures and analysis techniques is therefore indispensable.

**Standardization protocols should include the following:**

- Standardization of urine collection: endogenous mean cortisol levels fluctuate between 35% and 50% in one-week periods.
- Standardization of analysis procedures: different analysis methods give distinctly different results. As a standard method, the HPLC analysis is proposed in order to differentiate free cortisol from near metabolites.
- Taking metabolism processes into account: methods that involve cortisol metabolites offer a differentiation of chronic stress from acute stress.
- Longitudinal studies to be performed over a minimum of 6 weeks: this allows inclusion of circadian and circaseptanian endocrine rhythms.

These requirements are based upon today's view of noise/response activation as a process that is interconnected on many levels with physiological processes and a considerable variety of behavioural and personal experience. It is not sufficient, therefore, to measure only stress hormones, even when data collection is standardized, but in each evaluation several reaction levels have to be considered. To make correct and robust statements, it is our view that it is necessary to assess not only stress hormone level excretions, but also vegetative and EEG parameters.

Furthermore, it is essential to consider more closely the relationships between habituation and dishabituation or, in other words, sensitivity and insensitivity. This means that repeat studies are necessary in order also to determine the habitational capacities of individuals.

# References

Arguelles AE, Disisto MV (1970) Endocrine and metabolic effects of noise in normal, hypertensive and psychotic subjects. In BL Welch, AS Welch, (Eds) Physiological Effects of Noise. New York, London: Plenum Press.

Arguelles AE, Ibeas D, Ottone JP, Chekherdemian M (1962) Pituitary adrenal stimulation by sound of different frequencies. The Journal of Clinical Endocrinology & Metabolism. 22: 846f.

Aschoff J, Ceresa F, Halberg F (1974) Chronobiological aspects of endocrinology. Stuttgart-New York: Schattauer Verlag.

Babisch W, Fromme H, Beyer A, Ising H (1996) Katecholaminausscheidung im Nachturin bei Frauen aus unterschiedlich verkehrslärmbelasteten Wohngebieten [Catecholamine excretion in the night urine of women from differently traffic noise loaded residential areas]. WaBoLu Hefte 6/1996. Berlin: Institut für Wasser-, Boden- und Lufthygiene des Bundesgesundheitsamtes.

Balzer HU, Hecht K (1989) Ist Streβ( noninvasiv zu messen? [Is it non-invasive to measure stress?] Wiss Zeitschrift der Humboldt Universität zu Berlin 38(4): 456–60.

Basner M, Buess H, Luks N, Maaβ H, Mavet L, Müller EW, Müller U, Piehler C, Plath G, Quehl J, Rey E, Samel A, Schulze M, Vejvoda M, Wenzel J (2001) Nachtfluglärmwirkungen – eine Teilauswertung von 64 Versuchspersonen in 832 Schlaflabornmärchten [Effects of night flight noise: a partial evaluation of 64 subjects over 832 consecutive sleep laboratory nights]. Köln: Institut für Luft- und Raumfahrtmedizin.

Benschop RJ, Broschot JF, Godaert GL, De Smet MB, Geenen R, Olff M, Heinjen CJ, Ballieux RE (1994) Chronic stress affects immunologic but not cardiovascular responsiveness to acute psychological stress in humans. Amer J Physiol 266:R75–80.

Bondarev GL, Sinicina AD, Efimov IN (1970) Zur gleichzeitigen Einwirkung von niederfrequenten Schwingungen und Lärm auf den Zustand des Hypophysen Nebennierenrinden Systems [Effects of simultaneous low-frequency vibration and noise on the hypophysical adrenal cortex system]. Gig i Sanit: 35, 106f.

Bonneau RH, Brehm MA, Kern AM (1997) The impact of psychological stress on the efficacy of antiviral adoptive immunotherapy in an immunocompromised host. J Neuroimmunol 78(1–2): 19–33.

Born J, Fehm HL (2000) The neuroendocrine recovery function of sleep. Noise & Health, 2(7): 25–37.

Braun C (1999) Nächtlicher Straßenverkehrslärm und Stresshormon ausscheidung beim Menschen (Nightly traffic noise and stress hormone excretion in man) Thesis, Humboldt Universität zu Berlin.

Breznitz S, Ben-Zur H, Berzon Y, Weiss D, Levitan G, Tarcic N, Lischinsky S, Greenberg A, Levi N, Zinder (1988) Experimental induction and termination of acute psychological stress in human volunteers: effects on immunological, neuroendocrine, cardiovascular and psychological parameters. Brain Behav Immun 12(1): 34–52.

Cannon WB (1929) Bodily Changes in Pain, Hunger, Fear and Rage. New York: Appelton.

Carter NL, Hunyor SN, Crawford G, Kelly D, Smith AJM (1994) Environmental noise and sleep – a study of arousals, cardiac arrhythmia and urinary catecholamines. Sleep 17, 298–307.

Cavatorta A, Falzoi M, Romanelli A, Cigala F, Ricco M, Bruschi G, Franchini L, Borghetti A (1987) Adrenal response in the pathogenesis of arterial hypertension in workers exposed to high levels of noise. Journal of Hypertension, Supplement 5: S463–6.

Croiset G, Veldhuis HD, Ballieux RE, de Wied D, Heijnen CJ (1987) The impact of mild emotional stress induced by the passive avoidance procedure on immune reactivity. Ann NY Acad Sci 496: 477–84.

Evans GW, Bullinger M, Hygge S (1998) Chronic noise exposure and physiological response: a prospective study of children living under environmental stress. Amer Psychol Soc 9: 75–7.

Evans G, Lercher P, Meis M, Ising H, Kofler W (2001) Typical community noise exposure and stress in children. J Acoust Soc Am 109(3): 1023–7.

Fruhstorfer B, Pritsch MG, Ott P, Sturm G (1988a) Effects of daytime noise load on the sleep-wake cycle and endocrine patterns in man: II: 24 hours secretion of anterior and posterior pituitary hormones and of cortisol. Journal of Neuroscience 39 (3–4): 211–32.

Fruhstorfer B, Pritsch MG, MB, Clement HW Wesemann W (1988b): Effects of daytime noise load on the sleep-wake cycle and endocrine patterns in man: III:24 hours secretion of free and sulfate conjugated catecholamines. Journal of Neuroscience 43 (1–2): 53–62.

Haines MM, Stansfeld SA, Brentnall S, Head J, Berry B, Jiggins M, Hygge S (2001) The West London School Study: the effect of chronic aircraft noise exposure on child health. Psychol Med 31(8): 1385–96.

Harder J, Maschke C, Ising H (1988) Längsschnittstudie zum Verlauf von Streßreaktionen unter Einfluß, von nächtlichem Fluglärm (Longitudinal study on the course of stress reactions under the influence of nightly aircraft noise). Umweltbundesamt Berlin: Forschungsbericht. FKZ 506 01 003.

Harder J (1999) Streßreaktionen and deren Verlauf unter Einfluß von anhaltenden nächtlichen Fluglärm (Stress reactions and their course under influence of a persistent nightly aircraft noise). Thesis Technische Universität, Berlin.

Haus E, Lakatu DJ, Sackett-Lundeen L, Dumitriu L, Niclan G, Petrescu, E, Plinga L (1998) Interaction of circadian ultradian and infrandian rhythmus. In Y Touitou (Hrsg.) Biological Clocks. Mechanism and Applications. Proceedings of the International Congress on Chronobiology, Paris, 7–11 September, 1997, Amsterdam: Elsevier, Band V, 141–150.

Hecht K (2001) Chronopsychobiologische Regulationsdiagnostik (CRD) zur Verifizierung von funktionellen Zuständen und Dysregulationen (Chronic psychic biological regulation diagnostics (CRD) to the verification of functional conditions and dysregulations). In K Hecht, HP Scherf, O König (Hrsg.) (2001) Emotioneller Stress durch Überforderung und Unterforderung (Emotional Stress Through Excessive Eemand and Sub-demand). Berlin, Milow, Strasburg: Schibri Verlag: 193–252.

Hecht K, Maschke C, Balzer HU, Bärndal S, Czolbe C, Dahmen A, Greusing M, Harder J, Knack A, Leitmann T, Wagner P, Wappler I (1999) Lärmmedizinisches Gutachten (Expert Medical Opinion on Noise). DA-Erweiterung Hamburg. Institut für Stressforschung (ISF) Berlin, Band 2: "Theoretische Grundlagen psychobiologischer Funktionen des Menschen in Beziehung zu Lärmwirkungen" 1–185.

Heine H (1997) Gesundheit – Krankheit – Streβ( (Health – disease – stress). Biologische Medizin 26(5): S200–204.

Hellhammer D (2001) Wenn die Stressbremse nicht mehr funktioniert (What happens when the stress brake no longer works). Psychologie Heute 2: 52–7.

Hildebrandt G, Moser M, Kehofer M (1998) Chronobiologie und Chronomedizin (Chronobiology and Chronic Medicine). Stuttgart: Hippokrates.

Ising H, Braun C (2000) Acute and chronic endocrine effects of noise. Review of the research conducted at the Institute for Water, Soil and Air Hygiene. Noise & Health 7: 7–24.

Ising H, Ising M (2001) Stressreaktionen von Kindern durch LKW-Lärm (Stress reactions of children to truck noise). Umweltmedizinischer Informationsdienst 1: 12–14.

Ising H, Kruppa B (2001) VII-1 Lärm. In HE Wichmann, HW Schlipköter, G Fülgraff (eds.) Handbuch der Umweltmedizin: Toxikologie, Epidemiologie, Hygiene, Belastungen, Wirkungen, Diagnostik, Prophylaxe (Manual of Environmental Medicine: Toxicology, Epidemiology, Hygiene, Loads, Effects, Diagnostics and Prophylaxis). Landsberg am Lech: Ecomed Verlagsgesellschaft.

Lazarus RS, Baker RW, Broverman DM, Mayer J (1957) Personality and psychological stress. J of Personality 25: 559–77.

Levi L (1961) A new stress tolerance test with simultaneous study of physiological and psychological variables. Acta Endocr 37 (38).

Levi L (1967) Emotional Stress. Basel, New York: Karger.

Levi L (1974) Was ist und bedeutet Stress? (What is stress, and what does it mean?) Zschr für Praxis Klinik, Arbeitshygiene, Begutachtung, Rehabilitation 9: 210–11.

Lindsley DB (1951) Emotion. In SS Stevens (ed) Handbook of Experimental Psychology. New York: Wiley.

Linthorst AC, Flachskamm C, Hopkins SJ, Hoadley ME, Labeur MS, Holsboer F, Reul JM (1997) Long-term intracerebroventricular infusion of corticotropin-releasing hormone alters neuroendocrine, neurochemical, autonomic, behavioural and cytokine responses to a systemic inflammatory challenge. J Neurosci 17(11): 4448–60.

Maschke C (1992) Der Einfluß von Nachtsfluglärm auf den Schlafverlauf und die Katecholaminausscheidung (The influence of nocturnal aircraft noise on sleep course and catecholamine excretion). Thesis, Technische Universität Berlin.

Maschke C, Arndt D, Ising H, Laude G, Thierfelder W, Contzen S (eds) (1995) Nachfluglärmwirkungen auf Anwohner (The effects of night-time aircraft noise on residents). Schriftenreihe des Vereins für Wasser-, Boden- und Lufthygiene, 96: 1–140.

Maschke C, Hecht K, Balzer H-W (1998) Lärm – Belästigung – vegetativ / hormonelle Prozesse (Noise – Annoyance – Vegetative / Hormonal Processes) Zürich: DAGA.

Maschke C, Harder J, Ising H, Hecht K, Thierfelder W (2003) Stress hormone changes in persons exposed to simulated night noise. Noise & Health 5 (17): 35–45.

Melamed S, Froom P, Kristal-Boneh E, Gofer D, Ribak J (1997) Industrial noise exposure, noise annoyance and serum lipid levels in blue-collar workers – the Cordis Study. Arch Environ Health 52(4): 292–8.

Miki K, Kawamorita K, Araga Y, Musha T, Sudo A (1998) Urinary and salivary stress hormone levels while performing arithmetic calculation in a noisy environment. Ind Health 36(1): 66–75.

Nitsch JR (1981) Stress: Theorien, Untersuchungen, Maßnahmen (Stress: Theories, examinations and measures. ISBN: 3-456-80699-X. Bern: Huber (ua).

Perger F (1990) Die Therapeutischen Konsequenzen aus der Grundregulations forschung [The therapeutic consequences of basic regulation research] In A Pischinger, H Heine (eds) Das System der Grundregulation. 8. Auflage: Heidelberg: Karl F Haug Verlag.

Sapolsky RM (1998) Hormonal correlates of personality and social contexts: from non-human to human primates. In C Panter-Brick, CM Worthman (eds) Hormones, Health and Behaviour. Cambridge University Press.

Sapolsky RM, Krey LC, McEwen BS (1986) The neuroendocrinology of stress and aging: the glucocorticoid cascade hypothesis. Endocr Rev 7(2): 284–301.

Schandry R (1998) Lehrbuch Psychophysiologie (Textbook of Psychophysiology). Weinheim: Beltz, Psychologie Verlags Union.

Schöneshöfer M, Weber B, Oelkers W, Nahoul K, Mantero F (1986) Measurement of urinary free 20-dihydrocortisol in biochemical diagnosis of chronic hyper-corticoidism. Clin Chem 32(5): 808–10.

Selye H (1953) Einführung in die Lehre vom Adaptationssyndrom (Introduction to the Doctrine of the Adaptation Syndrome) Stuttgart: Thieme.

Slob A, Wink A, Radder JJ (1973) The effect of acute noise exposure on the excretion of corticosteroids, adrenalin and noradrenalin in man. Arch Arbeitsmed 31: 225.

Sokolow JN (1967) Die reflektorischen Grundlagen der Wahrnehmung (The reflectory bases of perception). In H Hiebsch (ed) Ergebnisse der sowjetischen Psychologie (Results of Soviet Psychology). Berlin: Akademie Verlag 61–93.

Sudo A, Nguyen AL, Jonai H, Matsuda S, Villanueva MB, Sotoyama M, Nguyen TC, Le VT, Hoang HT, Nguyen DT, Nguyen S (1996) Effects of earplugs on catecholamine and cortisol excretion in noise-exposed textile workers. Industrial Health 34(3): 279–86.

Zwiener U, Langhorst P (1993) Vegetatives Nervensystem [The vegetative nervous system]. In U Zwiener (ed) Allgemeine und Klinische Pathophysiologie (General and Clinical Pathophysiology). Jena, Stuttgart: Gustav Fischer Verlag.

# CHAPTER 25

# Noise and cognitive performance in children and adults

*Noise and Its Effects:* Edited by Linda Luxon and Deepak Prasher © 2007 John Wiley & Sons Ltd.

GARY W EVANS, STAFFAN HYGGE

This chapter is organized into three major sections. The first section provides brief overviews of what is currently known about the effects of noise on cognitive performance. Material on adults and children is presented separately. The second section examines possible mechanisms and underlying processes to explain why and how noise can affect cognitive performance. Finally, the third section notes limitations in the current knowledge base and offers suggestions for research priorities.

## Noise and cognition

### Adults

For children there is little research on basic cognitive processes such as memory and attention and considerable work on reading. The picture is reversed for adults. Veitch (1990), in a typical finding, indicates no main effects of noise on reading comprehension among adults. The results for memory and attention are complex and elaborate. We provide an overview of what we believe are representative studies to give a flavour of what we currently know.

### Memory

Early explanations for memory and noise relied on arousal models that suggested some enhancement of encoding created by noise (Hockey, 1979). However, these studies typically relied on paired associate learning and other simple forms of encoding with little or no meaning. Noise-induced elevations in arousal were hypothesized to enhance memory because of attentional narrowing or focusing (Easterbrook, 1959). Broadbent (1971) modified this model, arguing that enhanced arousal causes allocation of attention to the most dominant or salient information in a task. Several empirical studies support this allocation model (Broadbent, 1971; Hamilton, Hockey and Rejman, 1977; Smith, 1982; Smith and Broadbent, 1982). High arousal also appears to enhance the spontaneous encoding of order information (Hamilton, Hockey and Quinn, 1972; Broadbent, 1981; Banbury and Berry, 1997, 1998). The common finding that incidental memory is poorer under noise (Davies and Jones, 1975) can also be explained by an attentional allocation model of noise-induced focus on dominant cues.

## Factors relating noise and memory

- Arousal
- Attention allocation
- Influence of executive strategies

More recent work on noise and memory, although not denying the role of attention allocation, has adopted a more general position that what noise does is influence executive strategies about how information is processed. For example, under noise, adults appear to rely more on rehearsal rather than elaboration of material. Subjects in noise, for example, will often recall more physical details of stimuli but have less knowledge of meaning or the relationships or structure underlying the materials (Broadbent, 1981; Smith, Jones and Broadbent, 1981; Evans et al., 1984). One reason for this strategy could be the speeding up of processing under noise. People appear better able quickly to attend to and encode literal contents of material under noise but this may create a trade-off with deeper processing that would lead to better understanding and comprehension (Hamilton et al., 1977; Hockey, 1979).

Precisely how these strategy shifts occur is unclear. Efforts to provide a levels-of-processing explanation have proven moot. Smith and Broadbent (1981), for example, used instructions to manipulate how deeply materials were processed and found no interactions with noise. Similarly, examination of the degree of similarity of encoding and recall conditions (for example, noise at encoding, quiet at recall versus noise at both encoding and recall) also proved unsatisfactory as an explanation of strategy shifts (Bell et al., 1984; Hygge, Boman and Enmarker, 2003). Recent work suggests, however, some promise in examining memory processes requiring explicit, conscious elaboration and recall of semantic materials (episodic memory).

Hygge and colleagues (2003) with young adults, Enmarker (2005) with middle-aged and older adults, and Meis and colleagues (1998) with children find consistent patterns of deficits, indicating that implicit memory is largely impervious to noise whereas explicit memory tasks are vulnerable. For example, priming paradigms are unaffected by noise but recall of meaning and knowledge of underlying structures are vulnerable.

- Implicit memory resistant to noise
- Explicit memory vulnerable to noise

## Attention

Vigilance tasks that require sustained attention to low-frequency signals are generally robust with respect to noise unless processing demands are elevated by increasing the number, speed or ambiguity of salient signal cues (Broadbent, 1978; Hockey, 1979). Serial attention tasks that require sequential responses to variable targets indicate loss of accuracy (Broadbent, 1971; Hockey, 1979; Rabbit, 1979), especially at noise onset (Fisher, 1972). Visual search tasks in which target stimuli must be found in arrays are also sensitive to noise, especially when the memory load (number of targets) is high (Hockey, 1979; Cohen et al., 1986).

As mentioned earlier, Easterbrook and Broadbent both predicted that noise, as a result of elevated arousal, would cause greater allocation of attentional resources to central, more dominant cues. Several studies have directly examined this hypothesis with dual task paradigms in which attention must be divided among competing stimuli. Noise reliably interferes with whatever cues are less salient (as manipulated by instructions) and has little or slight facilitation effects on dominant cues (Boggs and Simon, 1968; Finkelman and Glass, 1970; Hockey, 1970a,b; Evans et al., 1996).

### Noise and cognitive performance in adults

- Memory impairment for meaning and comprehension, particularly for complex, difficult materials.
- Errors in memory for sequentially presented information.
- Deficits in attention to secondary (less important) information when competing signals must be attended to.

### Children

## Reading

The best-documented impacts of noise on children's performance is research showing negative effects on reading acquisition.

Close to 20 studies have found indications of negative relations between chronic noise exposure and delayed reading acquisition in young children (Evans and Lepore, 1993).

There are no contradictory findings and the few null results are probably due to methodological problems such as comparing children across school districts who have different reading curricula (Cohen et al., 1986). In addition to the near unanimity of the findings, several other aspects of the noise and reading research render definitive conclusions. The data include prospective, longitudinal effects (Hygge, Evans and Bullinger, 2002), evidence of a dose–response function (Lukas, Du Pree and Swing, 1981; Green, Pasternack and Shore, 1982), and results showing that sound attenuation interventions in three different situations reduced or eliminated the negative noise impacts on reading (Bronzaft, 1981; Cohen et al., 1986; Maxwell and Evans, 2000). Several of the studies have pretested children for hearing damage, showing none, as would be expected given the levels of ambient exposure. Furthermore, most of these studies had good controls for socioeconomic status. Finally some of the studies have carefully assessed children under quiet conditions, indicating that the effects of noise are due to chronic exposure rather than acute conditions during the testing phase. Recently, the largest study of noise and reading ever conducted (with approximately 11 000 children) found a relationship between noise and reading. However, after statistical controls for the percentage of low-income children attending each school, the association became non-significant (Haines et al., 2002). This same team of investigators found more recently, however, with more precise, individual level statistical controls, a significant relationship between noise levels and reading scores (Stansfeld et al., 2003). Furthermore, prospective (Hygge et al., 2002) and cross-sectional (Haines et al., 2001c) data reveal that not all reading tests are equally sensitive with an indication that more difficult items may be especially vulnerable.

Studies of acute noise on reading performance are much more mixed, which we attribute to the shorter duration of exposure. No effects have been found in several studies (Slater, 1968; Weinstein and Weinstein, 1979) along with a pattern of interactions suggesting that girls (Christie and Glickman, 1980) and lower ability children may be at some modest risk (Johansson, 1983). Kassinove (1972) found no impact of acute noise on mathematics performance but Zentall and Shaw (1980) uncovered an interaction indicating that hyperactive children might be at risk for adverse impacts on mathematics.

*Memory*

There are fewer studies of other cognitive processes and noise among children relative to reading. The most ubiquitous memory effects occur in chronic noise, particularly when complex, semantic materials are probed (Hygge, 2003). Several studies of both chronic (Evans, Hygge and Bullinger, 1995; Haines et al., 2001a; Hygge et al., 2002) and acute noise (Boman, 2004; Hygge, 2003; Hygge et al., 2003) have found adverse impacts of aircraft noise exposure on long-term memory for complex, difficult material. Stansfeld et al. (2003) replicate these effects on long-term memory for aircraft noise and extend prior work by showing adverse impacts on recall of details and conceptual meaning, as well as for recognition and prospective memory. The latter is assessed by asking the children beforehand to write their initials at several predefined points in the text. The Hygge (2003) study replicated the adverse impacts of simulated aircraft noise at both 66 dB (A) and 55 dB (A) $L_{eq}$. He also showed that the adverse impact of aircraft noise and road traffic noise exceeds noise in trains or irrelevant speech at comparable intensity levels.

Long-term recall of visual materials (Hambrick-Dixon, 1986) and recognition memory (Hambrick-Dixon, 1986; Hygge, 2003; Boman, 2004) are not impaired by chronic noise exposure. Both Hambrick-Dixon (1986) and Johansson (1983) found no memory effects of acute noise exposure on long-term memory. In both cases, however, they did not probe for complex, difficult material. Haines et al. (2001) did not replicate the effects of chronic noise on long-term memory for prose material, however.

Children's incidental memory for visual material may be adversely affected by chronic noise exposure (Heft, 1979; Lercher, Evans and Meis, 2003). The latter study is noteworthy in two respects. First, they used memory tests specifically developed to evaluate intentional and incidental memory and demonstrated, as predicted, stronger adverse effects on intentional memory. Second, they used typical community noise, not airport or high traffic noise sources. Hambrick-Dixon (1986) and Cohen et al. (1986) did not replicate these incidental memory effects but did not employ measures as sensitive to those relied on by Lercher et al.

Short-term memory does not appear to be sensitive to chronic noise (Hambrick-Dixon, 1986; Evans et al., 1995; Haines et al., 2001a,c) unless it is sufficiently loud to mask encoding stimuli (Fenton, Alley and Smith, 1974).

The differential sensitivity of information complexity or difficulty to noise effects could be related to the distinction between implicit and explicit memory. Meis et al. (1998) found that both chronic and simulated acute aircraft noise interfered with long-term recall but had no impact on word production.

Implicit memory tasks like word production are resistant to distraction or divided attention, whereas explicit memory tasks such as recall are more vulnerable to interference. This pattern of noise-and-task difficulty has also been found in the adult literature as described above.

*Attention*

Several studies have examined possible links between noise exposure and attentional deficits among young children with a mixed set of results. Studies in airport or train noise-impacted schools reveal that noise levels are sufficiently loud and intrusive to distract children as indexed by observers (Bronzaft and McCarthy, 1975; Kryter, 1994). Several investigators have uncovered relationships between chronic noise exposure and poorer visual search performance under controlled, quiet testing conditions (Karsdorf and Klappach, 1968; Heft, 1979; Moch-Sibony, 1981; Muller, et al., 1998).

Haines et al. (2001b) found analogous results with an auditory sustained attention task as did Kyzar (1977) with a series of clerical tasks, including proofreading. Several other studies of chronic noise (air and road traffic) have been unable to replicate these effects (Haines et al., 2001c; Lercher et al., 2003; Stansfeld et al., 2003). Furthermore, both Hambrick-Dixon (1986) and Evans et al. (1995) found no adverse effects of chronic noise on visual search tasks.

Other variables may moderate the relationships between chronic noise and visual attention or concentration. Cohen et al. (1986) found that duration of exposure to chronic noise may play some role. Fourth and fifth grade children were better on a visual search task during acute noise exposure if they had lived under chronic noise for 2 years or less, whereas the opposite pattern occurred for children chronically exposed to noise for more than 4 years. Heft (1979) found that young children from noisy homes were less negatively distracted by an auditory distracter during a visual matching task and Hambrick-Dixon (1986) found that a visual coding task was performed better under acute noise conditions by children attending noisy schools whereas they did worse, relative to well-matched quiet counterparts, when performing the task under quiet conditions. Hambrick-Dixon's data are difficult to compare with other studies because she assessed tachistoscopically presented stimuli whereas other investigators examined sustained attention in visual search tasks.

The findings suggesting differential resistance to auditory distraction as a function of personal history with ambient noise match work by Cohen, Glass and Singer (1973) and Moch-Sibony (1981), indicating that children chronically exposed to noise have poorer auditory discrimination (ability to detect differences between similarly sounding words). Cohen et al. suggested that noise-related deficits in auditory discrimination might be caused by children learning to ignore auditory stimuli (gate out distraction) as a way to cope with chronic noise. It is also interesting to note that two studies have found that young children chronically exposed to noise are less adept at picking out the optimum signal-to-noise ratio when meaningful stimuli are presented amongst a background of broadband continuous noise (Cohen et al., 1986; Evans et al., 1995).

Presentations of simulated noise in the laboratory can significantly mask speech (Glenn, Nerbonne and Tolhurst, 1978), degrade performance on visual attention tasks (Turnure, 1970; Steinkamp, 1980; Zentall and Shaw, 1980) and produce observable increases in child distraction and off-task time (Wyon, 1970). The simulated noise stimuli used in several of these studies were designed to be representative of classroom interior acoustic conditions (children talking, games, etc.). Data from Glenn et al. (1978) and Zentall and Shaw (1980) suggest that children with learning disabilities may be especially susceptible to attentional disruption by auditory distraction.

In three studies of children's reading and memory during acute noise (Hygge, 2003; Hygge et al., 2003; Boman, 2004), measures were also taken of attentional capacities but attention was not found to mediate memory deficits created by noise.

## Motivation

One laboratory study (Glass, 1977) and several field studies (Cohen et al., 1986; Evans et al., 1995; Bullinger et al., 1999; Maxwell and Evans, 2000) have found that children chronically exposed to noise are less motivated when placed in achievement situations where task performance is contingent upon persistence. Moch-Sibony (1981) also found that chronic noise was associated with deficits on a standardized index of frustration tolerance, and Wachs (1987) has reported that infants reared in noisier homes manifest lower mastery scores on a standardized developmental paradigm. Cohen et al. (1986) also found that a second index of motivation, abrogation of choice, was affected by chronic noise exposure. Children chronically exposed to noise, following a set of experimental procedures in quiet conditions, were more apt to relinquish choice over a reward to an experimenter, in comparison to their well matched quiet counterparts. Haines et al. (2001a) could not replicate the effects of aircraft noise on puzzle persistence in elementary schoolchildren although they administered the task in small groups rather than individually. Given the effects of competition and modelling on motivation, this procedural change may be consequential.

Most of these studies have good controls for Socioeconomic Status (SES) and the Bullinger et al. (1999) study is a prospective, longitudinal design. Furthermore, the Maxwell and Evans (2000) study is an intervention comparing motivation before and after acoustic renovations in a preschool. Both the Bullinger study and one of the Cohen et al. (1986) studies also found that, the longer the duration of noise exposure, the more negative the impact on motivation. Bullinger and her colleagues also assessed attributions for failure and found that children chronically exposed to noise were more likely to make attributions to stable, internal factors such as ability relative to controls from quiet areas. Teachers in noisy schools also report difficulties motivating their students (Crook and Langdon, 1974; Kyzar, 1977; Moch-Sibony, 1981). Haines et al. (2001a) did not replicate the link between aircraft noise and teacher reports about student motivation.

The pattern of motivational deficits in relation to chronic noise has been related to learned helplessness theory (Peterson, Maier and Seligman, 1993). Continuous exposure to aversive, uncontrollable stimuli has been shown across a wide variety of conditions, including noise, to induce feelings and behaviours indicative of helplessness. As one continues to struggle unsuccessfully with an uncontrollable, adverse stimulus, one eventually 'learns' that one is helpless to do anything about the situation, as manifested by feelings of hopeless and reduced persistence. It is worth reiterating that both experimental manipulations of control over stimuli and control-related personality beliefs are powerful moderators of these affective and motivational consequences of uncontrollable noise stimuli in a manner consistent with the learned helplessness model of motivation (Cohen, 1980; Evans, 2001).

### Noise and cognitive performance in children

- Deficits in reading acquisition from chronic exposure.
- Interference with long-term memory for complex, difficult materials.
- Problems in speech perception (for example, signal-to-noise discrimination, phonemes) in children chronically exposed to noise.
- Motivational deficits, indicative of learned helplessness. Acute and chronic exposure to uncontrollable noise leads to less persistence in problem solving.

# Mechanisms and underlying processes

Attempts to develop a unifying theoretical framework to understand why and under what conditions noise interferes with cognition have remained unfulfilled. We offer some tentative ideas and suggestions here but certainly do not provide a unifying theory.

### Auditory masking and speech perception

Some theories (Poulton, 1977) indicate that noise affects cognition because it interferes with speech perception directly (masking) or interrupts subvocalization processes (such as inner speech, auditory rehearsal, echoic memory). Several strands of data indicate that this theory cannot adequately account for all adverse noise impacts on cognition. As noted by Broadbent (1978), for example, non-semantic materials without linguistic content are also adversely impacted by noise. Studies of chronic noise find impacts at levels far below those necessary to produce hearing damage and several studies of reading, for example, pre-screened children with auditory damage. Since several of these same studies also tested children under quiet conditions, concurrent interference with auditory processing cannot explain these results.

On the other hand, several studies suggest that noise can interfere in important ways with speech perception or language acquisition that may in turn account for some of the harmful impacts of chronic noise on reading and other higher level processes (for example, long-term memory for complex, semantic material). Cohen et al. (1973) found that traffic noise levels in children with no auditory damage was significantly related to auditory discrimination of speech. Evans and Maxwell (1997) demonstrated that airport noise exposure was correlated with poorer speech perception. It is potentially important that they also showed that sound perception (for example, ability to recognize common, ambient sounds such as a church bell or a piano) was not related to ambient noise exposure. Both of these studies tested children under well-controlled, quiet conditions and ruled out auditory damage as an explanation. Two studies have also shown that children who attend schools in noisy areas are less adept at discriminating the optimum signal-to-noise ratio in an auditory task (Cohen et al., 1986; Evans et al., 1995). Deutsch (1964) theorized that perhaps children chronically exposed to noise develop a cognitive strategy of tuning out or ignoring noise as a way to deal with it. Unfortunately this tuning-out process may overgeneralize so that children learn to tune out not only ambient, background sound but also focal material such as speech.

Haines et al. (2001b), however, found no mediation of airport noise-related reading deficits and an auditory attention task. Note also that, in the adult literature, attempts to explain long-term memory deficiencies under noise as attentional deficits have proven futile (Hygge et al., 2003).

Three studies have attempted to examine whether speech perception could account for negative correlations between ambient noise levels and reading. Cohen et al. (1973) found that the significant relationship between ambient traffic noise and reading deficits in young children was largely accounted for by the co-variation between noise levels and auditory discrimination. Evans and Maxwell (1997) found partial mediation of negative noise impacts on reading by speech perception. Furthermore, as indicated sound perception was not adversely affected by chronic noise exposure. Hygge et al. (2002), in their prospective study of aircraft noise, reading and cognitive processes, found that speech perception did not mediate the link between noise exposure and reading deficits.

**Caregiver behaviours**

Some of the negative cognitive effects of ambient noise levels on children may be caused indirectly by effects on their caregivers. Many studies of aircraft and road traffic noise near to schools reveal significant interruptions, resulting in lost teaching time (Crook and Langdon, 1974; Bronzaft and McCarthy, 1975; Kryter, 1994). Bronzaft, for example, found that approximately 11% of teaching time was lost due to pauses in instruction when elevated trains passed next to classrooms on the noisy side of an elementary school in New York City. Fifty per cent of the teachers in Kryter's study of aircraft noise in San Diego reported regular interruptions (at least one every 10 minutes) in classroom teaching. Teachers in these schools also indicate moderate-to-high levels of their own annoyance and irritation with the noise (Crook and Langdon, 1974; Ko, 1979; Sargent et al., 1980) and themselves report dissatisfaction with their working environments, noting, for example, difficulties in concentration and mental fatigue (Ko, 1979; Sargent et al., 1980).

Parents in noisier homes are less responsive to their children (Wachs, 1989; Wachs and Camli, 1991) as are those who reside in homes judged as more chaotic (Matheny et al., 1995). The latter residential settings are characterized as high in ambient noise levels, distraction, and crowding. These three studies of residential noise assessed interior noise levels in low-income settings with most of the noise sources internally generated.

To our knowledge no one has examined parenting behaviours among those living near to airports or other high, ambient noise sources.

**Strategy shifts**

The well-established finding that task variables play a prominent role in understanding noise effects on performance raises problems and offers opportunities. The basic problem, akin to the arousal explanation of noise effects, is that lack of effects can simply be attributed to some amorphous variable like complexity or to an undefined process such as speed/accuracy tradeoffs. There is reasonable consensus (Broadbent, 1979; Hockey, 1979; Cohen et al., 1986; Smith and Jones, 1992) that noise leads to certain strategy preferences including greater attention to dominant strategies, faster processing of information, and the reduction in the flexibility and efficiency of executive control functions that allocate and track cognitive resources, particularly attention and episodic memory handling. There is some reason to believe that the manner in which noise affects attention or more immediate, perceptual processing is different to how it affects memory. Several studies showed that attentional shifts do not mediate noise-related memory effects. On the other hand, in children, apparent attentional strategy changes (tuning out) do appear related to deficits in reading acquisition. More effort is warranted to manipulating attentional and memory processes independently in the study of noise and performance.

The degree of selectivity and how much is lost when exposed to noise may be both a function of attention at intake (verbatim details, serial order versus linkages and underlying structure of materials) and how stored information is reorganized and elaborated in long-term memory (less spontaneous elaboration, poorer articulation of input to pre-existing structures and schema). Performance that requires flexibility, elaboration or in-depth comprehension and understanding of underlying structures and overarching connections appears most vulnerable to noise interference. Tasks that require judicious, flexible sharing and alteration of attentional strategies or those that require slower processing may be especially vulnerable to noise. The fact that noise can adversely impact both intentional and incidental memory, but seems to have more consistently negative effects on intentional memory suggests that encoding strategies may be especially salient.

**Underlying mechanisms to account for noise impacts on children**

- Interference with language acquisition (for example, speech perception deficits).
- Altered caregiver behaviours (for example, interruptions in teacher speech in noisy classrooms).
- Shifts in information processing strategies with focus on dominant information and less flexible use of alternative strategies.

# Limitations in current knowledge base and research priorities

## Measurement issues

At present several problematic measurement issues make it difficult to achieve the policy impact warranted by the quantity and quality of existing evidence for adverse noise impacts on cognition. For example, although there are nearly 20 studies demonstrating links between ambient noise exposure and delayed reading acquisition, we cannot say with certainty at what level of noise exposure this risk is serious. We only have two dose–response curves and both rely on aggregate (school) level estimates of exposure from noise contours.

The noise metrics available as well as their degree of precision are also problematic. Most transportation noise authorities rely upon $L_{dn}$ which is a 24-hour average with a 10 dB (A) night-time penalty. This metric, however, was developed for the purposes of predicting annoyance and may be inappropriate for cognitive impacts. As just one example, if some of the difficulties uncovered in children are related to problems in speech perception, then a metric that weights night-time exposure more heavily is, in fact, backwards since children's auditory processing with parents and teachers is obviously more critical during waking hours.

Estimates of exposure to noise are typically very crude, strongly influenced by geographical mobility, building attenuation properties and ongoing, internally generated noise sources. Nearly all of the chronic studies rely on noise contour maps generated for environmental impact studies and thus are focused on the external environment. We know from a few studies with children, for example, that home noise levels interact with school noise levels to increase the negative impact on reading (Lukas et al., 1981; Cohen et al., 1986). Wachs and Gruen (1982) and Michelson (1968) reported that the links between noise exposure in the home and cognitive outcomes in young children were weaker if the child had access to a quiet space or retreat within the home.

Use of averages and the decibel scale itself may also be problematic. A 24-hour average of 60 or even 50 $L_{eq}$ or $L_{dn}$ in fact means that for much of the day ambient levels are indeed very loud, with peaks probably exceeding 90 dB (A). This may mean that for much of the actual time that the individual is exposed to noise (while at school or work) the levels are rather loud whereas during other times (evening, at home) the intensity may be low. It is unclear what metrics would work better, but some guidance may be available from work on crowding and traffic congestion. Research on the former shows quite clearly that one's actual exposure rather than estimates prove potent. For example, the number of people per room in the residence is the critical density metric, whereas measures such as number of people per acre are largely irrelevant to human psychological health (Evans, 1999). For traffic congestion, average speed or average number of cars/hour has little or no linkage to human well being. The proportion of time one is exposed to high levels of congestion turns out to be the critical parameter (Evans, 1999).

It is also critical to keep in mind the temporal dimension of noise exposure. Several studies have indicated that duration of exposure amplifies the adverse impacts of noise on cognitive processing (Cohen et al., 1973, 1986; Bullinger et al., 1999; Hygge et al., 2002). Analogous duration-related impacts of noise on psychophysiology have also been noted among adults and children (Evans, 2001). Just as exposure estimation needs to take better account of intensity and temporal variables, Jones and Morris (1992) have raised the important issue of auditory content. Jones' work and that of others suggest that auditory stimuli with speech-like properties may have a special status in affecting cognitive processing. The content and timing of auditory stimuli may prove to be just as important as the intensity of sound levels in gaining a good understanding of how noise impacts human performance. Jones' work has identified the irrelevant speech effect (ISE). Sound with variation in pitch and timbre (even when holding intensity constant) is very disruptive of serial processing, particularly in short-term memory (Hughes and Jones, 2001). Interestingly, phonological structure as well as meaning have little role to play in the disruptive effects of ISE on short-term memory for order. When comprehension is assessed, however, meaning adds to the disruptive impacts of ISE.

Thus better exposure estimates, exploration of different summary descriptors (for example, percentage of time that some level is exceeded) and data on sound metrics where children live and learn, such as speech interference or transmission levels or reverberation time, are areas in need of further investigation. Consideration of the spectral parameters of noise, not just the level, are greatly needed. Researchers need to adopt a strategy, where possible, of sampling persons exposed across a range of noise levels so that we can begin to better inform policy-makers about thresholds and margins of safety. Nearly all of the current knowledge base emanates from quiet versus noisy comparisons. Of course without adequate financial support from granting agencies, these expanded types of research will not occur.

**Moderating factors**

Too much of the research on noise and cognition has focused solely on the main effects of noise, implicitly ignoring the important issue of other factors that can alter the manner in which noise affects human functioning. For example, both laboratory and field studies have indicated that children with learning disabilities are more adversely impacted by noise (Maser et al., 1978; Zentall and Shaw, 1980; Johansson, 1983). Use of overall average impacts while reasonable are not suitable for public policy because they do not provide a prudent margin of safety for vulnerable subgroups. Work with children also suggests that age may be a critical variable (Evans and Lepore, 1993). Other vulnerable subgroups among children, which it would seem vital to study, include learning to read in one's non-native language, children with temporary or permanent hearing loss, and those who are also exposed to other multiple sources of stress that often accompany high ambient noise levels (for example, crowding, poor-quality housing, family turmoil, high crime). To provide a sense of the potential importance of research on vulnerable subgroups, 40% of American elementary schoolchildren experience one or more incidents of temporary hearing loss from upper-ear infections during the school year. In several major American metropolitan areas the percentage of elementary children in school whose mother tongue is not English exceeds 33%.

**Mediating processes**

Despite 30 years of careful thinking and empirical work on noise and cognitive performance we still have very little in the way of a clear theoretical model of how noise affects performance. Research on noise tends to focus on the question of whether or not there is an effect, but ultimately real breakthroughs will come when we are able to specify with greater precision why and how these effects occur. This suggests a research strategy where more weight is put on thinking about the underlying processes and not just demonstrating an effect. Data need to be collected on speech perception, variable memory processes (for example, encoding, retrieval), attention, interference with acoustic rehearsal, motivation, etc., along with the particular target outcome variables of interest.

There are also a few cognitive processes that appear either especially resistant or even enhanced by noise. Here too we may have some possible insights into how noise operates. The latter approach is consistent with the idea that noise affects executive, cognitive functioning like the allocation of attention, the speed of processing and the integration of materials with existing networks (explicit memory paradigms).

With children more attention is probably warranted on adult caregivers' behaviours in the presence of noisy settings. A handful of studies suggest that parents are less responsive to their children in noisy settings. Perhaps their speech patterns, teaching and demonstration behaviours, or engagement in cognitive-related activities (for example, reading aloud), are adversely impacted by ambient noise. Some, but probably not all, of the adverse effects of noise on cognitive development are probably mediated by adult–child interactions.

Another potential area of insight that has not been fully explored is the dimension of time in noise studies. Memory studies indicate important temporal aspects of noise effects (for example, beginning versus middle or end of working memory span). Vigilance studies find exposure duration by noise interactions as well as time-related momentary lapses in performance. Reading acquisition deficits are sensitive to the age of the child during exposure. Progress has definitely been made in understanding under what conditions noise interferes with cognitive performance, but we still have a considerable amount of work ahead of us to provide a satisfactory explanation for why this occurs.

## Future research priorities

- More dose–response data are needed.
- Development of more appropriate noise metrics to study cognition.
- We need more precision for calibration of individual noise exposure over time and space.
- We know very little about qualitative aspects of noise in terms of human cognition. Recent work on speech spectrum characteristics of noise is especially promising.
- Application of psycholinguistic theory and measurement methods (for example, language acquisition and reading) may provide insight into how noise interferes with reading acquisition.
- Additional understanding of noise and children's cognition may come from examining noise-related changes in adult caregivers' behaviours. Prime candidates include adults' speech patterns and responsiveness to children under noisy conditions.
- Greater attention needs to be given to potentially vulnerable subgroups of the population (for example, children learning to read in their non-native language, individuals with hearing impariments) with respect to noise and cognition.

## References

Banbury S, Berry D (1997) Habituation and dishabituation to speech and office noise. Journal of Experimental Psychology: Applied 3: 187–95.

Banbury S, Berry D (1998) Disruption of office related tasks by speech and office noise. British Journal of Psychology 89: 499–517.

Bell P, Hess S, Hill E, Kukas S, Richards R, Sargent D (1984) Noise and context dependent memory. Bulletin of the Psychonomic Society 22: 99–100.

Boggs D, Simon J (1968) Differential effect of noise on tasks of varying complexity. Journal of Applied Psychology 52: 148–53.

Boman E (2004) The effects of noise and gender on children's attention episodic and semantic memory. Scandinavian Journal of Psychology: 45(5)407–16.

Broadbent DE (1971) Decision and Stress. London: Cambridge.

Broadbent DE (1978) The current state of noise research: reply to Poulton. Psychological Bulletin 85: 1052–67.

Broadbent DE (1979) Human performance in noise. In C Harris (ed.) Handbook of Noise Control, 2nd edn. New York: McGraw-Hill.

Broadbent DE (1981) The effects of moderate levels of noise on human performance. In JV Tobias, E Schubert (eds) Hearing Research and Theory. New York: Academic.

Bronzaft A (1981) The effect of a noise abatement program on reading ability. Journal of Environmental Psychology 1: 215–22.

Bronzaft A, McCarthy D (1975) The effect of elevated train noise on reading ability. Environment and Behaviour 7: 517–27.

Bullinger M, Hygge S, Evans GW, Meis M, Von Mackensen S (1999) The psychological costs of aircraft noise among children. Zentralblatt für Hygiene und Umweltmedizin 202: 127–38.

Christie D, Glickman C (1980) The effect of classroom noise on children: evidence for sex differences. Psychology in the Schools 17: 405–8.

Cohen S (1980) Aftereffects of stress on human performance and social behaviour: a review of research and theory. Psychological Bulletin 88: 82–108.

Cohen S, Glass DC, Singer JE (1973) Apartment noise, auditory discrimination and reading ability in children. Journal of Experimental Social Psychology 9: 407–22.

Cohen S, Evans GW, Stokols D, Krantz DS (1986) Behaviour Health and Environmental Stress. New York: Plenum.

Crook M, Langdon F (1974) The effects of aircraft noise in schools around London airport. Journal of Sound and Vibration 34: 221–32.

Davies D, Jones DM (1975) The effects of noise and incentives upon attention in short term memory. British Journal of Psychology 66: 61–8.

Deutsch D (1964) Auditory discrimination and learning: social factors. Merrill Palmer Quarterly 10: 277–96.

Easterbrook J (1959) The effect of emotion on cue utilization and the organization of behaviour. Psychological Bulletin 66: 183–201.

Enmarker I (2005) The effects of meaningful irrelevant speech and road traffic noise on teacher's attention, episodic and semantic memory. Scandinavian Journal of Psychology. 45: 393–405.

Evans GW (1999) Measurement of the physical environment as stressor. In SL Friedman, TD Wachs (eds) Assessment of the Environment across the Lifespan. Washington DC: American Psychological Association.

Evans GW (2001) Environmental stress and health. In A Baum, T Revenson, JE Singer (eds) Handbook of Health Psychology. Mahwah, NJ: Erlbaum.

Evans GW, Lepore SJ (1993) Nonauditory effects of noise on children. Children's Environments 10: 31–51.

Evans GW, Maxwell LM (1997) Chronic noise exposure and reading deficits: the mediating effects of language acquisition. Environment and Behaviour 29: 710–28.

Evans GW, Skorpanich MA, Garling T, Bryant K, Bresolin B (1984) The effects of pathway configuration landmarks and stress on environmental cognition. Journal of Environmental Psychology 4: 323–35.

Evans GW, Hygge S, Bullinger M (1995) Chronic noise and psychological stress. Psychological Science 6: 333–8.

Evans GW, Allen K, Tafalla R, O'Meara T (1996) Multiple stressors: performance psychophysiologic and affective responses. Journal of Environmental Psychology 16: 147–54.

Fenton T, Alley G, Smith K (1974) Effects of white noise on short-term memory of learning disabled boys. Perceptual and Motor Skills 39: 903–6.

Finkleman J, Glass DC (1970) Reappraisal of the relationship between noise and human performance by means of a subsidiary task measure. Journal of Applied Psychology 54: 211–13.

Fisher S (1972) A distraction effect of noise bursts. Perception 1: 223–36.

Glass DC (1977) Behaviour Patterns, Stress and Coronary Heart Disease. Hillsdale, NJ: Erlbaum.

Glenn L, Nerbonne G, Tolhurst G (1978) Environmental noise in a residential institution for mentally retarded persons. American Journal of Mental Deficiency 82: 594–97.

Green K, Pasternack B, Shore R (1982) Effects of aircraft noise on reading ability of school age children. Archives of Environmental Health 37: 24– 31.

Haines MM, Stansfeld SA, Job RFS, Berglund B, Head J (2001a) Chronic aircraft noise exposure, stress responses, mental health and cognitive performance in school children. Psychological Medicine 31: 265–77.

Haines MM, Stansfeld SA, Job RFS, Berglund B, Head J (2001b) A follow-up study of effects of chronic aircraft noise exposure on child stress responses and cognition. International Journal of Epidemiology 30: 839–45.

Haines MM, Stansfeld SA, Brenthall S, Head J, Berry B, Jiggins M et al. (2001c) The West London schools study: the effects of chronic aircraft noise exposure on child health. Psychological Medicine 31: 1385–96.

Haines MM, Stansfeld SA, Head J, Job RFS (2002) Multi-level modelling of aircraft noise on performance tests in schools around Heathrow, London Airport. International Journal of Epidemiology and Community Health 56: 139–44.

Hambrick-Dixon P (1986) Effects of experimentally imposed noise on task performance of black children attending daycare centers near elevated subway trains. Developmental Psychology 8: 259–64.

Hamilton P, Hockey G, Quinn J (1972) Information selection arousal and memory. British Journal of Psychology 63: 181–90.

Hamilton P, Hockey G, Rejman M (1977) The place of the concept of activation in human information processing In S Dornic (ed.) Attention and Performance, VI. Hillsdale, NJ: Erlbaum.

Heft H (1979) Background and focal environmental conditions of the home and attention in young children. Journal of Applied Social Psychology 9: 47– 69.

Hockey G (1970a) Effect of load noise on attentional selectivity. Quarterly Journal of Experimental Psychology 22: 28–36.

Hockey G (1970b) Signal probability and spatial location as possible bases for increased selectivity in noise. Quarterly Journal of Experimental Psychology 22: 37–42.

Hockey G (1979) Stress and cognitive components of skilled performance In V Hamilton, DM Warburton (eds) Human Stress and Cognition. New York: Wiley.

Hughes R, Jones DM (2001) The intrusiveness of sound: laboratory findings and their implications for noise abatement. Noise and Health 4: 51–70.

Hygge S (2003) Classroom experiments on the effects of different noise sources and sound levels on long term recall and recognition in children. Applied Cognitive Psychology 17: 895–914.

Hygge S, Evans GW, Bullinger M (2002) A prospective study of some effects of aircraft noise on cognitive performance in school children. Psychological Science 13: 469–74.

Hygge S, Boman E, Enmarker I (2003) The effects of road traffic noise and meaningful irrelevant speech on different memory systems. Scandinavian Journal of Psychology 44: 13–21.

Johansson C (1983) Effects of low intensity continuous and intermittent noise on mental performance and writing pressure of children with different intelligence and personality characteristics. Ergonomics 26: 275–88.

Jones DM, Morris N (1992) Irrelevant speech and cognition. In AP Smith, DM Jones (eds) Handbook of Human Performance, Vol. 1. London: Academic Press.

Karsdorf G, Klappach H (1968) The influence of traffic noise on the health and performance of secondary school students in a large city. Zeitschrift für die Gesamte Hygiene 14: 52–4.

Kassinove H (1972) Effects of meaningful auditory stimulation on children's scholastic performance. Journal of Educational Psychology 63: 526–30.

Ko N (1979) Responses of teachers to aircraft noise. Journal of Sound and Vibration 62: 277–92.

Kryter KD (1994) The Handbook of Hearing and the Effects of Noise. New York: Academic Press.

Kyzar B (1977) Noise pollution and schools: how much is too much? Council for Educational Facilities Planning Journal 4: 10–11.

Lercher P, Evans GW, Meis M (2003) Ambient noise and cognitive processes among primary school children. Environment and Behaviour 35: 725–35.

Lukas J, Du Pree R, Swing J (1981) Report of a Study on the Effects of Freeway Noise on Academic Achievement of Elementary School Children and a Recommendation for a Criterion Level for School Noise Abatement Programs. Sacramento, CA: California Department of Health Services.

Maser A, Sorensen P, Kryter KD, Lukas J (1978) Effects of Intrusive Sound on Classroom Behaviour. Data from a Successful Lawsuit. San Francisco, CA: Western Psychological Association.

Matheny A, Wachs TD, Ludwig J, Phillips K (1995) Bringing order out of chaos: psychometric characteristics of the confusion hubbub and order scale. Journal of Applied Developmental Psychology 16: 429–44.

Maxwell LM, Evans GW (2000) The effects of noise on preschool children's pre-reading skills. Journal of Environmental Psychology 20: 91–7.

Meis M, Hygge S, Evans GW, Bullinger M (1998) Effects of traffic noise on implicit and explicit memory: results from field and laboratory studies. In N Carter, RFS Job (eds) Proceedings of the Seventh International Congress on Noise as a Public Health Problem, Vol. 1. Sydney: Noise Effects 98 Ltd.

Michelson W (1968) Ecological Thought and its Application to School Functioning. Fourteenth Annual of the Eastern Research Institute of the Association for Supervision and Curriculum Development, New York City.

Moch-Sibony A (1981) Study of the effects of prolonged noise exposure on certain psychomotor and intellectual aspects and personality of children after a prolonged exposure: comparison between a soundproofed and a non-soundproofed school. Travail Humaine 44: 169–78.

Muller F, Pfeiffer W, Jilg M, Paulsen R, Ranft U (1998) Effects of acute and chronic traffic noise on attention and concentration of primary school children. In N Carter, RFS Job (eds) Proceedings of the Seventh International Congress on Noise as a Public Health Problem. Sydney: Noise 98 Ltd.

Peterson C, Maier S, Seligman MEP (1993) Learned Helplessness. New York: Oxford University Press.

Poulton C (1977) Continuous intense noise masks auditory feedback and inner speech. Psychological Bulletin 84: 977–1001.

Rabbit P (1979) Current paradigms and models in human information processing. In V Hamilton, DM Warburton (eds) Human Stress and Cognition. New York: Wiley.

Sargent J, Gidman M, Humphreys M, Utley W (1980) The disturbance caused to school teachers by noise. Journal of Sound and Vibration 70: 557–72.

Slater B (1968) Effects of noise on pupil performance. Journal of Educational Psychology 59: 239–43.

Smith AP (1982) The effects of noise on task priority and recall of order and locatio location. Acta Psychologica 51: 245–55.

Smith AP, Broadbent DE (1981) Noise and levels of processing. Acta Psychologica 47: 129–42.

Smith AP, Broadbent DE (1982) The effects of noise on recall and recognition of instances of categories. Acta Psychologica 51: 257–71.

Smith AP, Jones DM (1992) Noise and Performance. In AP Smith, DM Jones (eds) Handbook of Human Performance. Vol 1. London: Academic.

Smith AP, Jones DM, Broadbent DE (1981) The effects of noise on recall of categorized lists. British Journal of Psychology 72: 299–316.

Stansfeld SA, Berglund B, Lopez-Barrio I, Fisher P, Ohstrom E, Haines MM et al. (2003) Aircraft and road traffic noise and children's cognition and health: preliminary results from dose-response relationships from the RANCH study. In R DeJong (ed.) Noise as a Public Health Problem: Proceedings of the Eighth International Congress. Schiedam: Foundation ICBEN, pp. 134–9.

Steinkamp M (1980) Relationships between environmental distractions and task performance of hyperactive and normal children. Journal of Learning Disabilities 13: 40–5.

Turnure J (1970) Children's reactions to distracters in a learning situation. Developmental Psychology 2: 115–22.

Veitch J (1990) Office noise and illumination effects on reading comprehension. Journal of Environmental Psychology 10: 209–17.

Wachs TD (1987) Specificity of environmental action as manifest in environmental correlates of infants' mastery motivation. Developmental Psychology 23: 782–90.

Wachs TD (1989) The nature of the physical environment: an expanded classification system. Merrill Palmer Quarterly 35: 399–419.

Wachs TD, Camli O (1991) Do ecological or social characteristics mediate the influence of the physical environment upon maternal behaviour. Journal of Environmental Psychology 11: 249–64.

Wachs TD, Gruen G (1982) Early Experience and Human Development. New York: Plenum.

Weinstein N, Weinstein C (1979) Noise and reading performance in an open plan school. Journal of Educational Research 72: 210–13.

Wyon D (1970) Studies of children under imposed noise and heat stress. Ergonomics 13: 598–612.

Zentall S, Shaw J (1980) Effects of classroom noise on performance and activity of second grade hyperactive and control children. Journal of Educational Psychology 72: 830–40.

# CHAPTER 26

# Noise and sleep

*Noise and Its Effects:* Edited by Linda Luxon and Deepak Prasher © 2007
John Wiley & Sons Ltd.

BARBARA GRIEFAHN

## The nature and the function of sleep – sleep disturbances

People are complaining more about sleep disturbances which predominantly indicate an underlying health disorder. However, an increasing number of these disturbances are caused by environmental stimuli, particularly noise.

Sleep is not determined by reduced activity of the brain but by a qualitatively altered consciousness, reversible at any time. Sleep constitutes about one-third of human life but neither its cause nor its mechanisms or even its functions are well understood although its restorative effects are undisputed. Sleep is structured by a sequence of four to six cycles of 90–100 minutes each, which are characterized by increasing and decreasing sleep depth and that are terminated by rapid eye movement (REM) sleep, in which bursts of REMs occur (Figure 26.1). The successive cycles reveal the shape of a damped curve with gradually decreasing sleep depth (amplitude).

Sleep disturbances are regarded as the most deleterious effects of noise. They are increasingly often reported by residents who live in the vicinity of airports, in streets with heavy traffic, along railway tracks and in industrial areas (Griefahn, 2000). Traffic density and consequently the noises emitted are expected to continue to increase (European Commission, 1997), more during the night than during the day.

This chapter focuses on sleep disturbances – disturbance during the period that people spend in bed and during which they intend to sleep. It does not concern night-time annoyance, which usually refers to a broader time space and is determined by noise-induced disturbances of sleep and other activities (e.g. communication) (Hoeger et al., 2002).

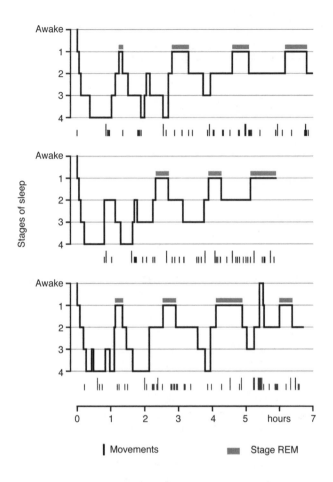

**Figure 26.1** Examples for normal sleep. REM, rapid eye movement. (From Dement and Kleitman, 1957.)

In the most general sense, sleep disturbances are measurable and/or subjectively experienced deviations from the usual or desired sleep behaviour.

**Three categories of sleep disturbance**

- Primary effects occur during the time in bed and include prolonged sleep latencies, intermittent and premature awakenings, alterations of sleep depth, body movements and autonomic responses.
- Secondary effects are the consequence of one or several disturbed nights and include alterations of self-estimated sleep quality, mood and performance.
- Tertiary effects or health disorders: primary and secondary effects are usually moderate and are tolerated for some time but, over time, they may contribute to the genesis of multifactorial diseases.

Due to the non-specific nature of the extra-aural effects, it is difficult to elucidate causal relationships, and this is especially true the greater the time lag between the onset of noise exposure and the manifestation of the effect in question. Alterations that occur shortly after stimulus onset (acute reactions) are obviously evoked by noise, whereas cumulative effects over the total night represent aggregated responses to a great variety of acoustic and non-acoustic stimuli. Uncertainty about causal linkages increases with secondary and more with health effects (Health Council of the Netherlands or HCN, 1999; Basner et al., 2004). However, adopting the World Health Organization (WHO) definition of health as 'a state of complete physical, mental and social well-being and not merely the absence of disease or infirmity' (WHO, 1968) sleep disturbances are clearly classified as health effects.

# Methods for recording and evaluating sleep

Many methods are available for recording and quantifying the primary effects. Acute alterations (awakening, sleep stage change, body movement, alterations of heart rate, etc.) are registered to evaluate the effects of distinct events; cumulative effects are used to describe the effects of more continuous noises over certain periods. Secondary effects are determined, for example, by self-estimated sleep quality, mood, performance and vigilance.

**Methods of recording and evaluating sleep**

- Polysomnogram
- Signalled awaking
- Body movements
- Autonomic responses
- Stress hormones
- Subjective questionnaires
- Performance tests
- Coping strategies

**Polysomnogram**

The simultaneous registration of the electroencephalogram (EEG), the electro-oculogram (EOG), and the electromyogram (EMG) is the only measure that reliably indicates whether a person is awake or asleep and provides information on sleep depth. The method requires electrodes to be fixed on the skull, the forehead and the chin, which creates an artificial situation, even in the normal home environment, and presupposes, therefore, the need for at least one adaptation night. The registration of the 'polysomnogram' requires the use of well-educated personnel and expensive electronic devices and evaluation software. This sophisticated method is, however, indispensable for laboratory studies.

Alternative methods have been applied in the field when the simultaneous influence of many non-acoustic environmental factors requires the observation of numerous subjects. As these measures, which include the registration of body movements or the urinary excretion of stress hormones, are less precise, it is reasonable to perform supplementary recordings of polysomnograms wherever possible.

### Signalled awakening

Noise-induced awakenings determine self-estimated sleep quality, mood and night-time annoyance and are regarded as most deleterious, in view of the hypothesized health disorders. To verify the awake state some researchers instruct their subjects to press a button whenever they wake up (Fidell et al., 1994, 1995; Passchier-Vermeer et al., 2002). False-positive signals are rare but missing signals are common. A disadvantage of this method might be that the required cooperation may make the subjects more alert, thus increasing their likelihood of being awakened by external stimuli.

### Body movements

Body movements, which usually accompany awakenings, are detected by actimeters, which are worn like wrist watches. As this scarcely bothers the subject and, as the actigrams are easy to evaluate, this method is preferred in field studies with numerous participants (Ollerhead et al., 1992; Fidell et al. 1998; Passchier-Vermeer et al., 2002; Griefahn et al., 2000). As body movements also occur during sleep, it is reasonable to combine this method with the registration of signalled awakenings.

### Autonomic nervous system

Responses of the autonomic nervous system, such as changes in heart rate and vasoconstrictions, indicate an increased sympathetic tone. They occur shortly after noise onset and last for a few seconds. These responses do not habituate and they are, therefore, assumed to contribute to health impairments in the long term (Muzet et al., 1981; Öhrström and Björkman, 1988; Carter, 1998; Whitehead and Hume, 2001).

### Stress hormones

Noise may provoke the release of stress hormones (cortisol, adrenaline and noradrenaline), which are measured by elevated urinary excretion of metabolites (Maschke et al., 1997; Carter, 1998). The urinary output is a cumulative response of the organism to various stimuli that occur during the sampling period, during which the contribution of noise cannot be quantified exactly (HCN, 1999). This method is, therefore, reliable only in highly controlled conditions.

## Subjective responses

Short questionnaires are usually completed just before bedtime and just after getting up. Evening questionnaires include questions on current tension and tiredness, physical, mental and emotional stress, tension and tiredness during the day, and consumption of alcohol and drugs. Morning questionnaires concern tension, tiredness, bedtime and rising time, sleep latency, intermittent and premature awakenings, sleep quality, window positions and so forth (Öhrström, 1999; Griefahn et al., 2000).

## Performance

Tests, which indicate the quality and quantity of performance (errors, speed) such as three- or four-choice tests that are usually completed every evening and every morning (Jurriëns et al., 1983; Griefahn and Gros, 1986; Öhrström and Björkman, 1988) are particularly suitable.

## Coping strategies

Several authors include in their questionnaires some questions on coping, particularly on the attenuation of noise by closing the windows (Öhrström, 1999; Griefahn et al., 2000).

# Noise-induced sleep disturbances – state of the art

The typical response to noise starts with a so-called K complex – a biphasic wave in the EEG, which is, dependent on the features of noise, the individual and the environment, followed by a more or less long-lasting-increase in brain activity – shallower sleep and even awakening. These responses are accompanied by body movements, autonomic responses and probably the release of stress hormones. Depending on the number of stimuli and the extent of the evoked responses, sleep becomes fragmented, and the total time awake and/or in shallow sleep increases at the expense of deep sleep and/or REM sleep.

Concerning after-effects, subjective evaluation of sleep is a complex problem and presupposes the recollection of the number, duration and courses of the periods awake. But despite occasionally reported large discrepancies between objective measures and subjective assessments, most people assess reliably sleep latency, total sleep time, and the number and duration of intermittent awakenings. After noisy nights, these quantitative sleep parameters are reported to be adversely affected and sleep quality is accordingly assessed as worse; the subjects feel less refreshed and even tired after final awakening, their mood decreases and night-time annoyance increases (Griefahn et al., 2006; Öhrström, 1999; Quehl, 2004).

Another consequence of disturbed sleep is impaired performance, where working speed decreases and/or the number of errors increases.

(Jurriëns et al., 1983; Öhrström and Björkman, 1988). Moreover, long-term residents in noisy areas revealed lower psychosocial well-being and more medical symptoms such as headaches, 'nervous' stomach disorders and tiredness (Öhrström, 1989, 1991).

The thresholds and the extent of noise-induced sleep disturbances vary in wide ranges due to acoustic features, personal characteristics and environmental conditions. Some of the most significant influences are listed below.

## Acoustic parameters

The influence of the sound pressure levels and the number of stimuli are among the acoustic parameters that have been studied most widely. Some papers examined the temporal distribution of noise and repetitive exposures over several days.

## Type of noise

With regard to the number of persons exposed, road traffic noise is most important, followed by noises from rail and air traffic. A meta-analysis based on 55 social surveys of approximately 58,000 interviews, revealed that aircraft, road traffic and rail noise cause the greatest to least annoyance, in that order (Miedema and Vos, 1998; Miedema and Oudshorn, 2001). As the brain can recognise properly the significance of a stimulus even while asleep and as individuals have been shown to react accordingly (e. g. Namba et al., 2004), it was hypothesized that the probability and the extent of human responses to transportation noise during sleep correspond to day-time annoyance. But an extended accordingly designed study has shown the largest effects under the influence of rail noise, i.e. more awakenings and less deep sleep as compared to the impact of aircraft and of road traffic noise (Griefahn et al., 2005, 2006), which is most likely related to the distinct acoustical feature of rail noise, namely the short rise times and the longer lasting periods of relatively high levels along with the characteristic variation of levels and frequencies.

### Intensity, sound pressure level

Acute effects as evoked by distinct noise events, for example awakenings, sleep stage changes and body movements, become more likely with increasing noise load. However, the thresholds and the ascents of dose–response curves that are derived from different studies vary greatly (Lukas, 1975; Griefahn, 1992; Pearsons et al., 1995; Basner et al., 2004).

Figure 26.2 shows dose-response curves that relate event-related awaken-ings to the maximum levels of aircraft noises, as ascertained in the worldwide largest study on noise-induced sleep disturbances (Basner et al., 2004). The upper curve presents EEG-defined awakenings recorded in the laboratory where 128 persons (18–65 yrs) were observed during 13 con-secutive nights each. Of those, 112 persons were exposed to 4 – 128 aircraft noises per night with maximum levels of 45 – 80 dBA during 9 con-secutive nights each. The curve below presents the probability of awakenings recorded in a complimentary field study at Cologne airport, where 64 residents were observed during 9 consecutive nights each, where maximum indoor levels varied between less than 30 and up to 73 dBA. After the awakening threshold of 33 dBA is surpassed, the likelihood of awakenings increases slowly and reaches 10% at a maximum level of 73 dBA. Similar results were reported from a field study where body move-ments of 418 residents in the vicinity of Schiphol Airport Amsterdam were registered during 11 nights each (Passchier-Vermeer et al., 2002).

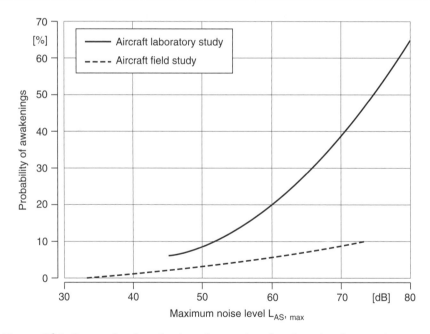

**Figure 26.2** Event-related awakenings due to aircraft noise related to maximum noise levels. Upper curve: Laboratory study 112 persons (18–65 years). Lower curve: field study 64 persons (18–64 years).

Cumulative responses, such as total time awake and in each sleep stage, were reported less often and the available data are insufficient for the derivation of dose–response curves. But the latter are plausible, as single studies have revealed that the total time awake and in shallow sleep increased at the expense of deep sleep and/or REM sleep, the higher the noise load (Jurriëns et al., 1983; Griefahn et al., 2006).

Contradictory results concern body movements, which were reported to increase and even to decrease with the noise dose, whereas frequently applied tones caused a redistribution, meaning that spontaneous movements decreased in favour of noise-related motions (Eberhardt and Akselsson, 1987; Öhrström and Björkman, 1988). An extended field study on the effects of aircraft noise revealed, however, clear close-response relationships between maximum noise levels and event-related awakenings (Passchier-Vermeer et al., 2002).

Responses of the autonomic nervous system occur earlier than when awake (at about 10 dB (A) lower levels) and their amplitudes increase with the maximum noise levels (Öhrström and Björkman, 1988; Muzet et al., 1981). Whether the excretion of stress hormones depends on the noise dose remains unresolved (Maschke et al., 1997; Basner et al., 2004).

Self-estimated sleep quality decreases with increasing noise load. Performance and mood showed similar trends – a worsening with higher noise levels (Öhrström and Rylander, 1982; Griefahn, 1986; Eberhardt and Akselsson, 1987; Griefahn et al., 2006).

Regarding coping strategies, it was reported that residents, who are exposed to rail or road noise, close their windows more often with higher outdoor levels (Figure 26.3) (Griefahn et al., 2000).

## Number of stimuli per night

The risk of being awakened by a distinct sound decreases with the total number of events during the night and the respective dose–response curve is

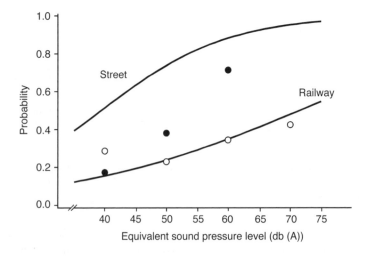

**Figure 26.3** Probability that residents living in streets with high traffic density and along railway tracks close the windows of their bedrooms as a function of the equivalent noise level.

determined by a gradually flatter ascent (Figure 26.4) that becomes negative beyond 35 events, at which point the difference between the equivalent sound pressure level and the maximum (the 'emergence') becomes less important (Eberhardt et al., 1987). Instead, as indicated by the linear increase of sleep-stage changes, it is most likely that sleep as a whole flattens – that the percentage of shallow sleep increases at the expense of deep sleep.

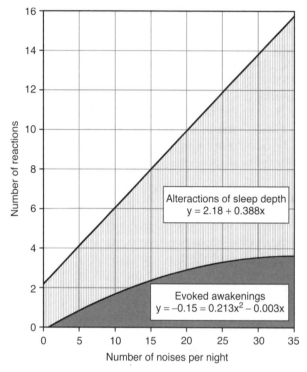

Alterations of sleep depth
$y = 2.18 + 0.388x$

Evoked awakenings
$y = -0.15 = 0.213x^2 - 0.003x$

**Figure 26.4** Noise-induced awakenings and sleep stage changes related to the number of noise events.

### Temporal distribution of noise

The temporal distribution of noise is decisive for the probability and the extent of responses. People are more disturbed by intermittent noises such as produced by air traffic, rail traffic and low-density road traffic, than by more continuous noises that are caused by heavy road traffic when noise levels fluctuate moderately during time. This was observed for sleep-stage changes, awakenings, body motions and subjective sleep quality; mood and performance revealed similar trends (Öhrström and Rylander, 1982; Eberhardt et al., 1987).

### Repetitive, long-term exposure and habituation

The probability and the extent of responses usually alter with repetitive long-term exposures. This is mainly related to the content of information, which is determined by the acoustic features of noise as well as by the experience of an individual with that sound. This implies, first, that the particular meaning of a particular noise varies between people, causing largely different responses and, second, that the meaning and, consequently, the extent of noise-induced reactions can alter with time for a particular person, thus providing the basic mechanism for habituation and sensitization as well. Sensitization – more and stronger responses with time – is expected for unpleasant noises. Habituation occurs more often but is limited, as indicated by field experiments, in which long-term residents in noisy areas still wake up more often, have less deep sleep or less REM sleep, assess their sleep quality as worse and perform less well in the morning. These people clearly benefit from the attenuation of noise levels, achieved by various measures (earplugs, sound-absorbing windows, tunnels, traffic deviation, etc.) (Jurriëns et al., 1983; Griefahn and Gros, 1986; Eberhardt and Akselsson, 1987; Öhrström, 2004). In contrast, responses of the autonomic nervous system do not habituate (Muzet et al., 1981; Whitehead and Hume, 2001) nor do body movements (Öhrström and Björkman, 1988).

**Other acoustic parameters**

Other acoustic features have only occasionally been studied. The probability and the extent of responses increase, for example, with bandwidth, duration of the stimuli and the intervals between them, and with emergence (the difference between maximum and equivalent sound level) (Eberhardt et al., 1987).

# Personal characteristics

The susceptibility of the organism to noise depends on several personal factors – on personality traits and on the periodically oscillating responses of the autonomic nervous system.

### Gender and age

Despite some contradictory reports, men and women seem to be equally susceptible to noise, whereas the significance of age is unclear. Few studies with a limited number of subjects revealed an age-related increase of awakenings (Griefahn 1985), but two recently published large scale studies with more than a hundred subjects each showed contradictory results. One study indicated that event-related awakenings are least frequent in persons between 40 and 50 years of age (Basner et al., 2004), the other revealed for this age group the highest rate of body movements (Passchier-Vermeer et al., 2002). The common belief that children are more sensitive to noise than adults has not yet been verified. On the contrary, their thresholds are about 10 dB (A) higher, which is probably related to their relatively high amount of deep sleep (Lukas et al., 1971; Eberhardt, 1990; Kahn, 2002).

**Personality traits**

Self-estimated sensitivity to noise, which most probably indicates an increased susceptibility to environmental pollutants in general, is clearly associated with stronger responses (Öhrström and Björkman, 1988). The significance of other personality traits for the perception and processing of noise have not been systematically studied but some authors routinely determine various traits and suspect that, for example, neuroticism, anxiety, introversion and dependency might be decisive. Poor sleepers revealed the same arousal thresholds as good sleepers, but once they are awake they have more difficulty in returning to sleep.

**Actual state and preceding noise exposure**

Physical and mental fatigue, as well as noise exposure during the previous day and particularly during the shoulder hours (the border between daytime and night time), are supposed to determine the responses to nocturnal disturbances.

**Biological rhythms**

The circadian rhythm that controls the fluctuations of the autonomic nervous system and enables the organism to perform well during the day and to recharge during the night is probably most significant. As this rhythm is almost impossible to invert, night workers sleep 1.5–2 hours less during the day than during the night even in sound-attenuated rooms. The real acoustic environment is, however, significantly worse during the day than during the night, the equivalent sound pressure level is then 8–15 dB (A) higher and determined by more meaningful and thus more disturbing noises (children, telephones, etc.). Experimental studies revealed accordingly greater susceptibilities to noises during the night than during the day (Knauth and Rutenfranz, 1972).

The probability and the extent of noise-induced responses are inversely related to sleep depth. The latter alters periodically during the night, when sleep depth decreases with successive cycles and when flatter stages and REM sleep increase gradually. The thresholds for the electrophysiological and the autonomic responses vary accordingly and, thus, decrease over the course of the night (Muzet et al., 1981; Basner et al., 2004; Griefahn et al., 2006).

# Environmental conditions – field studies versus laboratory studies

Apart from social surveys on community reactions, in which a few questions concerned sleep disturbances, the effects of noise were at first almost exclusively studied in the laboratory where the environmental conditions such as background noises, illumination and climate were strictly controlled. The usual environment at home is, however, determined by the simultaneous influence of many other factors. It is, therefore, debatable to evaluate residential settings on the basis of laboratory studies. Field studies performed within the last 15 years were concerned mainly the effects of aircraft noises (Ollerhead et al., 1992; Fidell et al., 1994, 1995; Passchier-Vermeer et al., 2002; Basner et al., 2004) and, less often noises emitted by road and rail traffic (Öhrström, 1999; Griefahn, 2000).

Pearsons et al. (1995) who pooled data from 21 studies have shown that the effects in field studies are much smaller than in the laboratory. Some possible reasons for these extensively debated discrepancies are listed below.

It is worthy of note that some field studies assume an intermediate position, for example, those in which noise levels are altered by the variation of window positions, the use of earplugs, the installation of sound-attenuating windows, and the construction of tunnels (Jurriëns et al., 1983; Öhrström, 2004). The results obtained fall between those registered in the laboratory and in the field. Another type of field experiment concerns the application of noises via loudspeakers in the subjects' own homes (Maschke et al., 1997; Whitehead and Hume, 2001).

## Assessment of the acoustic situation

Individual noise immission is precisely quantified in the laboratory but noise loads in the field are measured only at the source or at a representative point of a residential area and refer almost exclusively to the dominant noise source. Other acoustic influences are disregarded.

## Combined stress

Various non-acoustic stimuli influence the organism simultaneously and modify or even mask the responses to noise. Amplified responses have been shown in cases of simultaneous vibrations, which occur in dwellings near railway tracks or along roads with passing heavy trucks or in cases of elevated air temperatures (Eberhardt et al., 1987).

## Individual vulnerability

Experimental research has been almost exclusively performed on young and healthy persons, whereas in field studies age, personality traits, physical conditions, vulnerability, etc. vary across a large range and influence the responses to nocturnal noise.

## Habituation

Whereas experimental exposures take place only once or a very few times, exposures at home are repeated daily. Finegold (1993) assumed, therefore, that habituation is the main reason for the discrepancy between field and laboratory studies. Indeed, laboratory studies revealed a decrease in awakening responses over a couple of nights, whereas responses of the autonomic nervous system and body movements did not show habituation (Jurriëns et al., 1983; Griefahn, 1985; Eberhardt and Akselsson, 1987; Öhrström et al., 1998).

# Prediction of noise-induced sleep disturbances

As residents who live in the vicinity of airports, in streets with high traffic load or along railway tracks do not habituate completely to the impact of noise (Jurriëns et al., 1983; Griefahn and Gros, 1986; Öhrström, 1989, 1991) and as chronic sleep disturbances (of whatever origin) are expected to contribute to the genesis and the manifestation of multifactorial chronic diseases, directed appropriate prevention is strongly recommended (Figure 26.5).

Due to largely varying susceptibilities, it is, however, impossible to protect everybody completely against the deleterious effects of noise, meaning that the establishment of any limit excludes a certain percentage of people from full protection. Despite this, it has to be stated that any attenuation of noise improves the situation even for those most vulnerable people and makes their environment more acceptable.

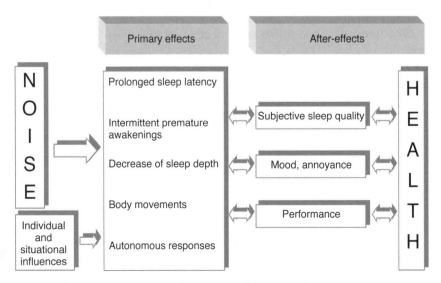

**Figure 26.5** Primary and secondary effects of noise on sleep.

Dose–response curves are a suitable basis for decision-making and predict the respective risk. For any defined risk it is then possible to calculate contours of equal risks, for example for airports or busy roads.

Dose–response curves presuppose the choice of relevant effects and of suitable acoustic metrics. Concerning the effects, awakenings are regarded as most deleterious. Their number and duration determine subjective sleep quality and mood; they are associated with impaired performance the next morning and supposed to contribute to multifactorial chronic diseases in the long term (Griefahn, 1992; Ollerhead et al., 1992; Pearsons et al., 1995; Passchier-Vermeer et al., 2002; Basner et al., 2004). Based on the WHO definition of health, awakenings are themselves classified as health effects.

Concerning noise metrics, two acoustic situations must be considered – intermittent and continuous noises where the first disturb more than the second (Öhrström and Rylander, 1982; Eberhardt et al., 1987). Accordingly, different noise metrics apply for the prediction of the respective effects. The equivalent sound pressure levels and other cumulative noise metrics are suitable for continuous noises. Additional effects are expected if continuous noises are interspersed with intermittent stimuli and, if the maximum levels exceed the equivalent noise levels by at least 8–10 dB (A). Maximum levels and sound exposure levels (SEL) are therefore appropriate for intermittent noises (Eberhardt et al., 1987; Finegold, 1993).

### Critical loads for continuous noises

Despite their frequency in real settings, dose–response curves for heavy road traffic and other essentially continuous noises are not yet available. However, results from both laboratory and field studies suggest that the critical equivalent sound pressure level is below 45 dB (A) (Eberhardt et al., 1987). With regard to self-estimated sleep quality (Griefahn, 1986) an upper limit of an equivalent noise level of 40 dB (A) is suggested, whereas Vallet et al. (1983) proposed a critical load of 37 dB (A) for cardiac responses.

### Critical load for intermittent noises

Noise pollution has become a serious problem worldwide and noise abatement is urgently required. Most decisions on limits are based on dose-response curves that are presented – mainly for aircraft – by several authors for awakenings or for body movements (FICAN 1997; Pearsons et al., 1995).

Decisions on this basis alone, however, merely consider the maximum levels and neglect the number of noises. Modern approaches define first admissible upper risks and calculate functions that relate the number of stimuli and the maximum noise levels for the same over-all risk, i.e. curves along which the noise-and-number-combinations do not exceed this predefined risk. The very first model is shown in Figure 26.6 based on the data of the then available 10 experimental studies that were comparable in method and evaluation (Griefahn, 1992). The upper risk was defined as a 10%-probability to be awakened after a short habituation period in the most sensitive sleep stage of the oldest tenth of the population. According to this curve the indoor maximum level must not exceed 61 dBA in case of a single event, or 55 dBA in case of 5 events. With increasing frequencies the maximum levels then approach 53 dBA.

A similar approach was chosen by Basner et al. (2005), who defined a single aircraft-induced awakening as the upper risk presupposing again the most sensitive sleep stage and a sensitive period of the night (middle of the second half of the night). This model was applied to protect the residents in the vicinity of the airport Leipzig/Halle.

A similar idea led to the development of a theoretical physiological model which, however, does not refer to awakenings but to an accu-mulated admissible noise-induced release of cortisol (Spreng 2002). The resulting curve relates numbers and levels of tolerable flights (Fig 26.7).

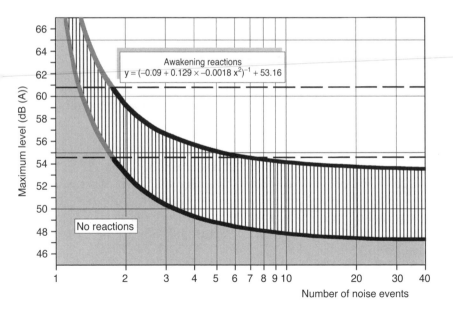

**Figure 26.6** Curves of equal risk of noise-induced awakenings and sleep-stage changes. Maximal allowable level for distinct noise events (flyover noises) as a function of overflights per night.

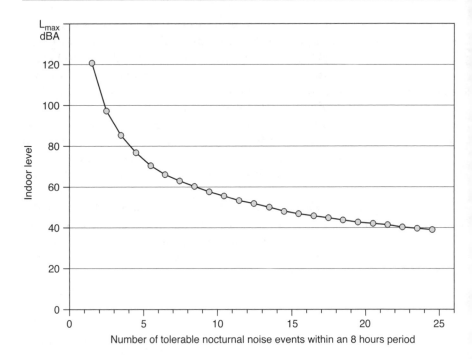

**Figure 26.7** Quantitative relationship between indoor peak level $L_{max}$ and the number of tolerable noise events within an 8-hour night (Spreng, 2002).

# Future research – unresolved problems

Despite extensive research in the past much remains to be done. Some main topics, which are also defined by other authors, are listed below.

### Noise effects

The majority of studies performed in the laboratory or in the field were restricted to the period between sleep onset and sleep offset where the time for falling asleep, premature awakenings, performance the next morning, and other possible after-effects on work performance, accident risk and social life were not or were insufficiently studied (Berry and Jiggins, 1999).

### Discrepancies between field and laboratory studies

The most striking reports of the last decade concerned the discrepancies between the effects observed in the laboratory and those observed in the field. Whether the much smaller responses in the field (Pearsons et al., 1995) are mainly related to habituation, as supposed by Finegold (1993), or rather to masking by other simultaneous environmental influences needs to be defined. The identification and quantification of the reasons is most important, particularly in view of the well-founded assumption that the extent of habituation is decisive in the development of long-term health effects.

### Prediction of noise effects

The development of predictive models must be pursued. It might be reasonable to create far-reaching realistic settings in the laboratory for the development of models, which then must be adapted to field situations.

### Combined stress

People in their residential settings are usually exposed to noise from different sources but previous studies were concerned almost exclusively with the dominant source. Man reacts to other simultaneous noises as well, so it is essential to evaluate the acoustic situation as a whole and to include noises from other sources. This is particularly the case for situations where various noises are related to each other, for example at airports where an increase in air traffic is accompanied by an increase in road and rail traffic. The same arguments apply for the simultaneous influence of non-acoustic influences (Berry and Jiggins, 1999; HCN, 1999).

### Time of day

The quality and quantity of sleep and the probability of disturbances depend on the timing of sleep. Night time is defined by legislation in most countries, but several reports stated that many persons sleep at least partly outside these hours (Passchier-Vermeer et al., 2002; Griefahn et al., 2000) and this behaviour becomes more frequent with increasing flexibility in working hours. Suitable concepts for the protection of those concerned – in particular for those who perform night work – must be developed (Carter, 1998; Berry and Jiggins, 1999).

### Shoulder hours

People want to relax and to communicate during their leisure time (Fields, 1986). However, whether, and to what degree, noise-induced disturbances of communication and of other activities during the evening hours impair the consecutive sleep period or increase the susceptibility against nocturnal noise is not yet known.

### Individual susceptibility

Experimental research has been almost exclusively performed on young and healthy individuals, which is justified as long as the identification of various responses and the respective mechanisms are the centre of attention. However, exposure limits deduced from those studies are only tentative. People who are particularly vulnerable were – apart from those with self-estimated sensitivity to noise – almost disregarded (Berry and Jiggins, 1999), although other personality traits, in particular neuroticism and anxiety as well as illness are supposed to determine the susceptibility to noise. It is also supposed that the individual circadian phase (morning types and evening types) plays a decisive role.

### Noise-induced sleep disturbances and health impairments

Whatever the reason may be, it is generally believed that chronic sleep disturbances contribute to the genesis and manifestation of several diseases, chronic annoyance and lasting behavioural alterations (Figure 26.5), but the assumed causal linkage between environmental noise, primary and secondary effects on the one hand and the hypothesized final outcomes, on the other, remain to be determined (Berry and Jiggins, 1999; HCN, 1994, 1999).

### Preventive measures and evaluation studies

Current knowledge is sufficient to claim that preventive measures must be established. The effects of attenuation (deviation of traffic, construction of tunnels, double glazing, etc.) must be evaluated by appropriately designed studies (Berry and Jiggins, 1999).

### Accumulation of data and cooperation between researchers

To date several hundred laboratory experiments have been performed and several hundred people have been observed in their homes, but, due to considerably varying concepts, different methodological procedures and shortcomings, only a few studies can be directly compared.

International cooperation between working groups is, therefore, urgently recommended. Researchers are requested to accept that their own individual studies are primarily essential elements in the achievement of a common goal and to develop guidelines and common elements for experimental and for epidemiological studies that might consist of a common protocol, a standardized questionnaire and the application of a 'reference' noise.

# References

Basner M, Buess H, Elmenhorst D, Gerlich A, Luks N, Maaß H, Mawet L, Müller EW, Müller U, Plath G, Quehl J, Samel A, Schulze M, Vejvoda M, Wenzel J (2004) Nachtflugwirkungen. Band 1, Zusammenfassung.
www.dlr.de/me/institut/abteilungen/flugphysiologie/fluglärm/fb2004-07-d.pdf.

Basner M, Isermann U, Samel A (2005) Die Umsetzung der DLR-Studie in einer nachtmedizinischen Beurteilung für ein Nachtschutzkonzept. Z Lärmbekämpfung 52:109–23.

Berry BF, Jiggins M (1999) An inventory of UK research on noise and health from 1994 to 1999. NPL Report CMAM 40. pp 1–47.

Carter NL (1998) Cardiovascular response to environmental noise during sleep. In N Carter, RFS Job (eds) Noise Effects '98, Sydney, pp. 439–44.

Dement W, Kleitman N (1957) Cyclic variations in EEG during sleep and their relation to eye movements, body motility, and dreaming. EEG Clinical Neurophysiology 9: 673–90.

Eberhardt J (1990) The disturbance of the sleep of prepubertal children by road traffic noise as studied in the home. In B Berglund, T Lindvall (eds) Proceedings of the Fifth International Congress on Noise as a Public Health Problem, Vol. V. Stockholm: Swedish Council for Building Research, pp. 65–9.

Eberhardt JL, Akselsson KR (1987) The disturbance by road traffic noise of the sleep of young male adults as recorded in the home. Journal of Sound Vibration 114: 417–34.

Eberhardt JL, Ståle LO, Berlin MHB 1987: The influence of continuos and intermittent traffic noise on sleep. J Sound Vib 116: 445–464

European Commission (1997) Green Paper on Future Noise Policy. COM 540 Final. Brussels, European Commission.

Federal Interagency Committee on Aviation Noise (1997) Effects of aviation noise on awakenings from sleep: www.fican.org/sleepdisturbance/sleepframe.html.

Fidell S, Pearsons K, Howe R, Tabachnik B, Silvati L, Barber DS (1994) Noise-induced Sleep Disturbance in Residential Settings. Wright Patterson Air Force Base, OH: Armstrong Laboratory, Occupational & Environmental Health Division.

Fidell S, Howe R, Tabachnik B, Pearsons K, Sneddon M (1995) Noise-induced Sleep Disturbance near Two Civil Airports. Langley Research Center: NASA.

Fidell S, Howe R, Tabachnik B, Pearsons K, Silvati L, Sneddon M, Fletcher E (1998) Field Studies of Habituation to Change in Night-Time Aircraft Noise and of Sleep Motility Measurement Methods. Canoga Park: BBN Technologies.

Fields JM (1986) The Relative Effect of Noise at Different Times of Day. An Analysis of Existing Survey Data. Langley Research Center: NASA.

Finegold LS (1993) Current Status of Sleep Disturbance Research and Development of a Criterion for Aircraft Noise Exposure. 126th Meeting of the Acoustical Society of America, Denver, CO.

Griefahn B (1985) Schlafverhalten und Geräusche. Stuttgart: Enke.

Griefahn B (1986) A critical load for nocturnal high density road traffic noise. American Journal of Industrial Medicine 9: 261–9.

Griefahn B (1992) Noise control during the night. Acoustics Australia 20: 43–7.

Griefahn B (2000) Noise-induced extraaural effects. Journal of Acoustical Society of Japan 21: 307–17.

Griefahn B, Gros E (1986) Noise and sleep at home, a field study on primary and after-effects. Journal of Sound and Vibration 105: 373–83.

Griefahn B, Schuemer-Kohrs A, Schuemer R, Moehler U, Mehnert P (2000) Physiological, subjective, and behavioural responses to noise from rail and road traffic. Noise Health 3: 59–71.

Griefahn B, Marks A, Kuenemund C, Basner M (2005) Awakenings by Road-, Rail- and Airtraffic Noise. Budapest: Forum Acusticum.

Griefahn B, Marks A, Robens S (2006) Noise emitted from road, rail and air traffic and their effects on sleep. JSV 295: 129–140

Health Council of the Netherlands (1994) Committee on Noise and Health. Noise and Health. The Hague: HCN.

Health Council of the Netherlands (1999) Committee on the Health Impact of Large Airports. Public Health Impact of Large Airports. The Hague: HCN.

Hoeger R, Schreckenberg D, Felscher-Suhr U, Griefahn B (2002) Night-time annoyance – state of the art. Noise Health 4: 19–25.

Jansen G (1970) Beeinflussung des natürlichen Nachtschlafes durch Geräusche. Forschungsbericht des Landes. Cologne: Westdeutscher Verlag. pp 1–42.

Jurriëns AA, Griefahn B, Kumar A, Vallet M, Wilkinson RT (1983) An essay in European research collaboration: common resuls from the project on traffic noise and sleep in the home. In G Rossi (ed.) Noise as a Public Health Problem. Milan: Edizioni Tecniche a cura del Centro Ricerche e Studi Amplifon, pp. 929–37.

Kahn A (2002) Noise exposure from various sources – sleep disturbance dose-effect relationships on children. WHO Technical Meeting on Exposure-response Relationships of Noise on Health. Paper 5038933-2002/7.

Knauth P, Rutenfranz J (1972) Untersuchungen zum Problem des Schlafverhaltens bei experimenteller Schichtarbeit. Internationales Archiv fur Arbeitsmedizin 30: 1–22.

Lukas JS (1975) Noise and sleep: a literature review and a proposed criterion for assessing effect. Journal of Acoustical Society of America 58: 1232–42.

Lukas JS, Dobbs ME, Kryter KD (1971) Disturbance of Human Sleep by Subsonic Jet Aircraft Noise and Simulated Sonic Booms. NASA, Contractor Report. Washington DC: NASA.

Maschke C, Ising H, Hecht K (1997) Schlaf – nächtlicher Verkehrslärm – Streß – Gesundheit: Grundlagen und aktuelle Forschungsergebnisse. Bundesgesundheitsblatt 40: 86–95.

Miedema HME, Vos H (1998) Exposure-response relationships for transportation noise. Journal of Acoustical Society of America 104: 3432–45.

Miedema HME, Oudshoorn CGM (2001) Annoyance from transportation noise: relationships with exposure metrics DNL and DENL and their confidence intervals. Environmental Health Perspectives 109: 409–16.

Muzet A, Ehrhart J, Eschenlauer R, Lienhard JP (1981) Habituation and age differences of cardiovascular responses to noise during sleep. In WP Koella (ed.) Sleep 1980. Fifth European Congress on Sleep Research. Basel: Karger, pp. 212–15.

Namba S, Kuwano S, Okamoto T (2004) Sleep disturbance caused by meaningful sounds and the effect of background noise. Joural of Sound and Vibration 277: 445–52.

Öhrström E (1989) Sleep disturbance, psycho-social and medical symptoms – a pilot survey among persons exposed to high levels of road traffic noise. Journal of Sound and Vibration 133: 117–28.

Öhrström E (1991) Psycho-social effects of traffic noise exposure. Journal of Sound and Vibration 151: 513–17.

Öhrström E (1999) Sleep disturbances caused by road traffic noise. Journal of Acoustical Society of America 105: 1218.

Öhrström E (2004) Longitudinal surveys on effects of changes in road traffic noise: effects on sleep assessed by general questionnaires and 3-day sleep logs. Journal of Sound and Vibration 276: 713–27.

Öhrström E, Björkman M (1988) Effects of noise-disturbed sleep – a laboratory study on habituation and subjective noise sensitivity. Journal of Sound and Vibration 122: 277–90.

Öhrström E, Rylander R (1982) Sleep disturbance effects of traffic noise – a laboratory study on after effects. Journal of Sound and Vibration 84: 87–103.

Öhrström E, Agge A, Björkman M (1998) Sleep disturbances before and after reduction in road traffic noise. In N Carter, RFS Job (eds) Noise Effects '98. Sydney, pp. 451–4.

Ollerhead JB, Jones CJ, Cadoux RE, Woodley A, Atkinson BJ, Horne JA et al. (1992) Report of a Field Study of Aircraft Noise in Sleep Disturbance. London: Department of Safety, Environment and Engineering.

Passchier-Vermeer W, Vos H, Steenbekkers JHM, van der Ploeg FD, Groothuis-Oudshoorn K (2002) Sleep disturbance and aircraft noise exposure. Exposure-effect relationship. TNO Prevention and Health. TNO-Report Nr 2002.027. Noise and Health. The Hague: Health Council of the Netherlands.

Pearsons K, Barber DS, Tabachnik B, Fidell S (1995) Predicting noise-induced sleep disturbance. Journal of Acoustical Society of America 97: 331–8.

Quehl J (2004) Effects of Nocturnal Aircraft Noise – Volume 4 – Psychological Effects. DLR Forschungsbericht 2004-10/E.

Skånberg A, Ohrström E (2004) Sleep disturbances from road traffic noise: a comparison between laboratory and field settings. Journal of Sound and Vibration 271: 279–96.

Spreng M (2002) Cortical excitations, cortisol excretion, and estimation of tolerable nightly over-flights. Noise Health 4: 39–46.

Vallet M, Gagneux JM, Blanchet V, Favre B, Labiale G (1983) Long term sleep disturbance due to traffic noise. Journal of Sound and Vibration 90: 173–91.

Whitehead C, Hume K (2001) A field experiment on the effect of aircraft noise on heart rate during sleep. Int Symp on Noise Pollution & Health. April 6-8. Cambridge: UK. Programme & Abstract Book. p 53.

World Health Organization (1968–69) Yearbook of International Organizations. Geneva: WHO.

# CHAPTER 27

# Measurements, standards and laws

*Noise and Its Effects:* Edited by Linda Luxon and Deepak Prasher © 2007
John Wiley & Sons Ltd.

RONALD HINCHCLIFFE

## Introduction

### Historical

The earliest civilizations would have needed systems of counting, for
example of livestock, and of measurement, for instance of land, and of produce to accommodate the requirements of trading and taxation. A legal
system would be required to define and endorse methods of mensuration
and to settle disputes. These developments would have been underpinned
by the concomitant emergence of a written language – indeed they would
have depended on it for any continuity.

Bottéro (1994) refers to the *rédaction notariale de documents offi-
cielles ou de 'papiers d'affaires'* (legal editing of official documents and
official papers) and to *textes juridique* (legal texts) in the ancient
Mesopotamian civilizations of Sumer and Babylon, which developed
5000–6000 years ago. *Assez complexe, mais forcément bien établi,
même si ses valeurs pouvaient changer de temps en temps, voire de ville
à ville, le système métrologique était normalement garanti par les pou-
voirs publics.* ('Very complex, but necessarily well established, even if
the values changed from time to time, seen from town to town, the system of weights and measures was in practice backed-up by the
authorities.') The Sumerian language became the prevailing speech of
the land. The people there developed the cuneiform script, a system of
writing on clay. This script was to become the basic means of written
communication throughout the Middle East for about 2000 years. It
ensured the concurrent development of metrology and of law with some
degree of permanence.

## Current

Countries vary in the way that metrology, standards and law are organized administratively. Slovenia has its Standards and Metrology Institute (in Ljubljana). The republic of Bosnia and Herzegovina has its Institute for Standards, Metrology and Intellectual Property (in Sarajevo). Gosstandart (State Committee of the Russian Federation on Standardization, Metrology and Certification) is a body of the federal authority of the Russian Federation. It comprises VNNIStandart (the All-Russian Research Institute for Standardization), VNIIS (the All-Russian Research Institute for Certification), VNIIKI (the All-Russian Research Institute for Classification, Terminology and Information on Standards and Quality), and VNIIMS (the All-Russian Research Institute for Metrology Services) (see www.bisnis.doc.gov/bisnis/isa/9903gos2.htm).

# Measurements

Metrology is that branch of science concerned with measurement. Legal metrology is covered later. Scales are a natural outcome of systems of measurement (Figure 27.1).

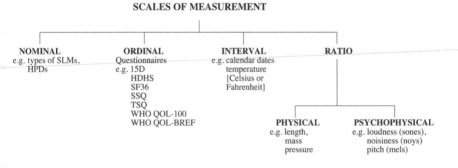

**Figure 27.1** Classification of measurement properties of data. The permissible statistical treatment of the data is governed by the class (Stevens, 1951; Hand, 1996; Svensson, 1997). See Appendix 1 for meaning of abbreviations. (Adapted from Stevens, 1951).

The question of uncertainties in measurements has been addressed by ISO/TAG 4/WG 3, an ISO working group supported by seven international organizations. This culminated in the 1995 Guide to the Expression of Uncertainty in Measurement (GUM). GUM states that the object of a measurement is to determine the value of the measurand, i.e. the value of the particular quantity to be measured. The result of a measurement can be considered an approximation only of the value of the measurand. The recorded value is thus only complete when accompanied by a statement of the uncertainty of that estimate.

The uncertainty in the result of a measurement generally consists of several components which may be grouped into two categories according to the way in which their numerical value is estimated, i.e. Type A (those which are evaluated by statistical methods) and Type B (those which are evaluated by other means). There is not always a simple correspondence between the classification into categories A or B and the previously used classification into 'random' and 'systematic' uncertainties. The term 'systematic uncertainty' can be misleading and should be avoided. Any detailed report of uncertainty should consist of a complete list of the components, specifying for each the method used to obtain its numerical value.

A companion definitions document to GUM was prepared by ISO/TAG 4/WG 1 and published in 1993 by ISO in the name of the same seven international organizations in whose name the GUM was published. It is entitled *Vocabulaire international des termes fondamentaux et généraux de métrologie* (International Vocabulary of Basic and General Terms in Metrology), or VIM, and gives the definitions of many important terms relevant to the field of measurement.

# Standards

### General

Standards are required to ensure (as far as possible) that measurements, *inter alia*, made by one individual in one place and at one time will be comparable to those made by another individual in another place at another time. This requires the provision of standards that bear upon the hardware for measuring, procedures for measurements, yardsticks for measurements, and the environment in which measurements are made.

British Standard BS 0: 1997 A Standard for Standards is relevant to understanding the whole global physical standardization system. The standard describes the context of standardization and, in particular, identifies the aims, principles and procedural safeguards that apply when standards are prepared. It explains how standards are used in trade descriptions and in contracts, and how they may be invoked in legislation. Although BS 0-1: 1997 has not yet been adopted by other standardization bodies one finds that these aims and indicated benefits are generally endorsed, e.g. by the Standardization Directorate of Malta (2004).

As opposed to laws and regulations, standards are voluntary application technical documents, drawn up by all of the economic players under the aegis of the standardization bodies. Although the application of standards is voluntary, a standards body may be created by a specific Act of a legislature. For example, the National Standards Authority of Ireland Act 1996 created the National Standards Authority of Ireland.

Many standards are constantly undergoing change, not only in what they specify, but also in their numbering. For example, depending on the frequency, the 1972 British Standard for the air conduction reference zero showed changes of up to 2.5 dB when compared to the 1954 standard (Haughton, 1980). In 1992 this standard was designated BS 2497: 1992. Now it is BS EN ISO 389-1:2000. The current BS EN ISO 389-3:1994 was previously BS 6950: 1988 (equivalent to ISO 7566-1987), and before that, BS 2497, Part 4: 1972. BS 6950: 1988 (equivalent to ISO 7566-1987) used a method of measurement different to that of BS 2497, Part 4: 1972. BS 6950: 1988 typically yielded bone conduction thresholds that were about 3 dB to 4 dB less acute averaged over 1, 2 and 3 kHz as compared to the previous standard, and about 5 dB to 8 dB less acute at 1 kHz in particular, depending on the date of manufacture of the mechanical coupler used for calibration (Coles, Lutman and Robinson, 1991).

The National Standards Systems Network (NSSN), now termed the National Resource for Global Standards, provides information on more than 600 national, foreign, regional and international standards bodies (www.nssn.org/index.html).

The names and the websites for the various standards bodies over the world are shown in Tables 27.1 and 27.2.

**Table 27.1** Some international standards bodies and their websites

| Standards body | Abbreviation | Website |
| --- | --- | --- |
| Comité Européen de Normalisation (European Committee for Standardization) | CEN | www.cenorm.be<br>www.cenorm.be/catweb |
| Comité Européen de Normalisation Eléctrotechnique | CENELEC | www.cenelec.org |
| European Telecommunications Standardization Institute | ETSI | www.etsi.org |
| International Electrotechnical Commission | IEC | www.iec.ch |
| International Organization for Standardization | ISO | www.iso.ch |

## International standards

The prefix ISO or IEC means that the standard is an international one (put out by the International Organization for Standardization or the International Electrotechnical Commission respectively). There currently exist 14 500 international standards (ISO and IEC). Those relevant to *Noise and Its Effects* are shown in Appendices 1 and 2.

**Table 27.2**  Some national standards bodies and their websites

| Country | Standards body | Abbrev. | Website |
|---|---|---|---|
| Australia | Standards Australia International Ltd | SA | www.standards.com. au/catalogue/script/ search.asp |
| Austria* | Österreichisches Normungsinstitut | ON | www.on-norm.at |
| Belgium* | Institut Belge de Normalisation/Belgisch Instituut voor Normalisatie | IBN/BIN | www.ibn.be |
| Canada | Standards Council of Canada – Conseil canadien des normes | SCC | www.scc.ca |
| Czech Republic* | Czech Standards Institute | CSNI | www.csni.cz |
| Denmark* | Dansk Standard | DS | www.ds.dk |
| Finland* | Suomen Standardisoimisliitto r.y. | SFS | www.sfs.fi |
| France* | l'Association française de normalisation. | AFNOR | www.afnor.fr |
| Germany* | Deutsches Institut für Normung e.V. | DIN | www.din.de |
| Greece* | Hellenic Organization for Standardization | ELOT | www.elot.gr |
| Iceland* | Stadlarad Islands (Icelandic Standards) | IST | www.stadlar.is |
| India | Bureau of Indian Standards | BIS | www.bis.org.in |
| Indonesia | Badan Standardisasi Nasional | BSN | www.bsn.go.id |
| Iran | Institute of Standards and Industrial Research of Iran | ISIRI | www.isiri.org |
| Ireland* | National Standards Authority of Ireland | NSAI | www.nsai.ie |
| Israel | The Standards Institution of Israel | SII | www.sii.org.il |
| Italy* | Ente Nazionale Italiano di Unificazione | UNI | www.uni.com |
| Japan | Japan Industrial Standards Committee | JISC | www.jisc.go.jp |
| Luxembourg* | Service de l'Energie de l'Etat Organisme Luxembourgeois de Normalisation | SEE | www.see.lu |
| Malta* | Malta Standards Authority | MSA | www.msa.org.mt |
| Netherlands* | Nederlands Normalisatie-instituut | NEN | www.nen.nl |
| New Zealand | Standards New Zealand | SNZ | www.standards.co.nz |
| Norway* | Standard Norge | SN | www.standard.no/sn |
| Peru | Instituto Nacional de Defensa de la Competencia y de la Protección de la Propiedad Intelectual | INDECOPI | www.indecopi.gob.pe |
| Portugal* | Instituto Português da Qualidade | IPQ | www.ipq.pt |
| Russia | State Committee of the Russian Federation for Standardization, Metrology and Certification | GOST-R | www.gost.ru/sls/ gost.nsf |
| South Africa | Standards South Africa | SABS | www.sabs.co.za |
| Spain* | Asociación Española de Normalización y Certificación | AENOR | www.aenor.es |
| Sweden* | Swedish Standards Institute | SIS | www.sis.se |
| Switzerland* | Schweizerische Normen-Vereinigung (Swiss Association for Standardization) | SNV | www.snv.ch |
| Thailand | Thai Industrial Standards Institute | TISI | www.tisi.go.th |
| Turkey | Türk Standardlari Enstitüsü | TSE | www.tse.org.tr |
| UK* | British Standards Institution | BSI | www.bsi-global.com |
| USA | American National Standards Institute | ANSI | www.ansi.org |

[a]Others are given at the World Standards Services Network Web site: www.wssn.net/WSSN/script-cache/ links_national.htm.
[b]All CEN (Comité Européen de Normalisation) members are listed here and denoted by an asterisk.

Each standard is given an alphanumeric descriptor with, perhaps, a Part number, which is unique to that standard. The numbering can help to indicate which standards are related to one another. Thus standards ISO 11200–11203 inclusive relate to noise emitted by machinery and equipment. ISO 389 concerns the reference zero for the calibration of audiometric equipment. The various parts of IEC 60318 provide standards for equipment used to calibrate the transducers used in the measurement of hearing.

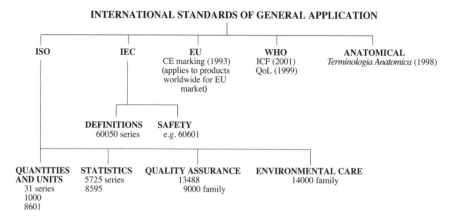

**Figure 27.2** Broad classification of international standards of general application.

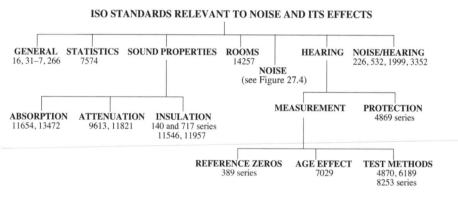

**Figure 27.3** Classification of ISO standards relevant to *Noise and Its Effects*.

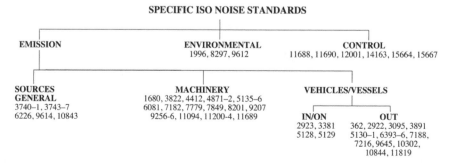

**Figure 27.4** Further classification of ISO standards relevant to *Noise and Its Effects*.

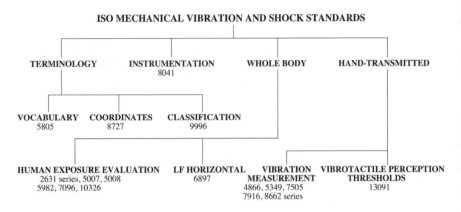

**Figure 27.5** Classification of ISO standards relevant to vibration.

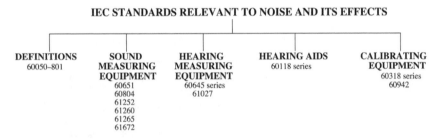

**Figure 27.6** Classification of IEC standards relevant to *Noise and Its Effects*.

An international standard prefixed by EN ('Euronorm') means that the standard has been adopted by the European Union; if an international standard is prefixed by, for example, BS or DIN it means that that standard has been adopted by the UK or Germany respectively and that BSI or DIN (Deutsches Institut für Normung) is providing the English or German language version of that standard respectively.

At international level, the voluntary standardization process is essentially operated and co-ordinated under the auspices of the International Electrotechnical Commission (IEC), the International Organization for Standardization (ISO), and the International Telecommunication Union (ITU). These three, that are termed the international apex organizations, have an extensive infrastructure which has its foundations at national level and extends into regional activities. This worldwide system is linked together via collaboration agreements between ISO, IEC and ITU at international level; by similar agreements between standardization organizations in certain regions; and, at the base, through an extensive array of cooperation arrangements between the national members of the three apex organizations.

The main stages of development of International Standards together with the abbreviations used for the various document types are given at www.usability.serco.com/trump/resources/standards.htm

**European standards**

There are three European standard organizations: Comité Européen de Normalisation (CEN), Comité Européen de Normalisation Eléctrotechnique (CENELEC) and European Telecommunications Standardization Institute (ETSI).

The alphanumeric identification of a European standard (CEN or CEN-ELEC standards) consists of the initial capital letters EN followed by a space and then a number without any spaces. A hyphen after the number is followed by a number that identifies the part of that standard (if any). A colon after the number sequence is followed by the year in which the standard became available.

The ETSI standards are preceded by the letters ETS, for example 'ETS 300 381 ed.1 (1994-12) – Telephony for hearing impaired people: inductive coupling of telephone earphones to hearing aids'.

European standards are intended to replace national standards to constitute the reference for defining technical requirements within the EU organizational framework. The harmonized standards have one method of showing conformity with European Directives and as a reference for the design of products, without, however, constituting intangible constraints.

European Standards (those relevant to *Noise and Its Effects* are shown in Appendices 2 and 3) must be implemented in their entirety as national standards by all participating countries and any conflicting national standards must be withdrawn. An example is provided by 'ISO 1680: 1999 Acoustics – Test code for the measurement of the airborne noise emitted by rotating electrical machines'. This international standard was adopted by CEN. It therefore now appears as national standard of all CEN member states. Thus in Germany it is 'DIN EN ISO 1680: 2000-02 Akustik – Verfahren zur Messung der Luftschallemission von drehenden elektrischen Maschinen'.

In general CEN and CENELEC take IEC and ISO standards and rubber stamp them as ENs, which are then adopted by national standards.

**National standards**

The vast majority of countries in the world now have their own standards organizations. These now include, for example, Albania with its General Directorate of Standardization (in Tirana). The administrative organization of national standards bodies varies with the country. For example, the Canadian General Standards Board (CGSB) is a standards development, certification and registration organization. It is a member of Canada's National Standards System, and is accredited by the Standards Council of Canada (SCC) (see www.pwgsc.gc.ca/cgsb/032_025/index-f.html).

A *code of practice* represents a standard of good practice. It may or may not be in the form of a national standard. For example, in the UK, BS 5228-1: 1997 is a code of practice for basic information and procedures for noise and vibration control on construction and open sites. BS 5228-3: 1997 (Noise and vibration control on construction and open sites) constitutes a code of practice applicable to surface coal extraction by opencast methods. The 1972 Code of Practice for Reducing the Exposure of Employed Persons to Noise has now been superseded by The Noise at Work Regulations 1989.

*Circulars* provide, *inter alia,* a means by which information on standards (or laws) can be disseminated by appropriate authorities to appropriate individuals or bodies. For example, in the UK, a HELA (Health and Safety Executive/Local Authorities Enforcement Liaison Committee) circular advises local authority enforcement officers that the British Standards Institution has published a British Standard Code of Practice for Safeguarding Woodworking Machines. It has been printed in two volumes:

- BS 6854: Part 1: 1987 – General recommendations (ISBN 0 580 15914 0).
- BS 6854: Part 2: 1988 – Circular sawing machines (sawing machines with rotating tools) (ISBN 0 580 16597 3).

Enforcement officers are reminded that whilst the use of a British Standard may assist the reader to comply with his legal obligations, fully implementing a British Standard does not necessarily imply full compliance with statutory requirements (see www.hse.gov.uk/lau/lacs/54-6.htm).

### Ongoing and future developments

*General comments*

New or amended standards are appearing at an enormous rate yet the development of new standards and codes of practice can be a complicated and time-consuming process.

*International*

The international standards organizations will need to address inconsistencies between their own standards. For example, ISO 389-3 quotes the mean value for the reference equivalent threshold force levels (RETFLs) for bone-conduction hearing levels, IEC 60645-3 clause 6 quotes median values in respect of hearing levels of short duration signals, and ISO 389-1 quotes the modal value for the reference equivalent threshold sound pressure levels (RETSPLs) for air-conduction hearing levels. Haughton (2002) points out:

> Although the distribution of hearing thresholds within the populace at large is highly skewed in the direction of impaired hearing, a far more symmetrical

distribution is found within the selected test populations used to establish the normal values. Accordingly it may make no difference whether the mean, the median or the modal value of threshold is taken as representative, but the lack of consistency in the standards is irksome.

## European

National standards are often *de facto* barriers to the free movement of goods in the EC. Achieving the single market requires the removal of these barriers. A 1985 Council of Ministers' resolution setting forth a 'new approach' to technical harmonization distinguished between EC legislative harmonization – in the form of Directives, which prescribe observance of 'essential requirements' of health and safety to users and consumers – and EC-wide technical standardization, a task entrusted to the European standards institutes, for example the European Committee for Standardization and the European Committee for Electrotechnical Standardization.

A 1989 EC Communication laid the foundations for possible EC directives designed to implement uniform principles of conformity assessment throughout the EC. This included the creation of a European Organization for Testing and Certification (EOTC).

A 1990 EC Green Paper (discussion document) reviewed the merits of establishing a single European standardization system, the component parts of which would include technical bodies (the EOTC, for example) and the national standards bodies. At the centre of this system would be the European Standardization Organization (Russotto, 1990).

An example of the complicated nature of producing new standards is illustrated by the approach of the European Commission to defining new and improved European standards for the measurement of, and defining testing methods for, the airborne transmission of noise from the intake/exhaust systems in road vehicles (www.cordis.lu/growth/calls/top-4.12.htm, accessed 3 August 2002). The focus of the EC project will be to conduct research for the development and validation of measurement and testing methods with respect to the airborne transmission of noise from the intake/exhaust systems in automotive vehicles, the scope being to define new and improved European standards through collaboration between car manufacturers and component suppliers and to promote the establishment of international equivalence of measurements. By applying the methodologies to be developed and validated during the course of the project it will be possible to optimize compatibility of subsystems and components related to the acoustic performance of vehicles, improve efficiency by avoiding duplication of effort, and introduce advantages from economies of scale to increase the general competitiveness of the European automotive industry. Furthermore, these methodologies will permit the qualification and benchmarking of vehicles in terms of noise generation and transmission, enabling the creation of technical data for the definition of performance requirements.

The aims of the project are also directly compatible with the general objectives of Key Action 3 for Land Transportation, particularly as regards the objective of reducing pass-by noise emission of vehicles to 70 dB (A) for cars and 74 dB (A) for commercial vehicles. Although the experimental methodologies to be developed could be considered to represent critical technology for improving product performance, particularly as concerns the production of more efficient and clean land transport vehicles, the actual state of the art in terms of currently used methods and existing test standards in directly related fields would favour an activity in support of European standardization.

# Legal metrology

### In general

Legal metrology is the entirety of the legislative, administrative and technical procedures established by, or by reference to, public authorities, and implemented on their behalf in order to specify and to ensure, in a regulatory or contractual manner, the appropriate quality and credibility of measurements related to official controls, trade, health, safety and the environment (see www.oiml.org, accessed 2 December 2002).

The Convention du Mètre was signed in Paris in 1875 by representatives of countries. As well as founding the Bureau International des Poids et Mesures (BIPM), the Convention du Mètre gave authority to the BIPM, the Conférence Générale des Poids et Mesures (CGPM or International Committee for Weights and Measures) and the Comité International des Poids et Mesures (CIPM) to act in matters of world metrology, particularly concerning the demand for measurement standards of ever-increasing accuracy, range and diversity, and the need to demonstrate equivalence between national measurement standards. The Convention, modified slightly in 1921, remains the basis of all international agreement on units of measurement. There are now fifty-one Member States, including all the major industrialized countries of the world (www.bipm.fr/enus/1_Convention, accessed 22 August 2002).

The Organisation Internationale de Métrologie Légale (OIML) is an intergovernmental treaty organization established in 1955 to promote the global harmonization of legal metrology procedures. The OIML develops model regulations (international recommendations) which provide members with an internationally agreed basis for the establishment of national legislation on various categories of measuring instruments. Given the increasing national implementation of OIML guidelines, more and more manufacturers are referring to OIML international recommendations to ensure that their products meet international specifications for metrological performance and testing. General performance and calibration requirements for audiometers are specified in OIML Document R 104.

Cooperative agreements are established between the OIML and certain institutions, such as the International Organization for Standardization (ISO) and the International Electrotechnical Commission (IEC), with the objective of avoiding contradictory requirements. Consequently manufacturers and users of measuring instruments, test laboratories, etc., may apply simultaneously OIML publications and those of other institutions.

The Eleventh CGPM adopted (1960) the name Système International d'Unités (International System of Units, international abbreviation SI), for the recommended practical system of units of measurement. That CGPM also laid down rules for prefixes, derived units and other matters. Base units included initially the metre, kilogram, second and ampere. Derived units are those formed by combining base units according to the algebraic relationships linking the corresponding quantities. The names and symbols of some of the units thus formed can be replaced by special names and symbols, which can themselves be used to form expressions and symbols of other derived units. The hertz (unit of frequency) and the pascal (unit of pressure) are derived units. Certain units, such as the bel (and therefore the decibel) are not part of the SI system, i.e. they are outside the SI, but are important and widely used. Consistent with the recommendations of the CIPM, the units in this category are accepted for use with the SI (www.bipm.fr/enus/3_SI, accessed 22-8-2002). ISO 1000: 1992 and technically equivalent national standards, such as BS 5555: 1993, are specifications for SI units and recommendations for the use of their multipliers.

In addition to the international OIML, there are regional and national metrological bodies. A list of National Metrological Laboratories is provided at www.nist.gov/oiaa/nat_pg3.htm (accessed 8 December 2002). The NPL (National Physical Laboratory) is the UK's national metrological laboratory.

**Metrological accreditation**

Accreditation is a formal recognition of competence. In the domain of metrology, accreditation of a laboratory is granted when measurement competence is demonstrated in all of the laboratory's technical practices. There are two international organizations for accreditation, the International Accreditation Forum Inc. (IAF) and the International Laboratory Accreditation Cooperation (ILAC), both of which are based in Australia, and at least two regional accreditation organizations, the European Cooperation for Accreditation and the EOTC. Each country should have its own accreditation organization. The United Kingdom Accreditation Service (UKAS) is the UK's national body responsible for assessing and accrediting the competence of organizations in the fields of calibration, measurement, testing, inspection, and the certification of systems, personnel and products. UKAS-accredited calibration laboratories represent the main focus for traceable calibration in the UK.

Thus audiometers and sound level meters in the UK should be calibrated by a UKAS-approved laboratory to provide an NAMAS (National
Accreditation of Measurement and Sampling) certificate. Certificates bearing the NAMAS logo are widely accepted in the UK and throughout the
world. There are multilateral agreements recognizing the equivalence of
accreditations.

Each country's national measurement system (NMS) is the technical and
organizational infrastructure that ensures confidence in the measurements
made in support of research and development, manufacturing, commerce,
and health and safety in that country. In the UK, the NPL is the focus of the
NMS with responsibility for developing, maintaining and disseminating
measurement standards. All activities in the NPL, excluding those accredited by the UKAS, are operated to a certified ISO 9001: 1994 quality system
standard. The NPL accredits calibration services to ISO/IEC 17025: 1999.

# Laws

### General comments

Basically, laws have been developed as a method of social control – to settle disputes and to ensure no harm comes to an individual or his society.
If this does happen then the law is there to ensure that the wrongdoer is
punished and amends made to the person who has been harmed. Thus
the development of the law is shaped by logic, history, custom and utility,
as well as the accepted standards of right conduct (Cardozo, 1921). There
is a complex interrelationship of custom, ethics, religion and law
(Hinchcliffe, 2003a). Consequently the laws of different countries differ
from each other.

A study of the law of the various countries of the world (for example,
David and Jauffret-Spinosi, 1992) indicates that there are broadly two
superfamilies of legal systems – the European and the Afro-Asian group.
Within the European grouping there are three broad families, i.e. the
Romano-Germanic, the Socialist and the Common Law families.

Romano-Germanic law, which dominates western Europe, is characterized by codification. Those legal systems that belong to the
Romano-Germanic group have a substantial input from Roman law. The
*law of delict* is based upon the second of the three precepts of Ulpian:
*iuris praecepta sunt haec: honeste vivere, alterum non laedere, suum
cuique tribuere* (the maxima of the law are these: to live honestly, to
harm no one, and to give everyone his due). Both Scottish law and
South African law derive from Roman–Dutch law. Consequently in both
these legal systems the law of delict governs civil legal wrongs, although
in Scotland it is referred to as the law of reparation. Under Roman law
a delict could be public (termed a 'crime' in modern legal systems) or

private. The latter covers what, under English law, is termed the 'law of tort'. Delict has shown considerable evolution since Roman times when it was essentially legalized vengeance. Delict has now been defined as an unlawful act that violates the subjective right(s) of a legal subject (Du Plessis, 1992).

Socialist law is derived from, and subordinate to, Marxist-Leninist doctrine. The common law is a uniquely English derivation. Following the end of the Roman occupation in AD 430, England saw invasions by a number of tribes (Angles, Jutes, Saxons and Vikings) from north-western Europe over the next six centuries. Each brought with them their own *customary law*. It was William the Conqueror's arrival from Normandy in AD 1066 that resulted in defining what these various customary laws had in common. Hence the designation of this collated law as the 'common law'. A more extended survey has been given previously (Hinchcliffe and Bellman, 1997). As well as being uncoded, the common law system is characterized by two other features: the method of acquisition of evidence (adversarial, as opposed to inquisitorial) and the practice of judicial precedent. It is the latter that gives rise to what is termed 'case law'. There are now some 400 000 case reports contained in 1000 volumes of law reports. The common law doctrine of abiding by precedent is known as *stare decisis* (short for *stare decisis et non quieta movere*). Thus for civil cases, the hierarchy of authority is House of Lords > Court of Appeal (Civil Division) > High Court of Justice > County Courts. It is thus a vertical, and not a horizontal, authority. Moreover, in 1966, the House of Lords declared that it would not be bound by its own decisions (Practice Statement). Consequently, the judgments of primary interest are those of the latest House of Lords and Court Appeal decisions relevant to the matter in question.

The *law of torts* (Hepple and Matthews, 1991; Jones, 1994) was a creation of the common law and it was evolved from the principle of providing a remedy for an unjustifiable injury done by one person to another. A tort is a civil wrong. As pointed out by Lord Denning, the province of tort is to allocate responsibility for injurious conduct. In the context of this chapter, the three most important torts are nuisance, negligence and trespass to person. As Atiyah (1970) pointed out, the concept of *fault* dominates the existing compensation systems under the law of torts. Although it has virtually no place in personal insurance compensation or in the social security system, it underlies almost the entire law of torts. The concept of the fault principle derives much from the writers on tort, particularly Sir John Salmond, at the beginning of this century. Salmond strove to reduce the whole law of torts to a set of moral principles around the concept of fault. But compensation payable bears no relation to the degree of fault.

With more than 200 sovereign states in the world the global legal scene can only be described as kaleidoscopic.

## United Kingdom

Many countries of the world have been, at one time or another, part of the British Empire, or the subsequent British Commonwealth of Nations. Consequently, many countries, including Singapore and the USA have, in some degree or another, inherited the English common law system. The UK's legal approach to 'noise and its effects', or any other matter, thus forms a model for the approach of many other countries to this subject.

Although the English common law is based on judicial decisions on cases, there is nevertheless, as in the civil law countries, a considerable body of law (statutes or Acts) enacted by the legislatures (the Westminster Parliament in England).

In the UK (and many other countries), there is also a considerable amount of what is termed *delegated* (or *subordinate*) legislation. In the UK a *statutory instrument* (abbreviation SI) is the most important form of delegated legislation. It may cover *Orders* and *Regulations*, e.g., Statutory Instrument 1996 No. 2219 (C.56) Environmental Protection: The Noise Act 1996 (Commencement No.1) Order, and The Noise at Work Regulations 1989 SI 1989 No. 1790 are based on EC Directive 86/188/EEC (for the control of hazardous occupational noise exposure). *Bye-laws* constitute another form of subordinate legislation.

## The European Community

The EC was an artificial creation by bureaucrats from certain countries of, initially, the western end of the western macropeninsula of Eurasia. Its legal system does not therefore follow Cardozo's evolutionary model. It relies on legislative measures adopted by its governing institutions, the four most prominent of which are the following:

1. The Commission, which is responsible for formulating policy, drafting legislative proposals and ensuring correct implementation.
2. The Council of Ministers, which represents the interests of the member states and which is responsible for adopting most EC legislation.
3. The European Parliament, whose directly elected members form the EC's principal consultative body.
4. The European Court of Justice, which is responsible for interpreting all issues of EC law; it is therefore comparable to the Supreme Court of the USA.

In the community's decision-making process, the Commission drafts proposed legislation, which is then submitted to the Council of Ministers and the European Parliament for review.

The community's *primary legislation* is the EEC Treaty (the Treaty of Rome), as amended in 1987 by the Single European Act. *Secondary legislation* includes *Regulations, Directives* and *Decisions*.

*Regulations* are binding acts that have direct, general and often immediate application in the member states and are often very specific with regard to the issues they address. *Directives* are also binding measures, but prescribe only the end result to be achieved; the means by which this result is obtained is left to the discretion of the member states. Thus, Directives have a built-in flexibility that is absent in other forms of EC legislation. For this reason, Directives are found to be the most widely used legal instrument as the community strives to harmonize the legislation of member states. Finally, *Decisions* may be made by the Council of Ministers or the Commission; decisions may consist of either legislative acts (for example, the proposed Council decision on a global approach to testing and certification) or executive measures (for example, Commission decisions relating to the competitive practice of companies under the EC rules of competition).

As signatories of the EEC Treaty, all member states are required to fulfil all obligations set forth in the treaty. This obligation includes the correct implementation of community legislation. Failure to do so is considered an infringement of community law, for which member states may be taken before the European Court of Justice (Russotto, 1990).

In the case of *Costa v ENEL* 1964, the European Court of Justice ruled, *inter alia:*

> The transfer by the States from their domestic legal system to the Community legal system of the rights and obligations arising under the Treaty carries with it a permanent limitation of their sovereign rights, against which a subsequent unilateral act incompatible with the concept of the Community cannot prevail.

Thus the European Court of Justice (ECJ) showed that EC provisions that do not specifically mention individuals may still create rights for them. Moreover, the ECJ indicated that the logic of EC law gives it supremacy over the domestic laws of its member states (Oppenheimer, 1994; Steiner, 1994).

## Psychological effects of noise

### General comments

Noise presents a pervasive and increasing nuisance. Noise caused by traffic and industrial or recreational activities is one of the main local environmental problems in Europe and the source of an increasing number of complaints from the public. There is therefore an increasing corpus of noise control law, whether in the form of legislation or, in common law countries, of case law.

### United Kingdom

Complaints about environmental noise were prominent more than a 100 years ago, with the same expectation that something would be done about it (by legislation): 'At last there appear some signs that in the course of the next few years or so some of the totally unnecessary noises of London may be checked . . . There is Mr Jacoby's Bill all ready; let the Government pass it, or if they do not like that Bill give the County Council powers to make the by-laws it wants' (Anon, 1896). No specific legislation was to appear until more than 60 years later.

The Committee on the Problem of Noise (Cmnd 2956) analysed the law relating to noise in the UK (as it was in 1963). Its conclusions were summarized in para. 74:

> We consider that the main aim of legislation against noise should be preven-
> tion . . . . There must, however, be remedy in law where prevention fails or is
> inapplicable for one reason or another. The law relating to nuisance is this
> remedy, and in general we can see no alternative to it. The factors which gov-
> ern whether or not a noise is a nuisance are so many and so subtle that it is
> possible in only a few instances to attempt to fix a quantitative limit to noise.

At the time that Cmnd 2956 conducted its review the Noise Abatement Act 1960 was in force. Since then the Environmental Protection Act 1990 (www.hmso.gov.uk/acts/acts1990/Ukpga_19900043_en_1.htm, accessed 28 July 2002) and the Noise Act 1996 (www.hmso.gov.uk/acts/acts1996/1996037.htm, accessed 18 August 2002) have appeared. Statutory Instrument 1996 No. 2219 (C.56) Environmental Protection: The Noise Act 1996 (Commencement No.1) Order brought Section 10(7) of that Act into force on 19 September 1996. This section provides that the power of a local authority under section 81(3) of the Environmental Protection Act 1990 to abate a statutory nuisance by virtue of section 79(1)(g) of that Act (noise emitted from premises), includes power to seize and remove any equipment used in the emission of that noise. Under Section 80 of the Environmental Protection Act 1990 local authorities have the power to serve Noise (or vibration) Abatement Notices on companies or individuals. The Noise and Statutory Nuisance Act 1993 amended the Control of Pollution Act 1974 and the Environmental Protection Act 1990 to make new provisions relating to the operation of loudspeakers in streets and roads and to audible intruder alarms.

A model noise control law for local authorities was set out in Appendix XVI of Cmnd 2956 as 'Model Byelaws Relating to Noise in Streets and Public Places'.

Ch III of Cmnd 2956 drew attention to the clarification of the nature a noise *nuisance* by Mr Justice Luxmoore in the case of *Vanderpant v. Mayfair Hotel Co* 1930:

> Apart from any right that may have been acquired against him by contract,
> grant or prescription, every person is entitled as against his neighbour to
> the comfortable and healthy enjoyment of the premises occupied by him
> and in deciding whether, in any particular case, his right has been interfered
> with and a nuisance thereby caused, it is necessary to determine whether

the act complained of is an inconvenience materially interfering with the ordinary physical comfort of human existence not merely according to elegant or dainty modes and habits of living but according to plain and sober and simple notions obtaining amongst English people.

The case clarified that intrusive noise need not be injurious to health. But it must incur substantial interference with comfort, convenience or health. Transitory upsets are excluded. Unlike trespass a nuisance does not require direct physical interference.

Both airborne noise (*Crump v Lambert* 1867) and structure-borne noise (*Hoare & Co v McAlpine* 1923) may constitute a nuisance.

Gunfire, especially when malicious, can be a cause for nuisance. A fox farmer was granted an injunction restraining his neighbour from firing guns so as to frighten the foxes during the breeding season (*Hollywood Silver Fox Farm v Emmett* 1936).

Noises other than those due to machinery or gunfire can also constitute a nuisance. In the case of *Tinkler v Aylesbury Dairy Co* 1888, it was held that noise resulting from moving milk churns when being loaded interfered with the personal comfort of the nearby residents and thereby constituted a common law nuisance. Noise from carts and shouts from their drivers during the night, so that they made the plaintiff unable to sleep, also constituted a common law nuisance (*Bartlett v Marshall* 1896).

Noisy animals can constitute a common law nuisance (*Leeman v Montagu* 1936). In the case of *Harrison v Metropolitan Police* 1972 the plaintiff obtained an injunction with respect to the howling and barking of dogs kept in a police station compound. These noises had disturbed his sleep and made it difficult for him to work in his study even when he wore earplugs and had installed both double glazing in the bedroom and internal shutters. 'Corky', a noisy cockerel, became a *cause célèbre* in a north Devon village (*Guardian,* 18 August 1994).

Malice may be a factor in an action for noise nuisance. In the case of *Christie v Davey* 1983, a music teacher was granted an injunction restraining a neighbour from knocking on the wall and otherwise creating a noise to interfere with professional teaching.

A landlord may be liable if he has authorized the creation of a nuisance expressly or by implication. Thus a landlord has been held liable for his tenant's blasting operations because he had let the property for that specific purpose (*Harris v James* 1876).

*Temporary noise,* for example that due to the demolition of a building, may not, if the operation is reasonably conducted and all proper reasonable steps taken to ensure that no undue inconvenience is caused to neighbours, form a basis for a successful action for nuisance at common law (*Andreae v Selfridge* 1938). Nevertheless, a teacher in New Zealand was successful in claiming damages in the New Zealand Supreme Court because nearby construction noise forced him to shout and this caused him to develop a tumour on the vocal folds (News Item, 1969 *The Times,* 4 September).

At common law, *prescriptive right* is a defence in an action for nuisance. This arises after 20 years. However, the time begins only when the act in fact becomes a nuisance. Thus it was held that the defendant had no prescriptive right in a case where he had used the machinery for more than 20 years but the vibrations caused by it became a nuisance only when the plaintiff, a physician, put up a consulting room at the end of his garden near the noise (*Sturges v Bridgman* 1879). This decision thus also upheld the principle, established in the case of *Bliss v Hall* 1838, that it is no defence to show that the plaintiff came to the nuisance.

In contrast to the statute law on noise, it is no defence for the defendant to show that he has taken all reasonable steps and care to prevent the noise (*Rushmer v Polsue and Alfieri Ltd* 1906). The judgment in this case was expressly approved by the House of Lords on appeal. With respect to this case, Lord Loreburn stated that 'It would be no answer to say that the steam hammer is of the most modern improved pattern and is reasonably worked.' This principle was upheld in the case of *Halsey v Esso Petroleum Co Ltd* 1961. The plaintiff was granted both damages for loss caused by acid smuts from the defendant's depot and injunctions to restrain the making of noise at night and the emission of pungent smells at any time. The action was also of note because in evidence the plaintiff brought noise level measurements to court.

An increasing number of disputes involving environmental noise and industry in the UK are now heard in the Technology and Construction Court (TCC) (Dyson, 1998). The TCC is comparable to the UK's Commercial Court. With a view to limiting the citation of previous authority to cases that are relevant and useful to the court, the Lord Chief Justice of England and Wales issued a Practice Direction in April 2001. This Practice Direction lays down a number of rules as to what material may be cited, and the manner in which that cited material should be handled by advocates. These rules are in large part such as many courts already follow in pursuit of their general discretion in the management of litigation. However, it is now desirable to promote uniformity of practice by the same rules being followed by all courts. It will remain the duty of advocates to draw the attention of the court to any authority not cited by an opponent which is adverse to the case being advanced (see www.courtservice.gov.uk/pds/tcc/pd_tcc.htm, accessed 28 July 2002).

*European Union*

Community environmental noise policy has long centred on legislation fixing maximum sound levels for vehicles, aeroplanes and machines with a single market aim, or to implement international agreements in the case of aircraft, linked to certification procedures to ensure that new vehicles and equipment are, at the time of manufacture, complying with the noise limits laid down in Directives. There are now a number of these Directives, such as EC Directive 89/392/EEC, which require all machinery (from small domestic appliances to large diesel engines) manufacturers to provide noise emission information as part of the process of CE marking and declaration of conformity.

*Other countries*

In general, legislation aimed at environmental noise control is embodied in environmental protection law rather than specific noise control Acts. Only a few examples will be cited in order to view the global scene.

After the move towards a liberal democracy in 1989, Albania began to enact a constellation of model laws, including one incorporating environmental noise control (www.pace.edu/lawschool/env/albanianlaw/albanianenvironmentalprotection.html, accessed 22 August 2002).

The Law of the People's Republic of China on the Prevention and Control of Pollution from Environmental Noise was adopted at the Twenty-second Meeting of the Standing Committee of the Eighth National People's Congress on 29 October 1996, promulgated by Order No. 77 of the President of the People's Republic of China on October 29, and became effective as of 1 March 1997. Article 1 of Chapter 1 states 'This Law is enacted for the purpose of preventing and controlling environmental noise pollution, protecting and improving the living environment, ensuring human health and promoting economic and social development' (www.china.org.cn/english/environment/34448.htm, accessed 21 August 2002).

In Japan, as part of the Basic Environmental Law, the Japanese Ministry of the Environment produced its Noise Regulation Law in November 1993. It was amended (specifically for community noise) in 1995. Chapter II provides regulations regarding specified factories, Chapter III regulations regarding specified construction work, Chapter IV maximum permissible levels of motor vehicle noise and Chapter VI penalties (www.env.go.jp/en/lar, accessed 21 August 2002).

In Nigeria Section 19 of the Federal Environmental Protection Act is concerned with noise control.

Noise law in the USA is summarized in Chapter 50 of Harris's *Handbook of Acoustical Measurements and Noise Control*. Section 4905 of the Noise Control Act 1972 covers noise emission standards for products distributed in commerce (www4.law.cornell.edu/uscode/42/ch65.html, accessed 22 August 2002).

## Damage to hearing from noise

*General comments*

A variety of injuries to the ear has been described after exposure to high levels of noise. Acute noise-induced damage to hearing (acoustic trauma) is the form that results from gunfire. Otic blast injury results from explosions. Cases of what has been described as an acoustic accident or industrial sudden deafness have also been reported. Chronic noise-induced damage to hearing (occupational noise-induced hearing loss or ONIHL) is associated with long-term exposure to high levels of noise in industry.

Military personnel are exposed to the risk of these types of hearing damage. Military regulations (particularly with regard to wearing hearing protective devices) are designed to reduce this risk. Various countries have different schemes for compensating military personnel who sustain damage to their hearing.

Civilians are also exposed to the risk of these types of hearing damage but ONIHL is dominant. Thus the law is concerned primarily with the prevention of ONIHL and with its compensation if it has occurred. Armourers in the ancient Roman Empire could receive compensation since it was recognized that working with metal could cause loss of hearing (Mackenzie, 1997).

*United Kingdom*

The Health and Safety at Work Act 1974 is the statute that governs the safety of workers and the prevention of industrial injuries and occupational diseases.

The Department for Work and Pensions' Health and Safety Executive (HSE) is the agency that is responsible for ensuring that risks to people's health and safety from work activities is minimized.

The Noise at Work Regulations 1989 SI 1989 No. 1790 (based on EC Directive 86/188/EEC) are aimed at the reduction of hazardous occupational noise exposures.

The Supply of Machinery (Safety) Regulations 1992 (as amended in 1994) ensures that the supplier of new machinery needs to provide the following:

- A 'Declaration of Conformity', usually supplied by the manufacturer; CE marking.
- Instructions for safe installation, use and maintenance of the machinery.
- Information on noise emissions, including:
  - sound pressure level at workstations where this exceeds 70 dB(A)
  - instantaneous sound pressure value at workstations, where this exceeds 63 Pa (equivalent to 130 dB (C) peak)
  - sound power level emitted by the machinery, where the sound pressure level at workstations exceeds 85 dB (A).

- Information about the operating conditions of the machinery during measurement and what methods have been used for the measurement of the noise emissions.

The Management of Health and Safety at Work Regulations 1999 (Statutory Instrument 1999 No. 3242 ISBN 0 11 085625) requires employers to assess the health and safety risks (including from hazardous noise or vibration exposure) to their employees.

There was official acceptance at the beginning of this century in the UK that 'boiler-makers' deafness was unquestionably a disease caused by employment (Departmental Committee on Compensation for Industrial Diseases, 1907). But it did not become a prescribed occupational disease until many years later (Department of Health and Social Security or DHSS, 1973). Since then compensation has been provided under social security law to workers with ONIHL. Common law claims may also be pursued in respect of the negligence of their employers (tort law).

The second sentence in paragraph 27 of the report by the Industrial Diseases Sub-Committee of the Industrial Injuries Advisory Council (DHSS, 1973), which led the government to recognize noise-induced hearing loss as a compensable occupational disease read: 'Relatively small departures from the audiometric baseline would not be apparent in practice so that it is only after the hearing loss has risen to about 30 dB or more, depending on frequency, that the subject himself is aware of deterioration to the point of seeking help.' This report was the product of a far-reaching enquiry to which acousticians, audiologists, general practitioners and otolaryngologists gave evidence individually and collectively as well as (through the Trade Union Congress) the country's noise-exposed workers. The latter were also represented (through Peter Jacques) on the subcommittee itself.

Compensation under social security law is related to the reduction in hearing sensitivity, impairment as measured in decibels. Yet hearing disability is a multifactorial quality of which hearing impairment is only one factor (Williams, 1992).

As far as common law actions are concerned there appears to be no 'low fence' concept that applies to the hearing sensitivity of claimants. Courts appear to have endorsed the doctrine that 'every decibel counts' (Merluzzi and Hinchcliffe, 1973).

Noise damage to the cochlea is multi-faceted (Stephens, 1976) so it is conceivable that (if symptomatic) there may be complaints related to other paracuses (Hinchcliffe, 2003c) and these may be compensable (Clement-Evans, 1998).

There is a component for tinnitus in the assessment of damages in common law actions.

With regard to the affect of noise on quality of life, the common law awards damages in respect of what it terms its 'loss of amenity'. This corresponds broadly to the medical concept of reduction in the quality of life.

The Court of Appeal has disposed of loss of amenity assessments based solely upon pure-tone audiograms in no uncertain terms (*per*

Stephenson LJ: 'a mere comparison of decibel loss is very misleading'; *per* Kerr LJ; in *Robinson v. British Rail Engineering* 1982 (Court of Appeal):

> . . . the learned judge was faced with the simple task – simple in one sense but not by any means simple in another – of quantifying, or putting into pounds and pence, the loss of amenity which the plaintiff has suffered as a result of noise-induced loss of hearing . . . insurers and trade unions . . . are interested in any guidance which the courts can give on the conventional figure which should be awarded for this kind of impairment of hearing, or this kind of interference with the quality of men's and women's lives . . . [Counsel for Plaintiff] says that it is wrong for a judge to look simply at decibels . . . and that the judge has to look at the effect on the particular plaintiff of that particular affliction, with the degree in decibels which it has reached.

---

**How British judges calculate compensation level**

'In this case Mr Justice Michael Davies referred to getting the feel of the case and feeling the right figure through the tips of his fingers. Of course, if he feels through the tips of his fingers a figure which excites the comment made years ago by Lord Justice Denning, as he then was, 'good gracious, as high as that?', you look again at the figure and this court may have to revise it . . . .' Lord Justice Stephenson in *Robinson v British Rail Engineering* 1982 (Court of Appeal).

---

With regard to diagnosis, retrognosis and prognosis, as the common law makes awards for any past, present and future loss of amenity resulting from an alleged hazardous occupational noise exposure, the examiner will need to construct a profile of such over the plaintiff's lifespan. Such a profile must be compared to the profile that would have been the case had that particular claimant *not* had that particular noise exposure. Thus the examiner will need to provide not only a diagnosis but also a retrognosis (going back over time) and a prognosis (going forward over time).

The clinical diagnosis by the medical examiner takes precedence over applications of statistical tables by the noise consultant (Tempest and Bryan, 1981). Clinical diagnosis, whether of noise damage to hearing or of any other disorder, is essentially one of pattern recognition (Abernathy and Hamm, 1994a,b; Dunea, 1997). The medical examiner therefore needs to be aware of both the clinical (Hinchcliffe, 2002) and the audiometric (Perlman, 1941; Robinson, 1976) pictures of ONIHL and of the conditions that come into the differential diagnosis. The latter encompass audiometric high tone notches resulting from various measurement artefacts (Coles 1967; Davis 1995; Mahoney and Luxon, 1996; Lutman and Qasem, 1998).

For estimations of *previous* hearing threshold levels (HTLs), a retrodiction exercise should be performed with the help of NPL Ac 61. Such an approach was specifically approved by a High Court Judge in the leading

English case of *Thompson, Gray and Nicholson v Smiths Ship Repairers (North Shields) Ltd*; *Blacklock and Waggott v Swan Hunter Shipbuilders Ltd*; *Mitchell v Vickers Armstrong Ltd and the Swan Hunter Shipbuilders Ltd* 1984. Lutman (1996) has shown how a retrodiction exercise may be performed for ISO 1999.

For estimations of *future* HTLs, it must be borne in mind that, if we live long enough, we may end up with the same HTL whether or not there had been any previous hazardous occupational noise exposure: 'the HTLs attained at the age of 60 or 65 years in the general population, when compared with those of noise-exposed persons of similar age, left little margin to account for the specific effects of noise' (Robinson 1987). It has, however, been said (without any supporting data) that this statement must be qualified as it only relates to the 3- to 4-kHz range where there is saturation due to the complete loss of cochlear amplifier gain.

A medical examiner's report will need to include information on a variety of matters (Hinchcliffe, 2000a). Appending Volume I of *Noise and Hearing* (Hinchcliffe, Luxon and Williams, 2001) to a medical report should reduce markedly the chances of lawyers manipulating medical and scientific knowledge that bears upon the case in question.

In the preface to Mark Cato's (1999) *magnum opus* on *The Expert*, The Right Honourable The Lord Saville of Newdigate, Chairman of the Judicial Committee of the Academy of Experts, tells us: 'The job of experts in litigation or arbitration is to give their independent, objective and unbiased opinions on the matter referred to them and falling within their area of expertise. The job of advocates is to present the best case they possibly can on behalf of their clients.'

In a joint document, the Law Society and the British Medical Association (1993) stated: 'It should be remembered that whether giving evidence as a witness of fact or as an expert witness, the role of the doctor is to assist the court and remain independent of the parties, regardless of the fact that the doctor will have been called to the court by one of them.'

In his *Access to Justice*, Lord Woolf (see later) considered the matter sufficiently important to draw attention to this manipulation of expert witnesses by lawyers by quoting from an editorial in *Counsel*: 'Expert witnesses used to be genuinely independent experts . . . . Today they are in practice hired guns.' At the Eleventh World Congress on Medical Law, the Right Honourable Lord Justice MacDermott (1997) expressed judicial concern regarding evidence provided by medical examiners in particular. But with whom does the fault lie? The lawyers, the medical examiners or the system? In his Presidential address to the Royal Statistical Society, Adrian Smith (1996) said 'It is somewhat paradoxical . . . that the procedures and protocols of UK law-courts seem so much at odds with the kinds of disciplined scientific reasoning that many of us would see as essential in an evidence-based society.' It is therefore not surprising that Lord Woolf summarized the current situation: 'There is now widespread support from judges, lawyers and academics, as well as from those who use the courts, for a new approach to civil litigation.' Removal of lawyers from the doctor–doctor interface should enable a more truthful and quicker resolution of disputes.

A solicitor (Clement-Evans, 1999) has drawn our attention to the words of Mr Justice Cresswell in a legal case (*Ikarian Reefer*) that included: 'Facts and assumptions upon which the opinion is based should be stated, with material facts which could detract from the expert's opinion being considered.' A barrister has pointed out 'that clinicians will now have to set out not only their own professional views, but also those of any other "relevant recognised body of opinion." This is likely to make the writing of medicolegal reports a lengthier and more demanding process, especially in view of the fact that the courts now expect reports to be well referenced and logical' (Friston, 1999). We are referred to the case of *Bolitho (Deceased) v City and Hackney HA* 1998.

*European Union*

There are a number of Directives that bear on the protection of workers from noise hazards:

- EC Directive 79/113/EEC: deals with determining sound power level.
- EC Directive 81/1051/EEC: deals with measuring operator position noise.
- EC Directive 86/188/EEC: deals with the protection of workers from the risks related to exposure to noise at work.
- EC Directive 89/392/EEC: requires all machinery (from small domestic appliances to large diesel engines) manufacturers to provide noise emission information as part of the process of CE marking and declaration of conformity.

*Other countries*

The Russian government was the first in modern times to recognize officially (in 1929) that noise damage to hearing was an occupational disorder and could be compensated. Now the governments of all developed countries recognize that noise can damage hearing and have laws aimed at the prevention of ONIHL and at compensation should it occur. Each sovereign state will have established its own protective measures and compensation criteria. Information on, for example, the position in Poland and the USA has been given by Sulkowski (1980) and Dobie (1993), respectively. The compensation schemes in Australia and Canada have been reported by Macrae and Piesse (1981) and by Alberti (1981) respectively.

**Ongoing and future developments**

A number of governments operate a continuing review of their laws. For example, the UK's Department for Environment, Food and Rural Affairs

(DEFRA) commissioned the University of Birmingham to undertake a review of the take-up and workings of the Noise Act 1996 in October 1999. The main objectives of the review were:

- to establish the effectiveness of the 1996 Act;
- to establish how far a common approach was developing by local authorities across England, Wales and Northern Ireland in handling noise complaints, specifically those occurring in the period covered by the Noise Act;
- to identify good practice in dealing with night noise whether or not an authority has chosen to adopt the 1996 Act.

The report is available on the DETR website at www.dtlr.gov.uk/consult. htm (accessed 18 August 2002).

*Medical scientific*

There is a singular lack of the use of appropriate controls by medical examiners. Controls are essential to the expert evidence (Hinchcliffe, 2000b). These are best drawn from the contemporaneous and situation-specific clinical and audiometric experience of the examiner (Hinchcliffe, 2003b).

An examination of the reports of medical examiners (Hinchcliffe, 2000b, 2003b) showed that it is more likely than not that they or their audiometricians would be unable to interpret their audiometric measurements. There are therefore good grounds for waiving a requirement of medical examiners to conduct audiometric tests. These could be conducted at a centre specializing in the testing of auditory function. The study showed that examiners would also more likely than not be unable to interpret the results of their clinical examinations. There are therefore good grounds for waiving the requirement of medical examiners to conduct clinical examinations. These could be conducted by a clinician experienced in this field who would be attached to the centre specializing in the testing of auditory function. The introduction of a new skill group (auditory function analysts) would ensure that a medical examiner/expert would be provided with the best possible information on which to base his report.

*Legal*

Legislating to provide permissible sound levels in order to reduce the risk of noise damage to hearing may be relatively simple. Legislating to provide permissible sound levels in order to reduce the nuisance risk is less so. The UK's NPL has shown that different acoustic features are responsible for annoyance at different sound levels: 'at low levels, the feature of tonality is dominant above absolute level. At higher noise levels, the feature of absolute level is more dominant than tonality' (Berry and Porter, 1994). Moreover, 'the wide variety of descriptions of the characteristics of the noise stimuli highlighted the large number of subjective descriptors for the perceived character of a noise resulting from a physical feature. It appears that a noise can be judged by different features by different listeners.' Furthermore, complaints may generate complaints (Porter, 1995):

> There is a strong possibility of hysteresis in the case of noise sources newly introduced into a community, in that they might have to be reduced to a greater extent once complaints have been generated, than would have been the case if the situation had never been allowed to develop to the complaint stage.

Moreover, as van Gunsteren (1999) has pointed out: 'annoyance is both a psychological and a political phenomenon.' If policy measures do not reflect this, policy itself may become a serious determinant of annoyance.

The European Union Network for the Implementation and Enforcement of Environmental Law (IMPEL) is an informal network of environmental authorities of the Member States of the European Union. Its objectives are to create the necessary impetus in the EC to make progress on ensuring a more effective and consistent application of environmental legislation as well as an exchange of information and experience (www.defra.gov.uk/environment).

The 1996 European Commission's Green Paper on Future Noise Policy is a discussion paper that marks the first step towards tougher anti-noise laws in the European Community (europa.eu.int/en/record/green/gp9611/noise.htm, accessed 22 August 2002).

A proposed European Directive will require the production of noise maps and noise reduction plans for conurbations with a population of more than 250 000 and for major roads, major railways and major airports. This requirement will later be extended to all centres of population above 50 000. The UK's Institute of Sound and Vibration Research (University of Southampton) has the experience and specialist knowledge to assist local authorities in developing noise management plans at all levels (www.isvr.co.uk/environm/noisemap.htm, accessed 18 August 2002).

The UK Government's Noise and Nuisance Policy, which is part of DEFRA's Air and Environmental Quality Division, is responsible for the development and promotion of initiatives to address noise and other statutory nuisance and manages research into noise. The team is responsible, amongst other things, for negotiating proposals for European legislation on environmental noise and implementing the legislation once it comes into force (www.defra.gov.uk/environment/noise, accessed 18 August 2002).

With regard to *procedural reform*, there have been considerable changes in the way litigation is conducted in the UK following the Right Honourable Lord Woolf's 1996 *Access to Justice – Final Report to the Lord Chancellor.*

It is now possible for the experts of opposing sides to meet and resolve differences in their reports without the intervention of lawyers.

The new Civil Procedure Rules are published by the Stationery Office Limited as Statutory Instrument 1998 No. 3132 L. 17 the Civil Procedure Rules 1998, ISBN 0 11 080378 7. The rules can also be downloaded from www.hmso.gov.uk/si/si1998/19983132.htm The rules dealing with Expert Witnesses contains the text: 'Experts - overriding duty to the court. 35.3 (1) It is the duty of an expert to help the court on the matters within his expertise. (2) This duty overrides any obligation to the person from whom he has received instructions or by whom he is paid.' (www.hmso.gov.uk/si/si1998/98313215.htm#35.3).

With regard to *the oath for an expert witness* one would think that taking an oath to 'tell the truth, the whole truth and nothing but the truth' (or words to that effect) would leave little room for differences in the reports of various experts that relate to a given claimant. In practice there are considerably more differences between expert witnesses than one would find at a medical or scientific meeting.

Lasch's (1908) seminal study showed that an oath to tell the truth existed from remote historical times. Such an oath remained essentially unchanged until Saint Thomas Aquinas in his *Summa Theologica* (1265–73) insisted that an oath to tell the truth did not oblige one to tell 'the whole truth' (Mellinkoff, 1963, p. 173). Consequently the witness's oath needed to be extended to swearing to 'tell the truth, the whole truth and nothing but the truth' (or words to that effect). But at least one American President, who was also a lawyer, maintained that even with such a format there was no requirement to volunteer everything. The witness's oath therefore needs to be extended with the words 'nought will be concealed, all will be revealed'. Even that format does not reflect developments in medicine and science over the past 100 years, which have been directed to establishing the truth of some observation or opinion. In particular there is the use of controls, especially those that are most appropriate. The suggested oath extension for medical experts should therefore be 'nought will be concealed; all will be revealed, including all information relating to relevant controls, particularly those drawn from my own clinical and audiometric contemporaneous and situation-specific experience'.

With regard to the issue of *changing sovereignty*, the law (and Standards) in an increasing number of European countries is changing as they progressively relinquish their sovereignty to the EU.

Parties to disputes have become increasingly dissatisfied with litigation as a means of resolving disputes, and resolution other than by litigation, *alternative dispute resolution* has been developed and implemented (Brown and Marriott, 1993). Alternative dispute resolution (arbitration, mediation or conciliation) allows the parties greater control over resolving the issues between them. It encourages problem-solving approaches and provides for more effective settlements.

With regard to the question of *other species,* one reads in national newspapers: 'Mammals such as whales and dolphins appear to use their hearing much as humans use sight – to find food and mates, to guard their young and to avoid predators . . . International shipping generates the most noise . . . Agencies should have the authority to regulate noise' (Whitworth, 1999). The EU has recognized that animals are 'sentient beings' (*New Scientist,* 28 June 1997, p. 11). We should therefore anticipate a future with standards and laws aimed at the protection of species other than humans from the effects of noise.

# Conclusion

This brief chapter indicates that there is a rapidly expanding ensemble of standards and a complexity of laws that are relevant to 'noise and its effects'. Harmonization policies, particularly those of the EU and OIML, are helping to attain a global consistency in measurements, standards and laws in this important field.

# Table of Cases

Andreae v Selfridge [1938] 3 All ER 255
Bartlett v Marshall [1896] 60 JP 104
Bliss v Hall [1838] 4 Bing (NC) 183
Bolitho (Deceased) v City and Hackney HA [1998] AC 232
Christie v Davey [1983] 1 Ch 316
Costa v ENEL Case 6/64 [1964] ECR585 European Court of Justice
Crump v Lambert [1867] LR 3 Eq 409
Halsey v Esso Petroleum Co. Ltd [1961] 2 All ER 145
Harris v James [1876] 45 LJQB 545
Harrison v Metropolitan Police [1972] The Times, 28 March, p. 4
Hoare & Co v McAlpine [1923] 1 Ch 167
Hollywood Silver Fox Farm v Emmett [1936] 1 All ER 825
Leeman v Montague [1936] 2 All ER 1677
Robinson v British Rail Engineering [1982] Court of Appeal (Civil Division) No.
     489 3 November
Rushmore v Polsue and Alfieri Ltd [1906] 1 Ch 234
Sturges v Bridgman [1879] 11 ChD 852
Thompson, Gray and Nicholson v Smiths Shiprepairers (North Shields) Ltd;
     Blacklock and Waggott v Swan Hunter Shipbuilders Ltd; Mitchell v Vickers
     Armstrong Ltd and the Swan Hunter Shipbuilders Ltd [1984] 1 All ER 881
Tinkler v Aylesbury Dairy Co. Limited [1888] The Times Law Report 52
Vanderpant v Mayfair Hotel Co [1930] 1 Ch 138

# References

Abernathy CM Hamm RM (1994a) Surgical Intuition. Philadelphia, PA: Hanley & Belfus.

Abernathy CM, Hamm RM (1994b) Surgical Scripts. Philadelphia, PA: Hanley & Belfus.

Albania: Law on Environmental Protection: www.pace.edu/lawschool/env/albanianlaw/albanianenvironmentalprotection.html (accessed 22 August 2002).

Alberti PW (1981) Compensation for industrial hearing loss: the practice in Canada. In HA Beagley (ed.) Audiology and Audiological Medicine, Vol. 2. Oxford: Oxford University Press, pp. 880–95.

American National Standards Association (1996) ANSI S3.44-1996. American National Standard Determination of Occupational Noise Exposure and Estimation of Noise-Induced Hearing Impairment. New York: ANSI.

Anon (1896) Street noises. Lancet 4 July: 36.

Atiyah PS (1970) Accidents, Compensation and the Law. London: Weidenfeld & Nicolson.

Barrow JD (1999) Impossibility: The limits of science and the science of limits. London: Vintage.

Bell J (1986) The acceptability of legal arguments. In N MacCormick, P Birks (eds) The Legal Mind: Essays for Tony Honoré. Oxford: Clarendon.

Beranek LL (1949) Acoustic Measurements. New York: Wiley.

Berry BF, Porter ND (1994) The evaluation of acoustic features in industrial noise. Proceedings of Inter-noise 94,Yokohama, 29–31 August, pp. 803–8.

Bottéro J (1994) Babylone: A l'aube de notre culture. Paris: Gallimard P 52.

British Medical Association (1981) Medical Evidence: The Report of a Joint Committee Representing the Legal and Medical Professions. London: BMA.

Brown H, Marriott A (1993) ADR Principles and Practice. London: Sweet & Maxwell.

Cardozo BN (1921) The Nature of the Judicial Process. New Haven, CT: Yale University Press.

Cato DM (1999) The Expert in Litigation and Arbitration. London: LLP.

Clement-Evans C (1998) New developments in noise-induced hearing loss. ENT News 7: 28–9.

Clement-Evans C (1999) Cenric Clement-Evans comments . . . . ENTNews 8: 29.

Coles RRA (1967) External meatus closure by audiometer earphone. Journal of Speech and Hearing Disorders 32: 296–7.

Coles RRA, Lutman ME, Robinson DW (1991) The limited accuracy of bone conduction audiometry: its significance in medicolegal assessments. Journal of Laryngology and Otology 105: 518–21.

Coles RRA, Lutman ME, Axelsson A, Hazell JWP (1991) Tinnitus severity gradings: cross-sectional studies. In JM Aran, R Dauman (eds) Tinnitus 91: Fourth International Tinnitus Seminar. Bordeaux: Kugler, pp. 453–5.

Committee on the Problem of Noise (1963) Noise: Final Report. Cmnd 2056. London: HMSO.

Cusack R (1969) Foreword. The Law on Noise. London: Noise Abatement Society.

David R, Jauffret-Spinosi C (1992) Les Grands Systèmes de Droit Contemporains. Paris: Dalloz.

Davis A (1995) Hearing in Adults. London: Whurr.

Davis AC, Roberts H (1996) Tinnitus and health status: SF36 profile and accident prevalence. In: GE Reich, JA Vernon (eds) Proceedings of the Fifth International Tinnitus Seminar. Portland, OR: American Tinnitus Association.

Department of the Environment, Food and Rural Affairs (UK) Review of Implementation of Noise Act 1996: www.defra.gov.uk/environment/consult/reviewofnoise, accessed 18 August 2002.

Department of the Environment, Transport and the Regions (UK) Report. The report is available on the DETR website at www.dtlr.gov.uk/consult.htm (accessed 18 August 2002).

Department of Health and Social Security (1973) Occupational Deafness: Report by the Industrial Injuries Advisory Council in accordance with Section 62 of the National Insurance (Industrial Injuries) Act 1965 on the Question whether there are Degrees of Hearing Loss Due to Noise which Satisfy the Conditions for Prescription under the Act. Cmnd 5461. London: HMSO.

Departmental Committee on Compensation for Industrial Diseases (1907) Report. London: HMSO.

Dobie RA (1993) Medical-Legal Evaluation of Hearing Loss. New York: Van Nostrand Reinhold.

Dunea G (1997) Diagnosing Trees and Men. British Medical Journal 315: 434.

Du Plessis LM (1992) Inleiding tot die Reg. Cape Town: Juta.

Dyson, Mr Justice (1998) Official referees: not that sort of match. The Times 13 October: 39.

Erlandsson SI, Hallberg LRM, Axelsson A (1992) Psychological and audiological correlates of perceived tinnitus severity. Audiology 31: 168–79.

European Commission (1996) Future Noise Policy: Green Paper (COM(96) 540 Final). Brussels: EC.

European Commission (2000) Proposal for a Directive of the European Parliament and of the Council relating to the Assessment and Management of Environmental Noise (COM(2000) 468 Final). Brussels: EC.

Friston M (1999) New rules for expert witnesses: the last shots of the medicolegal hired gun. British Medical Journal 316: 1365–6.

Gatehouse S, Noble W (2004) The Speech, Spatial and Qualities of Hearing Scale (SSQ). International Journal of Audiology 43: 85–99.

Gunsteren HR van (1999) When noise becomes too much noise . . . . Noise and Health 3: 3–5.

Hand DJ (1996) Statistics and the theory of measurement. Journal of the Royal Statistical Society Series A 159: 445–92.

Harris CM (1998) Handbook of Acoustical Measurements and Noise Control. New York: Springer.

Haughton PM (1980) Physical Principles of Audiology. Bristol: Adam Hilger.

Haughton PM (2002) Acoustics for Audiologists. New York: Academic Press P 329.

Hepple BA, Matthews MH (1991) Tort: Cases and Materials. London: Butterworths.

Hétu R, Getty L, Philbert L, Desilets F, Noble W, Stephens D (1994) Mise au point d'un outil clinique pour la mesure d'incapacités et de handicaps. Journal of Speech–Language Pathology and Audiology 18: 83–95.

Hinchcliffe R (2000a) Effects of noise on hearing – aspects of assessment: guidelines for giving advice to expert witnesses. Journal of Audiological Medicine 9: 1–18.

Hinchcliffe R (2000b) Expert witnesses need controls. Proceedings of 13th World Congress on Medical Law, Helsinki, Vol. I, pp. 486–96.

Hinchcliffe R (2002) The clinical picture of noise induced hearing loss – the historical perspective. Journal of Audiological Medicine 11: 63–74, 136–44.

Hinchcliffe R (2003a) Ethics, law and related matters. In L Luxon, A Martini, J Furman, D Stephens (eds) A Textbook of Audiological Medicine: Clinical aspects of hearing and balance. London: Martin Dunitz, Chapter 9.

Hinchcliffe R (2003b) The threshold of hearing. In L Luxon, A Martini, J Furman, D Stephens (eds) A Textbook of Audiological Medicine: Clinical aspects of hearing and balance. London: Martin Dunitz, Chapter 11.

Hinchcliffe R (2003c) Aspects of the paracuses. In L Luxon, A Martini, J Furman, D Stephens (eds) A Textbook of Audiological Medicine: Clinical aspects of hearing and balance. London: Martin Dunitz, Chapter 38.

Hinchcliffe R, Bellman S (1997) Legal and ethical matters. In D Stephens (ed.) Scott-Brown's Otolaryngology, 6th edn, Vol. 2. Adult Audiology. London: Butterworth-Heinemann, Chapter 7.

Hinchcliffe R, Luxon LM, Williams RG (2001) Noise and Hearing, Vol. 1. London: Whurr.

Hunt FV (1978) Origins in Acoustics. New Haven: Yale University Press.

Jenkinson C, Coulter A, Wright L (1993) Short form 36 (SF36) health survey questionnaire: normative data for adults of working age. British Medical Journal 306: 1437–500.

Jones MA (1994) Textbook on Torts. London: Blackstone.

Lasch R (1908) Der Eid. Seine Enstehung und Beziehung zu Glaube und Brauch der Naturvölker. Eine ethnologische Studie. Stuttgart: Von Strecker & Schröder.

Law Society and the British Medical Association (1993) Medical Evidence: Guidance for doctors and lawyers. London: The Law Society and the BMA.

Lutman ME (1996) Estimation of noise-induced hearing impairment for compound noise exposures based on ISO 1999. Journal of Audiological Medicine 5: 1–7.

Lutman ME, Qasem HYN (1998) A source of audiometric notches at 6 kHz. In D Prasher, L Luxon (eds) Advances in Noise Research, Vol. 1. London: Whurr.

Luxon LM (1998) The clinical diagnosis of noise-induced hearing loss. In D Prasher, L Luxon (eds) Advances in Noise Research, Vol. 1. London: Whurr.

MacDermott J (1997) A judicial point of view with regard to the testimony of medical experts. Medicine and Law 16: 635–42.

Mackenzie IJ (1997) Noise-induced deafness and compensation. Proceedings of WHO-PDH Informal Consultation on Prevention of Noise-induced Hearing Loss, Geneva 28–30 October 1997. Geneva: World Health Organization.

Macrae JH, Piesse RA (1981) Compensation for occupational hearing loss: the practice in Australia. In HA Beagley (ed.) Audiology and Audiological Medicine, Vol. 2. Oxford: Oxford University Press, pp. 896–909.

Mahoney CF, Luxon LM (1996) Misdiagnosis of hearing loss due to ear canal collapse: a report of two cases. Journal of Laryngology and Otology 110: 561–6.

Malta Standards Authority, www.msa.org.mt/standards/index.htm

Mellinkoff D (1963) The Language of the Law. Boston, MA: Little Brown.

Merluzzi F, Hinchcliffe R (1973) Threshold of subjective auditory handicap. Audiology 12: 65–9.

Oppenheimer A (1994) The Relationship Between European Community Law and National Law: The Cases. Cambridge: Cambridge University Press.

Perlman HB (1941) Acoustic trauma in man: clinical and experimental studies. Archives of Otolaryngology 34: 429–52.

Porter ND (1995) The Assessment of Industrial Noise – Subjective Listening Tests and Objective Assessment Procedures. NPL Report RSA(EXT) 0057A. Teddington, Middlesex: National Physical Laboratory, p 18.

Robinson DW (1976) Characteristics of noise-induced hearing loss. In D Henderson, RP Hamernik, DS Dosanjh, JH Mills (eds) Effects of Noise on Hearing. New York: Raven, pp 383–94.

Robinson DW (1987) Noise Exposure and Hearing: A New Look at the Experimental Data. HSE Contract Research Report No. 1/1987. London: Health and Safety Executive.

Robinson DW, Shipton MS (1977) Tables for the Estimation of Noise-induced Hearing Loss. NPL Acoustics Report Ac 61 (2nd). Teddington, Middlesex: National Physical Laboratory.

Russotto J (1990) The key role of standardization in the European Community. Journal of Medicine 42: 46.

Samuels G (1998) Medical truth and legal proof. Medical Journal of Australia 168: 84–7.

Silving H (1959) The oath. Yale Law Journal 68: 1329–90, 1527–77.

Sintonen H (2001) The 15D instrument of health-related quality of life: properties and applications. Annals of Medicine 33: 328–36.

Slapper G (1998) The curse of Clinton and Aitken. The Times 13 October: 39

Smith AFM (1996) Mad cows and ecstasy: chance and choice in an evidence-based society. Journal of the Royal Statistical Society A 159: 367–83.

Steiner J (1994) Textbook on EC Law. London: Blackstone.

Stephens SDG (1976) The input for a damaged cochlea. British Journal of Audiology 10: 97–101.

Stephens SDG (2003) Audiological rehabilitation. In LM Luxon, JM Furman, A Martini, D Stephens (eds) Textbook of Audiological Medicine. London: Martin Dunitz, pp. 513–31.

Sulkowski WJ (1980) Industrial Noise Pollution and Hearing Impairment. Warsaw: Foreign Scientific Publications Department of the National Center for Scientific, Technical and Economic Information.

Svensson E (1998) Ordinal invariant measures for individual and group changes in ordered categorical data. Statistics in Medicine 17: 2923–36.

Tempest W, Bryan ME (1981) Industrial Hearing Loss: Compensation in the United Kingdom. In HA Beagley (ed.) Audiology and Audiological Medicine Volume 2. Oxford: OUP.

Terminologia Anatomica (1998) Stuttgart: Thieme.

Ware JE (1993) The SF36 Health Survey: Manual and interpretation guide. Boston, MA: Nimrod Press.

Whitworth D (1999) Sea life is deeply troubled by noise. The Times 29 June: 14.

WHOQOL Group (1994) Development of the WHOQOL: rationale and current status. International Journal of Mental Health 23: 24–56.

Williams RG (1992) The evaluation of hearing impairment. Journal of Audiological Medicine 1: 156–60.

Wilson C, Lewis P, Stephens D (2002) The short form 36 (SF36) in a specialist tinnitus clinic. International Journal of Audiology 41: 216–20.

World Health Organization (1999) WHOQOL-100 and the WHOQOL-BREF. Geneva: The WHOQOL Group, Programme on Mental Health, WHO.

World Health Organization (2001) International Classification of Functioning, Disability and Health. Geneva: WHO (www.who.int/classification/icf).

# Appendix A: glossary (abbreviations and definitions)

15D: (Sintonen 2001)

accreditation: a formal recognition of competence

accreditation, metrological (of a laboratory): is granted when measurement competence is demonstrated in all of the laboratory's technical practices

accuracy of measurement: the closeness of the agreement between the result of a measurement and the true value of the *measurand* (VIM 3.5)

ADR: alternative dispute resolution

AFNOR: l'Association Française de Normalisation

ANSI: American National Standards Institute (successor to ASA); equivalent in the USA to BSI

APLMF: Asia-Pacific Legal Metrology Forum

Asia–Pacific Legal Metrology Forum: a grouping of legal metrology authorities in the Asia–Pacific Economic Cooperation (APEC) economies and other economies on the Pacific Rim founded in 1994, see www.aplmf.org

Association Française de Normalisation: the French standardization institute

BIML: Bureau International de Métrologie Légale

BIPM: Bureau International des Poids et Mesures

BS: British Standard

BSI: British Standards Institution (the national body in the UK dealing with Standards)

Bureau International de Métrologie Légale: the secretariat and headquarters of the OIML was established in 1955 in order to promote the global harmonization of legal metrology procedures

Bureau International des Poids et Mesures: the international secretariat and headquarters relating to weights and measures

Canadian General Standards Board: the Canadian standards development, certification and registration organization

CCN: Conseil Canadien des Normes (synonym SCC)

CD: (1) Compact Disc; (2) Committee Draft (an International Standards document type)

CDV: Committee Draft for Vote (IEC) (an International Standards document type)

CE: Conformité Européene (European Conformity). The CE marking on a product is a manufacturer's declaration that the product complies with the essential requirements of the relevant European health, safety and environmental protection legislations, in practice by many of the so-called Product Directives

CEN: Comité Européen de Normalisation (European Committee for Standardization)

CENELEC: Comité Européen de Normalisation Eléctrotechnique

CGPM: Conférence Générale des Poids et Mesures

CGSB: Canadian General Standards Board

CIPM: Comité International des Poids et Mesures

Code of Practice: a standard of good practice; it may or may not be in the form of a national standard

Comité Européen de Normalisation: European Committee for Standardization, which prepares European Standards (ENs) in the three official languages

(English, French and German); these standards must be implemented by all national member committees

Convention du Mètre: founded the Bureau International des Poids et Mesures (BIPM) and gave authority to the BIPM, the Conférence Générale des Poids et Mesures (CGPM) and the Comité International des Poids et Mesures (CIPM) to act in matters of world metrology, particularly concerning the demand for measurement standards of ever-increasing accuracy, range and diversity, and the need to demonstrate equivalence between national measurement standards

DEFRA: Department of the Environment, Food and Rural Affairs (UK)

DETR: Department of the Environment, Transport and the Regions (UK)

Deutsches Institut für Normung: the German Standardization Institute

DHSS: Department of Health and Social Security (subsequently split into the Department of Health and the Department of Social Security)

DIN: Deutsches Institut für Normung

Directive: an EC measure that is binding 'as to the results to be achieved, upon each member State to which it is addressed' but allows states a discretion as to the form and method of implementation. Directives are published in the *Official Journal of the European Communities* in the L series. A considerable number have now appeared on environmental noise, beginning with 70/157/EEC which applies to motor vehicles

DIS: Draft International Standard

dispersion: the spread of values obtained from a particular measurement

DSS: Department of Social Security (UK)

DTI: Department of Trade and Industry (UK)

EC: European Community/Communities (successor of EEC)

EEC: European Economic Community (succeeded by EC)

EFTA: European Free Trade Association. The Stockholm Convention establishing the Association came into force on 3 May 1960. With the accession of Austria, Denmark, Finland, Portugal, Sweden and the UK to the EU, EFTA has been reduced to Iceland, Liechstenstein, Norway and Switzerland

EMC: electromagnetic compatibility

EN: European Standard

ENV: European prestandard

EOTC: European Organization for Testing and Certification

ETSI: European Telecommunications Standards Institute (produces telecommunications standards that are needed for EU legislation)

EU: European Union

European Cooperation in Legal Metrology: founded in Switzerland in 1990 when a Memorandum of Understanding (MoU) was signed by representatives of 18 national legal metrology authorities in European Union and EFTA member states. Originally given the acronym WELMEC (Western European Legal Metrology Cooperation) but now extends beyond western Europe and includes representatives from central and eastern Europe

European prestandard: (Europäische Vornorm; Prénorme Européenne) is prepared as a prospective standard for provisional application in areas of technology where there is a high level of innovation or where an urgent need for guidance is felt and where safety of persons and goods is not involved

European standard: ('Euronorm'; Europäische Norm; Norme Européenne) a standard issued by CEN

FCAT: Federative Committee on Anatomical Terminology

FDIS: Final Draft International Standard (an International Standards document type)

Federative Committee on Anatomical Terminology: the body elected at the General Assembly of the Federative World Congress of Anatomy held in 1989 in Rio de Janeiro to: 'present the official terminology of the anatomical sciences after consultation with all the members (56) of the International Federation of Associations of Anatomists, thus ensuring a democratic input to the terminology.' Produced the *Terminologia Anatomica*

GUM: Guide to the Expression of Uncertainty in Measurement (ISO).

HA: (1) hearing aid; (2) health authority

harmonization document (Harmonisierungsdokument; document d'harmonisation): is drawn up in same way as a European Standard but its application is more flexible so that a particular national condition pertaining to some countries can be taken into account

harmonized standards: the technical specifications (European standards or harmonization documents) that have been established by several European standards agencies (CEN, CENELEC, ETSI)

HD: harmonization document

HDHS: hearing disabilities and handicap scale (Hétu et al., 1994)

HELA: Health and Safety Executive/Local Authorities Enforcement Liaison Committee (UK)

HL: hearing level

HPD: hearing protective device

HSE: Health and Safety Executive (UK)

HTL: hearing threshold level

IAF: International Accreditation Forum Inc.

IEC: International Electrotechnical Commission

ILAC: International Laboratory Accreditation Cooperation

IMPEL: European Union Network for the Implementation and Enforcement of Environmental Law, an informal network of environmental authorities of the member states of the EU

inspection: activities such as measuring, examining, testing, gauging one or more characteristics of a product or service and comparing these with specified requirements to determine conformity (ISO 9000-2000 3.14)

International Electrotechnical Commission: the international body that deals with setting standards in the field of electrical technology; based in Geneva

International Organization for Standardization: the international body including standards groups from many countries that develops standards for goods and services to facilitate international trade and exchange

International Recommendation: a model regulation issued by OIML, which provides members with an internationally agreed basis for the establishment of national legislation on one or other category of measuring instrument

ISO: International Organization for Standardization

legal metrology: the entirety of the legislative, administrative and technical procedures established by, or by reference to, public authorities, and implemented on their behalf in order to specify and to ensure, in a regulatory or contractual manner, the appropriate quality and credibility of measurements related to official controls, trade, health, safety and the environment

LF: low frequency

loudness: the subjective dimension of the objective (physical) dimension of sound (intensity, pressure); unit is the sone; as a rule of thumb, a 1-dB increase in the SPL of a noise gives a 10% increase in loudness; a 10-dB increase produces a doubling of the loudness

Malta Standards Authority: The national standards organization for Malta. The Standardization Directorate was set up under the Malta Standards Authority (MSA) Act 2000 by Legal Notice 213 of 2000 (Malta Standards Authority 2004)

mean: the arithmetic mean (colloquially termed the 'average') is the sum of all the observations divided by the number of observations. In hearing surveys, the difference between 'mean' and 'median' hearing level can be significant. The mean, however, gives a better description of the sample when supplemented with standard deviations. Mean HTLs are particularly sensitive to clinical rejection criteria

measurand: a particular quantity subject to measurement (VIM 2.6)

mel: the unit of pitch; 1000 mels is the pitch of a 1000-Hz tone at a sensation level of 40 dB

metrology: the branch of science concerned with measurement

MoU: Memorandum of Understanding

NAMAS: National Accreditation of Measurement and Sampling (an NPL-supervised calibration scheme)

National Physical Laboratory: the UK's national meteorological centre

noy: the unit (subjective) of noisiness, parallels the sone for loudness; thus a sound of 4 noys is four times as noisy as a sound of one noy

NPL: (1) National Physical Laboratory; (2) noise pollution level

NS: Norsk Standard (Norwegian Standard)

NSSN: originally termed the National Standards Systems Network, and now the National Resource for Global Standards (USA)

OIML: Organisation Internationale de Métrologie Légale

ONGC: L'Office des Normes Générales du Canada (synonym CGSB)

ONIHL: occupational noise-induced hearing loss

Organisation Internationale de Métrologie Légale: an intergovernmental treaty organization established in 1955 to promote the global harmonization of legal metrology procedures

Product Directives: the 'essential requirements' and/or 'performance levels' and 'Harmonized Standards' to which products must conform (EU)

quality: the totality of features and characteristics of a product or service that bear on its ability to satisfy stated or implied needs (ISO 9000-2000 3.1)

quality assurance: all those planned and systematic actions necessary to provide adequate confidence that a product or service will satisfy given requirements for quality (ISO 9000-2000 3.6)

quality loop: conceptual model of interacting activities that influence the quality of a product or service in the various stages, ranging from the identification of needs to the assessment of whether these needs have been satisfied (ISO 9000-2000 3.3)

quality of life: the degree to which an individual perceives himself able to function physically, emotionally and socially; it is thus a subjective measure

quality spiral: synonym quality loop

reference equivalent threshold force level: at a specified frequency, the *mean value of the equivalent threshold force levels* of a sufficiently large number of ears of *otologically normal persons*, of both sexes, aged between 18 and 30 years, expressing the hearing threshold in a specified mechanical coupler for a specified configuration of bone vibrator

reference equivalent threshold sound pressure level: at a specified frequency, the modal value of the *equivalent threshold sound pressure levels* of a sufficiently large number of ears of *otologically normal persons*, of both sexes, aged between 18 and 30 years inclusive, expressing the threshold of hearing in a specified *acoustic coupler* or *artificial ear* for a specified type of earphone

reference zero: a point on a scale of measurement to which all other measurements on that scale are referred; there will thus be values (at least in theory) both above (denoted as '+' values) and below (denoted as '−' values) that point; values other than zero do not necessarily denote values that are abnormal since the reference zero itself does not predicate a range of normality, let alone what is that range

reference zero, standard: a reference zero which has been set by one or other national or international standards institute, e.g. the British Standards Institution, the International Organization for Standardization; specifications exist for a standard reference zero for the calibration of pure-tone air (BS EN ISO 389-1:2000) and bone-conduction (BS ISO 389-3:1994) audiometers

RETFL: reference equivalent threshold force level (in dB re 1 (N))

RETSPL: reference equivalent threshold sound pressure level (in dB re 20 (Pa))

SCC: Standards Council of Canada

SF36: Short Form 36 health survey questionnaire (Jenkinson et al., 1993; Ware, 1993; Davis and Roberts 1996; Wilson et al., 2002)

SI: (1) the international abbreviation for Le Système International d'Unités; (2) statutory instrument

SLM: sound level meter

sone: the unit of loudness

specification: the document that prescribes the requirements with which the product or service has to conform (ISO 9000-2000 3.22)

SPL: sound pressure level

SSQ: Speech, Spatial and Qualities of Hearing Scale (Gatehouse and Noble, 2004)

Standard: a good definition has been given by the Malta Standards Authority (2004), i.e. a document defining the characteristics (for example, dimensions, safety aspects, performance requirements) of a product, process or service, in line with the technical/technological state-of-the art.

standard deviation: a measure of statistical dispersion. It is the square root of the variance. It is defined this way in order to give a measure of dispersion that is (a) a non-negative number; and (b) has the same units as the data.

standardization: activity of establishing, with regard to actual or potential problems, provisions for common and repeated use, aimed at the achievement of the optimum degree of order in a given context (BS 0−1: 1997).

statutory instrument: the most important form of delegated legislation (UK and other common law states)

Système International d'Unités: International System of Units; this international system, based on the MKS system, was initially proposed by the Italian physicist, Giorgi, in 1901, recommended by the IEC Advisory Committee on Nomenclature in 1935, and endorsed by the IEC and other international science bodies in 1938

TAG: Technical Advisory Group (ISO)

TC: technical committee

TCC: Technology and Construction Court (UK)

*Terminologia Anatomica*: (1998 successor of *Nomina Anatomica*)

traceability: the ability to trace the history, application or location of an item or activity, or similar items or activities, by means of recorded identification. (1) The term 'traceability' may have one of three main meanings: (a) in a distribution sense, it relates to a product or service; (b) in a calibration sense, it relates measuring equipment to national or international standards, primary standards or basic physical constants or properties; or (c) in a data collection sense, it relates calculations and data generated throughout the quality loop to a product or service. (2) Traceability requirements should be specified for some stated period of history or to some point of origin (ISO 9000-2000 3.15)

TSQ: tinnitus severity questionnaire (Coles, Lutman, Axelsson and Hazell, 1991; Erlandsson,Hallberg and Axelsson, 1992)

TUC: Trades Union Congress

UKAS: United Kingdom Accreditation Service

United Kingdom Accreditation Service: UK national body responsible for assessing and accrediting the competence of organizations in the fields of calibration, measurement, testing and inspection, and the certification of systems, personnel and products. The UKAS-accredited calibration laboratories represent the main focus for traceable calibration in the UK, acting as local guarantors of measurement quality. The NPL operates a UKAS-accredited calibration laboratory (No. 0478)(www. ukas.org.)

variance: the mean value of the squared deviations from the mean.

VIM: *vocabulaire international des termes fondamentaux et généraux de métrologie.*

*Vocabulaire international des termes fondamentaux et généraux de metrologie*: International vocabulary of basic and general terms in metrology. Geneva: International Organization for Standardization, 1993 (abbrev VIM)

WELMEC: European Cooperation in Legal Metrology

WG: working group

WHO: World Health Organization

WHOQOL-100: WHO's Quality-of-Life Scale – long form (WHO, 1999)

WHOQOL-BREF: WHO's Quality-of-Life Scale – short form (WHO, 1999)


# Appendix B: some ISO standards relating to noise and vibration control

ISO 16: 1975 Acoustics – Standard tuning frequency (Standard musical pitch).

ISO 31-7: 1992 Quantities and units – Part 7: Acoustics.

ISO 140-1: 1997 Acoustics – Measurement of sound insulation in buildings and of building elements – Part 1: Requirements for laboratory test facilities with suppressed flanking transmission.

ISO 140-2: 1991 Acoustics – Measurement of sound insulation in buildings and of building elements – Part 2: Determination, verification and application of precision data.

ISO 140-3: 1995 Acoustics – Measurement of sound insulation in buildings and of building elements – Part 3: Laboratory measurements of airborne sound insulation of building elements.

ISO 140-4: 1998 Acoustics – Measurement of sound insulation in buildings and of building elements – Part 4: Field measurements of airborne sound insulation between rooms.

ISO 140-5: 1998 Acoustics – Measurement of sound insulation in buildings and of building elements – Part 5: Field measurements of airborne sound insulation of façade elements and façades.

ISO 140-6: 1998 Acoustics – Measurement of sound insulation in buildings and of building elements – Part 6: Laboratory measurements of impact sound insulation of floors.

ISO 140-7: 1998 Acoustics – Measurement of sound insulation in buildings and of building elements – Part 7: Field measurements of impact sound insulation of floors.

ISO 140-8: 1997 Acoustics – Measurement of sound insulation in buildings and of building elements – Part 8: Laboratory measurements of the reduction of transmitted impact noise by floor coverings on a heavyweight standard floor.

ISO 140-9: 1985 Acoustics – Measurement of sound insulation in buildings and of building elements – Part 9: Laboratory measurement of room-to-room airborne sound insulation of a suspended ceiling with a plenum above it.

ISO 140-10: 1991 Acoustics – Measurement of sound insulation in buildings and of building elements – Part 10: Laboratory measurement of airborne sound insulation of small building elements.

ISO 140-12: 2000 Acoustics – Measurement of sound insulation in buildings and of building elements – Part 12: Laboratory measurement of room-to-room airborne and impact sound insulation of an access floor.

ISO 226: 2003 Acoustics – Normal equal-loudness contours.

ISO 266: 1997 Acoustics – Preferred frequencies.

ISO 362: 1998 Acoustics – Measurement of noise emitted by accelerating road vehicles – Engineering method.

ISO 389-1: 1998 Acoustics – Reference zero for the calibration of audiometric equipment – Part 1: Reference equivalent threshold sound pressure levels for pure tones and supra-aural earphones.

ISO 389-2: 1994 Acoustics – Reference zero for the calibration of audiometric equipment – Part 2: Reference equivalent threshold sound pressure levels for pure tones and insert earphones.

ISO 389-3: 1994 (Cor 1: 1995) Acoustics – Reference zero for the calibration of audiometric equipment – Part 3: Reference equivalent threshold force levels for pure tones and bone vibrators.

ISO 389-4: 1994 Acoustics – Reference zero for the calibration of audiometric equipment – Part 4: Reference levels for narrow-band masking noise.

ISO/TR 389-5: 1998 Acoustics – Reference zero for the calibration of audiometric equipment – Part 5: Reference equivalent threshold sound pressure levels for pure tones in the frequency range 8 kHz to 16 kHz.

ISO 389-7: 1996 Acoustics – Reference zero for the calibration of audiometric equipment – Part 7: Reference threshold of hearing under free-field and diffuse-field listening conditions.

ISO 389-8: 2004 Acoustics – Reference zero for the calibration of audiometric equipment – Part 8: Reference equivalent threshold sound pressure levels for pure tones and circumaural earphones.

ISO 532: 1975 Acoustics – methods for calculating the loudness of noises.

ISO 717-1: 1996 Acoustics – Rating of sound insulation in buildings and of building elements – Part 1: Airborne sound insulation.

ISO 717-2: 1996 Acoustics – Rating of sound insulation in buildings and of building elements – Part 2: Impact sound insulation.

ISO 1000: 1992 SI units and recommendations for the use of their multiples and of certain other units.

ISO 1680: 1999 Acoustics – Test code for the measurement of the airborne noise emitted by rotating electrical machines.

ISO 1683: 1983 Acoustics – Preferred reference quantities for acoustic levels.

ISO 1996-1: 1982 Acoustics – Description and measurement of environmental noise – Part 1: Basic quantities and procedures.

ISO 1996-2: 1987 (Amd 1: 1998) Acoustics – Description and measurement of environmental noise –Part 2: Acquisition of data pertinent to land use.

ISO 1996-3: 1987 Acoustics – Description and measurement of environmental noise –Part 3: Application to noise limits.

ISO 1999: 1990 Acoustics – Determination of occupational noise exposure and estimation of noise-induced hearing impairment.

ISO 2017: 1982 Mechanical vibration and shock – Isolators – Procedure.

ISO 2631-1: 1997 Mechanical vibration and shock – Evaluation of human exposure to whole-body vibration – Part 1: General requirements.

ISO 2631-2: 1989 Mechanical vibration and shock – Evaluation of human exposure to whole-body vibration – Part 2: Continuous and shock-induced vibrations in buildings (1 to 80 Hz).

ISO 2631-4: 2001 Mechanical vibration and shock – Evaluation of human exposure to whole-body vibration – Part 4: Guidelines for the evaluation of the effects of vibration and rotational motion on passenger and crew comfort in fixed-guideway transport systems.

ISO 2922: 2000 Acoustics – Measurement of airborne sound emitted by vessels on inland waterways and harbours.

ISO 2923: 1996 Acoustics – Measurement of noise on board vessels.

ISO 3095: 1975 Acoustics – Measurement of noise emitted by railbound vehicles.

ISO/TR 3352: 1974 Acoustics – Assessment of noise with respect to its effect on the intelligibility of speech.

ISO 3381: 1976 Acoustics – Measurement of noise inside railbound vehicles.

ISO 3382: 1997 Acoustics – Measurement of the reverberation time of rooms with reference to other acoustical parameters.

ISO 3534-1: 1993 Statistics – Vocabulary and symbols – Part 1: Probability and general statistical terms.

ISO 3534-2: 1993 Statistics – Vocabulary and symbols – Part 2: Statistical quality control.

ISO 3534-3: 1999 Statistics – Vocabulary and symbols – Part 3: Design of experiments.

ISO 3740: 2000 Acoustics – Determination of sound power levels of noise sources – Guidelines for the use of basic standards.

ISO 3741: 1999 Acoustics – Determination of sound power levels of noise sources using sound pressure – Precision methods for reverberation rooms.

ISO 3743–1: 1994 Acoustics – Determination of sound power levels of noise sources – Engineering methods for small, movable sources in reverberant fields – Part 1: Comparison method for hard-walled test rooms.

ISO 3743–2: 1994 Acoustics –Determination of sound power levels of noise sources using sound pressure – Engineering methods for small, movable sources in reverberant fields – Part 2: Methods for special reverberation test rooms.

ISO 3744: 1994 Acoustics – Determination of sound power levels of noise sources using sound pressure – Engineering method in an essentially free-field over a reflecting plane.

ISO 3745: 1977 Acoustics –Determination of sound power levels of noise sources – Precision methods for anechoic and semi-anechoic rooms.

ISO 3746: 1995 Acoustics – Determination of sound power levels of noise sources using sound pressure – Survey method using an enveloping measurement surface over a reflecting plane.

ISO 3747: 2000 Acoustics – Determination of sound power levels of noise sources using sound pressure – Comparison method for use in situ.

ISO 3822-1: 1999 Acoustics – Laboratory tests on noise emission from appliances and equipment used in water supply installations – Part 1: Method of measurement.

ISO 3822-2: 1995 Acoustics – Laboratory tests on noise emission from appliances and equipment used in water supply installations – Part 2: Mounting and operating conditions for draw-off taps and mixing valves.

EN ISO 3822-3: 1997 Acoustics – Laboratory tests on noise emission from appliances and equipment used in water supply installations – Part 3: Mounting and operating conditions for in-line valves and appliances.

EN ISO 3822-4: 1997 Acoustics – Laboratory tests on noise emission from appliances and equipment used in water supply installations – Part 4: Mounting and operating conditions for special appliances.

ISO 3891: 1978 Acoustics – Procedure for describing aircraft noise heard on the ground.

ISO 4412: 1991 Acoustics – Test code for the determination of airborne noise levels in pumps and motors.

ISO 4866: 1990 Mechanical vibration and shock – Evaluation and measurement for vibration in buildings. Guide for measurement of vibrations and evaluation of their effects on buildings.

ISO 4869-1: 1990 Acoustics – Hearing protectors – Part 1: Subjective method for the measurement of sound attenuation.

ISO 4869-2: 1994 Acoustics – Hearing protectors – Part 2: Estimation of effective A-weighted sound pressure levels when hearing protectors are worn.

ISO/TR 4869-3: 1989 Acoustics – Hearing protectors – Part 3: Simplified method for the measurement of insertion loss of ear-muff type protectors for quality inspection purposes.

ISO/TR 4869-4: 1998 Acoustics – Hearing protectors – Part 4: Measurement of effective sound pressure levels for level-dependent sound-restoration ear-muffs.

ISO/TR 4870: 1991 Acoustics – The construction and calibration of speech intelligibility tests.

ISO 4871: 1996 Acoustics – Declaration and verification of noise emission values of machinery and equipment.

ISO 4872: 1978 Acoustics – Measurement of airborne noise emitted by construction equipment intended for outdoor use – Method for determining compliance with noise limits.

ISO 5007: 1990 Mechanical vibration and shock – Agricultural wheeled tractors – Operator's seat – Laboratory measurement of transmitted vibration.

ISO 5008: 2002 Mechanical vibration and shock – Agricultural wheeled tractors and field machinery – Measurement of whole-body vibration of the operator.

ISO 5128: 1980 Acoustics – Measurement of noise inside motor vehicles.

ISO 5129: 2001 Acoustics – Measurement of sound pressure levels in the interior of aircraft during flight.

ISO 5130: 1982 Acoustics – Measurement of noise emitted by stationary road vehicles – Survey method.

ISO 5131: 1996 Acoustics – Tractors and machinery for agriculture and forestry – Measurement of noise at the operator's position – Survey method.

ISO 5135: 1997 Acoustics – Determination of sound power levels of noise from air-terminal devices, air-terminal units, dampers and valves by measurement in a reverberation room.

ISO 5136: 1990 Acoustics – Determination of sound power radiated into a duct by fans – In-duct method.

ISO 5349-1: 2001 Mechanical vibration – Measurement and evaluation of human exposure to hand-transmitted vibration – Part 1: General requirements.

ISO 5349-2: 2001 Mechanical vibration – Measurement and evaluation of human exposure to hand-transmitted vibration – Part 2: Practical guidance for measurement at the workplace.

ISO 5725-1:1994 Accuracy (trueness and precision) of measurement methods and results — Part 1: General principles and definitions.

ISO 5725-1:1994/Cor 1:1998.

ISO 5725-2:1994 Accuracy (trueness and precision) of measurement methods and results — Part 2: Basic method for the determination of repeatability and reproducibility of a standard measurement method.

ISO 5725-2:1994/Cor 1:2002.

ISO 5725-3:1994 Accuracy (trueness and precision) of measurement methods and results — Part 3: Intermediate measures of the precision of a standard measurement method.

ISO 5725-3:1994/Cor 1:2001.

ISO 5725-4:1994 Accuracy (trueness and precision) of measurement methods and results — Part 4: Basic methods for the determination of the trueness of a standard measurement method (available in English only).

ISO 5725-5:1998 Accuracy (trueness and precision) of measurement methods and results — Part 5: Alternative methods for the determination of the precision of a standard measurement method.

ISO 5725-6:1994 Accuracy (trueness and precision) of measurement methods and results — Part 6: Use in practice of accuracy values.

ISO 5725-6:1994/Cor 1:2001.

ISO 5805: 1997 Mechanical vibration and shock – Human exposure – Vocabulary.

ISO 5982: 2001 Mechanical vibration and shock – Range of idealized values to characterize seated-body biodynamic response under vertical vibration.

ISO 6081: 1986 Acoustics – Noise emitted by machinery and equipment; Guidelines for test codes requiring noise measurement at the operator's or bystander's position.

ISO 6189: 1983 Acoustics – Pure tone air conduction threshold audiometry for hearing conservation purposes.

ISO 6393: 1998 Acoustics – Measurement of exterior noise emitted by earth-moving machinery – Stationary test conditions.

ISO 6394: 1998 Acoustics – Measurement at the operator's position of noise emitted by earth-moving machinery – Stationary test conditions.

ISO 6395: 1988 Acoustics – Measurement of exterior noise emitted by earth-moving machinery – Dynamic test conditions.

ISO 6396: 1992 Acoustics – Measurement at the operator's position of noise emitted by earth-moving machinery – Dynamic test conditions.

ISO 6897: 1984 Mechanical vibration and shock – Guidelines for the evaluation of the response of occupants of fixed structures, especially buildings and off-shore structures, to low-frequency horizontal motion (0.063 to 1 Hz).

ISO 6926: 2000 Acoustics – Requirements for the performance and calibration of reference sound sources used in the determination of sound power levels.

ISO 7029: 2000 Acoustics – Statistical distribution of hearing thresholds as a function of age.

ISO 7096: 2000 Mechanical vibration and shock – Earth-moving machinery – Laboratory evaluation of operator seat vibration.

ISO 7182: 1984 Acoustics – Measurement at the operator's position of airborne noise emitted by chain saws.

ISO 7188: 1994 Acoustics – Measurement of noise emitted by passenger cars under conditions representative of urban driving.

ISO 7196: 1995 Acoustics– Frequency-weighting characteristic for infrasound measurements.

ISO 7216: 1992 Acoustics – Agricultural and forestry wheeled tractors and self-propelled machines – Measurement of noise emitted when in motion.

ISO 7235: 1991 Acoustics – Measurement procedures for ducted silencers – Insertion loss, flow noise and total pressure loss.

ISO 7505: 1986 Mechanical vibration and shock – Forestry machinery – Chain saws – Measurement of hand-transmitted vibration.

ISO 7574-1: 1985 Acoustics – Statistical methods for determining and verifying stated noise emission values of machinery and equipment – Part 1: General considerations and definitions.

ISO 7574-2: 1985 Acoustics – Statistical methods for determining and verifying stated noise emission values of machinery and equipment – Part 2: Methods for stated values for individual machines.

ISO 7574-3: 1985 Acoustics – Statistical methods for determining and verifying stated noise emission values of machinery and equipment – Part 3: Simple (transition) method for stated values for batches of machines.

ISO 7574-4: 1985 Acoustics – Statistical methods for determining and verifying stated noise emission values of machinery and equipment – Part 4: Methods for stated values for batches of machines.

ISO 7779: 1999 Acoustics – Measurement of airborne noise emitted by information technology and telecommunications equipment.

ISO/TR 7849: 1987 Acoustics – Estimation of airborne noise emitted by machinery using vibration measurement.

ISO 7916: 1989 Mechanical vibration and shock – Forestry machinery – Portable brush-saws – Measurement of hand-transmitted vibration.

ISO 7917: 1987 Acoustics – Measurement at the operator's position of airborne noise emitted by brush saws.

ISO 8041: 1990 Mechanical vibration and shock – Human response to vibration – Measuring instrumentation.

ISO 8041: 1990/Cor 1: 1993.

ISO 8041: 1990/Amd 1: 1999.

ISO 8201: 1987 Acoustics – Audible emergency evacuation signal.

ISO 8253-1: 1989 Acoustics – Audiometric test methods – Part 1: Basic pure tone air and bone conduction threshold audiometry.

ISO 8253-2: 1992 Acoustics – Audiometric test methods – Part 2: Sound field audiometry with pure tone and narrow-band test signals.

ISO 8253-3: 1996 Acoustics – Audiometric test methods – Part 3: Speech audiometry.

ISO 8297: 1994 Acoustics – Determination of sound power levels of multisource industrial plants for evaluation of sound pressure levels in the environment – Engineering method.

ISO 8595: 1989 Statistics – Interpretation of statistical data – Estimation of a median.

ISO 8601: 2000 Data elements and interchange formats – Information interchange – Representation of dates and times.

ISO 8662-1: 1988 Mechanical vibration and shock – Hand-held portable power tools – Measurement of vibrations at the handle – Part 1: General.

ISO 8662-2: 1992 Mechanical vibration and shock – Hand-held portable power tools – Measurement of vibrations at the handle – Part 2: Chipping hammers and riveting hammers.

ISO 8662-3: 1992 Mechanical vibration and shock – Hand-held portable power tools – Measurement of vibrations at the handle – Part 3: Rock drills and rotary hammers.

ISO 8662-3: 1992/Amd 1: 1999.

ISO 8662-4: 1994 Mechanical vibration and shock – Hand-held portable power tools – Measurement of vibrations at the handle – Part 4: Grinders.

ISO 8662-5: 1992 Mechanical vibration and shock – Hand-held portable power tools – Measurement of vibrations at the handle – Part 5: Pavement breakers and hammers for construction work.

ISO 8662-5: 1992/Amd 1: 1999.

ISO 8662-6: 1994 Mechanical vibration and shock – Hand-held portable power tools – Measurement of vibrations at the handle – Part 6: Impact drills.

ISO 8662-7: 1997 Mechanical vibration and shock – Hand-held portable power tools – Measurement of vibrations at the handle – Part 7: Wrenches, screwdrivers and nut runners with impact, impulse or ratchet action.

ISO 8662-8: 1997 Mechanical vibration and shock – Hand-held portable power tools – Measurement of vibrations at the handle – Part 8: Polishers and rotary, orbital and random orbital sanders.

ISO 8662-9: 1996 Mechanical vibration and shock – Hand-held portable power tools – Measurement of vibrations at the handle – Part 9: Rammers.

ISO 8662-10: 1998 Mechanical vibration and shock – Hand-held portable power tools – Measurement of vibrations at the handle – Part 10: Nibblers and shears.

ISO 8662-12: 1997 Mechanical vibration and shock – Hand-held portable power tools – Measurement of vibrations at the handle – Part 12: Saws and files with reciprocating action and saws with oscillating and rotating action.

ISO 8662-13: 1997 Mechanical vibration and shock – Hand-held portable power tools – Measurement of vibrations at the handle – Part 13: Die grinders and tests.

ISO 8662-14: 1996 Mechanical vibration and shock – Hand-held portable power tools – Measurement of vibrations at the handle – Part 14: Stone-working tools and needle scalers.

ISO 9000: 2000 Quality management systems – Fundamentals and vocabulary.

ISO 9001: 2000 Quality management systems – Requirements.

ISO 9053: 1991 Acoustics – Materials for acoustical applications – Determination of airflow resistance.

ISO 9207: 1995 Acoustics – Manually portable chain-saws with internal combustion engine. Determination of sound power levels. Engineering method (grade 2).

ISO 9295: 1988 Acoustics – Measurement of high-frequency noise emitted by computer and business equipment.

ISO 9296: 1988 Acoustics – Declared noise emission values of computer and business equipment.

ISO 9611: 1996 Acoustics – Characterization of sources of structure-borne sound with respect to sound radiation from connected structures – Measurement of velocity at the contact points of machinery when resiliently mounted.

ISO 9612: 1997 Acoustics – Guidelines for the measurement and assessment of exposure to noise in a working environment.

ISO 9613-1: 1993 Acoustics – Attenuation of sound during propagation outdoors – Part 1: Calculation of the absorption of sound by the atmosphere.

ISO 9613-2: 1996 Acoustics – Attenuation of sound during propagation outdoors – Part 2: General method of calculation.

ISO 9614-1: 1993 Acoustics – Determination of sound power levels of noise sources using sound intensity – Part 1: Measurement at discrete points.

ISO 9614-2: 1996 Acoustics – Determination of sound power levels of noise sources using sound intensity – Part 2: Measurement by scanning.

ISO 9614-3: 2002 Acoustics – Determination of sound power levels of noise sources using sound intensity – Part 3: Precision method for measurement by scanning.

ISO 9645: 1990 Acoustics – Measurement of noise emitted by two-wheeled mopeds in motion – Engineering method.

ISO 10302: 1996 Acoustics – Method for the measurement of airborne noise emitted by small air-moving devices.

ISO 10326-1: 1992 Mechanical vibration – Laboratory method for evaluating vehicle seat vibrations – Part 1: Basic requirements.

ISO 10534-1: 1996 Acoustics – Determination of sound absorption coefficient and impedance in impedance tubes – Part 1: Method using standing wave ratio.

ISO 10534-2: 1998 Acoustics – Determination of sound absorption coefficient and impedance in impedance tubes – Part 2: Transfer-function method.

ISO 10843: 1997 Acoustics – Methods for the description and physical measurement of single impulses or series of impulses.

ISO 10844: 1994 Acoustics – Specification of test tracks for the purpose of measuring noise emitted by road vehicles.

ISO 10846-1: 1997 Acoustics and vibration – Laboratory measurement of vibro-acoustic transfer properties of resilient elements – Part 1: Principles and Guidelines.

ISO 10846-2: 1997 Acoustics and vibration – Laboratory measurement of vibro-acoustic transfer properties of resilient elements – Part 2: Dynamic stiffness of elastic supports for translatory motion – Direct method.

ISO 10846-3: 2002 Acoustics and vibration – Laboratory measurement of vibro-acoustic transfer properties of resilient elements – Part 3: Indirect method for determination of the dynamic stiffness of resilient supports for translatory motion.

ISO 10847: 1997 Acoustics – In-situ determination of insertion loss of outdoor noise barriers of all types.

ISO 11094: 1991 Acoustics – Test code for the measurement of airborne noise emitted by power lawn mowers, lawn tractors, lawn and garden tractors, professional mowers, and lawn and garden tractors with mowing attachments.

ISO 11200: 1995 (Cor 1: 1997) Acoustics – Noise emitted by machinery and equipment – Guidelines for the use of basic standards for the determination of emission sound pressure levels at a work station and at other specified positions.

ISO 11201: 1995 (Cor 1: 1997) Acoustics – Noise emitted by machinery and equipment – Measurement of emission sound pressure levels at a work station and at other specified positions – Engineering method in an essentially free field over a reflecting plane.

ISO 11202: 1995 Acoustics – Noise emitted by machinery and equipment – Measurement of emission sound pressure levels at a work station and at other specified positions – Survey method in situ.

ISO 11203: 1995 Acoustics – Noise emitted by machinery and equipment – Determination of emission sound pressure levels at a work station and at other specified positions from the sound power level.

ISO 11204: 1995 (Cor 1: 1997 – applies to French version only) Acoustics – Noise emitted by machinery and equipment – Measurement of emission sound pressure levels at a work station and at other specified positions – Method requiring environmental corrections.

ISO 11546-1: 1995 Acoustics – Determination of sound insulation performances of enclosures – Part 1: Measurements under laboratory conditions (for declaration purposes).

ISO 11546-2: 1995 Acoustics – Determination of sound insulation performances of enclosures – Part 2: Measurements in situ (for acceptance and verification purposes).

ISO 11654: 1997 Acoustics – Sound absorbers for use in buildings – Rating of sound absorption.

ISO/TR 11688-1: 1995 Acoustics – Recommended practice for the design of low-noise machinery and equipment – Part 1: Planning.

ISO/TR 11688-2: 1998 Acoustics – Recommended practice for the design of low-noise machinery and equipment – Part 2: Introduction to the physics of low-noise design.

ISO 11689: 1996 Acoustics – Procedure for the comparison of noise-emission data for machinery and equipment.

ISO 11690-1: 1996 Acoustics – Recommended practice for the design of low-noise workplaces containing machinery – Part 1: Noise control strategies.

ISO 11690-2: 1996 Acoustics – Recommended practice for the design of low-noise workplaces containing machinery – Part 2: Noise control measures.

ISO/TR 11690-3: 1997 Acoustics – Recommended practice for the design of low-noise workplaces containing machinery – Part 3: Sound propagation and noise prediction in workrooms.

ISO 11691: 1995 Acoustics – Measurement of insertion loss of ducted silencers without flow – Laboratory survey method.

ISO 11819-1: 1997 Acoustics – Measurement of the influence of road surfaces on traffic noise – Part 1: Statistical pass-by method.

ISO 11820: 1996 Acoustics – Measurements on silencers in situ.

ISO 11821: 1997 Acoustics – Measurement of the in situ sound attenuation of a removable screen.

ISO 11904-1: 2002 Acoustics – Determination of sound immission from sound sources placed close to the ear – Part 1: Technique using a microphone in a real ear (MIRE technique).

ISO 11957: 1996 Acoustics – Determination of sound insulation performance of cabins – Laboratory and in situ measurements.

ISO 12001: 1996 Acoustics – Noise emitted by machinery and equipment – Rules for the drafting and presentation of a noise test code.

ISO 1214: 2001 Acoustics – Procedures for measurement of real-ear acoustical characteristics of hearing aids.

ISO 13472-1: 2002 Acoustics – Measurement of the sound absorption properties of road surfaces in situ – Part 1: Extended surface method.

ISO 13475-1: 1999 Acoustics – Stationary audible warning devices used outdoors – Part 1: Field measurements for determination of sound emission quantities.

ISO/TS 13475-2: 2000 Acoustics – Stationary audible warning devices used outdoors – Part 2: Precision methods for determination of sound emission quantities.

ISO 13488: 1996 Quality systems – Medical devices – Particular requirements for the application of ISO 9002. Specifies, in conjunction with the application of ISO 9002, the quality system requirements for the production and, when relevant, installation and servicing of medical devices.

ISO 14000 family is primarily concerned with 'environmental management'. This means what the organization does to:
– minimize harmful effects on the environment caused by its activities, and to
– achieve continual improvement of its environmental performance.

ISO 14163: 1998 Acoustics – Guidelines for noise control by silencers.

ISO 14257: 2001 Acoustics – Measurement and parametric description of spatial sound distribution curves in workrooms for evaluation of their acoustical performance.

ISO 15664: 2001 Acoustics – Noise control design procedures for open plant.

ISO 15667: 2000 Acoustics – Guidelines for noise control by enclosures and cabins.

# Appendix C: some IEC standards

IEC 60050-801 (1994-08) International Electrotechnical Vocabulary Chapter 801: Acoustics and electroacoustics.

IEC 60126: 1973 IEC reference coupler for the measurement of hearing aids using earphones coupled to the ear by means of ear inserts (will become IEC 60318-5).

IEC 60268-7 (1996-02) Sound system equipment – Part 7: Headphones and earphones.

IEC 60268-16 (1998-03) Sound system equipment – Part 16: Objective rating of speech intelligibility by speech transmission index.

IEC 60318-1 (1998-07) Electroacoustics – Simulators of human head and ear – Part 1: Ear simulator for the calibration of supra-aural earphones.

IEC 60318-2 (1998-08) Electroacoustics – Simulators of human head and ear – Part 2: An interim acoustic coupler for the calibration of audiometric earphones in the extended high-frequency range.

IEC 60318-3 (1998-08) Electroacoustics – Simulators of human head and ear – Part 3: Acoustic coupler for calibration of supra-aural earphones used in audiometry.

IEC 60318-4 Electroacoustics – Simulators of human head and ear – Part 4: Occluded ear simulator for the measurement of earphones coupled to the ear by ear inserts (will succeed IEC 60711).

IEC 60318-6 Electroacoustics – Simulators of human head and ear – Part 6: Mechanical coupler for measurements on bone vibrators (will succeed IEC 60373 (1990-01)).

IEC 60373 (1990-01) Electroacoustics – Simulators of human head and ear – Part 6: Mechanical coupler for measurements on bone vibrators (will become IEC 60318-6).

IEC 60645-1 (2001-06) Audiological equipment – Part 1: Pure tone audiometers.

IEC 60645-2 (1993-11) Audiometers – Part 2: Equipment for speech audiometry.

IEC 60645-3 (1994-10) Audiometers – Part 3: Auditory test signals of short duration for audiometric and neuro-otological purposes.

IEC 60645-4 (1994-10) Audiometers – Part 4: Equipment for extended high-frequency audiometry. (Specifies requirements for equipment in the frequency range 8 kHz to 16 kHz.)

IEC 60645-5 (2002) Audiological Equipment – Part 5: Instruments for the measurement of aural acoustic impedance/admittance (successor of IEC 61027 (1991)).

IEC 60651:1979 (Amendment 2000.) Specification for sound level meters.

IEC 60711: 1981 Occluded-ear simulator for the measurement of earphones coupled to the ear by means of ear inserts (will become IEC 60318-4).

IEC 60804 (2000-10) Integrating-averaging sound level meters.

IEC 60942 (1997-11) Electroacoustics – Sound calibrators.

IEC 61027 (1991-04) Instruments for the measurement of aural acoustic impedance/admittance.

IEC 61252 (2002-03) Electroacoustics – Specifications for personal sound exposure meters.

IEC 61260 (1995-08) Electroacoustics – Octave-band and fractional-octave-band filters.

IEC 61265 (1995-04) Electroacoustics – Instruments for measurement of aircraft noise – Performance requirements for systems to measure one-third-octave band sound pressure levels in noise certification of transport-category aircraft.

IEC 61672 – 1 (2002-05) Electroacoustics – Sound Level Meters – Part 1: Specifications (supersedes IEC 651 and IEC 804).

IEC 61672 – 2 (2002-11) Electroacoustics – Sound Level Meters – Part 2: Pattern evaluation tests.

## Appendix D: an ISO/IEC Joint Standard

ISO/IEC 17025:1999 General requirements for the competence of testing and calibration laboratories.

# CHAPTER 28

# Preventing hearing loss by sound conditioning

*Noise and Its Effects:* Edited by Linda Luxon and Deepak Prasher © 2007 John Wiley & Sons Ltd.

BARBARA CANLON, XIANZHI NIU

## Introduction

Sound conditioning is an established means of protecting the cochlea against the morphological, functional and molecular consequences induced by acoustic trauma. The purpose of this chapter is to discuss those mechanisms that are most likely to be involved in sound conditioning, including the middle-ear muscles, the medial efferents and the lateral efferents reflex systems.

## Preventing hearing damage induced by acoustic trauma

Unfortunately, the sensory hair cells in mammals do not regenerate following degeneration. Thus, we are left with the hope of discovering strategies to prevent hearing loss. The success of these strategies is being awaited by more than 10% of the global population who have significant hearing loss due to noise, ototoxic drugs, ageing, genetic factors and infection. This amounts to nearly 600 million people who are suffering from hearing loss and communication problems. The economic toll for these disorders is enormous as is the tremendous reduction in the quality of life for the afflicted individuals. Hearing research has recently benefited tremendously from the progress of molecular and pharmacological studies, yet the abundance of information generated from these studies has far surpassed the rate at which it has been clinically implemented. The vital challenge of the coming decade will be the application of these new therapeutic strategies to restore hearing in humans.

Numerous studies have shown that there are a variety of means by which cochlear sensitivity can be either increased or decreased in response

**Table 28.1** Factors that modify cochlear sensitivity to acoustic trauma

| Factor | Effector | Reference |
|--------|----------|-----------|
| Ageing | The young are more sensitive than the old | Henry (1984), Li (1992), Ohlemiller, Wright and Heidbreder (2000) |
| Body temperature | Lowered protects, raised exacerbates | Drescher (1976), Henry and Chole (1984) |
| Preconditioning stressors (heat shock, ischaemia, physical restraint) | Protect | Yoshida, Kristiansen and Liberman (1999), Koga et al. (2003), Wang and Liberman (2002) |
| Medial efferent | Activation protects | Rajan (1988), Cody and Johnstone (1982), Reiter and Liberman (1995), Liberman and Gao (1995), Zheng et al. (1997a) |
| Lateral efferent | Activation protects afferent dendrites | Pujol et al. (1993), Gil-Loyzaga et al. (1994), Gaborjan, Lendvai and Vizi (1999) |
| Blood flow | Lowered exacerbates | Hansen (1988) |
| Sound conditioning | Protects | Canlon, Borg and Flock (1988), McFadden, Henderson and Shen (1997), Ryan et al. (1994), Kujawa and Liberman (1997), Yoshida and Liberman (2000) |
| Stapedius reflex | Activation protects | Margolis (1993) |
| Genetic susceptibility | More sensitive | Li (1992), Gates, Couropmitree and Myers (1999), Erway et al. (1996) |
| Pharmacological substances | Protects | D'Aldin et al. (1995b), Agerman et al. (1999), Duan et al. (2000) |

to acoustic trauma (Table 28.1). For example, young subjects are more sensitive to acoustic trauma than old subjects with normal hearing (Henry, 1984; Li, 1992; Ohlemiller, Wright and Heidbreder, 2000). Altering body temperature modifies the susceptibility of the inner ear to acoustic trauma such that lowered body temperature protects against hearing loss and increased body temperature worsens the effects (Drescher, 1976; Henry and Chole, 1984). It is believed that generalized metabolic processes are the underlying cause for these temperature effects. Whole body heat stress has been shown to increase heat shock protein mRNA in the mouse cochlea and simultaneously to protect against noise trauma (Yoshida, Kristiansen and Liberman, 1999). This finding suggests that sound conditioning can be induced by systemic means and direct activation of cochlea processes may not be necessary. There are two efferent reflex pathways controlling the cochlea. One is the medial efferent system that innervates the contralateral outer hair cells, and the other is the lateral efferent system that innervates primarily the ipsilateral inner hair cells. The medial olivocochlear efferent system is known to protect against noise trauma (Cody and Johnstone, 1982; Rajan, 1988; Reiter and Liberman, 1995). In addition, the lateral efferent system inhibits the excitotoxic effects of glutamate release from the inner hair cells during acoustic overstimulation (Pujol et al., 1993 ). As a consequence, these two efferent reflex pathways are potential candidates for controlling the magnitude of protection against acoustic trauma by sound conditioning. Acoustic overexposure is also known to affect cochlear blood flow through the stria vascularis and these changes will alter intracellular ion concentrations and redox status, which can thereafter elicit an array of stress responses. Finally, pharmacological strategies aimed at oxidative stress, neurotrophic factors and antagonists to glutamate have proven successful in protecting against acoustic trauma.

This chapter will focus on sound conditioning, another example of protecting against noise-induced hearing loss. Sound conditioning consists of exposing animals to a low-level, non-damaging sound exposure prior to an acoustic trauma.

## Sound conditioning

- It is a well-established means of protecting against noise-induced hearing loss.
- It protects against both temporary and permanent noise-induced hearing loss.
- It has also been shown to protect against heredity-related hearing loss.

The phenomenon of sound conditioning is found across a range of mammalian species – guinea pigs, rats, mice, gerbils, chinchillas and, of most interest, humans – and a wide spectrum of sound conditioning paradigms have been established (Table 28.1). The physiological consequence of this preconditioning is protection of the inner ear against an acoustic damage, or hearing loss induced by hereditary factors (Canlon, Borg and Flock, 1988; Miyakita et al., 1992; Kujawa and Liberman, 1997; Zheng et al., 1997a; Yamasoba and Dolan, 1998; Willott and Turner, 1999). As shown in Table 28.2, the most commonly used paradigms for sound conditioning consist of relatively long-term stimuli that are either continuous or intermittent, and presented before the traumatic exposure (Canlon, Borg and Flock, 1988; Ryan et al., 1994; Kujawa and Liberman, 1997; McFadden, Henderson and Shen, 1997). A sound conditioning paradigm as short as 15 minutes has been shown to protect mice against a subsequent hearing loss (Yoshida and Liberman, 2000). Effective conditioning stimuli can include octave band noise (OBN), broadband noise (BBN), pure tones or music. At present, the mechanisms responsible for sound conditioning are not yet known, and focus has been centred around the likely candidates such as the middle-ear muscles, and the medial and the lateral efferent systems. An overview of how these candidates are involved in sound conditioning is presented.

**Table 28.2** Examples of sound conditioning paradigms

| Species | Conditioner | Pause | Trauma | Reference |
|---|---|---|---|---|
| Cat | BBN, 115 dB, 7.5 min, 16 days | 24 hr | | Miller, Watson and Covell (1963) |
| Chinchilla | OBN 0.5 kHz, 95 dB, 6 h/d 10 days | 5 days | Impulse noise, 150 dB | Henselman et al. (1994) |
| Chinchilla | OBN 0.5 kHz, 95 dB, 6 h/days, 10 days | Max 60 days | OBN 0.5 kHz, 106 dB, 48 h | McFadden et al. (1997) |
| Gerbil | OBN (1414–5656 Hz) | Max 3 weeks | OBN (1.4–5.6 Hz) 110 dB, 1 h | Ryan et al. (1994) |
| Gerbil | OBN at 2 kHz, 74 dB, 10 days | 2 hr | OBN at 2 kHz, 107 dB, 48 h | White et al. (1998) |
| Guinea pig | 1kHz, 81 dB, 24 days | none | 1 kHz, 105 dB, 72 h | Canlon, Borg and Flock (1988), Canlon and Fransson (1995), Canlon, Ryan and Boettcher (1999) |
| Guinea pig | 6.3 kHz, 78 dB, 13 days | none | 6.3 kHz, 100 dB, 24 hr | Canlon, Borg and Flock (1988), Canlon and Fransson (1995), Canlon, Ryan and Boettcher (1999) |
| Guinea pig | BBN, 85 dB, 5 h/days, 10 days | 5 days | 2–20 kHz, 110 dB, 5 h | Yamasoba, Dolan and Miller (1999) |
| Rat | OBN at 4 kHz, 55–95 dB, 10 h | 10 h | OBN at 4 kHz, 105 dB, 13 h | Pukkila et al. (1997) |
| Rabbit | OBN at 1 kHz, 95 dB, 3 weeks | | 4.215 kHz, 95 dB, 5 min | Franklin et al. (1991) |
| Mouse | OBN (8–16 kHz), 89 dB, 15 min | 24 h | OBN (8–16 kHz) 100 dB, 2 h | Yoshida, Kristiansen and Liberman (1999), Yoshida and Liberman (2000) |
| Mouse | Heat stress (41.5°C) | 6 h | OBN (8–16 kHz) 100 dB, 2 h | Yoshida, Kristiansen and Liberman (1999), Yoshida and Liberman (2000) |
| Mouse | BBN (4–25 kHz), 70 dB, 12 h | | Hereditary hearing loss | Willott and Turner (1999) |
| Human | Music, 70 dBA, 6 h/days, 5 days | None | OBN 2 kHz, 105 dB, 10 min | Miyakita et al. (1992) |

BBN, broad-band noise; OBN, octave-band noise.

# Middle-ear muscles

While the mechanisms underlying sound conditioning have not been clarified, it is believed that the stapedius muscle, known to afford sound
attenuation, is not involved (Henderson et al., 1994; Ryan et al., 1994;

Dagli and Canlon, 1997). The acoustic reflex has been shown to attenuate the transmission of sound through the middle ear of humans and experimental animals. The middle-ear reflex can afford maximal attenuation for frequencies below approximately 2 kHz. Avan et al. (1992) tested the response of the middle-ear muscles to acoustic stimulation in awake guinea pigs and rabbits. Sound-induced activation of the stapedius reflex greatly attenuated the amplitude of the cochlear microphonic potential in awake rabbits. In contrast, attenuation was not found for the awake guinea pig, despite the fact that electromyographic measurements demonstrated sound-induced contraction of the stapedius muscle. The primary role of the stapedius muscle in the guinea pig may therefore not be solely for the attenuation of loud sounds. However, this does not mean that the middle-ear muscles are not involved in sound conditioning since their role needs to be directly tested.

Three different investigations have shown that the middle-ear muscles are most probably not involved in protecting against acoustic trauma by sound conditioning.

After sectioning the middle-ear muscles in the gerbil (Ryan et al., 1994) or in the chinchilla (Henderson et al., 1994), or paralysing the middle-ear muscles in the guinea pig (Dagli and Canlon, 1995), protection against a subsequent noise trauma in sound-conditioned animals was still found. Thus, it appears that the stapedius muscle in these species does not contribute to the protection afforded by sound conditioning.

The mechanisms underlying the phenomenon of sound conditioning include a role of either the medial efferents or the lateral efferents. There appears to be no participation of the middle-ear muscles.

# Medial efferent system

The medial olivocochlear efferent system, innervating the outer hair cells, is another candidate because the efferent system can reduce the damaging effects of noise trauma resulting in either temporary (Cody and Johnstone, 1982; Rajan, 1988; Reiter and Liberman, 1995) or permanent hearing loss (Handrock and Zeisbertg, 1982; Liberman and Gao, 1995; Kujawa and Liberman, 1997; Zheng et al., 1997b). When the medial olivocochlear efferent system is electrically activated a decrease in a variety of physiological responses from the cochlea, including the compound action potential, single afferent fibres (Wiederhold and Kiang, 1970), intracellular responses from hair cells (Brown and Nuttall, 1984), otoacoustic emissions (Mountain, 1980) and motion of the basilar membrane (Murugasu and Russell, 1996).

Even though the medial efferent system has been shown to protect against noise-induced damage, a direct role of these efferents in sound conditioning has not been demonstrated (Kujawa and Liberman, 1997; Yamasoba and Dolan, 1998; Rajan, 2001). Yamasoba and Dolan (1998) treated cochleas with strychnine, a toxin that results in the degeneration of the medial efferent system. These authors showed a protective role of the medial efferents in noise-induced hearing loss. However, strychnine treatment did not alter the protective effect against acoustic trauma by sound conditioning. In contrast to Yamasoba and Dolan (1998), Zheng et al. (1997b) found that an intact medial efferent reflex was necessary for obtaining protection against acoustic trauma by sound conditioning.

Zheng et al. (1997b) compared a temporary threshold shift (TTS) in control and chronically de-efferented animals. In the efferent-intact (control) animals, TTSs were successively reduced during the 10-day conditioning paradigm. In the de-efferented animals, the TTS reductions were eliminated suggesting a role of the olivocochlear system in the sound-conditioning phenomenon. Kujawa and Liberman (1997) sectioned the olivocochlear bundle and found an increased vulnerability to acoustic injury compared with the intact animals. However, when the de-efferented animals were sound conditioned and then traumatized, a greater threshold shift was found compared with the trauma-alone animals. An interesting finding from that study was that animals who had sham surgery showed protection against noise exposure independent whether they received the conditioning stimulus or not. The authors suggest that a generalized stress response may be sufficient to elicit protection. Thus, these findings make it difficult to conclude that the medial efferent system is participating in the sound conditioning. Brown et al. (1998) measured physiological features of olivocochlear neurons during monaural and binaural stimulation in a group of animals that were sound conditioned and a group that was not sound conditioned. The olivocochlear neurons from the sound-conditioned animals showed an increased firing rate relative to the control animals. These increases were largest for neurons with best characteristic frequencies above the conditioning frequency band and these neurons showed long-term changes. Long-term persistence from sound conditioning has also been found in the chinchilla (McFadden et al., 1997). Protection against noise trauma was found even 2 months after the cessation of sound conditioning.

## Lateral efferent system

The cochlea receives a second efferent innervation from the brain stem through the lateral olivocochlear system (LOS) that forms axodendritic synapses with the afferent dendrites of the inner hair cells. Pharmacological lesions to the LSO caused a reduction of the compound action potential and degeneration of the lateral efferent innervation under the inner hair cells (Le Prell et al., 2003). These findings demonstrate that the lateral efferent innervation to the cochlea can modulate auditory nerve activity. There are numerous neurotransmitters and peptides contained within the lateral efferents including acetylcholine, γ-aminobutyric acid (GABA), dopamine, dynorphin, enkaphalin and calcitonin-gene-related peptide (Eybalin, 1993). Cochlear dopamine is thought to be involved in the modulation of noise trauma by inhibiting the activity of the afferent dendrites under the inner hair cells (Gil-Loyzaga and Pares-Herbute, 1989; Gil-Loyzaga et al., 1994; d'Aldin et al., 1995 a, b; Gil-Loyzaga, 1995; Safieddine, Prior and Eybalin, 1997; Gáborján, Lendvai and Vizi, 1999). Such a hypothetical role has been illustrated by showing dopamine receptor mRNA modifications in auditory neurons after acoustic trauma (Safieddine, Prior and Eybalin, 1997), and reductions in noise damage by dopamine antagonists (Gil-Loyzaga et al., 1994; d'Aldin et al., 1995b; Gil-Loyzaga, 1995). Tyrosine hydroxylase is the key enzyme of the dopamine synthesis and cochlear tyrosine hydroxylase has been immunohistochemically localized within the varicosities of the inner and tunnel spiral bundles in the guinea pigs (Eybalin et al., 1993; Niu and Canlon, 2002).

Considering the suggestion that protection against trauma is associated with dopamine activity, investigations were performed to determine if the lateral efferents play a role in sound conditioning. 6-Hydroxydopamine is a toxin that disrupts the synthesis of tyrosine hydroxylase, which is abundant in the lateral efferent terminals under the inner hair cells. As shown in Figure 28.1, the protection afforded by sound conditioning was blocked by the administration of 6-hydroxydopamine (Niu and Canlon, 2002). Furthermore, tyrosine hydroxylase immunoreactivity was upregulated both by sound conditioning alone and by the combined treatment of sound conditioning and acoustic trauma. In contrast, acoustic trauma alone resulted in a reduction in tyrosine hydroxylase immunoreactivity compared with unexposed controls. These findings are the first demonstration that tyrosine hydroxylase in the lateral efferents is upregulated during sound conditioning and suggests a role for the lateral efferent system in protecting against acoustic trauma by sound conditioning. In both immunocytochemical and western blot studies, tyrosine hydroxylase levels in the cochleas were increased by sound conditioning, and decreased either by trauma alone or by pretreatment with 6-hydroxydopamine. These changes in tyrosine hydroxylase levels in the cochlea indicate that dopaminergic transmission can modulate the sensitivity of the cochlea to acoustic trauma. A variety of stimuli is known to produce increases in tyrosine hydroxylase activity via phosphorylation of pre-existing enzymes. In the present study, the 24-hour sound-conditioning paradigm may lead to increased cAMP (adenosine cyclic 3':5'-monophosphate) synthesis and protein kinase activity in the lateral efferent system. In turn, gene expression in the cell nucleus may trigger an increased synthesis of tyrosine hydroxylase. In this way, the lateral efferent would have the capacity to release more dopamine and thereby protect the afferent dendrites from the excitotoxic actions of glutamate overstimulation from the inner hair cells. It is well known that glutamate excitotoxicity, leading to the swelling and degeneration of afferent dendrites, is one mechanism underlying hearing loss induced by acoustic trauma.

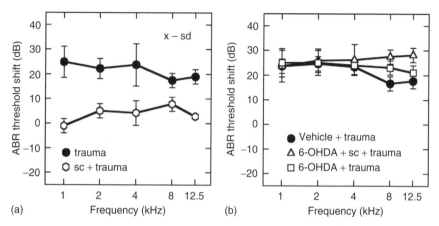

**Figure 28.1** (a) Auditory brain-stem response (ABR) threshold shifts obtained from acoustic trauma (filled circles), and a group who were pretreated with sound conditioning (open circles). Pretreatment with sound conditioning provided significant protection against the same acoustic trauma. (b) Pretreatment with 6-hydroxydopamine (6-OHDA) (open triangles) prevented the protective effects of sound conditioning on ABR thresholds.

Another issue that is addressed is whether protection against acoustic trauma by sound conditioning is governed by central mechanisms, or if the lateral efferent synapses under the inner hair cells in the cochlea are locally activated by sound conditioning. Neurons in the lateral olivocochlear system (LOC) regulate the peripheral expression of tyrosine hydroxylase in the cochlea and were identified by employing retrograde tracing techniques (Niu, Bogdanovic and Canlon, 2004). Retrogradely labelled neurons were found predominantly in the ipsilateral LOC system including lateral superior olive (LSO), and the surrounding periolivary regions (dorsal periolivary nucleus (DPO), dorsolateral periolivary nucleus (DLPO) and lateral nucleus of trapezoid body (LNTB)). Acoustic trauma (without sound conditioning) decreased the number of tyrosine hydroxylase-positive neurons in the LSO and the surrounding DLPO, and caused a reduction of fibre immunolabelling in these regions. Sound conditioning protected against the decrease of tyrosine hydroxylase immunolabelling by acoustic trauma and increased the fibre staining for tyrosine hydroxylase in the LSO and DLPO (Figure 28.2). Changes were not noted in the DPO or the LNTB after acoustic trauma or after the combined treatment of sound conditioning and acoustic trauma. These results provide evidence that tyrosine hydroxylase-positive neurons in the LOC system are protected by sound conditioning. In addition, these findings demonstrate that protection against acoustic trauma by sound conditioning has a central component that is governed by tyrosine hydroxylase in the LSO and the surrounding DLPO region.

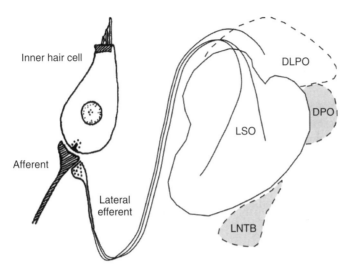

**Figure 28.2** Sound conditioning upregulates tyrosine hydroxylase immunolabelling in the lateral superior olive (LSO) and the dorsolateral periolivary nucleus (DLPO), but not in the dorsal periolivary nucleus (DPO) or the lateral nucleus of trapezoid body (LNTB). An increase in the fibre staining in the LSO and the DLPO was also noted after sound conditioning.

## Conclusions

Protection by sound conditioning is of clinical interest since noise-induced hearing loss and overexposure to sound stimulation are a common feature in our society. Although the biological mechanisms underlying protection are poorly understood, three candidates are possibly responsible for the sound conditioning phenomenon. These candidates include the middle-ear muscle reflex, and the medial and lateral efferent reflexes. However, several studies have shown that protection by sound conditioning is unaffected under conditions where the muscles are inactivated. It is generally agreed upon that the middle-ear muscle reflex is not a primary mechanism underlying protection by sound conditioning. At present, the role that the medial efferent reflex plays in sound conditioning is less well established. There are investigations showing that the medial efferent system may influence the resistance to acoustic trauma, or increase the firing patterns of the medial olivocochlear neurons, while other studies have not detected any change in the medial efferents by sound conditioning.

There is increasing evidence, both direct and indirect, that the lateral efferent system may be contributing to sound conditioning.

Sound conditioning may increase the inhibitory action of the lateral efferents and protect the afferent dendrites under the inner hair cells against excitotoxicity. Future studies are required to characterize the role that the medial and lateral efferent systems may be playing during sound conditioning.

To achieve these goals additional electrophysiological, pharmacological and molecular studies are needed.

## Acknowledgements

Supported by grants from the Swedish Research Council, AMF Trygghetsförsäkring, Tysta Skolan, Royal National Institute for Deaf People and the Karolinska Institute.

## References

Agerman K, Canlon B, Duan M, Ernfors P (1999) Neurotrophins, NMDA receptors, and nitric oxide in development and protection of the auditory system. Annals of the New York Academy of Sciences 884: 131–42.

Avan P, Loth D, Menguy C, Teyssou M (1992) Hypothetical roles of middle ear muscles in the guinea pig. Hearing Research 59: 59–69.

Brown MC, Nuttall AL (1984) Efferent control of cochlear inner hair cell responses in the guinea pig. Journal of Physiology 354: 625–46.

Brown MC, Kujawa SG, Liberman MC (1998) Single olivocochlear neurons in the guinea pig. II. Response plasticity due to noise conditioning. Journal of Neurophysiology 79: 3088–97.

Canlon B, Fransson A (1995) Morphological and functional preservation of the outer hair cells from noise trauma by sound conditioning. Hearing Research 84: 112–24.

Canlon B, Borg E, Flock Å (1988) Protection against noise trauma by pre-exposure to a low level acoustic stimulus. Hearing Research 34: 197–200.

Canlon B, Ryan A, Boettcher FA (1999) On the factors required for obtaining protection against noise trauma by prior acoustic experience. Hearing Research 127: 158–60.

Cody AR, Johnstone BM (1982) Temporary threshold shift modified by binaural acoustic stimulation. Hearing Research 6: 199–205.

Dagli S, Canlon B (1995) Protection against noise trauma by sound conditioning in the guinea pig appears not to be mediated by the middle ear muscles. Neuroscience Letter 194: 57–60.

Dagli S, Canlon B (1997) The effect of repeated daily noise exposure on sound-conditioned and unconditioned guinea pigs. Hearing Research 104: 39–46.

D'Aldin C, Eybalin M, Puel JL, Charachon G, Ladrech S, Renard N et al. (1995a) Synaptic connections and putative functions of the dopaminergic innervation of the guinea pig cochlea. European Archives of Oto-Rhino-Laryngology 252: 270–4.

D'Aldin C, Puel JL, Leduqc R, Crambes O, Eybalin M, Pujol R (1995b) Effects of a dopaminergic agonist in the guinea pig cochlea. Hearing Research 90: 202–11.

Drescher DG (1976) Effect of temperature on cochlear response during and after exposure to noise. Journal of the Acoustical Society of America 59: 401–7.

Duan M, Agerman K, Ernfors P, Canlon B (2000) Complementary roles of neurotrophin 3 and a $N$-methyl-D-aspartate antagonist in the protection of noise and aminoglycoside-induced ototoxicity. Proceedings of the National Academy of Sciences of the USA 97: 7597–602.

Erway LC, Shiau YW, Davis RR, Krieg EF (1996) Genetics of age-related hearing loss in mice. III. Susceptibility of inbred and F1 hybrid strains to noise-induced hearing loss. Hearing Research 93: 181–7.

Eybalin M (1993) Neurotransmitters and neuromodulators of the mammalian cochlea. Physiology Review 73: 309–73.

Eybalin M, Charachon G, Renard N (1993) Dopaminergic lateral efferent innervation of the guinea-pig cochlea: immunoelectron microscopy of catecholamine-synthesizing enzymes and effect of 6-hydroxydopamine. Neuroscience 54: 133–42.

Franklin DJ, Lonsbury-Martin BL, Stagner BB, Martin GK (1991) Altered susceptibility of 2f1-f2 acoustic-distortion products to the effects of repeated noise exposure in rabbits. Hearing Research 53: 185–208.

Gáborján A, Lendvai B, Vizi ES (1999) Neurochemical evidence of dopamine release by lateral olivocochlear efferents and its presynaptic modulation in guinea-pig cochlea. Neuroscience 90: 131–8.

Gates GA, Couropmitree NN, Myers RH (1999) Genetic associations in age-related hearing thresholds. Archives of Otolaryngology – Head and Neck Surgery 125: 654–9.

Gil-Loyzaga P (1995) Neurotransmitters of the olivocochlear lateral efferent system: with an emphasis on dopamine. Acta Otolaryngologica 115: 222–6.

Gil-Loyzaga P, Pares-Herbute N (1989) HPLC detection of dopamine and noradrenaline in the cochlea of adult and developing rats. Brain Research, Developmental Brain Research 48: 157–60.

Gil-Loyzaga P, Vicente-Torres MA, Fernandez-Mateos P, Arce A, Esquifino A (1994) Piribedil affects dopamine turnover in cochleas stimulated by white noise. Hearing Research 79: 178–82.

Handrock M, Zeisberg J (1982) The influence of the effect system on adaptation, temporary and permanent threshold shift. Archives of Oto-Rhino-Laryngology 234: 191–5.

Hansen S (1988) Postural hypotension – cochleo-vestibular hypoxia – deafness. Acta Otolaryngologica (Supplementum) 449: 165–9.

Henderson D, Subramaniam M, Papazian M, Spongr VP (1994) The role of middle ear muscles in the development of resistance to noise induced hearing loss. Hearing Research 74: 22–8.

Henry KR (1984) Cochlear damage resulting from exposure to four different octave bands of noise at three ages. Behavioral Neuroscience 98: 107–17.

Henry KR, Chole RA (1984) Hypothermia protects the cochlea from noise damage. Hearing Research 16: 225–30.

Henselman LW, Henderson D, Subramaniam M, Sallustio V (1994) The effect of 'conditioning' exposures on hearing loss from impulse noise. Hearing Research 78: 1–10.

Koga K, Hakuba N, Watanabe F, Shudou M, Nakagawa T, Gyo K (2003) Transient cochlear ischemia causes delayed cell death in the organ of Corti: an experimental study in gerbils. Journal of Comparative Neurology 456: 105–11.

Kujawa SG, Liberman MC (1997) Conditioning-related protection from acoustic injury: effects of chronic deefferentation and sham surgery. Journal of Neurophysiology 78: 3095–106.

Le Prell CG, Shore SE, Hughes LF, Bledsoe SC Jr (2003) Disruption of lateral efferent pathways: functional changes in auditory evoked responses. Journal of the Association for Research in Otolaryngology 4: 276–90.

Li HS (1992) Influence of genotype and age on acute acoustic trauma and recovery in CBA/CA and C57BL/6J mice. Acta Otolaryngologica 112: 956–67.

Liberman MC, Gao WY (1995) Chronic cochlear deefferentation and susceptibility to permanent acoustic injury. Hearing Research 90: 158–68.

McFadden SL, Henderson D, Shen Y-H (1997) Low-frequency 'conditioning' provides long-term protection from noise-induced threshold shifts in chinchillas. Hearing Research 103: 142–50.

Margolis RH (1993) Detection of hearing impairment with the acoustic stapedius reflex. Ear and Hearing 14: 3–10.

Miller JD, Watson CS, Covell WP (1963) Deafening effects of noise on the cat. Acta Otolaryngologica (Supplementum) 176: 1–91.

Miyakita T, Hellström PA, Frimanson E, Axelsson A (1992) Effect of low level acoustic stimulation on temporary threshold shift in young humans. Hearing Research 60: 149–55.

Mountain DC (1980) Changes in endolymphatic potential and crossed olivocochlear bundle stimulation alter cochlear mechanics. Science 210: 71–2.

Murugasu E, Russell IJ (1996) The effect of efferent stimulation on basilar membrane displacement in the basal turn of the guinea pig cochlea. Journal of Neuroscience 16: 325–32.

Niu X, Canlon B (2002) Activation of tyrosine hydroxylase in the lateral efferent terminals by sound conditioning. Hearing Research 174: 124–32.

Niu X, Bogdanovic N, Canlon B (2004) The distribution and the modulation of tyrosine hydroxylase immunoreactivity in the lateral olivocochlear system of the guinea-pig. Neuroscience 125: 725–33.

Ohlemiller KK, Wright JS, Heidbreder AR (2000) Vulnerability to noise-induced hearing loss in middle-aged and young adult mice: a dose-response approach in CBA, C57BL, and BALB inbred strains. Hearing Research 149: 239–47.

Pujol R, Puel JL, d'Aldin C, Eybalin M (1993) Pathophysiology of the glutamatergic synapses in the cochlea. Acta Otolaryngologica 113: 330–4.

Pukkila M, Zhai S, Virkkala J, Pirovola U, Ylikoski J (1997) The 'toughening' phenomenon in rat's auditory organ. Acta Otolaryngologica 529: 59–62.

Rajan R (1988) Effect of electrical stimulation of the crossed olivocochlear bundle on temporary threshold shifts in auditory sensitivity. I. Dependence on electrical stimulation parameters. Journal of Neurophysiology 60: 549–68.

Rajan R (2001) Noise priming and the effects of different cochlear centrifugal pathways on loud-sound-induced hearing loss. Journal of Neurophysiology 86: 1277–88.

Reiter ER, Liberman MC (1995) Efferent-mediated protection from acoustic overexposure: relation to 'slow effects' of olivocochlear stimulation. Journal of Neurophysiology 73: 506–14.

Ryan AF, Bennett TM, Woolf NK, Axelsson A (1994) Protection from noise-induced hearing loss by prior exposure to a nontraumatic stimulus: role of the middle ear muscles. Hearing Research 72: 23–8.

Safieddine S, Prior AM, Eybalin M (1997) Choline acetyltransferase, glutamate decarboxylase, tyrosine hydroxylase, calcitonin gene-related peptide and opioid peptides coexist in lateral efferent neurons of rat and guinea-pig. European Journal of Neuroscience 9: 356–67.

Wang Y, Liberman MC (2002) Restraint stress and protection from acoustic injury in mice. Hearing Research 165: 96–102.

White DR, Boettcher FA, Miles LR, Gratton MA (1998) Effectiveness of intermittent and continuous acoustic stimulation in preventing noise-induced hearing and hair cell loss. Journal of Acoustical Society of America 103: 1566–72.

Wiederhold ML, Kiang NYS (1970) Effects of electric stimulation of the crossed olivocochlear bundle on single auditory-nerve fibers in the cat. Journal of the Acoustical Society of America 48: 950–65.

Willott JF, Turner JG (1999) Prolonged exposure to an augmented acoustic environment ameliorates age-related auditory changes in C57BL/6J and DBA/2J mice. Hearing Research 135: 78–88.

Yamasoba T, Dolan DF (1998) The medial cochlear efferent system does not appear to contribute to the development of acquired resistance to acoustic trauma. Hearing Research 120: 143–51.

Yamasoba T, Dolan DF, Miller JM (1999) Acquired resistance to acoustic trauma by sound conditioning is primarily mediated by changes restricted to the cochlea, not by systemic responses. Hearing Research 127: 31–40.

Yoshida N, Liberman MC (2000) Sound conditioning reduces noise-induced permanent threshold shift in mice. Hearing Research 148: 213–9.

Yoshida N, Kristiansen A, Liberman MC (1999) Heat stress and protection from permanent acoustic injury in mice. Journal Neuroscience 19: 10116–24.

Zheng XY, Henderson D, McFadden SL, Hu BH (1997a) The role of the cochlear efferent system in acquired resistance to noise-induced hearing loss. Hearing Research 104: 191–203.

Zheng XY, Henderson D, Hu BH, McFadden SL (1997b) The influence of the cochlear efferent system on chronic acoustic trauma. Hearing Research 107:147–59.

# CHAPTER 29

# Industrial noise control

*Noise and Its Effects:* Edited by Linda Luxon and Deepak Prasher © 2007
John Wiley & Sons Ltd.

TPC BRAMER

Before exploring the various methods of controlling noise in industry, it is important to appreciate the principles of how noise is produced and propagated in an industrial situation. This can be simplified by considering the characteristics of the source of the noise, how it is propagated and how the subject receives it. Noise control can be applied to each or all of these separate stages and this chapter will cover the first two – the noise source and the propagation path. The last – hearing protection – is covered in Chapter 30.

It is essential that the exact cause of the noise problem should be recognized so that the appropriate cost-effective action can be applied. In many cases, time and effort have been wasted by inexperienced practitioners not recognizing this at the beginning.

## Sources of noise

**The most common sources of noise in industry are:**

- *Aerodynamic from air movement,* such as compressed air release or fan noise;
- *Impact,* such as from hammering, components falling into bins or gear noise;
- *Stick-slip friction* such as from lathe tools cutting or brake noise;
- *Vibration* and associated radiation from surfaces.

## The propagation path

In a typical industrial situation, noise is produced by a multitude of sources – machines or associated items – in a semi-reverberant or acoustically 'live' space with little acoustic absorbent present. In the opposite situation, a noise source in the open air ('free-field'), the radiated noise level reduces with distance away from the source, according to the inverse square law. In simplified terms, this means that the noise falls off at the rate of 6 dB every time the distance is doubled – for example, if the level at 1 m from a small noise source is 93 dB, then it will have reduced to 87 dB at 2 m and to 81 dB at 4 m. The levels at other distances can be calculated with the appropriate logarithmic relationship, or read off from a table. The resultant noise is called the 'direct level'.

## Noise reduction according to the inverse square law

*Simply:*
The noise falls off at the rate of 6dB every time the distance is doubled.

In a typical factory building this is modified by the tendency for the noise level to fall only as far as a 'plateau' of reverberant noise produced by the sum of all the noise sources in the area. This 'reverberant level' of noise depends on the noise levels and layout of the noise sources, and the acoustic characteristics of the space. In a much-simplified form, this is illustrated in Figure 29.1. There are obviously many configurations of this basic situation, depending on the exact layout and type of machines, and the acoustics of the space.

The resultant noise level at any point in the building is made up of the contribution from the direct and reverberant levels from the various noise sources.

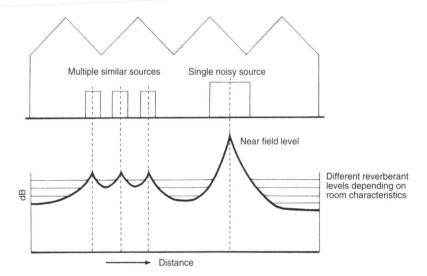

**Figure 29.1** Noise levels against distance from source in reverberant surroundings. Reproduced with permission of Sound Research Laboratories from 'Internal Factory Noise' in *Noise Control in Industry*. London, Taylor Francis, 1991.

# Noise-control principles

A factory operator at a machine in a typical industrial situation tends to be affected by noise arising from three reasonably distinct causes:

1. the direct noise from the machine only, plus possibly others in the immediate vicinity;
2. the reverberant noise from other machines further away;
3. in a less than perfect reverberant situation, a combination of the direct noise from the nearest machine(s) and the reducing reverberant noise from others in the building at greater distances.

These are shown diagramatically in Figures 29.2 and 29.3.

The problem is complicated by the need to select carefully the correct approach to noise control in a particular situation. If, for example, the subject is working close to a single noisy machine, then it would be inappropriate to attempt noise control by adding absorbent to walls or roof to reduce the general reverberant level. At position (a) in Figure 29.2, it can be seen that this would not produce any significant noise reduction. This approach is generally only appropriate if the subject works in an area remote from noisy machines – for example, positions (b) or (c) in Figure 29.2.

In a very reverberant area, with a multitude of similarly noisy machines, significant noise reduction may be achieved only by dealing with all of the sources. This is illustrated in Figure 29.3. A typical example of this is

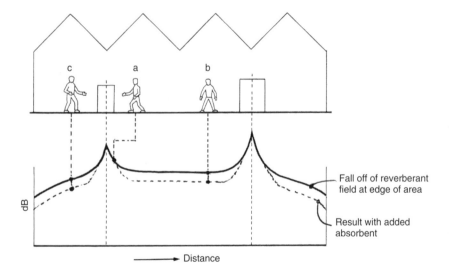

**Figure 29.2** Operator noise levels from individual machines in reverberant surroundings. Reproduced with permission of Sound Research Laboratories from 'Internal Factory Noise' in *Noise Control in Industry*. London, Taylor Francis, 1991.

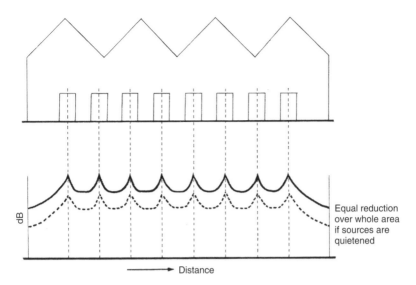

**Figure 29.3** Noise levels from multiple identical machines in reverberant surroundings, showing the effect of noise reduction at source. Reproduced with permission of Sound Research Laboratories from 'Internal Factory Noise' in *Noise Control in Industry*. London, Taylor Francis, 1991.

found in a machine shop with a large number of lathes, milling machines, grinders, etc.

Another problem is in correctly identifying what to deal with first. In a typical industrial situation, there may be a number of sources and/or propagation paths contributing to the combined noise at a particular position. If one of these is dominant compared with the others, then this must be tackled first. If this is ignored and the less dominant ones are reduced first, by however much, there is likely to be little or no effect on the noise reaching the subject.

In this context, 'dominant' means more than approximately 5 dB higher than the other sources.

Table 29.1 puts matters into perspective. It is a simple table of noise reductions with a comment about the practical subjective and objective significance of each step in an industrial situation.

**Table 29.1** Noise reductions and their effects

| Noise reduction (dB) | Effect |
| --- | --- |
| 1 | Imperceptible |
| 2 | Barely detectable |
| 5 | Definite improvement, worth spending money on |
| 10 | Striking improvement, worth considerable cost |
| 20 | Outstanding improvement |
| 25 | Equivalent to 'switching off' the noise |

# Practical noise control

Starting from the noise source, there are a number of methods of noise control available in practice:

## Methods of noise control

- change process or redesign machine;
- control noise of machine or process;
- enclose machine;
- noise refuge;
- acoustic treatment of building.

### Change the process or the design of the machine

It is not often practicable to switch the noise source off completely but it may be possible to change the process from a noisy one to a quieter one. This is obviously a fundamental change and is not usually applicable to an existing situation. It is often the case that this is done more from the economic point of view but the result can be a worthwhile additional noise reduction. An example often quoted is the change from old-fashioned reciprocating air compressors to modern rotary or screw compressors. Not only is the reciprocating compressor noisier but the predominant noise is at low frequency and more difficult to reduce without large and expensive silencers. The modern rotary or screw compressor is smaller, quiet enough to be easily sited inside the factory and more efficient (Figures 29.4 and 29.5).

It may be possible to replace noisy press forming of metal components with extrusion or hydraulic forming.

Care must obviously be taken that one noisy process is not replaced by another. For example, the old-fashioned method of building boilers or ship hulls was by hand riveting, which involved heavy hammering and was very noisy indeed. This has now been replaced by welding, which is obviously much quieter. However, this is not the complete story as the edges of the

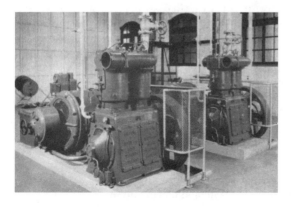

**Figure 29.4** Obsolescent reciprocating air compressors. Reproduced with permission of CompAir UK.

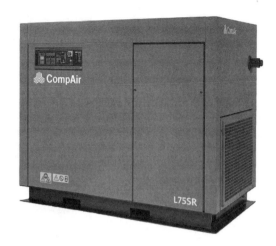

**Figure 29.5** A modern rotary
screw air compressor.
Reproduced with permission of
CompAir UK.

plates have to be prepared for the welding by bevelling them off. This is commonly done with an angle grinder or an air operated chisel, both of which are very noisy tools typically producing over 100 dB (A) at the operator's ear.

### Noise control of the machine or process

This is a very large subject and it is possible in this book to cover only a few of the most important examples.

#### Machine/process sources of noise

- high-velocity air release via exhausts;
- compressed air jets;
- air movement, e.g. fans;
- impact noise, e.g. dropping metal components;
- gear noise;
- motor noise;
- steam/gas passing through pressure-reducing valve.

One of the most common sources of noise in a typical factory where components are machined and assembled is the use of compressed air. This is universally used in industry to operate actuators on production lines, to operate hand tools and to remove debris from machined components. In the first case, the air release from the actuator is often exhausted directly to atmosphere through an open port. The multiple and frequent high-velocity air releases produce a large amount of high-frequency noise, the *direct level* of which affects the immediate operator, and combines to increase the *reverberant level* in the factory. This problem can be alleviated very easily and cheaply by fitting dissipative silencers to the individual exhaust ports, or by piping the combined exhaust away to one or more larger silencers (Figures 29.6 and 29.7). Air-operated hand tools are often noisy and this can also be dealt with by

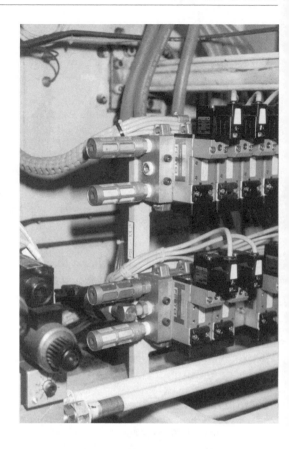

**Figure 29.6** Individual
silencers on air exhausts.

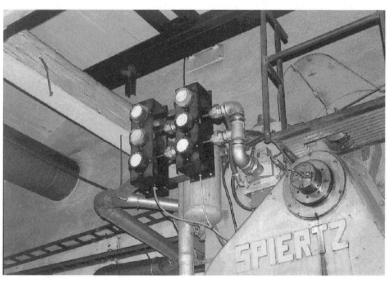

**Figure 29.7** Bank of silencers on pneumatic exhaust. Reproduced with permission
of Silvent UK. Ltd.

adding exhaust silencers. There is a new generation of air-operated tools now available, which are significantly quieter than their predecessors.

The high level of noise from the use of compressed air for blowing away the debris from machining operations is more difficult to deal with. The common problem is that the noisy, high-velocity jet of air is perceived as necessary to remove debris from small holes and crevices. Nevertheless, there are specialist blowing guns available (Figures 29.8 and 29.9), which are considerably quieter than the simple straight piece of copper tube that is commonly used for this purpose. As well as being quieter, they can be arranged to be safer from misuse than normal nozzles. A similar application is the 'air knife' used to remove liquids or debris from material moving past on a conveyor. Specialist blowing nozzles can be fitted, which work effectively and give a significant noise reduction.

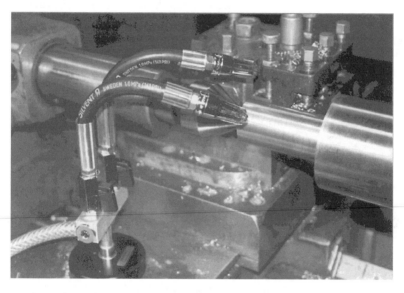

**Figure 29.8** Silenced nozzles on lathe to clear swarf. Reproduced with permission of Silvent UK. Ltd.

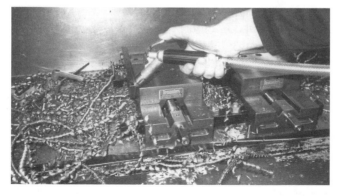

**Figure 29.9** Silenced blowing nozzle for hand use. Reproduced with permission of Silvent UK. Ltd.

The noise produced by fans and air movement on ovens, fume extracts etc., can be reduced by appropriate use of duct attenuators, casing lagging and vibration isolation, but care must be taken to identify the correct source of the noise. For example, fan noise radiated from the inlet or outlet of a fan will not be reduced by lagging the fan casing or the addition of vibration isolators.

A completely different approach must be used where noise arises from impact between items. This can range from the dropping of metal components from a pressing operation into a collection or storage bin to the manipulation of metal beer kegs on a loading or unloading dock.

In the case of the press and metal bin, noise can be reduced by arranging for the components to slide relatively gently into the bin, and/or by applying resilient rubber cushioning to the inside surfaces or treating the external surfaces with vibration damping material. This latter approach can also be used to deal with the problem of impact noise produced in a frozen food factory by the movement of frozen peas or sprouts and so forth along the vibrating stainless steel trough conveyors that are commonly used. Resilient material cannot be used on the top surface as this would reduce the effectiveness of the desired movement. Vibration damping compound must be used on the underside of the thin metal conveyors, but care must be taken to choose an appropriate material. The problem is that the low temperature promotes water to freeze under or inside the material and this eventually causes it to flake off. Another problem is that the hygiene aspects common to all food factories must be taken into account.

In a brewery or beer warehouse, a common problem is the impact noise from the kegs (especially when empty) being moved around on a hard-surfaced loading or unloading bay. Covering the essential floor area with thick rubber matting can largely alleviate this. In other situations where raw materials or finished goods are moved around, the use of plastic or wooden, instead of metal, pallets, etc., will reduce noise. Where they can be used, electric fork lift trucks are quieter than diesel or gas-powered trucks. A common problem that can cause excessive noise exposure for forklift truck drivers is carrying metal bins or similar loads that rattle and bang when driven over a rough, pot-holed yard or factory floor.

Gear noise is often a common problem in high-speed machines in factories. This is largely caused by the continuous series of impacts between the teeth of straight spur gearing, and occurs at a frequency depending on the speed and the number of teeth on the gear. It tends to be worse from poorly finished or worn gears. It can be reduced in some cases by the substitution of helical for straight gearing. A related problem arises from the use of toothed belts, instead of smooth vee belts, to drive machines. There are quieter versions of toothed belts available, which have a carefully shaped tooth form designed to minimize this noise.

High levels of discrete frequency impact noise are produced by woodworking machinery – circular saws, routers and planers. All of these can be reduced by appropriate design of the cutting tool. Quieter, damped saw blades, and helical bladed cutter blocks for planers, are available and can be used in most circumstances.

It may be beneficial to the correct operation of machinery to install it on resilient vibration-isolated mounts and this is often done additionally in an attempt to reduce noise levels. However, it generally only has an effect if machinery vibration is being transmitted to other structures that vibrate and radiate noise. It does not usually have much effect on the radiation of noise from the machine itself.

A large proportion of industrial machinery is powered by individual electric motors. The normal standard type of fully enclosed motor has not been designed with low noise in mind. The usual dominant source of noise on a standard motor is the cooling fan at one end of the shaft, which is a relatively crude device designed to work equally well at the movement of cooling air for either direction of rotation. It is possible to specify a motor with a unidirectional fan for a particular direction of rotation and this is significantly quieter. A motor with a larger frame size than the minimum for a particular power can be specified, and this should be quieter. In both cases, of course, the cost will be higher but this approach may obviate more expensive noise control at a later stage. To put this into perspective, the cost of electricity used in the first month for a motor running continuously 24 hours a day is of the same order as the original cost of the motor.

Steam or other gases passing along pipes can be a potent source of noise, particularly when passed through a pressure-reducing valve. The noise propagates along the pipe downstream of the valve, to be radiated as high-frequency noise from a considerable length of the pipe. This can be reduced by choosing a type and size of valve designed for lower noise, adding an in-line silencer or by appropriately lagging the valve and pipe.

**Enclosure of machines**

It is possible to build a sound-resistant enclosure around some machines on the factory floor. If this enclosure can be complete, and almost airtight, then the theoretical noise reduction can be up to about 35 dB for a purpose-built heavy box with an acoustically absorbent lining. Unfortunately, it is almost always necessary to have openings for passing in materials for processing, and for taking out the finished product. In addition, ventilation or cooling is invariably needed, and this compromises the final effect. Both of these problems can be overcome with careful attention, but the enclosure will obviously need to be removed or dismantled at some stage when the machine needs repair or adjustment. This factor is probably the most important in practice, as it is rare for a demountable sound-resistant enclosure to be built robustly enough to withstand the attentions of the average maintenance department for very long.

It is sometimes possible to build a complete sound-resistant enclosure around something as large as a newspaper press or a cardboard corrugating machine, with the operating personnel remaining outside at the

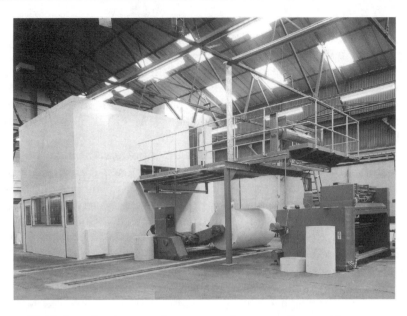

**Figure 29.10** Sound-resistant enclosure around a corrugating machine.
Reproduced with permission of Hodgson and Hodgson Group Ltd.

control console (Figures 29.10 and 29.11). If it is necessary in the short
term to go inside for adjustment, etc., then hearing protection can be
worn. This is obviously an expensive solution to the problem and must be
properly considered at the design stage.

Simpler versions of sound-reducing enclosures can be fitted around noisy
sections of, for instance, bottling lines or food production lines. These are
often constructed of transparent plastic sheeting such as polycarbonate, with
hinged access panels. These rarely provide more than 5 dB (A) or 10 dB (A)
of attenuation but this may well be sufficient in the circumstances.

If only a small amount of noise reduction is needed to alleviate problems from one area of a factory then it is possible to use acoustic screening.
This would normally consist of a barrier partly or completely around the
area, without a roof. In the open air, or very dead acoustic conditions, such
a barrier can provide up to about 10 dB (A) or 12 dB (A) of attenuation.
However, in the reverberant or semi-reverberant conditions of the typical
factory environment this is not so effective in practice, as noise from inside
the barrier tends to spread over the top and affect the surrounding areas.

### Noise refuges

The previous section has dealt with the case of an enclosure around the
noisy machine or process but it is possible to reverse the situation and put
the enclosure or screen around the operating personnel – to produce a

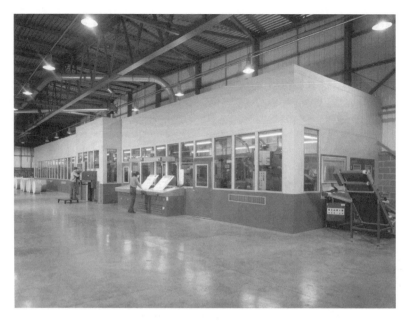

**Figure 29.11** Sound-resistant enclosure around a printing press. Reproduced with permission of Hodgson and Hodgson Group Ltd.

sound-resistant control room, for instance (Figure 29.12). Similar rules apply, with hearing protection being worn when it is required to venture outside for any reason.

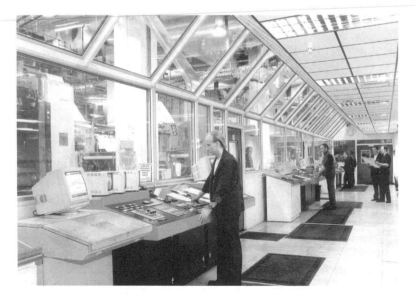

**Figure 29.12** Noise refuge alongside newspaper printing press. Reproduced with permission of Hodgson and Hodgson Group Ltd.

# Acoustic treatment to the building

There are some circumstances where applying acoustic absorbent treatment to the building surfaces is of value.

It must be appreciated that applying acoustic absorbent treatment to the building surfaces reduces only the reverberant noise and will have little or no effect on the noise reaching the operator from a machine close by. The exception is where a large number of similarly noisy machines are distributed around a large area. In such cases it is often found that the direct noise from each machine does not extend very far from the machine and merges into the reverberant field after only a short distance. Another case where acoustic treatment to the room can be beneficial is where there is a group of particularly noisy machines in one area and a potentially quiet area elsewhere. The provision of acoustic treatment to the roof (and possibly the walls close to these machines) will considerably reduce the noise reaching the quieter area.

In practice, it is only usually worthwhile adding absorbent treatment to the roof or ceiling of an industrial building as this is the largest area normally available and is near all of the machines below. Adding treatment to a wall is normally only useful if a machine is close to it, and it is required to reduce reflection of noise back to nearby personnel.

There are basically two ways of applying this acoustic absorbent treatment to the roof or ceiling of an industrial building – actually adding absorbent material to the surface or hanging 'modular acoustic absorbers' from the roof.

Surface treatment can be added by fixing panels of absorbent, such as glass fibre or mineral wool slab in a suspension frame, to the underside of the roof (Figure 29.13), or by applying a sprayed absorbent finish (Figures 29.14 and 29.15). In both these cases, the treatment may also be useful in providing improved thermal insulation to the building.

The modular absorbers typically consist of panels of glass fibre or mineral wool slab 600 mm × 1200 mm × 50 mm, enclosed in a frame or covered with a thin film of plastic. They are hung vertically on wires or rods from the roof, in a grid pattern at a typical spacing of one per square metre. They should be hung as low as possible above the machinery, commensurate with lighting and fire sprinkler requirements (Figure 29.16).

This acoustic treatment does not, as mentioned earlier, have a significant effect on the direct noise reaching the operator of a machine. Nevertheless, in practice it often has a very beneficial subjective noise-reducing effect, rather better than the theory would seem to predict. In a typical semi-reverberant factory building there tends to be an objectionable 'jumble' of noise assailing personnel from all sides. This is subjectively very tiring. The addition of the reverberant acoustic treatment often transforms the situation and makes it far less objectionable to work in.

In a typical food or pharmaceutical factory the building surfaces are often covered with washable hard and shiny materials for hygiene reasons. In such cases the areas can be very reverberant indeed, and unpleasant to work in, as only one noisy machine will tend to fill the whole room with noise. If at least the roof can be treated with an appropriate absorbent material, it will produce a large improvement in the

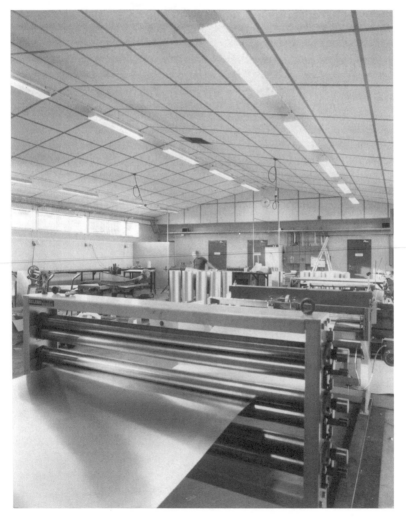

**Figure 29.13** Production area with acoustic absorbent material on ceiling. Reproduced with permission of Hodgson and Hodgson Group Ltd.

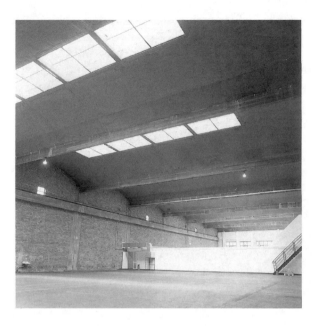

**Figure 29.14** Original roof in a reverberant factory. Reproduced with permission of Asona Nederland b.v.

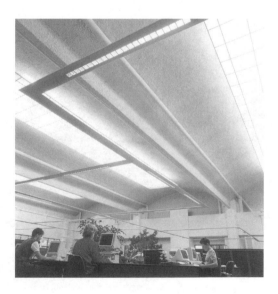

**Figure 29.15** The same area after conversion to open-plan office with absorbent finish. Reproduced with permission of Asona Nederland b.v.

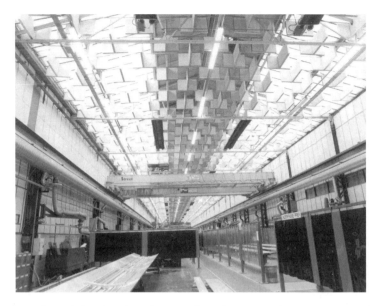

**Figure 29.16** Modular absorbers hanging from factory roof. Reproduced with permission of Hodgson and Hodgson Group Ltd.

acoustic working conditions. It is important that the materials used should be compatible with the hygiene requirements. Unfortunately, covering acoustic absorbent with an impervious finish to withstand washing down, for instance, can unacceptably reduce the acoustic absorbent effect. However, it is possible to obtain effective acoustic materials that meet these hygiene requirements.

## Conclusions

It is essential to identify and appreciate the different ways in which noise from machines and so forth in an industrial situation affects personnel in the area. If the wrong method of noise reduction for a particular situation is applied then there may be little or no useful effect. For example, adding surface absorbent to a factory roof to reduce the reverberant noise level is unlikely to reduce significantly the direct noise reaching an operator immediately next to a noisy machine.

Successful noise control in industry often depends more on practical engineering skills rather than on purely acoustic expertise. Will the proposed treatment be practicable in the particular situation? Will the machine in question still operate efficiently at the same production rate? Will it still be adequately ventilated and cooled?

# Further reading

Noise at Work – Guidance for employers on the Control of Noise at Work Regulations 2005. Health and Safety Executive Booklet – INDG 362 (rev1) 10/05 C1400.

Health and Safety Executive (1995) Sound Solutions: Techniques to Reduce Noise at Work. London: HMSO.

Sound Research Laboratories (1991) Noise Control in Industry. Third Edition. London, Taylor Francis.

# CHAPTER 30

# Hearing protectors

*Noise and Its Effects:* Edited by Linda Luxon and Deepak Prasher © 2007
John Wiley & Sons Ltd.

JUKKA STARCK, ESKO TOPPILA, ILMARI PYYKKÖ

## Legislative approach to protection of workers

In the European community the protection against noise is controlled by
Directives 86/188/EEC, which sets the noise protection requirement of the
workplaces, 89/656/EEC, which sets the requirements concerning the use
of personal protective equipment (PPE), and 89/686/EEC, which sets the
requirement to test the PPE (Figure 30.1). The seventeenth individual
Directive 2003/10/EC specifies exposure limit values (87 dB, 200 Pa) and
exposure action values (upper values 85 dB, 140 Pa and lower values

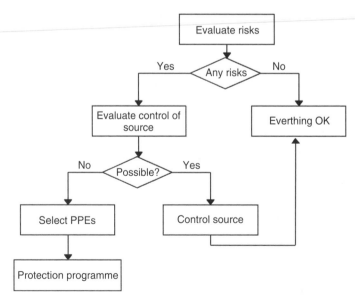

**Figure 30.1** The general approach to the protection programme of workers against
noise risks in the workplace. PPEs, personal protective equipment.

80 dB, 112 Pa) for 8 hours of daily exposure and peak sound pressure. When applying exposure limit values, the determination of the worker's effective exposure should take account of the attenuation provided by the individual hearing protectors. The exposure to action values should not take account of the effect of any such protectors. The employer should give special attention to ensure the availability of hearing protectors (hearing protection devices or HPDs) with adequate attenuation characteristics and proper fitting where the noise exposure exceeds the lower action value. When the noise exposure level matches or exceeds the upper exposure level, individual HPDs should be used. The individual HPDs should be selected so as to eliminate the risk to hearing or to reduce the risk to a minimum.

These guidelines are insufficient for practical purposes, as too many uncertainties exist concerning:

**Difficulties surrounding use of HPDs**
- how to guarantee that the HPDs are used properly;
- identification of the workplaces or tasks with the highest risks;
- addressing countermeasures against the correct noise source, especially if the major exposure occurs out of the workplace.

In the prevention of noise-induced hearing loss (NIHL), the use of HPDs should be considered a last resort, but when they are used the selection and use have to be planned carefully to achieve appropriate protection. Inadequate use of HPDs, which commonly occurs, leads to a very rapid and drastic decrease in the level of protection, which is far below that which it is possible to achieve. This emphasizes the importance of training and motivation of the workers. However, the role of HPDs in noise-control programmes is always secondary as their use does not decrease the noise in the work place, but merely protects a person wearing such a device.

Hearing protectors are required when the noise exposure level exceeds the national action level of 85 or 90 dB, in European countries. The assessment should be based on the measurements of noise in order to define A-weighted equivalent noise level over the exposure period, corresponding also to the usage period of HPDs. It is preferable that the impulsiveness of the noise should be considered. Information on the frequency content of noise is also needed for the selection of HPD. The most sophisticated method will use octave-band analysis data, but other methods use C- and A-weighted level data either together or separately depending on the selected method, as shown below.

## Models of hearing protectors

Passive HPDs include earmuffs and earplugs; active HPDs include sound restoration systems and noise cancellation systems. The main models of hearing protectors are earmuffs and earplugs (Table 30.1).

**Types of HPDs**

- Passive
  - Earmuffs
    - Headband
    - Integral to safety helmet
  - Earplugs
    - Disposable
    - Reusable
- Active
  - Sound generation systems
  - Noise cancellation systems

Earmuffs cover the entire pinna with a force in the headband, determined by the standard. The cup of the earmuff is supplied with a soft cushion ring to allow firm and tight fitting on the head of the user with no air leakage. The attenuation of the earmuff generally depends on the volume and mass of the cup, properties of the cushion ring, and the force or pressure provided by the headband (or neckband) on the head. Alternatively, the earmuffs can be fitted to a safety helmet using a special mounting device. Typically, the attenuation is dependent on the frequency content of noise – earmuffs attenuate high frequencies more effectively than low frequencies. This property generally allows good attenuation against industrial impulse noise, as impulses represent high-frequency components in the noise spectrum (Pekkarinen, 1987).

**Table 30.1** Benefits and disadvantages of earmuffs and earplugs

| Earmuffs | Earplugs |
| --- | --- |
| Communication problems may arise | Communication problems may arise |
| Problems with hearing warning signals | Problems with hearing warning signals |
| Sweat in warm environment | Sensation of pressure in ear canal |
| Effective earmuffs are heavy | Disposable earplugs cause waste |
| Need maintenance | Get lost easily |

There are several types of earplugs, which are either disposable or reusable, intended for long-term use. They are usually made of soft material that is easy to insert into the ear canal. In general, the attenuation of earplugs is less frequency dependent than earmuffs and, thus, they attenuate low-frequency components of noise more effectively than earmuffs.

In addition to the earmuffs and earplugs, where the attenuation of noise is based on a passive mode of function, there are earmuffs that

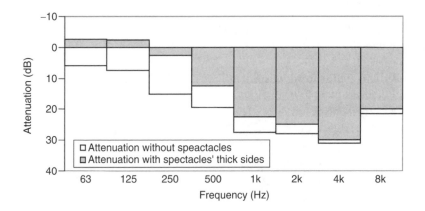

**Figure 30.2** Effect of wearing spectacles on the attenuation of earmuffs (Starck, Pekkarinen and Aatola, 1987).

are supplied with electronics in order to achieve level-dependent functions of sound attenuation. Two main types of function can be separated: sound restoration and noise cancellation systems. The first one transfers external sound signals in order to improve communication facilities. This can be done by microphones that are mounted outside the earmuffs and by small loudspeakers that are inside the earmuffs. The other possibility is to use a wireless technique to listen to local broadcasting so the device can also act as a radio set. The maximum level for the transmitted sound has to be limited to 80 dB to meet the basic safety requirements. Noise cancellation systems are constructed to produce sound that is in the opposite phase to the external noise inside the cup of the earmuff. By the interference of these two noises, some attenuation will be achieved, which in practice will take place most effectively at low frequencies below 1000 Hz resulting typically in 20 dB attenuation.

Against very high-level impulses coming from blasts and explosions, it is preferable to wear earplugs and earmuffs simultaneously. The sum attenuation will not be the sum of both HPDs, but additional protection can still be achieved as shown in Figure 30.3.

Acoustic helmets may provide proper attenuation as these cover large part of the head as well as the outer ear. They additionally reduce the transmission of an airborne sound to the skull and, therefore, reduce bone conduction of the sound to the inner ear. The fitting has to be made very carefully to avoid leakage between the skull and the helmet in order to get good attenuation.

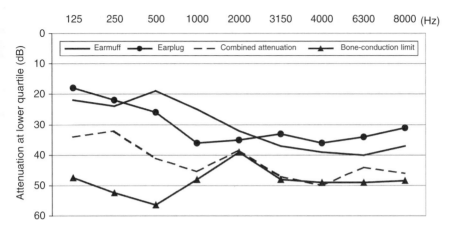

**Figure 30.3** Attenuation of an earplug and earmuff measured separately and in combination. Bone-conduction limit is to show the maximum possible attenuation possible to get with hearing protectors.

## Testing of HPDs

The personal protective devices Directive 89/686/EEC sets the basic health and safety requirements that in turn provide the requirements for the hearing protectors, in the revised standard series EN 352, and the test methods in the standard series EN 13819. At present EN 352-1 for earmuffs, EN 352-2 for earplugs and EN 352-3 for helmet-mounted earmuffs are available. Hearing protectors supplied with electronic circuits are covered by standards EN 352-4, -5, -6 and 7-2002.

When testing in accordance with EN 352 the mechanical tests serve also as preconditioning. The earmuffs and the helmet-mounted muffs are cycled 1000 times with a 25-mm movement in the width of the head band, the cup rotation and size are evaluated, and a drop test is performed. Optionally the drop test can be performed after preconditioning to a temperature of –25°C. The head-band force and the pressure of the cushions are measured. The change in head-band force is measured after conditioning, during which the protectors are set in a 40°C water bath for 24 hours. The acoustic tests comprise an objective test, according to ISO 4869-3, and a subjective test, according to ISO 4869-1. Finally, the ignitability of protectors is tested (EN 13819-1).

The objective test, intended for quality control purposes, is an insertion loss measurement and is done using an artificial test fixture. The subjective measurement is obtained using 16 test persons as a threshold measurement with and without hearing protectors. H, M, L and SNR indices, and the assumed protection values (APVs), are given as results. The H-, M- and

L-indices describe the performance in industrial noise tuned to high, medium and low frequencies. The signal:noise ratio (SNR) index describes the performance in average industrial noise. The APV values are the performances of the protectors at octave bands with frequencies from 125 Hz to 8000 Hz. All the figures have a statistical character, that is 84% of the people get better protection than that indicated by the indices. In addition, the standard sets requirements for the user information and its availability. The comfort index issue, which is emphasized in annex II of the Directive 89/686/EEC, is not covered in the standard. This issue has been studied by many groups (Lataye et al., 1983; Mimpen, 1987; Ming-Young et al., 1991) but still none of the methods is generally approved.

## Use of HPDs

The attenuation results obtained using EN 352-1 should be used in the selection of hearing protectors. The selection criteria are given in standard EN 458-1993, covering the selection, use and maintenance of protectors. According to EN 458 the selection of hearing protectors should be made in such a way that usage rate is as high as possible. EN 458 recommends that the lightest possible protectors should be used, as long as they provide adequate protection. To do this the sound pressure level inside the protector must be evaluated. Moreover, EN 458 recommends that several models should be available for the users to select between them.

**Table 30.2** Attenuation requirements for HPD

| Frequency (Hz) | 125 | 250 | 500 | 1000 | 2000 | 4000 | 8000 |
|---|---|---|---|---|---|---|---|
| APV$f$ (dB) | 5 | 8 | 10 | 12 | 12 | 12 | 12 |

APV$f$ = M$f$ – SD$f$. APV is the assumed protection value, $M$ is a mean attenuation in a subjective test of 16 individuals, SD is the standard deviation for the given frequency $f$.

As shown above, some statistical safety limits are included to facilitate the selection of the HPD. In practice the protection values defined in type tests can only seldom be achieved in the workplace. The level of protection can be lower due to the many work-related factors, such as wear and tear of HPDs, movement of the worker, and simultaneous use of other PPE, such as safety glasses and helmets. Thus the real protection level is difficult to determine in the workplace.

EN 458 gives four methods for using these indices to evaluate the level inside the HPD:

- In the *octave band method*, the octave spectrum of noise is measured, and, from each octave band, the APV is subtracted to get the noise spectrum inside the HPD. Finally, the levels inside the HPD are summed up to obtain the noise level inside the protector ($L_A$).

- In the *HML method* the A and C weighted noise levels ($L_A$ and $L_C$) are measured. The difference ($L_C - L_A$) provides an estimate of the noise frequency characteristics. Positive values indicated low-frequency noise and negative values high-frequency noise. Based on the difference and given H, M and L values an estimate of the attenuation of the HPD can be obtained.
- In the *HL-check method* the noise is divided into low, medium and high frequency. In the case of low-frequency noise, the L value, and, in the case of medium- and high-requency noise, the M value is used as an underestimate of the attenuation of the HPD.
- In the *SNR method,* the SNR value is directly subtracted from the noise level.

The *octave band method* is the most accurate method, although the HML method is almost as accurate, while the HL-check method provides a reasonable estimate for attenuation. The SNR method gives a reasonable estimate in typical industrial environment, but a considerable underestimation occurs in low-frequency noise.

# Example of the selection procedure for the given noise environment

The EN 458 recommendation for selection, use, care and maintenance gives four methods to guide selection of an HPD, depending on the level of information available about the noise in the workplace concerned. The appropriate method of hearing protector should be chosen according to Table 30.3.

**Table 30.3** Information of the workplace noise and the appropriate method for assessing sound attenuation

| Method | Information needed |
| --- | --- |
| Octave band | Octave band sound pressure level |
| HML | A weighted sound pressure level $L_A$ and $L_C - L_A$ |
| HML check | A weighted sound pressure level $L_A$ |
| SNR | C weighted sound pressure level $L_C$ |

HML, see text; SNR, signal:noise ratio.

For example, shipyard platers' exposure to noise was measured resulting in $L_A$ = 100 dB (A) and $L_C$ = 101 dB (C). Based on the measured results, the HML method can be applied using Figure 30.4.

To use Figure 30.4, the first task is to calculate $L_C - L_A$ = 101 dB (C) – 100 dB (A) = 1 dB.

An HPD with H = 28 dB, M = 23 dB and L = 17 dB is available. As the difference between $L_C$ and $L_A$ is 1 dB, the HM area will be used. The next task

| | H | | | | | | | | M | | | | | | | | L | | | | | |
|---|---|---|---|---|---|---|---|---|---|---|---|---|---|---|---|---|---|---|---|---|---|---|
| | **40** | 40 | 40 | 40 | 40 | 40 | 40 | 40 | **40** | 40 | 40 | 40 | 40 | 40 | 40 | 40 | **40** | 40 | 40 | 40 | 40 | 40 |
| | **39** | 39 | 39 | 39 | 39 | 39 | 39 | 39 | **39** | 39 | 39 | 39 | 39 | 39 | 39 | 39 | **39** | 39 | 39 | 39 | 39 | 39 |
| | **38** | 38 | 38 | 38 | 38 | 38 | 38 | 38 | **38** | 38 | 38 | 38 | 38 | 38 | 38 | 38 | **38** | 38 | 38 | 38 | 38 | 38 |
| | **37** | 37 | 37 | 37 | 37 | 37 | 37 | 37 | **37** | 37 | 37 | 37 | 37 | 37 | 37 | 37 | **37** | 37 | 37 | 37 | 37 | 37 |
| | **36** | 36 | 36 | 36 | 36 | 36 | 36 | 36 | **36** | 36 | 36 | 36 | 36 | 36 | 36 | 36 | **36** | 36 | 36 | 36 | 36 | 36 |
| | **35** | 35 | 35 | 35 | 35 | 35 | 35 | 35 | **35** | 35 | 35 | 35 | 35 | 35 | 35 | 35 | **35** | 35 | 35 | 35 | 35 | 35 |
| | **34** | 34 | 34 | 34 | 34 | 34 | 34 | 34 | **34** | 34 | 34 | 34 | 34 | 34 | 34 | 34 | **34** | 34 | 34 | 34 | 34 | 34 |
| | **33** | 33 | 33 | 33 | 33 | 33 | 33 | 33 | **33** | 33 | 33 | 33 | 33 | 33 | 33 | 33 | **33** | 33 | 33 | 33 | 33 | 33 |
| | **32** | 32 | 32 | 32 | 32 | 32 | 32 | 32 | **32** | 32 | 32 | 32 | 32 | 32 | 32 | 32 | **32** | 32 | 32 | 32 | 32 | 32 |
| | **31** | 31 | 31 | 31 | 31 | 31 | 31 | 31 | **31** | 31 | 31 | 31 | 31 | 31 | 31 | 31 | **31** | 31 | 31 | 31 | 31 | 31 |
| | **30** | 30 | 30 | 30 | 30 | 30 | 30 | 30 | **30** | 30 | 30 | 30 | 30 | 30 | 30 | 30 | **30** | 30 | 30 | 30 | 30 | 30 |
| | **29** | 29 | 29 | 29 | 29 | 29 | 29 | 29 | **29** | 29 | 29 | 29 | 29 | 29 | 29 | 29 | **29** | 29 | 29 | 29 | 29 | 29 |
| | **28** | 28 | 28 | 28 | 28 | 28 | 28 | 28 | **28** | 28 | 28 | 28 | 28 | 28 | 28 | 28 | **28** | 28 | 28 | 28 | 28 | 28 |
| | **27** | 27 | 27 | 27 | 27 | 27 | 27 | 27 | **27** | 27 | 27 | 27 | 27 | 27 | 27 | 27 | **27** | 27 | 27 | 27 | 27 | 27 |
| | **26** | 26 | 26 | 26 | 26 | 26 | 26 | 26 | **26** | 26 | 26 | 26 | 26 | 26 | 26 | 26 | **26** | 26 | 26 | 26 | 26 | 26 |
| | **25** | 25 | 25 | 25 | 25 | 25 | 25 | 25 | **25** | 25 | 25 | 25 | 25 | 25 | 25 | 25 | **25** | 25 | 25 | 25 | 25 | 25 |
| | **24** | 24 | 24 | 24 | 24 | 24 | 24 | 24 | **24** | 24 | 24 | 24 | 24 | 24 | 24 | 24 | **24** | 24 | 24 | 24 | 24 | 24 |
| | **23** | 23 | 23 | 23 | 23 | 23 | 23 | 23 | **23** | 23 | 23 | 23 | 23 | 23 | 23 | 23 | **23** | 23 | 23 | 23 | 23 | 23 |
| | **22** | 22 | 22 | 22 | 22 | 22 | 22 | 22 | **22** | 22 | 22 | 22 | 22 | 22 | 22 | 22 | **22** | 22 | 22 | 22 | 22 | 22 |
| | **21** | 21 | 21 | 21 | 21 | 21 | 21 | 21 | **21** | 21 | 21 | 21 | 21 | 21 | 21 | 21 | **21** | 21 | 21 | 21 | 21 | 21 |
| | **20** | 20 | 20 | 20 | 20 | 20 | 20 | 20 | **20** | 20 | 20 | 20 | 20 | 20 | 20 | 20 | **20** | 20 | 20 | 20 | 20 | 20 |
| | **19** | 19 | 19 | 19 | 19 | 19 | 19 | 19 | **19** | 19 | 19 | 19 | 19 | 19 | 19 | 19 | **19** | 19 | 19 | 19 | 19 | 19 |
| | **18** | 18 | 18 | 18 | 18 | 18 | 18 | 18 | **18** | 18 | 18 | 18 | 18 | 18 | 18 | 18 | **18** | 18 | 18 | 18 | 18 | 18 |
| | **17** | 17 | 17 | 17 | 17 | 17 | 17 | 17 | **17** | 17 | 17 | 17 | 17 | 17 | 17 | 17 | **17** | 17 | 17 | 17 | 17 | 17 |
| | **16** | 16 | 16 | 16 | 16 | 16 | 16 | 16 | **16** | 16 | 16 | 16 | 16 | 16 | 16 | 16 | **16** | 16 | 16 | 16 | 16 | 16 |
| | **15** | 15 | 15 | 15 | 15 | 15 | 15 | 15 | **15** | 15 | 15 | 15 | 15 | 15 | 15 | 15 | **15** | 15 | 15 | 15 | 15 | 15 |
| | **14** | 14 | 14 | 14 | 14 | 14 | 14 | 14 | **14** | 14 | 14 | 14 | 14 | 14 | 14 | 14 | **14** | 14 | 14 | 14 | 14 | 14 |
| | **13** | 13 | 13 | 13 | 13 | 13 | 13 | 13 | **13** | 13 | 13 | 13 | 13 | 13 | 13 | 13 | **13** | 13 | 13 | 13 | 13 | 13 |
| | **12** | 12 | 12 | 12 | 12 | 12 | 12 | 12 | **12** | 12 | 12 | 12 | 12 | 12 | 12 | 12 | **12** | 12 | 12 | 12 | 12 | 12 |
| | **11** | 11 | 11 | 11 | 11 | 11 | 11 | 11 | **11** | 11 | 11 | 11 | 11 | 11 | 11 | 11 | **11** | 11 | 11 | 11 | 11 | 11 |
| | **10** | 10 | 10 | 10 | 10 | 10 | 10 | 10 | **10** | 10 | 10 | 10 | 10 | 10 | 10 | 10 | **10** | 10 | 10 | 10 | 10 | 10 |
| | **9** | 9 | 9 | 9 | 9 | 9 | 9 | 9 | **9** | 9 | 9 | 9 | 9 | 9 | 9 | 9 | **9** | 9 | 9 | 9 | 9 | 9 |
| | **8** | 8 | 8 | 8 | 8 | 8 | 8 | 8 | **8** | 8 | 8 | 8 | 8 | 8 | 8 | 8 | **8** | 8 | 8 | 8 | 8 | 8 |
| | **7** | 7 | 7 | 7 | 7 | 7 | 7 | 7 | **7** | 7 | 7 | 7 | 7 | 7 | 7 | 7 | **7** | 7 | 7 | 7 | 7 | 7 |
| | **6** | 6 | 6 | 6 | 6 | 6 | 6 | 6 | **6** | 6 | 6 | 6 | 6 | 6 | 6 | 6 | **6** | 6 | 6 | 6 | 6 | 6 |
| | **5** | 5 | 5 | 5 | 5 | 5 | 5 | 5 | **5** | 5 | 5 | 5 | 5 | 5 | 5 | 5 | **5** | 5 | 5 | 5 | 5 | 5 |
| | **4** | 4 | 4 | 4 | 4 | 4 | 4 | 4 | **4** | 4 | 4 | 4 | 4 | 4 | 4 | 4 | **4** | 4 | 4 | 4 | 4 | 4 |
| | **3** | 3 | 3 | 3 | 3 | 3 | 3 | 3 | **3** | 3 | 3 | 3 | 3 | 3 | 3 | 3 | **3** | 3 | 3 | 3 | 3 | 3 |
| | **2** | 2 | 2 | 2 | 2 | 2 | 2 | 2 | **2** | 2 | 2 | 2 | 2 | 2 | 2 | 2 | **2** | 2 | 2 | 2 | 2 | 2 |
| | **1** | 1 | 1 | 1 | 1 | 1 | 1 | 1 | **1** | 1 | 1 | 1 | 1 | 1 | 1 | 1 | **1** | 1 | 1 | 1 | 1 | 1 |
| | **0** | 0 | 0 | 0 | 0 | 0 | 0 | 0 | **0** | 0 | 0 | 0 | 0 | 0 | 0 | 0 | **0** | 0 | 0 | 0 | 0 | 0 |
| $L_C - L_A$ | **-2.0** | -1.5 | -1.0 | -0.5 | 0 | 0.5 | 1.0 | 1.5 | **2** | 3 | 4 | 5 | 6 | 7 | 8 | 9 | **10** | 11 | 12 | 13 | 14 | 15 |

**Figure 30.4** Protector attenuation predicted noise reduction (dB).

is to connect the corresponding H and M values and read from the 1-dB row the PNR (= 24 dB (A)), which is the predicted noise reduction that can be achieved by the selected HPD in the noise concerned. The effective sound pressure level inside the HPD is: $L_A$ – PNR = 100 dB (A) – 24 dB = 76 dB (A).

The selection of the HPD is rated based on the noise level inside the HPD, which should meet the criteria in Table 30.4.

**Table 30.4** The rating of the attenuation according to EN 458

| Rating | Criteria |
|---|---|
| Insufficient | $L' > L_{AL}$ |
| Satisfactory | $L_{AL} - 5 < L' < L_{AL}$ |
| Good | $L_{AL} - 10 < L' < L_{AL} - 5$ |
| Satisfactory | $L_{AL} - 15 < L' < L_{AL} - 10$ |
| Overprotection | $L' < L_{AL} - 15$ |

Where $L_{AL}$ is the national action level and L' is the effective sound pressure level inside the hearing protector affecting the ear.

The selection is good when it is between 75 dB and 80 dB in the countries where the action level is 85 dB (A).

In working conditions, the attenuation of HPDs also depends on environmental factors. In a cold environment, as in forest work, the hardening of the cushion rings causes a slight, but systematic, deterioration in the attenuation. Worn-out cushions and reduction in the head-band force also affect the attenuation to such an extent that it is difficult to assess protectors in continuous use. In the winter time forest workers use helmet liners, which in some cases nullify the attenuation of the hearing protectors (Starck, Pekkarinen and Aatola, 1987).

## Protection efficiency at workplaces

The attenuation performance given in the type tests is based on the 84% probability that can be achieved for the population in laboratory conditions. In practice, we may suppose that this corresponds to the maximum attenuation that it is possible to obtain in field conditions.

**Causes of lower attenuation**
- the earmuff is old and the worn protector may not provide the same attenuation as the new one;
- the fitness and mounting of the earplug is not as good as in a laboratory;
- movement at work may decrease the attenuation;
- earmuffs are used together with spectacles.

Moreover the variation in attenuation was shown to be clearly higher at workplace measurements than in laboratory measurements. Figure 30.5 shows the measurement obtained at 21 different working places from 238 workers. The curves show that the mean difference between laboratory and field measurement is 7 dB (Toppila, 1998).

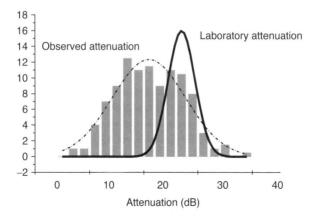

**Figure 30.5** Distribution of observed attenuation in 238 measurements at working places in comparison to the laboratory measurements of the same type of protectors.

Fitness and insertion of an earplug may result in variation in earplug protection efficiency of up to at least 10 dB (Figure 30.6). Figure 30.6 was obtained in a study performed in the laboratory by providing an EN 352-2 test first to naive test persons without any guidance from the operator, and then repeating the test after personal guidance by the operator. The effect seemed to be most prominent at low frequencies below 1 kHz, whereas at high frequencies the difference was about 5 dB (Toppila et al., 1997).

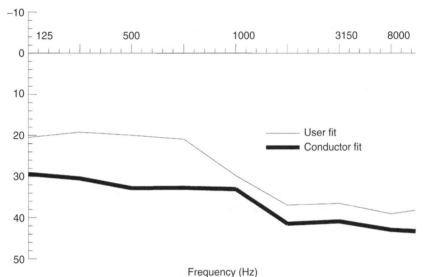

**Figure 30.6** The effect of education to protection efficiency of earplugs. The test was performed before and after the guidance of the operator.

# Effect of usage rate

The protection efficiency of HPDs decreases very rapidly if HPDs are not worn full time. Figure 30.7 shows the protection efficiency of three HPDs

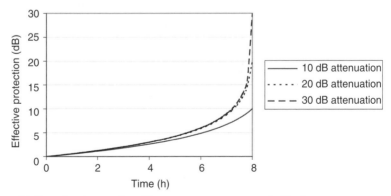

**Figure 30.7** Reduction in the effective protection provided by hearing protectors with decreased wearing time in noisy environment for the protectors of 10, 20 and 30 dB attenuation.

providing nominal attenuation of 10 dB, 20 dB and 30 dB, as a function
of usage rate in noisy environment. The nominal protection performance
is achieved if protectors are worn full time in the noisy environment, but
if worn for only 4 hours out of an 8-hour day the effective protection provided by any HPD will not be more than 3 dB (EN 458).

# Hearing deterioration and usage of HPDs

Figure 30.8 shows the results from a case study performed among paper
mill workers ($n = 400$) exposed to 91-dB to 94-dB noise levels in their
work. The workers were divided into three groups: those who never used
HPDs, those who were casual users and used HPDs about 50% of the
exposure duration, and those who were full-time users. According to the
audiograms, workers in the groups were divided into four categories
(Starck et al., 1995).

Normal hearing was observed among 73% of full-time users whereas
among non-users only 50% had normal hearing. Among casual users the
cases of mild hearing losses were elevated. Non-users were the dominant
group in the moderate and severe hearing loss groups.

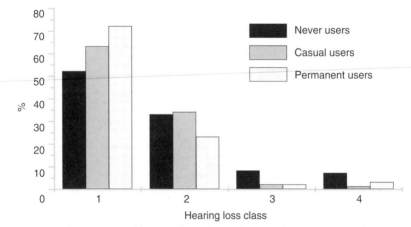

**Figure 30.8** The severity of hearing loss depending on the usage rate of HPDs
among paper mill workers: 1 = normal hearing, 2 = minor hearing loss, 3 =
moderate hearing loss and 4 = severe hearing loss.

# Protection against shooting impulses

Military service is mandatory in many European countries but the prevalence of exposure to gunfire noise is country dependent. In England,
Smith et al. (2000) found that about 3% of young people were exposed to
gunfire noise whereas in Finland the corresponding prevalence is about
10% (Toppila et al., 1997). During military service, young men are

exposed to gunfire and explosive noises where peak levels are clearly above 140 dB peak level, presented as a threshold level for instantaneous sound peak levels (EEC/188/89). The attenuation of HPDs has to be investigated in field conditions applying a miniature microphone method, in which small-size microphones are mounted outside and inside the earmuff. Table 30.5 shows that the higher the peak level outside the HPD the lower the attenuation. This can, in part, be explained by amplitude non-linearity. However, the main degradation of attenuation is strongly related to the frequency content of the impulse. Large-calibre weapons like cannons generate lower-frequency impulses than small calibre weapons such as pistols and rifles (Starck et al., 1987).

**Table 30.5** Average peak sound pressure levels and standard deviations outside ($P_{peakout}$) and inside ($L_{peakin}$) the earmuff and the attenuation of the peak levels in an earmuff intended for military use.

| Weapon | $n$ | $L_{peakout}$ (dB) | $L_{peakin}$ (dB) | Attenuation (dB) |
|---|---|---|---|---|
| Pistol 9 mm | 5 | 159±0.5 | 129±0.5 | 30±0.5 |
| Pistol 22 cal | 5 | 149±1 | 121±1 | 29±1.5 |
| Attack rifle 7.62 mm | 30 | 157±1 | 139±0.5 | 17±1 |
| Ordinary rifle | 25 | 155±0.5 | 139±1 | 16±1.5 |
| Bazooka | 7 | 171±1 | 162±2 | 8±2 |
| Cannon 130 mm | 3 | 176±1 | 172±0.5 | 4±1 |

$n$ = number of impulses.

## Conclusion

Hearing protectors have to be used all the time during a noise exposure period. To meet this requirement, HPDs have to be put on before entering noise areas or before switching on a noisy machine. Figure 30.7 demonstrates that even very short periods without using HPDs will decrease the protection efficiency very significantly. Care and maintenance of the protectors is also very important. Decreased head-band force, broken cushion rings and simultaneous use of spectacles with thick side arms causing leakage also decrease protection efficiency. Comfort of the HPD is not included in the evaluation but is important and may affect the usage rate. Therefore, workers should have the opportunity to select from several models and types of HPD, so that they can choose which fits them best. Earplugs have to be mounted deep enough into the ear canal and exactly according to the instructions. Thus, their size should be selected to correspond with ear-canal dimensions. Motivation of the workers is included in the hearing conservation programme. It means that workers have to be informed and educated about the risks of exposure to noise and about the preventive measures available. Importantly, this should include information not only about the workplace noise but also about any noise in other aspects of the environment, and especially leisure noise.

# References

Lataye R, Damongeot A, Lievin D, Englert M (1983) Efficacité et confort des protecteurs individuels control le bruit. Travail et Securité 10: 551–77.

Ming–Young Park, Casali J6 (1991) An empirical study on comfort afforded by various protection devices: laboratory versus field results. Applied Acoustics 34: 151–79.

Mimpen AM (1987) Field study on the comfort of eight types of earmuffs. Report No. IZF 1987-5E. Soesterberg, Netherlands: TNO Institute for Perception.

Pekkarinen J (1987) Industrial noise, crest factor and the effect of earmuffs. American Industrial Hygiene Association Journal 48: 861–6.

Pekkarinen J, Iki M, Starck J, Pyykkö I (1993) Hearing loss risk from exposure to shooting impulses in workers exposed to occupational noise. British Journal of Audiology 27: 175–82.

Smith PA, Davis A, Ferguson M, Lutman ME (2000) The prevalence and type of social noise exposure in young adults in England. Noise Health 6: 41–56.

Starck J, Pekkarinen J, Aatola S (1987) Attenuation of earmuffs against low frequency noise. Journal of Low Frequency Noise and Vibration 6: 167–74.

Starck J, Pyykkö I, Toppila E, Pekkarinen J (1995) Do the models assess noise-induced hearing loss correctly? ACES 7(3–4): 21–6.

Toppila E (1998) What kind of protectors are used in the EU and is their use mandatory? In D Prasher, L Luxon, I Pyykkö (eds) Advances in Noise Research, Vol. 2. Protection against noise. London: Whurr, pp. 164–6.

Toppila E, Starck J, Pyykkö I, Pihlström A (1997) Free time and military noise in the evaluation of total exposure to noise. In B Das, W Karwowski (eds) Advances in Occupational Ergonomics and Safety II. Proceedings of the Annual International Occupational Ergonomics and Safety Conference, 1–4 June. Washington: IOS Press and Ohm-Sha, pp. 533–7.

# Appendix A

2003/10/EC (2003) Council Directive on the minimum health and safety requirements regarding to the exposure of workers to the risks arising from physical factors (noise). Brussels: European Commission.

86/188/EEC (1986) Council Directive on the protection of workers from the risks related to exposure to noise at work. Brussels: European Commission.

89/656/EEC (1989) Council Directive on the minimum requirements for the use by workers of personal protective equipment. Brussels: European Commission.

89/686/EEC (1989) Council Directive on the approximation of the laws of the member states relating to personal protective equipment. Brussels: European Commission.

EN 352-1 (2002) Hearing protectors – General requirements – Part 1: Ear muffs. Brussels: CEN.

EN 352-2 (2002) Hearing protectors – General requirements – Part 2: Earplugs.

Brussels: CEN.

EN 352-4 (2002) Hearing protectors – Safety requirements and testing – part 4: Level dependent ear muffs. European draft standard. Brussels: CEN.

EN 352-5 (2002) Hearing protectors – Safety requirements and testing – part 5: Active noise reduction ear muffs. European draft standard. Brussels: CEN.

EN 352-6 (2002) Hearing protectors – Safety requirements and testing – part 6: Audio communication ear muffs. European draft standard. Brussels: CEN.

EN 352-7 (2002) Hearing protectors – Safety requirements and testing – part 7: Level dependent earplugs. European draft standard. Brussels: CEN.

EN 458 (1993) Hearing protectors – Recommendations for selection, use, care and maintenance – Guidance document. Brussels: CEN.

EN 352-3 (2003) Hearing protectors – General requirements – part 3: Helmet mounted ear muffs. Brussels: CEN.

EN 13819-1 (2002) Hearing protectors – Testing – Part 1: Physical test methods. European draft standard. Brussels: CEN.

EN 13819-2 (2002) Hearing protectors – Testing – Part 2: Acoustic test methods. European draft standard. Brussels: CEN.

ISO 4869-1 (1990) Acoustics-hearing protectors. Subjective method for the measurement of sound attenuation. Geneva: International Organization for Standardization.

ISO 4869-3 (1989) Acoustics – Hearing protectors. Part 3. Simplified method for the measurement of insertion loss of earmuff type protectors for quality inspection purposes. Geneva: International Organization for Standardization.

# CHAPTER 31

# Audiological rehabilitation programmes and the ICF

*Noise and Its Effects:* Edited by Linda Luxon and Deepak Prasher © 2007 John Wiley & Sons Ltd.

HOLGERS KM, BARRENÄS ML

For people with noise-induced hearing loss (NIHL), conventional audiology rehabilitation programmes (ARPs) focus mainly on the individual with hearing impairment, aiming at reducing the hearing problems by fitting hearing aids, prescribing additional technical devices and functional training courses including lip reading. The role of the environment is often overlooked, even though environmental adjustments are crucial. Such demands have now been put forward by the World Health Organization (WHO). The objective of this chapter is to describe, from the perspective of the WHO (2001), the activity limitations and participation restrictions experienced by our patients and their spouses and the coping strategies that they use to solve such problems. Our recent group-rehabilitation model is described and also the questionnaires and scales used to evaluate the outcome of the intervention.

## Audiological rehabilitation and the WHO

Recently, the WHO replaced the previous *International Classification of Impairment, Disability and Handicap* with the *International Classification of Functioning, Disability and Health* (ICF: WHO, 2001).

- 'Functioning' is used as an umbrella term for *body functions* and *structures,* and *activities and participation in normal life.*
- 'Disability' is used as an umbrella term for *impairment, activity limitations* (the difficulties that an individual with a hearing impairment may have in executing activities) and *participation restrictions* (nonauditory problems an individual may experience in the involvement in different life situations).

The ICF also describes the contextual factors, divided into environmental and personal factors. Personal factors include:

- age;
- gender;
- race;
- educational background;
- social background;
- profession;
- past and current experiences;
- personality;
- character style;
- attitudes;
- other health conditions;
- fitness;
- lifestyle;
- habits;
- upbringing;
- coping styles.

Environmental factors include:

- the physical world and its features;
- other people in different relationships and their roles;
- attitudes and values;
- different services;
- social systems in a society and its policies, rules and laws.

To improve quality of life, the ultimate aim of an ARP is to reinstate satisfactory listening and communication abilities. Besides technical solutions and hearing tactics, psychosocial skills such as coping strategies for reducing problems and negative emotions should be practised. ARPs should also improve self-acceptance and the self-esteem. Moreover, if individuals with hearing impairment are to participate in activities as other people, then the environment and society must adjust accordingly.

## Facets of ARP

- Technical solutions
- Hearing tactics
- Psychosocial skills
- Raise self-acceptance/self-esteem
- Adjustment of society/environment
- Involvement of family
- Involvement of 'significant others'

Consequently, the significant others should be addressed in an ARP as adjustments are necessary from their side, too. Finally, as all family members bear several consequences of an NIHL in the working husband, attention should be paid to the impact on the total life situation of other family members apart from the hearing-impaired person.

# Activity limitations, participation restrictions and consequences for the family due to NIHL

The perceived problems as expressed by our patients are in accordance with Lalande, Lambert and Riverin (1988) and Hétu and Getty (1991), who summarized the activity limitations due to NIHL (hearing disability) as 'reduced listening and communication abilities' (Figure 31.1). The participation restrictions due to NIHL (hearing handicap) are presented, including precursors to the activity limitations and participation restrictions. Consequently, it is important that these mechanisms are discussed in detail with the ARP participants. Two obstacles for success must be highlighted:

- the reluctance to acknowledge hearing difficulties;
- the illusive sensorineural high-frequency hearing loss.

### Reluctance and unwillingness to acknowledge any hearing difficulty

It is known, both from research, clinical practice and spouses, that men with NIHL are reluctant, or even unwilling to acknowledge their hearing difficulties (Blakie and Guthrie, 1984; Hétu et al., 1990; Hallberg and Barrenäs, 1993).

Surprisingly, when asking what difficulties they relate to their NIHL, the most common answer is that they experience no problems, but regard their hearing as normal. 'I have no problems with poor hearing. It is my wife who experiences problems, not me.' 'She is the one who should receive the insurance compensation, because she has suffered the most.'

Note the projection from the husband towards the spouse. Only when questions are asked about very specific situations, such as speech intelligibility during group conversations or watching TV with others, will the patient reveal his hearing disability: 'I have my own TV set.' 'At meetings and parties I can hear nothing.' 'I feel left out at conversations.' 'Since I can hear nothing I rather stay at home, but this is not a problem for me.'

Some authors suggest that this denial is a coping strategy helping the individual to avoid the fear of being rejected as a handicapped person. Or of being discredited by appearing prematurely old, abnormal, bizarre and stigmatized. Or of lowering one's self-image by admitting an impairment or imperfection (Jones, 1987; Jones, Kyle and Wood, 1987; Hétu and Getty,

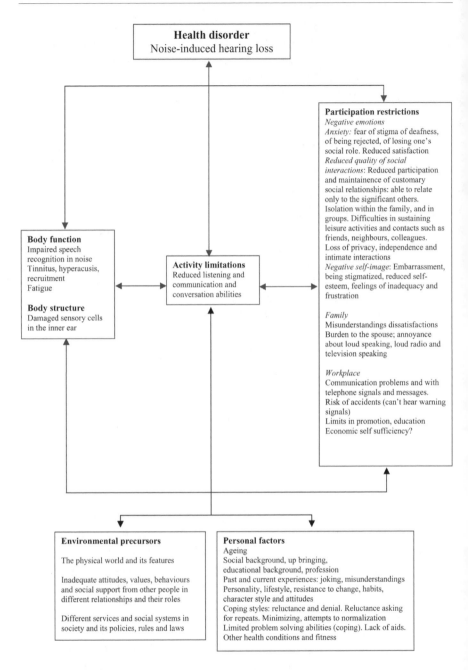

**Figure 31.1** International Classification of Functioning, Disability and Health (ICF) (WHO, 2001) applied to noise-induced hearing loss.

1991). Denial is a normal part of one's work, when coping with a daily danger to one's health in a situation essential to one's living. Trying to protect one's social image means not only reluctance to acknowledge one's hearing problems, but also a lack of attempts to solve them.

All ARP participants, both men and spouses, must learn to identify the psychosocial problems typically induced by NIHL. Meeting others with NIHL helps the person to realize that he is normal and not 'deviant'. The psychosocial support from a group allowing and sharing the negative experiences of NIHL will also improve self-esteem and the self-acceptance of the hearing loss necessary to start a continuously ongoing rehabilitation process.

## The illusive sensorineural high-frequency hearing loss

Even though NIHL is severe, one-to-one communication in a quiet surrounding is seldom troublesome. However, the slightest background noise may induce severe speech intelligibility problems even to individuals with a mild NIHL. According to Aniansson (1974), speech recognition scores were 98% in quiet and 75% in noise if hearing was normal. If the 3-kHz frequency is damaged, then 90% correct answers in quiet were achieved, but only 40% in noise, whereas only a 65% score in quiet and 10% in noise were obtained if 2 kHz was also affected. Usually, as NIHL develops slowly, the fact that the husband's speech intelligibility is dependent mainly upon the level of the prevailing background noise or whether or not the wife is turned towards the husband when addressing him stays more or less unacknowledged. The illusive sensorineural high-frequency hearing loss induces an inconsistent behaviour from the person with the hearing impairment, creating some almost compulsory negative interpretations by the significant others, even in families who have received insurance compensation for NIHL. A situation distressing to most couples is the opinion of the spouse that the husband 'understands [hears] whenever he wants to', or 'is interested in the matter'. One common adjustment is that the husband uses a separate room with his own TV set, while the rest of the family watch TV in the living room. One could say that the significant others and the environment dictate whether a person with a hearing impairment can participate in a social gathering or not, and not the hearing-impaired person himself.

There is also a remarkable discrepancy between the knowledge of the experts and the opinions of NIHL as expressed by workers. Workers believe that hearing is lost – they expect to hear nothing. Instead, the recruitment phenomenon is perceived as 'sensitive' hearing. Therefore, the workers regard their hearing as normal. Moreover, as one-to-one communication in quiet surroundings is seldom troublesome, even though the NIHL is severe, the workers believe it is 'normal' not to recognize speech in noisy conditions. A better expression for hearing loss would be 'loss of hearing clarity'. Thus an ARP requires not only adequate information about the high-frequency hearing loss but also support to cope with the tension and irritation that arise because of the communication difficulties. In this latter regard, there is a need to search actively for solutions.

**Individual and environmental precursors to communication difficulties**

Factors that predispose an individual to communication difficulties include:

- poor socioeconomic conditions;
- poor education;
- low self-esteem;
- a limited acceptance of the problem;
- stigmatization;
- a difficult work environment.

Factors associated with poor adaptation to NIHL include:

- unsupportive family;
- overzealous, inappropriate social support;
- tinnitus;
- background noise;
- poor articulation/phonation of companion(s).

Poor socioeconomic standards, a low level of education, low self-esteem and poor understanding/acceptance of the hearing problem relate to the use of resignation as a coping strategy. This may in turn reduce ability to solve communication problems using instrumental aids or active verbal coping strategies, such as asking others to adapt. This is because active coping increases the possibility of being stigmatized and identified as hearing impaired. On the other hand, increased self-knowledge of a hearing problem makes one recognize the disadvantages due to the hearing loss. Moreover, white-collar workers, in contrast with blue-collar workers, are required to participate in more meetings, discussions and communication with customers, which are very stressful situations for people with hearing impairment. Complaints or blame from the family appears to create feelings of being useless and inadequate. These factors represent serious psychosocial disadvantages both to the worker and to the family which require attention. Tinnitus often further increases the hearing disability. Other unfavourable environmental predictors include too much social support, inappropriate support, negative attitudes, inadequate behaviours, disturbing background noise, and poor articulation and phonation from others.

One way to reduce the fear of stigmatization and participation restrictions is to improve self-acceptance, self-esteem and self-image, and to increase the understanding of 'reduced listening and communication abilities'. The rehabilitation process can start only when the hearing loss is integrated into the self-image of the person's mind. Specific problem-solving coping styles are initiated by sorting out misunderstandings, negative attitudes and unhelpful social support. In order to train couples to adopt and use effective coping strategies, the group leaders must recognize the coping strategies that people with NIHL and their spouses adopt in different stressful situations.

# Coping strategies adopted by people with NIHL and their spouses

Coping includes different strategies or tactics used by a person to handle stressful situations. For people with hearing impairment, coping means the strategies used to handle auditorily demanding situations. The driving force of coping is defined as the person's desire to pass as normal in social interactions and to avoid being regarded as deviant in order to maintain a positive self-image.

In general, there are two types of coping strategies: *active* and *avoiding* strategies:

* Avoiding strategies: consequently, the person avoids demanding hearing situations such as social gatherings or meetings. Further, he minimizes his disability by not admitting his hearing difficulties to anyone including himself. He guesses and pretends to understand while keeping silent.
* Active strategies: strategies defined as 'active' require the need to structure demanding auditory situations by preparing and planning beforehand and to control the environment by instructing others. Social interactions are maintained by being tolerant and by making the best of the situation, which often means acceptance of missing conversations. *Active verbal communication strategies* include asking for repeats, informing others about one's hearing loss, and monopolizing or leading the conversation. *Active non-verbal strategies* include positioning oneself so that it is possible both to hear and to see the speaker or to look for a quieter area in which to talk.

Depending upon the situation, a person shifts between avoiding and active strategies. For example, if important information is given at meetings, at work or if speaking to only a few familiar persons, active coping strategies are adopted more frequently than at home or at social gatherings (Hallberg and Barrenäs, 1995).

Three strategies used, regardless of preference for active or avoiding behaviour, are space to recover from fatigue and physical tension caused by the NIHL, adaptations to work by working alone or by changing to a less noisy workplace, and the use of technical aids.

Spouses also use coping strategies to handle the impact of the husband's hearing loss upon the family. Four different coping styles are described by Hallberg and Barrenäs (1993) of how spouses cope with the husband's reluctance to acknowledge hearing difficulties, the influence of the hearing loss on the couple's close relationship and the consequences of the NIHL on their daily living:

- The *co-acting wife* does not admit any impact of the NIHL upon the family life. 'Everything at home works well. You just have to adjust to each other. As a spouse you must be patient.'
- The *minimizing wife* admits some influence of the NIHL on the intimate relationship, even though she minimizes the communication problems related to her husband's hearing loss. 'During the last years I have become more and more silent . . . there is no use in discussing the problem with him . . . it does not work, it always ends up in a conflict and you want to avoid that . . . especially me.' The minimizing wife often 'clenches her teeth' in order to maintain domestic peace. The suspicion that the husband might be mentally altered was also expressed.
- The *mediating wife* controls the situation by listening for both herself and the husband and she carefully navigates him away from demanding auditory situations. She also advises him how to behave. During social gatherings, she works hard to keep up the image of the couple as normal.
- The *distancing wife* expresses a severe impact both on the close relationship and on the communication ability. The pair often live side by side without participating in each other's lives. 'It is hard to get in touch with one another . . . we are on different levels, so to speak . . . sometimes it is almost impossible to reach each other.'

According to our research and clinical experience, men with a severe audiometric NIHL experience severe hearing problems, and often feel hearing disabled, while hearing handicap is perceived only seldom or sometimes. Non-verbal communication strategies are used more often than verbal strategies, while the avoiding strategies (avoiding auditory demanding situations, guessing or pretending that you have understood) are used more seldom than the other two. As the hearing problems worsen from slight to moderate the use of the avoiding strategies increases from 'seldom' to 'every now and then', the verbal strategies from 'every now and then' to 'every other time' and the non-verbal strategies from 'every now and then' to 'often'. By using the right coping strategy at the right moment, communication ability can be improved.

Due to their denial and reluctance to acknowledge and verbalize their hearing difficulties and also their use of avoiding coping strategies, the life situation of workers with NIHL will probably remain unexplored. Thus, proper preventive action is not put in place, which constitutes a problem both for themselves and for society.

## Measurement scales (assessment I–IV)

To estimate the effect of intervention, many different scales or questionnaires are used (for a review, see Table 31.1). Besides those listed below another four items designed by Lutman, Brown and Coles (1987) are used (see Appendix A).

**Table 31.1** Review of hearing handicaps scales

| Scale | Design | Subjects | Response-format | Administration | Correlation to pure-tone audiometry | Correlation to speech discrimination | Total variance |
|---|---|---|---|---|---|---|---|
| Hearing Handicap Scale<br>1. High et al. (1964)<br>2. Blumenfeld et al. (1969)<br>3. Speaks et al. (1970)<br>4. Marcus-Bernstein (1986) | 20 items relating to hearing ability for speech and situational difficulties | 1. 50 (conductive HL)<br>2. 55 (elderly)<br>3. 60 (elderly)<br>4. 100 (elderly) | Almost always/usually/sometimes/rarely/almost never | 1, 2. Paper and pencil/self-administered<br>4. Face-to-face interview | 1. $r = 0.7$<br><br>4. $r = 0.5$ | 1. $r = 0.2$<br>2. $r = 0.3$–$0.5$ quiet<br>$r = 0.3$–$0.6$ noise<br>3. $r = 0.3$–$0.5$<br>4. $r = 0.5$–$0.6$ | 1. Pearson coefficient $= 0.96$<br>4. Total variance $= 46\%$ |
| Hearing Measurement Scale<br>1. Noble and Atherley (1970)<br>2. McCartney et al. (1976)<br>3. Tyler and Smith (1983)<br>4. Eriksson-Mangold et al. (1992) | 42 weighted items relating to speech perception, non-speech sounds, and hearing handicaps | 1. 46 men with NIHL.<br>2. 36 (elderly) 60 year olds<br>3. 30<br>4. 133 (elderly) | 5-point response format:<br>always/nearly always/sometimes/hardly ever/ever | 1–4. Face-to-face interview | 1. Speech: 0.6–0.8<br>Localization 0.4<br>Handicap 0.5<br>2. $r = 0.5$<br>3. $r = 0.7$–$0.8$<br>4. $r = 0.4$–$0.5$<br>Emotional response: 0.3<br>Location: 0.2 | 1. Speech: 0.6<br>Localization: 0.4<br>Emotional response: 0.4<br>2. $r = 0.4$<br>3. Speech: 0.7<br>Localisation: 0.3<br>Handicap: 0.5 | 1. Pearson coefficient $= 0.9$<br>1. Coefficient $\alpha$ emotional $= 0.9$<br>disability $= 0.9$ |
| Hearing Handicap Inventory for the Elderly<br>1. Ventry and Weinstein (1982)<br>2. Marcus-Bernstein (1986) | Disability (12 items), and emotional consequences (13 items) | 1. 100 (elderly)<br>2. 100 (elderly) | 3-point response format:<br>yes/sometimes/no | Face-to-face interview | 1. $r = 0.6$<br>2. Disability: 0.4<br>Handicap: 0.3 | 2. Disability: 0.4–0.5<br>Handicap: 0.3–0.4 | 2. Total variance $= 23\%$ |
| Lutman et al. (1987) | Everyday speech (4 items), localization (1 item), and hearing handicap (4 items) | 1470 subjects from the general population | 3- or 4-point response format:<br>never/rarely/quite often/very often<br>no/some/great difficulty | Self-administered | Everyday speech: 0.6<br>Localization: 0.3<br>Hearing handicap: 0.6 | Not analysed | Total variance $= 68\%$ |

**Table 31.1** continued

| Scale | Design | Subjects | Response format | Administration | Correlation to pure-tone audiometry | Correlation to speech discrimination | Total variance |
|---|---|---|---|---|---|---|---|
| Lalande et al. (1988) | Quality of life at home/work (14 items), isolation and self-esteem (8 items) and telephone + leisure activities (3 items) | 65 workers with NIHL | Different alternatives | Self-administered followed by a semi-structured interview | Quality of life: 0.42 Self-esteem: 0.54 Telephone: 0.3 | Not investigated | Total variance = 68% |
| The Hearing Disability and Handicap Scale 1. Hétu et al. (1994) 2. Hallberg (1998) 3. Barrenäs and Holgers (1999) | 20 items/3 factors; speech perception (5 items), non-speech sounds (5 items) and hearing handicaps (10 items) | 1. 242 cases 2. 101 men with NIHL 3. 168 men with NIHL | 4-point response format never/ seldom/often/ always | Self-administered | 1,3. Disability 0.5–0.6 Handicap 0.3–0.4 2. Disability 0.3 Handicap 0.2 | 1. Disability: 0.3 Handicap: 0.1 3. Disability: 0.4 Handicap: 0.3 | 1. Coefficient $\alpha = 0.88$ 2, 3 Total variance = 65% |
| Hearing Handicap and Support Scale Hallberg et al. (1993) | 25 items/3 factors. attitude of others, social support, and handicap (8 items) | 89 workers with NIHL. | 5-point response format: ranging from 'strongly agree' to 'strongly disagree' | Self-administered | Not evaluated | Not evaluated | Total variance = 56% |
| Social Hearing Handicap Index 1. Brainerd and Frankel (1985) 2. Tyler and Smith (1983) | 21 items on speech hearing | 1. 430 (adults) 2. 30 (adults and elderly) | 4 alternatives Yes/(yes)/no/(no) | Self-administered, mailed | 1. $r = 0.4$ 2. $r = 0.7–0.8$ | 2. $r = 0.5–0.7$ | |

HL, hearing loss; NIHL, noise-induced hearing loss.

## The Hearing Handicap and Support Scale (HHSS)

The HHSS, which includes 21 items in a five-point response format, ranging from (1) 'strongly disagree' to (5) 'strongly agree', is used to assess negative attitudes from others, social support and disability/handicap. Illustrative items include 'My hearing loss makes my relatives upset', 'People around know that I am hearing impaired and they try to help me' and 'Almost everything I do is affected by my hearing disability'. The Swedish version was previously used in studies on patients with NIHL by Hallberg, Johnsson and Axelsson (1993).

## The Communication Strategies Scale (CPHI/CSS)

The CPHI/CSS is a 25-item subscale of the Communication Profile for the Hearing Impaired (Demorest and Erdman, 1986, 1987). The individuals respond in a five-point response format, ranging from (1) 'rarely/almost never' to (5) 'generally/almost always'. The CSS assesses avoiding, and active verbal and non-verbal communication coping strategies. Avoiding behaviour was defined as 'strategies detracting from or inhibiting the communication process' such as avoiding stressful situations or pretending or guessing that one had understood. Active verbal and non-verbal strategies were intended to 'enhance communication or at least to minimize the effects of the hearing loss' by asking for repeats or by sitting close to the speaker.

## The Hearing Disability and Handicap Scale (HDHS)

The HDHS is a short version of the Hearing Measurement Scale (Noble and Atherly, 1970). HDHS assesses disability and perceived handicap (10 + 10 items; Hétu et al., 1994; Barrenäs and Holgers, 2000; see Appendix B). The four-point response format includes 'never', 'seldom', 'often' and 'always'.

## The Nottingham Health Profile (NHP)

The NHP is a non-disease specific questionnaire widely used for health assessment, which has been adapted also to Swedish conditions (Wiklund, Herlitz and Hjalmarsson, 1989). The questionnaire consists of 45 items, divided into two parts. NHP I includes 38 items that describe the relative functional limitations across six specified areas within everyday living: energy, pain, emotional reactions, sleep, social isolation and mobility. NHP II comprises seven items referring to health-related problems in daily life. Dichotomous response choices are present (yes/no). For each NHP domain, a relative scale score is calculated and expressed as a percentage of total possible dysfunction, where a score of 0 means no reported dysfunction, while a score of 100 indicates maximum dysfunction. The psychometric properties of the NHP and the suggested scales have been proved to be satisfactory (Hunt et al., 1980, 1981).

**The Tinnitus Severity Questionnaire (TSQ)**

The severity of tinnitus was assessed by the TSQ (Baskill et al., 1991; Coles et al., 1991). The questionnaire is designed for self-administration and includes 10 items. Single items can be aggregated into three subscales – Q 1; Q 2–7 and Q 8–10 – or into a total score (TSQ all). All items are scored on a five-point scale (0 = not affected to 4 = always affected). The maximum score is 40. A higher score indicates greater perceived severity of tinnitus.

# An audiological group-rehabilitation programme

The intervention consists of four weekly, 3-hour sessions scheduled at the Rehabilitation Centre in Göteborg. Our ARP is broadly in line with that of Getty and Hétu (1991). The inclusion criterion for the programme is NIHL with a pure-tone average in the better ear > 35 dB HL at 2 kHz and 3 kHz and simultaneously a pure-tone average at 4 kHz and 6 kHz > 45 dB or worse. Additional inclusion criteria are age between 40 and 65 years and participants had to be Swedish speaking.

The programme aims at offering the couples psychosocial support, adequate knowledge on the nature of NIHL and its consequences on the daily life and to provide training in effective coping strategies, hearing tactics and speech therapy. Another objective is to strengthen the hearing-impaired individual's self-esteem and to initiate an active problem-solving rehabilitation process aimed at reducing the communication difficulties and the psychological distress within the family. Finally, the rehabilitation programme is intended to facilitate the mutual acceptance of the hearing disability by family, friends and person affected. In order to achieve this, the participant's own experiences and questions are continuously brought into focus for discussion at all sessions and both men and spouses are always encouraged to share their experiences of dealing with problems related to the hearing loss. The coffee breaks offer important opportunities for spontaneous interactions between the participants and must be allowed to take their time, sometimes 20 minutes or longer.

The intervention is evaluated by pre- and post-intervention assessments of the variables: disability, negative emotions/perceived handicap, acceptance of the hearing disability, and social support and attitudes from the significant others. Assessment I is conducted before intervention. The short-term evaluation of the effects (assessment II) is made at the end of the fourth group session. Six months and also one year after intervention, the long-term effects are evaluated (assessments III and IV). The same measurement scales (described below) are used at all assessments.

**Session 1: adequate knowledge**

Session 1 focuses mainly on medical information about NIHL and its consequences for daily life for the husband, the spouse and other family members. After having introduced the group leaders, the participants and the aims of the project, all participants are given a simple hearing device to test. Information is then given by a physician on the functioning of the ear and how it is affected by noise. The logarithmic decibel scale is exhaustively explained and examples of different noise levels are given. The individual pure-tone audiogram and speech recognition scores in noise are described to each couple. Hearing difficulties as experienced by the participants are then highlighted and both men and spouses are asked to share with the group how they think, feel and manage their communication difficulties. The group leaders simultaneously make notes about the different situations coming up. The coping strategies described by the participants are categorized into verbal, non-verbal or avoiding on the black board. The three coping styles are structured and described according to Hétu et al. (1987) and Hallberg and Barrenäs (1993, 1995).

---

**Components of session 1: education**

(Assessment I completed before any intervention)

- Medical information
- Provision of simple hearing aid
- Explanation of sound and logarithmic decibel scale
- Interpretation of individual pure-tone audiogram and speech discrimination results
- Individual description of hearing difficulties to group
- Coping strategies identified and categorized
- Coping strategies explained
- Homework:
  - identify $L_{eq}$ at work
  - bring hearing protectors to meeting
  - practise face-to-face communication with spouse
- Homework given
- Practise a 10-minute relaxation session

---

The first home assignment is to report the actual $L_{eq}$ level at one's workplace and also to bring one's personal hearing protectors to the forthcoming group session. This task is aimed at increasing the awareness of the noise hazards at work and at facilitating the ability to choose adequate hearing protectors. The second home assignment is to adopt the speech to-and-through-faxing strategy: to always demand face-to-face contact and repeats when asking the significant other for something. The husband must verify having received the correct message by sending it back to the sender saying: 'Did you say, you want me to buy you an orange?' Finally, the spouse must confirm her message, for example by nodding her head or some other body language. The third home assignment is to recognize and compare the efficacy of face-to-face contact to that of not having face-to-face contact.

The session ends by practising a 10-minute relaxation programme. In this ARP, different techniques for relaxation as recovery are regarded as major active non-verbal coping strategies.

## Session 2: Active coping strategies, social support and attitudes from others

Session 2 addresses hearing aids and assistive listening devices. An audiologist participates as a lecturer. Information about various aids for communicating in the car, television listening, for telephone both at home and at work and also for mobile telephones is compulsory. The benefits and shortcomings of hearing aids are described and all participants receive appointments with the project audiologist to discuss their need for technical rehabilitation. The feelings created by seeing oneself wearing a hearing aid are discussed.

**Components of session 2: support**

- Information on communication aids
- Detailed information on hearing aids
- Individual appointment with project audiologist
- Previous homework results presented and discussed
- 'Homework' – diary of participant and spouse of day-by-day coping strategies
- Relaxation session

The outcome of the previous home assignments is presented. The different active verbal and non-verbal coping strategies are described in detail, having the participant's experiences from the previous home assignments in focus. The noise levels at the workplace are explained and discussed.

The aim of the next home assignment is to have both the man and the spouse identify their own coping style in order to learn the most efficient coping strategies. They are asked to write a diary each day about one event at home and at work when active verbal or non-verbal strategies were used. The participants are also asked to consider which active verbal and non-verbal strategies they use in different situations. In what way did the coping strategy of choice work out and in what way did it not? How may one's coping strategies be improved?

The relaxation programme ends the session.

## Session 3: avoiding coping strategies and speech training

**Components of session 3: self-development**

- Couples develop own problem-solving strategies
- Advice on effective strategies and hearing tactics given

- Review of previous 'homework'
- Information on importance of environmental noise provided
- Information on voice/speech production provided
- Information on body language
- 'Homework' – identify and problem solve three most severe communication problems at home
- Relaxation session

Session 3 focuses on encouraging the couples to start their own problem-solving rehabilitation process to decrease negative emotions and reduce the psychological distress in the family. The lecturers are a hearing therapist and a speech therapist. Effective coping strategies and useful hearing tactics of how to improve communication abilities in specific auditory demanding situations (job meetings, lectures, shop and restaurant visits, car and bus travelling, etc.) are highlighted having the previous home assignment as a background. The importance of the acoustic environment for speech recognition and the responsibility of the speaker are also stressed.

Awareness about voice function is essential if the sending part of communication is to improve. Among both the men and the spouses, voice problems occur as a consequence of vocal hyperfunction and fatigue. The speech therapist gives instruction on how to avoid such hoarseness and how to improve the voice and speech quality. The importance of body language, eye contact, proper pronunciation and speech clarity, pausing, etc., is always stressed and all participants take part in a speech-training programme. In this ARP, speech training is regarded as a major active coping strategy. Benefits and shortcomings of the passive avoiding strategies are discussed in detail.

The new home assignment is to identify and deal with the three most important communication problems at home in need of improvement. It identifies and optimizes the present coping strategies, speech tactics and avoiding behaviours included.

The session ends with the 10-minute relaxation programme.

**Session 4: tinnitus**

**Components of session 4: tinnitus**

- Information on tinnitus and its treatment
- Completion of tinnitus questionnaires to identify those needing specific rehabilitation
- Video on hearing disability and hearing tactics shown
- Review of previous 'homework'
- 'Homework' – identify the next three major issues at work or socially to be resolved over 6 months

Assessment II is undertaken for comparison of before and after.

Session 4 elucidates problems related to, and treatment of, noise-induced tinnitus. The Tinnitus Severity Questionnaire and the Nottingham Health Profile are used to identify high-risk tinnitus patients, who will be referred to the aetiologically based tinnitus therapy rehabilitation team. Information on local resources for the hearing impaired is an important section. Insurance items are clarified. A video concerning hearing disability problems and hearing tactics summarizes the content of the four group sessions. The results from the previous home assignment are discussed. Advice is given from all other participants on which strategies to use or avoid. The next home assignment also includes the identification and improvement of the three most important communication problems at work and/or socially that participants wish to solve during the 6 months to come. The aim is to continue the problem-solving process.

An oral evaluation by the participants of the sessions so far is tape-recorded. Speech therapy and the relaxation tape are practised as in previous sessions. The participants fill in assessment II.

## Visits at the workplace and to the audiologist

Most participants discuss the need for technical devices in the workplace, noise measurements and information about NIHL with their workmates. All participants also visit the project audiologist to discuss hearing aids or assistive hearing devices to use at home.

## The 6-month session

This session deals with noise exposure levels at the workplace, hearing protectors (HPs) and safety limitations. The outcome of the visits to the workplaces, noise-level measurements and also the benefit or limits of different technical rehabilitation solutions are discussed.

An important misunderstanding to clarify with the participants is the worker's belief that the human ear is capable of differentiating between damaging and non-damaging noise levels and that this also applies to ears with NIHL.

Most workers design their own noise-level scale by relating the perceived noise level in their present workplace to what they remember from previous workplaces. Many workers argue: 'I got my NIHL when I was working in the shipyard in the 1950s and 1960s. HPs were not available then. Today, noise levels are lower today than before. I need to hear the telephone ringing and what my boss says. Therefore, I use HP only when necessary.' In a survey in Gothenburg, 87% did not think that HPs were properly used in their workplace, 44% took their HP off when it was 'less noisy', 33% when speaking and 20% for comfort reasons, 33% didn't use the HP because they could not hear their mobile telephone. As workers use their HP in the same way as their workmates, most workers believe they use the HP correctly. In order to improve HP usage at a workplace, the worker's beliefs must be replaced by correct knowledge. This includes, as a minimum, the safety limits, the meaning of the decibel scale and the 'noise factor'.

**The noise factor: use an HP if you work:**

40 hours/week in 85 dB
20 hours/week in 88 dB
10 hours/week in 91 dB
5 hours/week in 94 dB
2½ hours/week in 97 dB
1 hour/week in 100 dB
30 min/week in 103 dB
15 min/week in 106 dB

The outcome of the last home assignment is reported. The last home assignment is to continue the previous one with other stressful events using a more effective coping style.

Speech therapy and the relaxation tape are practised as in previous sessions. Assessment III is collected.

**The 12-month session**

This session summarizes the participant's experiences, benefits and shortcomings from the group-rehabilitation intervention and suggestions for future improvements.

Usually, as the knowledge about NIHL increases among the participants, their sense of responsibility grows stronger towards their workmates, especially the younger ones. 'This knowledge should be compulsory at all noisy workplaces, to the working leaders and in schools' is a common suggestion.

Probably, discussions about the hazards of noise, and its impact on life quality and on one's self-esteem seem more relevant and trustworthy if presented by an older workmate of one's own trade than from nurses from the occupational health service centre. Noise levels should label noisy work places and machinery, like other hazards. The workers also request a renewal of the old noise information, starting from the perspective of the users, not from that of the experts. The decibel scale and the safety limitations must be made available and comprehensible to the workers.

The spouses often report improvements of communication ability and also the husband's self-esteem. 'He now feels more confident with himself.' 'I'm more concerned with addressing him properly. I often touch his arm before I say anything, so that he can look at me.' Usually, the active coping strategies have improved: 'He has told his workmates that they must speak up because he has an NIHL.' Also other family member had learnt how to facilitate the communication. One spouse said 'My 3-year-old granddaughter now says to me: "Granny, you must push grandfather like this. Then he can listen to you."'

Speech therapy and the relaxation tape are practised as in previous sessions. Assessment IV is collected.

# Tinnitus rehabilitation

The suffering associated with tinnitus may enhance the perception of being handicapped substantially. As approximately one-third of workers with NIHL also suffer from tinnitus this matter should be highlighted in rehabilitation. In tinnitus rehabilitation it is important to make the patients identify the situations in which tinnitus becomes worse, the difficulties related to tinnitus and the patient's coping strategies. Different programmes are used, such as individual or group cognitive–behavioural therapy, relaxation, counselling and sound stimulation, together with individual directive counselling (tinnitus retraining therapy (TRT), developed by Jastreboff and Hazell (1993). This concept states that persistent tinnitus and suffering from tinnitus are a conditioned response to the perceived tinnitus sound, involving both the limbic and the autonomic nervous systems and TRT is aimed at decreasing this response by habituation. Sound stimulation may also be given together with group sessions ('tinnitus school'), influenced by cognitive–behavioural therapy ('physiological tinnitus treatment') of Holgers (Holgers, Eliasson and Olsson, 2002). Tinnitus rehabilitation may also include individual or group psychotherapy or physiotherapy.

## Identification of profiles of tinnitus sufferers

When evaluating results from 'classic' tinnitus rehabilitation by Axelsson (1995), it was found that 23% of the tinnitus patients developed severe tinnitus according to the definition by Holgers, Erlandsson and Barrenäs (2000) – absence from work, related to tinnitus.

Negative predictors for tinnitus include:

- somatic disorder;
- depression;
- anxiety.

The most important predictors for this negative development were somatic disorders, depression or anxiety disorders (Holgers, Erlandsson and Barrenäs, 2000). In another study including consecutive tinnitus patients seeking help at an audiological clinic during a 6-month period, 75% had depression and/or anxiety disorders, according to the American Psychiatric Association *Diagnostic and Statistical Manual of Mental Disorders* (APA, 199?), but the great majority had never sought help for psychological or psychiatric symptoms. Other medical conditions, as well as depression and somatic disorders' may trigger tinnitus symptoms, and medical treatment should be offered.

Tinnitus suffering can be described in different ways, such as how often tinnitus occurs, the annoyance or intrusiveness of tinnitus, limitations in daily life or how tinnitus affect the patient mentally.

We have chosen reduced working capacity due to tinnitus symptoms as one end-point of the severity of tinnitus. Many of these symptoms may reflect an underlying anxiety or depression, so a basic knowledge in diagnosing and treating these disorders is essential in the management of tinnitus. It is also possible that the same aetiological mechanisms causing symptoms in a depressive disorder can also lead to tinnitus suffering (Zöger et al., 2001). Antidepressant drugs that modulate serotoninergic functions in the brain have been used in a clinical trial by Sullivan et al. (1993) and they reported on the positive effect of nortriptyline in the treatment of patients with tinnitus and depressive symptoms. Their result showed a reduction in depression parameters, functional disability and actually also the psychoacoustic measurement of tinnitus loudness and frequency. In our clinic today (2003), a double-blind, parallel, randomized study on the effect of selective serotonin re-uptake inhibitor (SSRI) (sertraline) on severe tinnitus sufferering is ongoing.

**Rehabilitation based on aetiological factors of the suffering**

In the clinical management of tinnitus patients it is essential to have reliable tools to examine the tinnitus symptoms in order to analyse the effect of different therapies. It is of great importance to identify high-risk patients early, before they develop a severe refractory tinnitus and in order to treat this condition its aetiology must be diagnosed (Figure 31.2). Usually, different aspects of tinnitus are assessed by clinical gradings and/or by questionnaires (see Holgers, Eliasson and Olsson, 2000; see

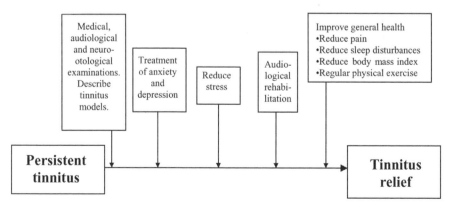

**Figure 31.2** Aetiologically based tinnitus therapy. (Adapted from Holgers (1999), reproduced with permission.)

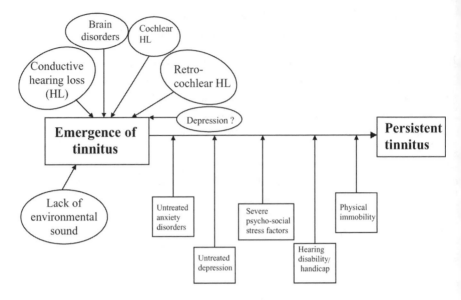

**Figure 31.3** Emergence and persistence of tinnitus. (Adapted from Holgers (1999) reproduced with permission.)

also Chapter 12). According to our clinical experience and research, the main predictors for severe suffering, defined as absence from work related to tinnitus of more than 1 month during the first 18 months, were physical immobility and depression/anxiety-related symptoms. Hearing levels had only a minor impact. The type of rehabilitation programme is determined by the most important factor for each patient (Figure 31.3).

# Outcome of ARP and aetiologically based tinnitus therapy

Audiological rehabilitation should be directed specifically to people with NIHL, and not only in programmes for elderly people, especially as this latter group constitutes one of the largest populations in the industrialized part of the world with acquired preventable hearing loss. At the oral evaluation of our ARP, the topics highlighted during the sessions seem to be relevant to the participants. Both males and spouses were grateful for the psychosocial support from the other group members. 'It is easier to talk in front of others with the same difficulties, who understand the problems', one participant said.

It is obvious that the spouse is a very important key person if rehabilitation efforts are to be successful. She often takes the first step to have an appointment with the audiologist. She also distributed information to others and educates the children about noise, its effects on hearing and the value of HP usage, for example at discos. This is a very important aspect, since education about noise in school hardly exists. However, some spouses may also be a hindrance. In our pilot study, we observed that all spouses participating in the group rehabilitation programme seemed to use either the mediating or minimizing strategies. We could not identify any couples where the spouse used the co-acting or distancing coping strategies. All the males had been very enthusiastic when invited to the programme so we suspect that it is the spouse who decides if the couple should participate or not. Consequently, it is possible that the males most in need of rehabilitation are those who do not attend. Dropouts might need rehabilitation individually.

In the recently developed tinnitus rehabilitation programme in Sweden (Holgers, 1999), the patients were categorized according to a risk-profile analysis. The patients with depression or anxiety symptoms as their main predictor were included in a psychotherapy programme, led by two therapists, one of them a psychologist. Patients with physical immobility as their main predictor were recommended to a physiotherapy programme led by a physiotherapist.

All group interventions included eight sessions with five to eight patients in each group. The sessions were 1.5 hours long and held on the same day, each week, over 8 consecutive weeks.

The outcome from aetiologically based tinnitus therapy compared with waiting list controls were that the intervention gave significant reduction in:

- the self-assessed evaluation of tinnitus annoyance and loudness;
- how often tinnitus was perceived;
- sleep disturbances related to tinnitus and concentration problems related to tinnitus;
- an increased ability to mask tinnitus (Holgers, 1999).

Significant differences between the outcome of the TSQ at the first visit and the follow-up were correlated to changes in the outcome of the patient's health profile according to the NHP. A significant correlation was found between maskability of tinnitus and anxiety levels – the lower the level of anxiety, the easier it was to mask tinnitus. These correlations underscored the importance of designing rehabilitation programmes, resulting in changes in the areas that are of importance for the awareness of tinnitus.

# References

American Psychiatric Association (1980) Diagnostic and Statistical Manual of Mental Disorders, 4th edn revised. Washington DC: APA.
Aniansson G (1974) Methods for assessing high frequency hearing loss in everyday listening situations. Acta Otolaryngologica Supplement 320: 1–50.
Axelsson A (1995) Vårdprogramme för Tinnitus. Stockholm: National Board of Health and Welfare.

Barrenäs ML, Holgers KM (2000) A clinical evaluation of the hearing and disability scale. Noise and Health 6: 67–78.

Baskill JL, Coles RRA, Lutman ME, Axelsson A (1991) Tinnitus severity grading: longitudinal studies. In JM Aran, R Dauman (eds) Proceedings of the Fourth International Tinnitus Seminar. Amsterdam: Kugler, pp. 457–60.

Blakie NWH, Guthrie RV (1984) Noise and the Family, An Enquiry into Some Effects of Noise-induced Deafness. Prepared for the Deafness Foundation (Victoria). Melbourne: Department of Social Science.

Blumenfeld VG, Bergman M, Millner E (1969). Speech discrimination in an aging population. J Speech Hear Res 12: 210–17.

Brainerd SH, Frankel BG (1985). The relationship between audiometric and self-report measures of hearing handicap. Ear and Hearing 2(6): 89–92.

Coles RRA, Lutman ME, Axelsson A, Hazell JWP (1991) Tinnitus severity gradings; cross sectional studies. In JM Aran (ed.) Tinnitus 91, Fourth International Tinnitus Seminar. Amsterdam: Kugler.

Demorest ME, Erdman SA (1986) Scale composition and item analysis of the Communication Profile for the Hearing Impaired. Journal of Speech and Hearing Research 29: 515–35.

Demorest ME, Erdman SA (1987) Development of the Communication Profile for the Hearing Impaired. Journal of Speech and Hearing Disorders 52: 129–43.

Eriksson-Mangold M, Hallberg LR-M, Ringdahl A, Erlandsson SI (1992). The development of a shortened Hearing Measurement Scale: the HMS-25. J Audiol Med 1: 161–75.

Getty L, Hétu R (1991) The development of a rehabilitation programme for people affected by occupational hearing loss. II: results from group intervention with 48 workers and their spouses. Audiology 30: 317–29.

Hallberg LR-M, Barrenäs ML (1993) Living with a male with noise-induced hearing loss: experiences from the perspective of spouses. Br J Audiol 27: 255–61.

Hallberg LR-M, Barrenäs ML (1994) Group rehabilitation of middle-aged males with noise-induced hearing loss and their spouses: evaluation of short- and long-term effects. British Journal of Audiology 28: 71–9.

Hallberg LR-M, Barrenäs ML (1995) Coping with noise-induced hearing loss: experiences from the perspective of male victims. British Journal of Audiology 29: 219–30.

Hallberg LR-M, Carlsson SG (1991) A qualitative study of strategies for managing a hearing impairment. British Journal of Audiology 25: 201–11.

Hallberg LR-M, Johnsson T, Axelsson A (1993) Structure of perceived handicap in middle-aged males with noise induced hearing loss with and without tinnitus. Audiology 32: 137–52.

Hallberg LRM (1998). Evaluation of a Swedish version of the hearing disabilities and handicaps scale, based on a clinical sample of 101 men with noise-induced hearing loss. Scand Aud; 27: 21–29.

Hétu R, Getty L (1991) The development of rehabilitation programme for people affected by occupational hearing loss. I: a new paradigm. Audiology 30: 305–16.

Hétu R, Riverin L, Getty L, Lalande NM, Cyr C (1990) The reluctance to acknowledge hearing difficulties among hearing-impaired workers. British Journal of Audiology 24: 265–76.

Hétu R, Getty L, Philibert L, Noble WG, Stephens D (1994) Development of a clinical tool for the measurement of severity of hearing disabilities and handicaps. Journal of Speech and Language Pathology and Audiology 18: 83–95.

Hetu R, Lalonde M, Getty L (1987). Psychosocial disadvantages associated with occupational hearing loss as experienced in the family. Audiology 26(3):141–52.

High WS, Fairbanks G, Glorig A (1964). Scale for self-assessment of hearing handicap. J Speech Hear Disord 29: 215–30.

Holgers KM (1999) Tinnitus Vårdprogramme 2000. Stockholm: National Board of Health and Welfare.

Holgers KM, Erlandsson SI, Barrenäs ML (2000) Predictive factors for auditory, somatic and depression/anxiety related tinnitus. Audiology 39: 284–91.

Holgers KM, Eliasson AC, Olsson P (2000) 'Tinnitus school' and sound enrichment – a pilot study. Seventh International Tinnitus Seminar. Freemantle, Australia, 5–9 March.

Holgers K, Eliasson A, Olsson P (2003) Cognitive Behavioral Therapy and sound stimulation - a preliminary report. J. Psychosomatic Research 55(2): 160–161.

Hunt SM, McKenna SP, McEwen J, Backett EM, Williams J, Papp E (1980) A quantitative approach to perceived health status: a validation Study. Journal of Epidemiology and Community Health 34: 281–6.

Hunt SM, McKenna SP, Williams J (1981) Reliability of a population survey tool for measuring perceived health problems: a validation study. Journal of Epidemiology and Community Health 35: 297–300.

Jastreboff PJ, Hazell JWP (1993) A neurophysiological approach to tinnitus: clinical implications. British Journal of Audiology. 27: 7–17.

Jones L (1987) Living with hearing loss. In JG Kyle (ed.) Adjustment to Acquired Hearing Loss: Analysis, change and learning. Chippenham: Antony Rowe, pp. 126–39.

Jones L, Kyle J, Wood PL (1987) Losing your Hearing as an Adult. Words apart. Padstow: TJ Press.

Lalande NM, Lambert J, Riverin L (1988) Quantification of the psychosocial disadvantages experienced by workers in a noisy industry and their nearest relatives: perspectives for rehabilitation. Audiology 27: 196–206.

Lutman ME, Brown EJ, Coles RRA (1987) Self-reported disability and handicap in the population in relation to pure-tone threshold, age, sex and type of hearing loss. British Journal of Audiology 21: 45–58.

Marcus-Bernstein C (1986). Audiologic and nonaudiologic correlates of hearing handicap in black elderly. J Speech Hear Res 29: 301–12.

McCartney JH, Maurer JF, Sorenson FD (1976). A comparison of the Hearing Handicap Scale and the Hearing Measurement Scale with standard audiometric measures on a geriatric population. J Aud Res 16: 51–58.

Noble WG, Atherley GRC (1970) The Hearing Measurement Scale: a questionnaire for the assessment of auditory disability. Journal of Audiology Research 16: 51–8.

Speaks C, Jerger J, Trammel J (1970). Measurement of hearing handicap. J Speech Hear Res 13: 768–76.

Sullivan M, Katon W, Russo J, Dobie R, Sakai CA (1993) Randomized trial of nortriptyline for severe chronic tinnitus. Effects on depression, disability, and tinnitus symptoms. Archives of Internal Medicine 153: 2251–9.

Tyler RS, Smith PA (1983). Sentence identification in noise and hearing-handicap questionnaires. Scand Audiol 12(4):285–92.

Tyler S, Smith PA (1983). Sentence identification in noise and hearing-handicap questionnaires. Scand Aud; 12: 285–92.

Ventry IM, Weinstein BE (1982). The Hearing Handicap Inventory for the Elderly: A new tool. Ear Hear; 3(3): 128–34.

Wiklund I, Herlitz J, Hjalmarsson Å (1989) Quality of life five years after myocardial infarction. European Heart Journal 10: 464–72.

World Health Organization (2001) International Classification of Functioning, Disability and Health. Geneva: WHO.

Zöger S, Svedlund J, Holgers KM (2001) Psychiatric disorders in tinnitus patients without severe hearing impairment: 24 months follow-up of patients at an audiological clinic. Audiology 40: 133–40.

# Appendix A: items used by Lutman et al. (1987)

1. How difficult do you usually find it to follow somebody's conversation when other people are talking close by? Great difficulty/some difficulty/no difficulty.
2. How often does any hearing problem you may have restrict your enjoyment of social and personal life, compared with others around you? Never/rarely/quite often/very often.
3. Do you get a feeling of being cut off from things because of difficulty in hearing? Never/rarely/quite often/very often.
4. Do any hearing difficulties you might have lead to embarrassment? Never/rarely/quite often/very often.

# Appendix B: items included in the Hearing Disability and Handicap Scale (HDHS: Hétu et al. 1994)

1. Do you have difficulty following a conversation normally in any of the following situations: at work, in a bus or a car, or when shopping?
2. Can you hear the sound of the door opening when you're inside the room?
3. Do you worry that people will find out you have a hearing problem?
4. Is it difficult for you to ask people to repeat themselves?
5. Do you have difficulty hearing what's being said on TV if someone other than yourself adjusts the volume?
6. Can you hear the water boiling in the pan when you're in the kitchen?
7. Do you get upset if you give the wrong answer to someone because you've misheard them?
8. Does your hearing condition restrict your social or personal life?
9. Do you have difficulty hearing what's being said on the radio if someone other than yourself adjusts the volume?
10. Can you hear the footsteps of someone coming into the room without you seeing them?
11. Does it bother or upset you if you are unable to follow a conversation?
12. Do you find that you are more tense and tired because of your hearing difficulty?

13. Do you have difficulty hearing in group conversations?
14. Do you hear when someone rings the doorbell or knocks on the door?
15. Do people avoid you because of your hearing difficulties?
16. At present, would you say that you lack self-confidence because of your hearing difficulty?
17. Do you find that, although you can hear someone speaking, you cannot understand what they're saying?
18. Do you hear the telephone ringing from another room?
19. Do you ever get the feeling of being cut off from things because of your hearing difficulty?
20. Do you feel that your hearing condition has an influence on the relationship you have with your spouse or a person close to you?

# CHAPTER 32

# Target groups in prevention of health effects from listening to music

*Noise and Its Effects:* Edited by Linda Luxon and Deepak Prasher © 2007 John Wiley & Sons Ltd.

B PETTERSSON

## Introduction

Training and information on noise and its effects are absolutely crucial in coping with the high sound levels to be found at, in particular, discotheques and concerts (Artists and Musicians Against Tinnitus, 2002). The immediate effects of noise are relatively rare, which means that the risk of hearing impairment is underestimated. The long-term effects of noise are equally intangible and a great deal of information is required for people to be able to understand the link between noise and hearing impairment. Health effects that manifest themselves in the long term are always difficult to establish, and the propensity to take measurements now to avoid effects in perhaps 30 or 40 years' time is not especially high.

Nevertheless, anxiety among the population that high sound levels may cause harm has grown as the sound levels of music played in discotheques and elsewhere have risen (National Board of Health and Welfare, 1996). Many people can logically grasp the fact that high sound levels may be harmful but an understanding of how this harm arises and at what sound levels it may occur is very superficial. Those who require this knowledge, such as young people, disc- jockeys, etc., often have a poor idea, and as often as not are not worried that the music may cause hearing loss. On the other hand, politicians seem to have grasped that the anxiety among the general population is high and there is, therefore, a broad political acceptance about the need to 'do something about it'. The far-reaching information initiative that is needed to spread knowledge of the risks posed by high noise levels should therefore be started now.

## Occupational noise versus leisure noise

The effects of noise in working life have been perceived for a long time and this has contributed to progress in reducing the number of cases of hearing loss (Johansson and Arlinger, 2001). As a result, a great deal would be lost if training about noise, high sound levels and the detrimental effect was not to be extended to cover leisure noise as well. Of course, not all occupational groups in society have a detailed understanding of the effects of various kinds of noise. Society has, via various regulations, often protected workers from being exposed to excessive sound levels (Swedish National Board of Occupational Safety and Health, 1992). The requirements for measures at workplaces have often been followed by information on the risks of hearing impairment. The authorities then find it easier to get a range of measures accepted. Employers have been compelled to take measures to protect employees, including the enforced use of various forms of ear protectors. The long-term effects on hearing have been attributed to cooperation of authorities, employers and employees. Unlike noise at work, leisure noise has not been the subject of regulations from the authorities. Nor have many countries structured the monitoring of various risks in society in such a way that it is possible to monitor any hearing loss risks in society outside of workplaces. What has been won in the battle against harmful noise at work has been lost in the growth of noise in the leisure environment.

Music at discotheques and pop/rock concerts is delivered at excessive sound levels. Loudspeaker equipment technology has developed so that very high sound levels can be delivered without the music sounding cracked and false. The tuning before and during a concert can occasionally be technically complex. During 'soundchecks' the musical equipment can emit unexpected and very high sound levels. Sometimes this can also happen during the show in the presence of the audience. The sound level at a concert or disco is often raised gradually during the evening in order to reach the highest volume as a crescendo at the end of the show.

Knowledge about leisure noise and possible hearing impairment is, in many respects, completely non-existent among not only the groups who expose others to high sound levels but also among those exposed. In certain cases, myths about high sound levels exist that have to be corrected before correct information can be given. One such myth is that music cannot be harmful since 'it is enjoyed'. People have more of an understanding that other sound sources such as gunshot noise or noise from firecrackers may be harmful, but there too gaps in understanding are evident.

Moreover, the high sound levels of music at discotheques and concerts are also desired by those exposed to them. The volume of the music is used for competitive purposes so that the operator of a discotheque does not dare to reduce the volume of the music because of the risk of losing customers. A change in attitude is needed to achieve the objective of reducing sound levels and, to a certain extent, this has already started. Many more people are using ear protectors at concerts than in the past (Artists and Musicians Against Tinnitus, 2002).

Sound at cinemas has also increased. New kinds of sound equipment in which the sound is guided in multichannel systems around the cinema auditorium have given film makers new opportunities of incorporating sound as an artistic part of the film. Sound levels have consequently been raised to achieve greater effects, often to such high levels that they are found to be painful by some cinema goers.

## Protection

There are actually only two ways of coping with high sound levels:

1. use ear protectors;
2. reduce the sound levels.

The target groups who should be encouraged to use heavy protection are children and young adults, who are exposed to loud sounds. However, a major objective should still be that leisure noise must decrease so that it is unnecessary to protect oneself against it. To reduce the sound levels in society, the target groups are completely different, and can also be subdivided into the following:

- Those who can influence regulations in society, such as politicians, other decision-makers and authorities entrusted with providing politicians with information that is to serve as the basis for decisions on regulations.
- Those who have to comply with the regulations but are not usually directly in contact with the activity – these may be discotheque owners, concert organisers, etc.
- Those who play music in various forms may be musicians, disc jockeys, sound engineers and others involved in practising music in some way; this group also includes those who use music in other contexts, e.g. at the gym or in a similar context.

## Target groups

The target groups for information initiatives can essentially be subdivided into three kinds: those exposed to the high sound levels, those who expose others, and those with the power to lay down rules and make sure that they are followed. The various target groups must be reached in various ways but are nevertheless not completely independent of each other, in as much as different target groups, such as young people and politicians, have, for example, the shared principle that there must be a certain level of acceptance to be able to force through requirements concerning maximum permissible limits, etc.

The various target groups are best reached with different forms of content which are specifically tailored to each group. The more the message can be adapted to a specific target group, the easier it is to get across the fact that measures must be taken to lower sound levels.

The starting point for information for those who listen to music and play should be positive and attempt to draw attention to the fact that the 'intense' effect of sound thumping into the body can be achieved without the sound levels being able to cause hearing impairment. Those who already have tinnitus will also be reached by the message concerning the risks of high sound volumes; there is therefore a reason to point out, not too categorically, that tinnitus is an irreversible condition.

## Young people

Young people are probably the group in society in most need of information on the risks of high sound levels as they are the most exposed. The high sound levels to which they are exposed come from various sources but very often from music in various forms. Young people often listen to music at extremely high levels for a large part of their leisure time, or at work if they have the opportunity. The really high sound levels usually affect young people via headphones or at discotheques and concerts (National Board of Health and Welfare, 2003). Music at gyms is also found at extremely high volumes.

Many theories exist about how a message should be conveyed to young people and how they should be induced to alter or never adopt a form of behaviour. The common aim in most of these theories is to try to provide information on the risks from various directions in a form that is recognized or attractive to take in. Most people who have been to a concert or discotheque are aware of a buzzing in their ears when they go home or even on the next day. This 'warning' can be understood by most young people. Many campaigns involving the distribution of earplugs together with information on the risks of high sound levels have been conducted at concerts. Moreover, brochures explaining the hazards of loud music exist in many countries. Experiments have been carried out using various 'idols', generally musicians, who have presented information on the risks of hearing impairment. Newer forms of information technology can and should be used. References to the internet can make the dissemination of this information both more cost-effective and attractive, and at the same time link together a campaign with a number of different approaches.

## Children

Children may be exposed to the high sound levels to which teenagers and young adults are subjected, albeit not on the same scale. Children are also more grateful about being told about risks than other young people. The easiest way of reaching children with information is probably via their teachers. This often requires the teacher to be briefed first. Competition for the favours of the teaching profession is stiff, with many other information providers wanting to reach children via their teachers with campaigns of varying expense. A good way of reaching children may be to draw up various teacher guides that can be used in normal teaching.

The provision of information to children is also an excellent way of reaching parents. Children who are exposed to high sound levels from music are exposed because parents or organizers of children's activities do not understand the risks. It may therefore be effective to target the information directly at parents of this well-defined age group.

## Decision-makers

Decision-makers in society require clear links between various forms of behaviour and ill health in order to lay down limits. Links that produce effects on, for instance, hearing only after a long time have less of a chance than other risks of receiving the support of politicians when it comes to laying down limit values and guidelines. Arguing for greater caution can sometimes be difficult in a society in which many interested parties want politicians to listen to them. In addition, it can be difficult to substantiate decisions on limit values if groups in society do not want them. Decision-makers exist at various levels in society: at a central level they have scope to create regulations for coping with high sound levels, whereas at the local level decision-makers often have the scope to prioritize between different initiatives and in this way can ensure that high sound levels come on to the agenda.

Information that is directed at politicians and other decision-makers must be formulated differently depending on the objective. If the objective is to put the question of the effects of high sound levels on the agenda and thereby encourage debate, individual politicians can be informed about the risks. The media also play a major role. Decision-makers who have opportunities to create regulations must be given adequate information on the risks of high sound levels but also what consequences such regulations may have, be they positive or negative. A positive consequence may be the number of cases of hearing loss, tinnitus, etc. prevented. Other information that should be put across is expected compliance and any costs associated with the introduction of regulations. Local politicians who can prioritize the matters in relation to other important issues must be given more information on the risks of hearing impairment if no measures are taken in their own region. It is also local politicians who decide whether, for example, individual rock concerts are to be allowed and what requirements are to be imposed during the performance.

## Authorities

Authorities who are charged with ensuring compliance with sound limits and other objectives essentially need information on how they must carry out monitoring and what measures can be taken. At the same time, the authorities must have sufficient information to be able to inform local politicians about the issues involved but also so that they are able to reach the general public with information on the risks of high sound levels. The authorities need information on where they may be expected to find high sound levels and how they are to be able to measure these. Of course, they must also have sufficient information on medical effects, to be able to motivate their own contribution and anyone who, for example, runs a campaign to reduce volumes. Information for the authority must be both extensive and detailed. The authority is, however, expected to be able to take on board relatively complicated information.

Other forms of support from which authorities may derive benefit are information sheets, which may be passed on to those responsible for ensuring that specified sound levels or other regulations are observed – those who run various kinds of activities in which high sound levels may occur, such as discotheque owners and concert organizers. Authorities greatly value 'good examples' or experience that other authorities have gained so that they avoid having to reinvent the wheel.

## Music teachers

Music teachers are an important group for those who subsequently become practising musicians. The ability to listen is, after all, at the very heart of music. Music teaching has, like other forms of education, attempted to make the teaching more appealing. People often want to give, for example, guitar or piano lessons on 'pop or rock bands', which means that the drums also appear. Premises are often small and the volume deafening. Information on the effects of high sound levels on hearing must form a natural part both of how music teachers teach skills on the instrument and of how students must be able to protect themselves and others when practising music. This probably requires information on hearing and high sound levels to be incorporated into music teaching.

## Musicians

Musicians expose both themselves and others to high sound levels. They are therefore an important group to reach with information on the effects of high sound levels. At the same time, musicians are far from being a homogeneous group. The group that needs to be reached if sound at concerts is to be reduced essentially comprises pop/rock musicians, whose listeners are chiefly young people. Information can be difficult to get across to such a heterogeneous grouping as musicians. There are national associations for musicians who have been affected by hearing loss and tinnitus. Information on the risks of hearing loss can be provided advantageously to various interest groups within the profession via such organizations.

## Organizers/owners

Organizers/owners sometimes have scope for setting limits for sound levels at concerts, discotheques and other places where music is played. Ultimately, the organizer/owner of the premises or business is responsible for the activity carried on within the premises. The party responsible for the activity is also the party to whom the authority turns and on whom it imposes requirements. Organizers and owners, or those who carry on activities in which high sound levels may be expected, are usually more susceptible to pressure from authorities or the general public than those who play music. Since the organizer/owner runs a business in which the volume of the music has become a means of competition, he or she is very interested in not losing customers if the sound level is lowered. One way of guaranteeing these groups an even playing field is if intervention on the part of the authorities is directed at all interested parties on the market. Similarly, trade associations should work to ensure that any voluntary reductions in sound levels take place neutrally in terms of competition. The owner must also safeguard the staff who are also exposed to risks of hearing loss. Information on risks of hearing loss and what scope exists for avoiding this can be provided via trade associations or the relevant authority.

### Disc jockeys

Disc jockeys often control what sound levels prevail at the discotheque. The disc jockey is frequently someone who is himself an attraction and 'celebrity'. The discotheque operator often uses well-known disc jockeys to attract customers to the discotheque. Various attempts have been made to provide information on effects of high sound levels. One viable way of making sure that the disc jockey is aware of the risks of hearing loss may be to have the professional group of disc jockeys trained in health aspects of noise exposure and given 'noise control' certificates. Attempts at developing certification on a voluntary basis have been made but obligatory certification should be considered. One way for the authority to reduce sound levels at discotheques has been to demand the use of so-called sound guards. If the disc jockey plays music too loudly the music is turned off or lowered automatically. The mere threat that such a measure may be employed may be enough for the disc jockey not to play too loudly.

### Sound engineers

Sound engineers who control the output of the sound at concerts are also those who control the entire effect. Sound engineers are the most important groups to reach with information in relation to reducing sound levels at concerts. The sound engineer often sits in the middle of the audience and controls the sound level from every single instrument, and the singing from the stage, from his sound console. The object of the engineer's work is for the sound to be as good as possible. Instruments and singing should preferably be heard constantly so that nothing sticks out and disturbs the whole. It is common for those appearing on the stage to signal to the sound engineer to raise the volume of their particular instrument. If sound engineers accede to the desires of one individual musician they are soon forced to raise the volume for the others as well. The consequence is that sound levels increase.

Sound engineers are also those who build up loudspeaker systems. It is important that the equipment is tested well before the show so that unexpected excessive noise does not occur during the show, when it can have a directly adverse effect on hearing. A system consisting of large loudspeakers on the stage must have a high output to reach those at the back. If such a system has to be used, greater requirements are imposed on individual loudspeakers not being too close to the audience's seats. Loudspeakers that distribute the sound over the larger area do not need the same output and the requirement concerning distance from the audience is not the same.

The information that sound engineers require is of course medical in order to understand what the reasons are for keeping sound levels down. Nevertheless, the emphasis of information is placed on how the technical system can be built up without the 'intense' effects being lost, how loud-speakers and other equipment can be positioned, etc. For sound engineers, too, a certification system or some form of certificate proving that they have the necessary understanding of what harm they can cause may be possible.

### Gym instructors etc.

Gym instructors and others who provide fitness training and run gyms often also use music as an aid, partly to make the rhythm easier and partly to encourage extra exertion. Many gyms have music systems that can raise the volumes to levels that impair hearing. The music, together with the instructor's electronically amplified voice, usually produces the highest levels. With regard to music that is intended only to make the rhythm for the exercises easier, the levels can be easily lowered. In the case of physical training with weights and the like, a number of gym instructors consider that the extremely high music volume helps people to exert themselves even more and thus obtain even more effective training.

## Conclusion:

In order to reduce the risks of hearing damage, a wide variety of different social groups need to be informed and educated about the risks of high sound levels in discotheques and concert halls. Those who need to be reached include users, owners, employees and politicians, authorities, administrators and decision-makers.

## References

Artists and Musicians against Tinnitus (2002) Hearing and Safety in Music Education and High Sound Levels: Young people's behaviour, knowledge and attitudes. Stockholm: National Board of Health and Welfare.

Johansson M, Arlinger S (2001). The development of noise-induced hearing loss in the Swedish County of Östergötland in the 1980s and 1990s. Noise and Health 3:15–28.

National Board of Health and Welfare (1996) Höga ljudnivåer (high sound levels) SOSFS 2005:6, p 1–4.

National Board of Health and Welfare (2003) Investigation of High Sound Levels. Report to the Swedish Government. Stockholm: National Board of Health and Welfare page 1–43.

Swedish National Board of Occpational Safety (1992) Statue Book of the Swedish Work Environment Authority, Ordinance (AFS 2005:16) on Noise, p 1–37.

# CHAPTER 33

# Agencies involved with noise

*Noise and Its Effects:* Edited by Linda Luxon and Deepak Prasher © 2007
John Wiley & Sons Ltd.

DIETRICH H SCHWELA, ANDREW W SMITH

## Introduction

This chapter focuses on global agencies, especially those that are part of the United Nations' family of organizations. These include the United Nations itself, the World Health Organization (WHO), the International Labour Organization (ILO), the World Bank and the World Trade Organization. The European Community has been included because of its extensive work on noise and its specific cooperation between its Commission in the field of environment and health and the WHO. Various international organizations that deal with certain specific or technical aspects of noise are covered, as are international non-governmental organizations (NGOs) that have at least part that is specifically involved in noise.

Although many national organizations are involved in noise these are too numerous and too country specific to warrant inclusion here.

### Global Agencies

- United Nations
- World Health Organization
- International Labour Organization
- World Bank
- World Trade Organization
- The European Community

## United Nations

The United Nations has six main organs: the General Assembly, the Security Council, the Economic and Social Council (ECOSOC), the Trusteeship Council and the Secretariat, based at UN Headquarters in New York, and the International Court of Justice in The Hague (United Nations 2000).

Subsidiary bodies of ECOSOC that may occasionally deal with aspects of noise would include the UN Conference on Trade and Development (UNCTAD) and the UN Environment Programme (UNEP). However, most of the work in this field is dealt with by the so-called 'specialized agencies', which are linked to the UN through cooperative agreements. For issues related to noise, these include the WHO, the ILO and the World Bank group.

Bodies within the UN itself that deal directly with noise are the Regional Economic Commissions, and some of the Functional Commissions, all part of ECOSOC. For example, the Working Party on Noise, under the auspices of the Economic Commission for Europe, deals mainly with standards for motor vehicle noise control. In addition, the UN, through a special Rapporteur, deals somewhat indirectly with the effects of noise in the process of monitoring *the Standard Rules on the Equalization of opportunities for persons with disabilities*: such persons would include those with a hearing disability due to noise. The special Rapporteur reports to the Commission for Social Development. The Commission on Human Rights has also addressed noise through the International Covenant on Economic, Social and Cultural Rights in relation to the prevention of accidents in the workplace, through the International Covenant on Civil and Political Rights in relation to effects of noise on individual health, and through the Convention on the Rights of the Child in relation to noise affecting families.

The UN Environment Programme (UNEP), following the UN Conference on Environment and Development in Rio de Janeiro, 1992, put together a set of programme of tasks for the coming century called

A programme on noise is included in Agenda 21, of the UN Environment Programme for development in the 21$^{st}$ century.

Agenda 21. One of these, on noise, recognized the need to develop criteria for maximum permitted safe noise exposure levels and promote noise assessment and control as part of environmental health programmes. The recent report on the global environment outlook, GEO-2000 (UNEP, 1999) referred to reports from various regions which state that maximum acceptable noise level is regularly exceeded in most cities to levels that may cause hearing loss (Organization for Economic Co-operation and Development, European Conference of Ministers of Transport or OECD-ECMT, 1995). The global overview mentioned noise as one of the many environmental problems that reinforce one another in small, densely populated areas and turn these areas into environmental hot spots.

In June 1994, the first inter-agency Earthwatch Working Party agreed on the mission statement for the revitalized Earthwatch, which was first introduced by UNEP in 1973. The mission of the UN system-wide Earthwatch is to coordinate, harmonize and integrate observation, assessment and reporting activities across the UN system in order to provide environmental and appropriate socioeconomic information for national and international decision-making on sustainable development and for early warning of emerging problems requiring international action. This should include timely information on the pressures on, status of and trends in key global resources, variables and processes in both natural and human systems and on the response to problems in these areas (UNEP, 2001). Noise is considered as an omnipresent, yet underestimated, form of pollution, the long-term exposure to which can cause adverse effects on human health (UNEP, 2001).

Since 1958, the UN Economic Commission for Europe (ECE) has installed a Working Party on the Construction of Vehicles (WP.29). The mission of this Working Party is to harmonize vehicle construction standards throughout Europe. A Working Party on Noise is subsidiary to WP.29 and its activities relate to various amendments to existing ECE Regulations on noise limit levels and noise abatement measures such as the new draft ECE Regulation on tyre noise, the ECE Reg. 51 (Noise Emissions from Category M and N vehicles) and ECE Reg. 59 (replacement mufflers) (UNECE, 2001).

The main interactions between international agencies involved in noise are depicted in Figure 33.1.

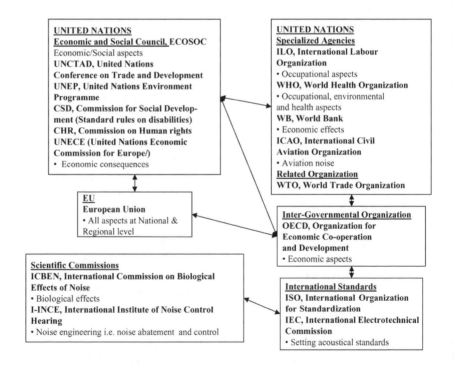

**Figure 33.1** Main interactions between agencies involved in noise (extracted from www.un.org/aboutun/chart.html).

# World Health Organization

The objective of the WHO is the attainment by all people of the highest possible level of health, defined as a state of complete physical, mental and social well-being.

The WHO works to reduce mortality, morbidity and disability, especially in poor and marginalized populations, and to promote healthy lifestyles and reduce risk factors to human health that arise from environmental, economic, social and behavioural causes.

In support of its main objective, the WHO promotes the improvement of nutrition, housing, sanitation, recreation, economic or working conditions and other aspects of environmental hygiene. It has considered health impacts of occupational and environmental noise an important problem since the 1970s. The deliberations of a WHO Task Group on Environmental Health Criteria for Noise were published in the Environmental Health Criteria Series of the International Programme for Chemical Safety (WHO, 1980). Building upon the recommendations of this early publication, the WHO Regional Office for Europe, in its Environmental Health Series, published a report on the assessment of noise impact on the urban environment (WHO, 1986a). The WHO Regional Centre for Environmental Health Activities (CEHA) in Amman, Jordan, organized an Informal Consultation on Noise Pollution in 1991, with selected presentations published in 1995 (WHO, 1995a). In 1992, a WHO Task Force meeting largely expanded the noise document of 1980 (WHO, 1993). A corresponding report by the Karolinska Institute, Stockholm, on behalf of the WHO, recommended guidelines for levels of community noise in different environments (Berglund and Lindvall, 1995). In a WHO Expert Task Force meeting in 1999, this report was revised, updated and largely expanded to include, besides guidelines and guideline values, the topics of environmental noise assessment and management. The deliberations of this meeting constitute the new WHO Guidelines for Community Noise (WHO, 2000a) which are described in the next section.

## WHO Initiatives

- Environmental Health Criteria for Noise (1980)
- Assessment of noise impact on the urban environment (1986)
- WHO report on the prevention of deafness and hearing impairment (1986)
- Consultation on Noise Pollution (1995)
- Recommended guidelines for levels of community noise in different environments (1995)
- 48th World Health Assembly passed resolution on prevention of hearing impairment (1995)

- WHO guidelines for community noise (2000)
- Links with NGOs

In addition to what is covered in the Guidelines for Community Noise, WHO has also considered, in greater depth, the role of noise as an important cause of deafness and hearing impairment. Thus a WHO report on prevention of deafness and hearing impairment was submitted to the Thirty-ninth World Health Assembly (WHO, 1986b). This listed noise as causing a moderate proportion of hearing impairment and stated that noise-induced hearing loss is one of the commonest work-related diseases. In 1991 an informal WHO working group on programme planning considered methods for primary, secondary and tertiary prevention of important causes of deafness and hearing impairment, which included excessive noise. It recommended as a priority the collection of data on the incidence and prevalence of communication disorders, including those related to noise (WHO, 1991).

The Forty-eighth World Health Assembly passed a resolution on prevention of hearing impairment in 1995 (WHO, 1995c). This stated that 120 million people in the world were estimated to have disabling hearing difficulties and that the Assembly was aware of the significant public health aspects of avoidable hearing loss related to causes including exposure to excessive noise. It urged Member States to prepare national plans for prevention and to introduce appropriate legislation for the proper management of particularly important causes of deafness and hearing impairment. These included harmful exposure to noise, such as noise in the work environment and loud music.

Following on from this resolution, a series of consultations of experts on strategies for prevention of deafness and hearing impairment was commenced, and the third of these, on prevention of noise-induced hearing loss, was held in Geneva in 1997 (WHO, 1998). This affirmed that exposure to excessive noise is the major avoidable cause of permanent hearing impairment worldwide, and in many countries is the biggest compensable occupational hazard. Occupational noise and urban, environmental noise (especially traffic noise) in developing countries and social noise in young people in developing countries are increasing risk factors for hearing impairment.

**The WHO consultation defined noise-induced hearing loss, for survey purposes only, according to the following:**

- Noise exposure history: 100 dB (NI) or 83 dB (A) $L_{aeq,40}$ for a 50-year lifetime (equivalent exposure);
- Audiometric criteria: sensorineural but not unilateral hearing loss, 0.5-kHz threshold less than 50 dB HL, and at least a 15-dB difference between high- and low-frequency threshold averages in under 50 year-olds.

The WHO plans to produce guidelines for countries setting up programmes for the prevention of noise-induced hearing loss.

In 2001, WHO revised upwards its global estimates of all causes of disabling hearing impairment[a] to 250 million people in 2000 (WHO, 2001a). This figure is approximately 4.2% of the world's population in 2000; two-thirds are in the developing world and 11% are children under the age of 15 years.

WHO regional offices have also addressed the effects of noise. For example the WHO Regional Office for Europe (EURO) hosted the Third Ministerial Conference on Environment and Health in London in 1999, attended by 54 countries. One outcome was the Charter on Transport, Environment and Health, which stated that ambient noise levels in Europe are increasing due to the increase in number of vehicles, and called for various measures to reduce exposure to noise from transport (WHO, 1999a). A steering group meets regularly to address implementation of the charter. The WHO Programme on Transport, Environment and Health provides recent evidence on the health effects of transport (WHO, 2000b) including noise and facilitates the integration by Member States of health considerations into planning and investment decisions affecting transport and mobility. The implementation of activities that achieve health gains when included in the transport agenda was assessed in a survey in the WHO European Healthy Cities network in 1997–8 (WHO, 2002). However, only in 4% of cities was reducing noise a priority for action. The WHO European Centre for Environment and Health is developing a system of indicators to support the monitoring of environmental and public health policies in Member States. This initiative includes the effects of noise on health; the most recent reports are available on the internet (see, for example, WHO, 2001c).

The WHO Regional Office for the Eastern Mediterranean has the Centre for Environmental Health Activities, based in Amman, Jordan. This has addressed the subject of noise in 1995 (Figure 33.2).

The WHO Regional Office for the Western Pacific (WPRO) considered environmental air quality and noise in its 'Healthy Cities – Healthy Islands' programme. The effects of occupational noise and measures to deal with it are included in the WPRO Regional Guidelines for the Development of Healthy Workplaces (WHO, 1999b).

A small number of international NGOs, which deal specifically or partly with deafness and hearing impairment, as one of the consequences of excessive noise, have links with the WHO. These are focused from the point of view of persons with the impairments and of professionals who

---

[a]WHO definition of disabling hearing impairment: 'The permanent unaided hearing threshold level for the better ear of 41 or 31 dB or greater in age over 14 or under 15 years respectively; for this purpose the "hearing threshold level" is to be taken as the better ear average hearing threshold level for the four frequencies 0.5, 1, 2, and 4 kHz.' (From: WHO (1991) with adaptations from WHO (1997).)

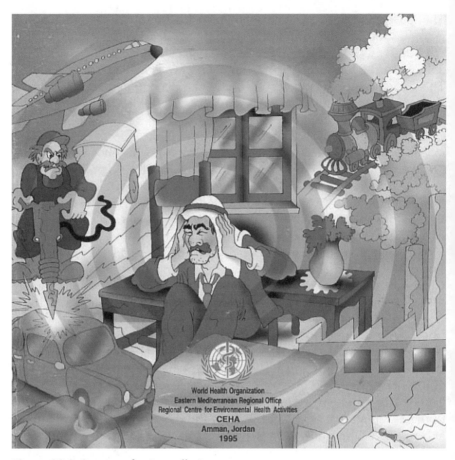

**Figure 33.2** Sources of noise pollution.

deal with them and include the International Federation of Hard of Hearing People (IFHOH), and the World Federation of the Deaf (WFD) in the first category, and the International Federation of Oto-Rhino-Laryngological Societies (IFOS), the International Association of Logopaedics and Phoniatrics (IALP), the International Society of Audiology (ISA) and the International Association of Physicians in Audiology (IAPA) in the second category. Hearing International (HI) spans both these categories. Another international NGO, the Christoffelblindenmission (CBM), gives support to programmes and projects against deafness and hearing impairment, as part of their mandate.

One of the international NGOs previously mentioned, the IFOS, has a standing committee on noise-induced hearing disorders. It is a federation of national and international otorhinolaryngological societies and associations from more than 120 countries. The standing committee is working towards prevention of hearing loss caused by noise and conservation of hearing. It endeavours to obtain information on regulations in various countries for assessing the degree of occupational noise-induced hearing loss and the resulting hearing handicap.

## WHO Guidelines for Community Noise (WHO, 2000a)

Environmental noise is considered in the WHO Guidelines for Community Noise (hereafter called the Guidelines) to include noise emitted from outdoor and indoor sources except noise at the industrial workplace (occupational noise). Sources of outdoor noise include road, rail and air traffic, industries, construction and public work, and the neighbourhood. The main indoor sources are ventilation systems, office machines, home appliances and neighbours. Typical neighbourhood noise comes from premises and installations related to the catering trade (restaurant, cafeterias, discotheques, etc.), live or recorded music, sports events including motor sports, playgrounds, car parks, and domestic animals such as barking dogs. Many countries have regulations on community noise from road, rail and rail traffic, construction machines and industrial plants through applying emission standards, on the construction of barriers and on the acoustic properties of buildings. In contrast, few countries have regulations on community noise from the neighbourhood, probably due to lack of methods to define and measure it, and the difficulty of controlling it.

Noise is a problem that affects everybody. Most people are typically exposed to several noise sources or combinations of noise exposure from more than one source, including several types of community noise. In contrast to many other environmental problems, noise pollution continues to grow accompanied by an increasing number of complaints by noise-exposed persons.

**The growth in noise pollution is unsustainable because it involves (Berglund, 1998):**
- direct as well as cumulative adverse health effects;
- adverse effects on future generations;
- sociocultural, aesthetic and economic effects.

These consequences of noise pollution call for precautionary action in any environmental planning situation. Therefore, the new Guidelines also address, for the first time, noise monitoring and noise management.

The Guidelines describe the main sources of noise in some detail.

- *Mechanized industry*, with machinery of all kinds, subjects a significant proportion of the working population to potentially harmful sound pressure levels of noise. The characteristics of industrial noise vary considerably, depending on specific equipment. Rotating and reciprocating machines generate sound that is dominated by tonal and harmonic components; air-moving equipment tends to generate sounds with a wide frequency range and a large component of low frequencies. The highest sound pressure levels are usually caused by components or gas flows that move at high speed (fans, steam pressure relief valves) or by operations involving mechanical impacts (stamping, riveting, road breaking).

- *Transport*: the noise of road vehicles is mainly generated from the engine and from frictional contact between the vehicle and the ground and air. Special problems can arise in areas where the traffic movements involve a change in engine speed and power, such as at traffic lights, hills and intersecting roads. Railway noise depends primarily on the speed of the train but variations are present depending upon the type of engine, wagons and rails. Impact noises can be generated in stations and marshalling-yards because of shunting operations. The introduction of high-speed trains has created special noise problems, as at speeds greater than 250 km/h, the proportion of high-frequency sound energy increases. Aircraft operations have caused severe community noise problems since the 1970s. Aircraft takeoffs are known to produce intense noise including vibration and rattle, but landings also cause noise annoyance especially when reverse thrust is applied. An aircraft in supersonic flight trails a sonic boom (a shock wave at flying speed slightly above the speed of sound) that can be heard up to 50 km on either side of its ground track depending upon the flight altitude and the size of the aircraft.

- *Building work and services*: building construction and earth works are activities that can cause considerable noise emissions. A variety of sounds are present from cranes, cement mixers, welding, hammering, boring and other work processes. Construction equipment is often poorly silenced and maintained and building operations are sometimes carried out without considering the environmental noise consequence. Street services such as garbage disposal and street cleaning can cause considerable disturbance if carried out at sensitive times of day. Building service noise can affect people both inside and outside the building. Ventilation and air conditioning plants and ducts, heat pumps, plumbing systems and lifts, for example, can compromise the internal acoustic environment and upset nearby residents.

- *'Neighbour' noise*: noise from neighbours is often one of the main causes of noise complaints. These complaints are largely due to the inconsiderate or thoughtless use of powered domestic appliances (vacuum cleaners, washing machines, lawn mowers, etc.), systems for music reproduction, TV sets or hobby activities. Substantial societal problems, less frequent but nevertheless important, are caused by disturbing noise emanating from neighbours and their social activities.

- *Leisure noise*: the possibilities of using powered machines in leisure activities are increasing all the time. For example, motor racing, off-road vehicles, motorboats, water skiing, snowmobiles, and so forth, can all contribute significantly to sound pressure levels in previously quiet areas. Shooting activities not only have considerable potential for disturbing nearby residents but can also damage the hearing of those performing this activity. Discotheques and rock concerts may exceed hearing damage risk criteria for the musicians, employees and audience. This sometimes applies also to outdoor concerts. Careful attention to the design of buildings can substantially eliminate neighbourhood noise problems caused by discotheques. But there can still be a noise problem outdoors due to customers arriving and leaving.

The Guidelines extensively discuss the different measures used to describe environmental noises and mention the limitations to these simple measures, but also stress the many practical advantages including economy and the benefits of a standardized approach.

Health impacts considered in deriving the Guidelines include noise-induced hearing impairment, interference with speech communication, sleep disturbance, cardiovascular and physiological effects, mental health effects, performance effects, and effects on residential behaviour and annoyance.

Table 33.1 presents the WHO Guideline values structured according to specific environments and appropriate critical effects. Guideline values given consider all identified adverse health effects for specific environments, the specific values being set according to the specific effect with the lowest effect level (critical health effect).

For the first time, the Guidelines address questions related to noise management. The goal of noise management is stated as achievement and maintenance of noise levels that protect human health. The fundamental principle for noise management is to develop criteria for maximum permitted safe noise exposure levels and promote noise assessment and control as part of environmental health programmes.

**Table 33.1** Guideline values for community noise in various environments

| Specific environment | Critical health effect(s) | $L_{Aeq}$ (dB (A)) | Time base (h) | $L_{Amax}$fast (dB) |
|---|---|---|---|---|
| Outdoor living area | Serious annoyance, daytime and evening | 55 | 16 | – |
| | Moderate annoyance, daytime and evening | 50 | 16 | – |
| Dwelling, indoors | Speech intelligibility and moderate annoyance, daytime and evening | 35 | 16 | |
| Bedrooms, indoors | Sleep disturbance, night-time | 30 | 8 | 45 |

**Table 33.1** continued

| Specific environment | Critical health effect(s) | $L_{Aeq}$ (dB (A)) | Time base (h) | $L_{Amax}$fast (dB) |
|---|---|---|---|---|
| Outside bedrooms | Sleep disturbance, window open (outdoor values) | 45 | 8 | 60 |
| School classrooms and pre-schools, indoors | Speech intelligibility, disturbance of information extraction, message communication | 35 | During class | – |
| Pre-school Bedrooms, indoor | Sleep disturbance | 30 | Sleeping-time | 45 |
| School, playground outdoor | Annoyance (external source) | 55 | During play | – |
| Hospital, ward rooms, indoors | Sleep disturbance, night-time | 30 | 8 | 40 |
| | Sleep disturbance, daytime and evenings | 30 | 16 | – |
| Hospitals, treatment rooms, indoors | Interference with rest and recovery | [a] | | |
| Industrial, commercial, shopping and traffic areas, indoors and outdoors | Hearing impairment | 70 | 24 | 110 |
| Ceremonies, festivals and entertainment events | Hearing impairment (patrons: < 5 times/year) | 100 | 4 | 110 |
| Public addresses, indoors and outdoors | Hearing impairment | 85 | 1 | 110 |
| Music through headphones/earphones | Hearing impairment (free-field value) | 85[b] | 1 | 110 |
| Impulse sounds from toys, fireworks and firearms | Hearing impairment (adults) | – | – | 140[c] |
| | Hearing impairment (children) | – | – | 120[c] |
| Outdoors in parkland and conservation areas | Disruption of tranquillity | [d] | | |

[a]As low as possible; [b]Under headphones, adapted to free-field values; [c]Peak sound pressure level, not LAF, max, measured 100 mm from the ear; [d]Existing quiet outdoor areas should be preserved and the signal to noise ratio should be kept low;

**Noise management includes:**

- noise problem identification;
- environmental noise impact assessment;
- noise control options;
- decisions on, and operation and evaluation of, noise regulations.

The Guidelines emphasize that politically important variables of noise-induced health impacts include hearing impairment leading to social handicap, reduced productivity, decreased performance in learning, workplace and school absenteeism, increased drug use and accidents. Recommendations on the implementation of the Guidelines are given to governments, municipalities, international organizations and the scientific community.

The WHO now undertakes a major effort to collect information on exposure–response relationships between noise and health impacts from international databases in a harmonized holistic approach. In 2002, a meeting was convened to clarify some gaps using new scientific and medical studies about the exposure to noise and different responses, in order to establish exposure–response relationships functions between noise and subsequent effects on human health.

**The following health end-points consequent upon noise were covered during the meeting:**

- sleep disturbance;
- hearing impairment;
- annoyance;
- loss of productivity in adults;
- loss of productivity in children (learning difficulties, loss of concentration).

Proposals for exposure–response relationships for children and for adults were discussed for each of these topics. Thus, the main outcome of the meeting was exposure–response relationships (curves) for different levels and sources of noise in children and adults. These curves are intended as guidance for decision-makers to derive noise standards in a transparent way and enable them to estimate the potential health impacts and the success of mitigation measures applied in noise management (WHO, 2003)

In addition to this activity, the WHO, in collaboration with the Federal Institute for Occupational Safety, Germany, published in 2001 a special report on exposure to noise in the occupational environment (WHO, 2001b). This book, with a CD-ROM, is intended for occupational hygienists and other occupational and safety personnel as a handbook. It provides an overview of the evaluation, prevention and control of exposure to noise at the workplace, with a view to preventing noise-induced hearing loss.

## International Labour Organization

The ILO is the UN-specialized agency that seeks the promotion of social justice and internationally recognized human and labour rights. It was founded in 1919 and is the only major surviving creation of the League of Nations. It became the first specialized agency of the UN in 1946. The ILO formulates international labour standards in the form of conventions and recommendation, setting minimum standards of basic labour rights including in the field of occupational safety and health.

The General Conference of the ILO adopted the Working Environment (Air Pollution, Noise and Vibration) Convention, 1977 (ILO, 1977a), which deals with the obligations of member states in the prevention and control of and protection against these occupational hazards. The term 'noise' covers all sound that can result in hearing impairment or be harmful to health or otherwise dangerous. It also adopted a recommendation with regards to the implementation of the Convention (ILO, 1977b).

**ILO Initiatives**

- Working Environment (Air Pollution Noise and Vibration) Convention 1977
- Code of Practice *'Protection of Workers Against Noise and Vibration in the Working Environment'* 1997
- Code of Practice *'Ambient factors in the Work Place'* 2001
- 'Managing Disability in the Workplace' 2001

Under its Safe Work Programme, the ILO publishes standards and codes of practice on safety and health. The ILO published the code of practice *Protection of Workers against Noise and Vibration in the Working Environment* in 1977 to underpin the Convention. In 2001 the ILO published the code of practice entitled *Ambient Factors at the Workplace* (ILO, 2001a), which updates the 1997 code of practice, and one on occupational exposure to airborne substances harmful to health, and contributes to the practical implementation of the provisions of the Convention. The provisions of this new code are the basis for eliminating or controlling exposure to hazardous airborne chemicals, ionizing and non-ionizing radiation, ultraviolet, infrared and (in some circumstances) visible radiation, electric and magnetic fields, noise, vibration, high and low temperatures, and humidity.

A draft code of practice on *Managing Disability in the Workplace* (ILO, 2001b) refers to the 1977 Convention and includes recommendations for hearing impairment such as in improving accessibility for people with hearing impairment and in the use of sign language in the workplace.

The ILO convened a meeting of experts on workers' health surveillance in 1997 and the resulting report included a section on 'Hearing impairment caused by noise' as an occupational disease (ILO, 1997).

Another useful resource is the *Encyclopaedia of Occupational Health and Safety.* Volume II focuses on all types of hazards including a chapter on noise. Other parts of the encyclopaedia, such as Chapter 11 on sensory systems and sections on different industries, would also be relevant. An online version is available for which a subscription is required (ILO, 1998).

# International Civil Aviation Organization

The International Civil Aviation Organization (ICAO) is a specialized agency of the UN and serves as a means to secure international cooperation for the highest possible degree of uniformity in regulations and standards, procedures and organization regarding civil aviation matters. In 2001, the ICAO Assembly endorsed the concept of a 'balanced approach' to aircraft noise management. Identifying the noise problem at an airport and and analyzing the various measures available to reduce noise, ICAO has developed policies on reduction at source (quieter aircraft), land-use planning and management, noise abatement operational procedure and operating restrictions. The noise emission of aircraft is limited by ICAO Annex 16, Chapters 2 and 3, which estimate maximum potential sound emissions under certification procedures (ICAO, 1993). Aircraft following the norms of Chapter 3 represent the state of the art of noise control of the 1970s. In many countries, non-certified aircraft (aircraft not fulfilling the ICAO requirements) are not permitted and Chapter 2 aircraft may not be registered again. In June 2001, ICAO adopted a new Chapter 4 noise standard, more stringent than that contained in Chapter 3. Commencing 1 January 2006, the new standard will apply to newly certificated aeroplanes and to Chapter 3 aeroplanes for which re-certification to Chapter 4 is requested (ICAO, 2005)

# World Bank

The mission of the World Bank is to fight poverty with passion and professionalism for lasting results, to help people help themselves and their environment by providing resources, sharing knowledge, building capacity, and forging partnerships in the public and private sectors.

Environmental Assessment (EA) is used in the World Bank to examine the environmental risks and benefits associated with the Bank's lending operations (World Bank, 1999). In project assessment, an environmental review will include consideration of issues related to noise, its environmental and social impact, and recommendations for noise reduction. The Bank's *Environmental Assessment Sourcebook and Updates 1991* provide guidance and information on the procedural requirements and practical aspects of environmental assessment in various sector- and location-specific contexts (World Bank, 1991, 1994).

For example, a project review for World Bank funding of a power station in a developing country stated that the power station would be designed to meet World Bank ambient noise guidelines of 75 dB (A) (day) and 70 dB (A) (night) at the property boundary. It described how this would be achieved. It also stated that one of the most problematic occupational health and safety concerns associated with plants of this type is hearing protection and that full ear protectors would be worn by all employees in the facility (World Bank, 1995a). A more recent assessment addresses similar considerations in the environmental review of a tyre factory in a developing country (World Bank, 2002).

The World Bank's *Environment, Health and Safety Guidelines for Mining and Milling* include a brief section on the minimization of workplace noise and a recommendation that personnel must use hearing protection when exposed to noise levels above 85 dB (A) (World Bank, 1995b). The *Handbook on Roads and the Environment* includes chapters on impacts on the noise environment and on human health and safety (World Bank, 1997). The *Pollution Prevention and Abatement Handbook* (World Bank, 1998) includes some recommendations on noise abatement in industrial settings.

Excessive noise and its health effects also receive a mention in a website presentation of the policy issues related to urban poverty (World Bank, 2002).

# World Trade Organization

The WTO is the only international organization dealing with the global rules of trade between nations. Its main function is to ensure that trade flows as smoothly, predictably and freely as possible. The goal is to improve the welfare of the peoples of the member countries.

World Trade Organization transparency provisions support the proper functioning of the multilateral trading system, by helping to prevent unnecessary trade restrictions. Technical regulations and product standards applied for environmental purposes are subject to the WTO Agreement on Technical Barriers to Trade (WTO, 2000a). Where suitable international standards exist they must be used unless a country adopts higher environmental standards. National measures notified under the agreement, which are used to implement international environmental agreements, include those for air, water, and noise pollution among others.

Countries may make notifications to the WTO Committee on Technical Barriers to Trade. For example, a country reported on draft orders for the fixing of sound levels on the ground to be respected by aircraft using airports with the stated objective of protecting the health of those living close to airports (WTO, 2000b).

Any state or customs territory having full autonomy in the conduct of its trade policies may become a member of ('accede to') the WTO. In this process potential members make various commitments, which include undertakings to provide market access and national treatment for particular service activities on specified terms and conditions. Sector-specific commitments include environmental services which in many cases include noise abatement services (WTO, 2002a).

The WTO Committee on Trade in Civil Aircraft meets regularly and has discussed issues relating to European Communities' regulation on aircraft noise in 2000 (WTO, 2001), and the status of implementation of ICAO stage 4 aircraft noise standards in 2001 (WTO, 2002b).

The WTO Committee on Trade and Environment recently discussed the issue of environmental goods and services (those 'used to measure, prevent, limit or correct environmental damage to water, air, and soil, as well as problems related to waste, noise and eco-systems, and may also include clean technologies, processes, products and services which reduce environmental risk and minimize pollution and material use'). This is part of a process for developing coverage for an agreement on environmental goods (WTO, 2002c)

# European Union

The European Community has considered the source control of noise since the 1960s.

For road vehicles, the maximum permissible noise levels range from 69 dB (A) for motor vehicles to 77 dB (A) for cars, and from 83 dB (A) for heavy two-wheeled vehicles to 84 dB (A) for trucks. A number of European Directives give permissible sound levels for motor vehicles and motorcycles (EC, 1970; EC, 1973; EC, 1978; EC, 1984a, b; EC 1996; EC, 1997 – see Appendix A). In addition to noise level limits for new vehicles (type test), noise emissions of vehicles already in use should be controlled regularly. Limits on the sound pressure levels for vehicles reduce the noise emission from the engines.

Particular categories of aircraft (such as helicopters, rotorcraft and supersonic aircraft) pose additional problems that require appropriate controls. For subsonic airplanes two EU Directives give the permissible sound levels (EC, 1980; EC, 1989 – see Appendix A) and a Council Directive adopted in 1992 limits the operation of certain aircraft in Community airports (EC, 1992 – see Appendix A). Another Council Regulation (EC, 1999) deals with modified and recertificated aircraft ('hushkits'). In 2002, this Regulation was modified by a Council Regulation on the registration and operation within the community of certain types of subsonic jet aeroplanes (EC, 2002a). In the same year, Directive 2002/49/EC on the assessment and management of environmental noise was adopted. The aim of this Directive was to define a common approach to avoid, prevent or reduce adverse effects due to exposure to environmental noise by applying a day-evening-night level $L_{den}$ and a night-time noise indicator $L_{night}$ as defined in ISO 1996-2:1987 standard (EC 2002b).

Until the year 2000, within the European Union, 'permissible sound levels' and 'sound power levels' had to be stated for several groups of machines; e.g. lawn mowers, construction machines and household equipment according to regulations adopted in the mid-1980s (EC 1984c–h; EC 1986b,c – see Appendix A). In 2000, Directive 2000/14/EC of the European Parliament and the Council of 8 May 2000, on the approximation of the laws of the Member States relating to the noise emission in the environment by equipment for use outdoors (EC, 2000a), was adopted. This Directive supersedes previous ones related to noise emitted by machines, for example, lawn mowers, construction machines and household equipment (EC 1984a–f; EC 1986b,c – see Appendix A). For many groups of machines and equipment sound level data have been compiled and are 'state of the art' with respect to noise control (EC, 2000a).

A comprehensive overview of the noise situation in Europe and an analysis of existing noise abatement actions is given in the European Commission Green Paper titled *Future Noise Policy* (EC, 1996), which was established to give noise abatement a higher priority in policy making and public discussion.

*Future Noise Policy* **outlines a new framework for noise policy in Europe with the following options for future action:**

- Harmonizing the methods for assessing noise exposure, and encouraging the exchange of information among member states.
- Establishing plans to reduce road traffic noise by applying newer technologies and fiscal instruments.

- Paying more attention to railway noise in view of the future extension of rail networks.
- Introducing more stringent regulation on air transport and using economic instruments to encourage compliance.
- Simplifying the existing nine regulations on outdoor equipment by proposing a Framework Directive that covers a wider range of equipment, including construction machines and others.

Following the analysis of the Green Paper, the European Commission published, in 2000, a proposal for a Directive of the European Parliament and of the Council relating to the assessment and management of environmental noise (COM(2000)468 final, see EC, 2000b). The objective of this proposal is to establish a common EU framework for the assessment and management of exposure to environmental noise. The aim of this Directive is to define a common approach intended to combat the effects of exposure to environmental noise. With harmonized noise indicators and assessment methods, noise maps shall be established by Member States. These will give a basis for public information on noise effects and for the implementation of action plans by the Member States. In a second phase of implementation of this Directive, the Commission shall establish a report assessing the need for further Community actions for environmental noise, on aspects such as the reduction of the number of people affected or the reduction of noise emitted by specific sources. It has to be noted, however, that the EC definition of environmental noise is slightly narrower than that of the WHO as it does not include noise from domestic activities, noise created by neighbours, and noise in discotheques and at open air concerts, toys and fireworks.

In 1999 the Council of the European Union published Council Regulation (EC) No. 925/1999 on restriction of the registration of recertificated subsonic aeroplanes, which do not comply with the noise performance requested in ICAO Annex 16, Chapter 3 (EC, 1999). Recently, the European Parliament and the Council of the European Union have adopted Directive 2002/30/EC, which establishes rules and procedure with regard to the introduction of noise-related operating restrictions at Community airports (EC, 2002a). This Directive supersedes (EC) No 925/1999.

The European Commission funds research and related demonstration projects related to noise. An example is the recent concerted action 'Protection against Noise' funded by Directorate General Research and Development. The evidence for environmental effects on children's health, including noise, has recently been reviewed in a joint report by WHO-EURO and the European Environment Agency (EEA, 2002).

# Organization for Economic Co-operation and Development

The Organization for Economic Co-operation and Development (OECD) groups 29 member countries in an organization that, most importantly, provides governments with a setting in which to discuss, develop and perfect economic and social policy. Exchanges between OECD governments flow from information and analysis provided by a Secretariat in Paris. Parts of the OECD Secretariat collect data, monitor trends, analyse and forecast economic developments, whereas others research social changes or evolving patterns in trade, environment, agriculture, technology, taxation and more.

As early as 1978, and later in 1985, the OECD recommended that its member countries undertake a significant improvement in their noise abatement policies by (OECD, 1978, 1985):

**OECD suggested noise abatement policies**

- ensuring a more effective enforcement of existing noise abatement regulations;
- progressively strengthening noise control regulations, and in particular noise emission limits on products;
- complementing existing regulations with incentives and measures designed to promote the production and use of quieter products;
- developing measures to finance noise abatement policies;
- protecting the most exposed members of the population by means such as traffic management, the construction of noise barriers, the insulation of buildings; and preventing the creation of new noise situations by appropriate land-use planning, especially in urban areas.

The OECD also advocated the continuation of the exchange of information between member countries in the field of noise abatement policies and to assess the policies adopted by member countries pursuant to this recommendation.

The OECD, in collaboration with the World Resources Institute, publishes reports on the state of the environment. The third report (OECD, 1991a) focuses on the environment in OECD countries, assessing the progress achieved over the previous two decades and identifying remaining problems. The report draws attention to the relationship between the state of the environment and economic growth and structural changes in OECD countries, and discusses economic and international responses to environmental problems.

The OECD fixes noise-related financial taxes in order to give incentives for reduction of aircraft noise. Examples of systems for noise-related financial charges are given in OECD (1991b) and OECD-ECMT (1995). Recently, the OECD has developed the 'Project on Environmentally Sustainable Transport (EST)'. This project (OECD, 2000) is an attempt of eight OECD member countries (Austria, Canada, France, Germany, Norway, Sweden, Switzerland and the Netherlands) to develop a sustainable transport system. Such a system is defined as one where 'transportation does not endanger public health or ecosystems'. Noise is one of the six criteria regarded as being the minimum number required to address the wide range of health impacts from transport. The EST requests that noise caused by transport no longer result in outdoor levels that present a health concern or serious nuisance. Depending on local and regional conditions this may entail a reduction of transport noise to no more than a maximum of 55 dB–65 dB (A) during the day and 45 dB (A) at night and indoors. The OECD also extends this project, in collaboration with UNEP and the Federal Ministry for Environment, Youth and Family (FMEYF), Austria to sustainable transport in countries of the Central European Initiative (FMEYF, 1999).

# International Institute of Noise Control Engineering

The International Institute of Noise Control Engineering (I-INCE) is a worldwide consortium of professional societies concerned with noise control and acoustics. It is the sponsor of the series of International Congresses on Noise Control Engineering (INTER-NOISE) and publishes, with the Institute of Noise Control Engineering of the USA, the quarterly magazine *Noise/News International*.

In 1991 the Board of Directors decided that 'there is urgent need for a long-range international noise control policy'. In 1992 and 1994 the I-INCE General Assembly established four Working Parties, which were expected to produce reports on the following topics:

- noise limits at the workplace;
- noise emission of flowing traffic;
- effectiveness of noise walls;
- community noise.

Three final reports (I-INCE, 1997, 1999, 2001) were produced.
Currently I-INCE has adopted six technical study groups (TSG: I-INCE, 2004):

1. I-INCE TSG No. 1 on Outdoor Recreational Activities;
2. I-INCE TSG No. 2 on Noise Labels for Products;
3. I-INCE TSG No. 3 on Noise Policies and Regulations;
4. I-INCE TSG No. 4 on Noise Control for Schoolrooms;

5. I-INCE TSG No. 5 on Noise as a Global Policy Issue.
6. I-INCE TSG No. 6 on Community Noise: Environmental Noise Impact Assessment and Mitigation.

The TSG has produced four work reports in 2001 and five work reports in 2002 (I-INCE, 2004).

# International Commission on Biological Effects of Noise

The object of the International Commission on Biological Effects of Noise (ICBEN) is: to encourage international cooperation in the study of the biological effects of noise; to promote communication among research scientists, governmental agencies, industrial workers and managers, and other parties and entities concerned with noise and noise effects; and to stimulate the exchange and dissemination of information about the biological effects of noise (ICBEN, 2002). The ICBEN is sponsoring and conducting the series of noise effects Congresses that are convened every fifth year. ICBEN has organized an International Congress on Noise as a Public Health Problem at 5-yearly intervals: Washington (1968), Dubrovnik (1973), Freiburg (1978), Turin (1983), Stockholm (1988), Nice (1993) Sydney (1998) and Rotterdam (2003). The next Congress will take place in Connecticut in 2008 (ICBEN, 2004). The primary aim of all of these Congresses has been to provide a forum for reporting, discussing and critically evaluating recent work in the nine subject areas covered by ICBEN international noise teams.

International noise teams study and communicate information about a special aspect of the biological effects of noise. Each team is responsible for the portion of the Congress programme that is dedicated to surveys, reviews and studies of that special aspect for which it was formed. It is also responsible for communications with governments, industries, workers, scientists, and other concerned parties and entities both as part of the Congress programme and as part of the team's work during the period between Congresses.

**International teams in the following areas have been formed:**

- noise-induced hearing loss;
- noise and communication;
- non-auditory physiological effects induced by noise;
- influence of noise on performance and behaviour;
- effects of noise on sleep;
- community responses to noise;
- noise and animals;
- effects of noise combined with other agents;
- regulations and standards.

The main goal of the ICBEN is to promote a high level of scientific research concerning all the aspects of noise-induced effects on human beings and on animals including preventive regulatory measures, and to sustain a lively communication among the scientists working in that field. This responsibility is delegated primarily to the international noise teams, in particular to the experts who are appointed at the beginning of each 5-year term. As these experts are familiar with the state of the art in their respective research area they are expected to build and to chair a team of highly qualified scientists actively working in that field.

# International Organization for Standardization

The International Organization for Standardization (ISO) is a worldwide federation of national standards bodies from some 130 countries, one from each country. ISO is an NGO established in 1947. The mission of the ISO is to promote the development of standardization and related activities in the world with a view to facilitating the international exchange of goods and services, and to developing cooperation in the spheres of intellectual, scientific, technological and economic activity.

The ISO's work results in international agreements, which are published as International Standards.

In the International Standards (see Appendix B) many fields of noise problems are considered from noise emissions to noise management. These include:

- standards for noise test codes (e.g. ISO 1680: 1999; ISO 3740: 2000; ISO 230-5: 2000; ISO 4412-1: 1991; ISO 4412-2: 1991; ISO 4412-3: 1991; ISO 12001: 1996);
- a majority of standards for measurements of sound power levels at sources (e.g. ISO 362: 1998; ISO 2151: 1972; ISO 2922: 1975; ISO 3095: 1975; ISO 3740: 2000; ISO 3741: 1999; ISO 3743-1: 1994; ISO 3743-2: 1994; ISO 3744: 1994; ISO 3745: 1977; ISO 3746: 1995; ISO 3747: 2000; ISO 3822-1: 1999; ISO 3822-2: 1995; ISO 3822-3: 1997; ISO 3822-4: 1997; ISO 5130: 1982; ISO 6190: 1988; ISO 6395: 1988; ISO 6396: 1992; ISO 6798: 1995; ISO 6926: 1999; ISO 7188: 1994; ISO 7216: 1992; ISO 7574-1: 1985; ISO 7574-2: 1985; ISO 7574-3: 1985; ISO 7574-4: 1985; ISO 7960: 1995; ISO 8960: 1991; ISO 9295: 1988; ISO 9614-1: 1993; ISO 9614-2: 1996; ISO 9645: 1990; ISO 10302: 1996; ISO 10494: 1993; ISO 10996: 1999; ISO 11094: 1991; ISO 11200: 1995; ISO 11201: 1995; ISO 11202: 1995; ISO 11203: 1995; ISO 11204: 1995; ISO/TR 11688-1: 1995; ISO/TR 11688-2: 1998; ISO 11689: 1996);
- noise immission standards were also developed (e.g. ISO 4872: 1978; ISO 7779: 1999; ISO/TR 7849: 1987; ISO 8528-10: 1998; ISO 8687: 1987;

ISO 9568: 1993); indoor spaces standards are also in existence (e.g. ISO 2923: 1996; ISO 3381: 1976; ISO 5128: 1980; ISO 5129: 1987);

- environmental noise has also been considered an important but difficult issue by the ISO (e.g. ISO 1996-1: 1982; ISO 1996-2: 1987; ISO 1996-3: 1987);
- quite recently, mitigation and management of noise have become important issues in the ISO as well, particularly for the workplace (e.g. ISO 7235: 1991; ISO 10847: 1997; ISO 11690-1: 1996;ISO 11690-2: 1996; ISO/TR 11690-3: 1997; ISO 14163: 1998; ISO 15667: 2000);
- occupational exposure is considered in several standards (e.g. ISO 1999: 1990; ISO 5131: 1996; ISO 6394: 1998; ISO 6396: 1992; ISO 7182: 1984; ISO 7917: 1987; ISO 9612: 1997);
- in a few standards human exposure to noise and vibrations is considered (e.g. ISO/TR 3352: 1974; ISO 2631-1: 1997; ISO 2631-2: 1989; ISO 5805: 1997; ISO 8041: 1990);
- a few ISO standards relate to attenuation of sound during propagation (e.g. ISO 9613-1: 1993; ISO 9613-2: 1996; ISO 11821: 1997);
- and sound insulation performance (e.g. ISO 11546-1: 1995; ISO 11546-2: 1995; ISO 11957: 1996).

The ISO collaborates with all major national agencies on standardization with respect to noise issues. These contributors include the American National Standards Institute (ANSI), the British Standards Institute (BSI), the Danish Institute of Dansk Standards (DS), the German Agency of Deutsche Industrie Normen (DIN), the Swedish Institute for Standards (SIS), the French Association for Normalization (Association Française de Normalisation (AFNOR) and the Netherlands Normalisatie Instituut (NNI).

# International Electrotechnical Commission

The International Electrotechnical Commission (IEC) is the world organization that prepares and publishes international standards for all electrical, electronic and related technologies.

The membership consists of more than 50 participating countries, including all of the world's major trading nations and a growing number of industrializing countries.

The mission of the IEC is to promote international cooperation on all questions of electrotechnical standardization and related matters, such as the assessment of conformity to standards, in the fields of electrotechnologies including electronics, magnetics and electromagnetics, electroacoustics, telecommunication, energy production and distribution, and related technologies. The IEC charter embraces all electrotechnologies as well as associated general disciplines such as terminology and symbols, measurement and performance, dependability, design and development, safety and the environment.

The IEC has constituted about 100 Technical Committees (TCs). The work of the TCs is published in International Standards documents, Technical Reports and Guides. Standards are publications resulting from international consensus on a particular area of technology with the prime objective of promoting international trade.

Important IEC publications regarding noise are listed in Appendix C. Standards refer to:

- noise from rotating electrical machines (e.g. IEC 60034-9: 1997);
- electronic tubes and valves (e.g. IEC 60151: 1968; IEC 60235-1A: 1975; IEC 60235-2A: 1974; IEC 60235-2D: 1976);
- resistors (e.g. IEC 60195: 1965);
- industrial-process control valves (e.g. IEC 60534-8-1: 1986; IEC 60534-8-2: 1991; IEC 60534-8-3: 2000; IEC 60534-8-4: 1994);
- household and similar electrical appliances (e.g. IEC 60704-1: 1997; IEC 60704-2-1: 2000; IEC 60704-2-2: 1985; IEC 60704-2-3: 2001; IEC 60704-2-4: 2001; IEC 60704-2-5: 1989; IEC 60704-2-6: 1994; IEC 60704-2-7: 1997; IEC 60704-2-8: 1997; IEC 60704-2-9: 2003; IEC 60704-2-10: 2004; IEC 60704-2-11: 1998; IEC 60704-2-13: 2000; 60704-3: 1992);
- steam turbines (e.g. IEC 61063: 1991), aircraft (e.g. IEC 61265: 1995);
- and wind turbine generator systems (e.g. IEC 61400-11: 1998).

# Conclusion

A large number of international agencies deal with different aspects of noise, although for all of them this subject represents only a small or very small part of their mandate. They can be grouped according to the type of organization, i.e. UN and linked organizations, other intergovernmental organizations, NGOs, and various scientific and technical organizations. They may also be grouped according to subject area, thus variously covering environmental, occupational, biological, human rights, transport, economic, measurement and control aspects. Noise generally began to be addressed internationally as a significant problem in the 1970s especially by the WHO, ILO, EU, ISO and IEC. Economic and human rights aspects were increasingly addressed from the late 1980s and the importance and methods of noise control during the 1990s. As developed and developing countries become increasingly urbanized, the problem of occupational and environmental noise assumes ever greater importance, and more and more organizations, both international and national, are realizing the need to address it.

# References

Berglund B, Lindvall T (1995) Community Noise. Archives of the Centre for Sensory Research, Vol. 2, Issue 1. Stockholm: Stockholm University and Karolinska Institute.

Berglund B (1998) Community noise in a public health perspective. In VC Goodwin, DC Stevenson (eds) Inter Noise 98. Sound and Silence: Setting the Balance. Vol. 1. Auckland: New Zealand Acoustical Society, pp. 19–24.

EC (1996) Future Noise Policy – European Commission Green Paper. Report COM (96) 540 final. Brussels: Commission of the European Communities.

EC (1999) Council Regulation (EC) No 925/1999 on the registration and operation within the Community of certain types of civil subsonic jet aeroplanes which have been modified and recertified as meeting the standards of Volume I, Part II, Chapter 3 of Annex 16 to the Convention on International Civil Aviation (3rd edn, July 1993). Official L 115, 4/5/1999, pp. 1–4. Corrigenda: Official Journal L 120, 8/5/1999; Official L 262, 8/10/1999.

EC (2000a) Directive 2000/14/EC of the European Parliament and of the Council of 8/5/2000 on the approximation of the laws of the Member States relating to the noise emission in the environment by equipment for use outdoors. Official Journal L 162, 3/07/2000, pp. 1–78.

EC (2000b) Proposal for a Directive of the European Parliament and of the Council relating to the Assessment and Management of Environmental Noise. COM(2000) 468 final, 2000/0194/(COD), 26/7/2000. Brussels: Commission of the European Communities.

EC (2002a) Directive 2002/30/EC of the European Parliament and of the Council of 26/3/2002 on the establishment of rules and procedures with regard to the introduction of noise-related operating restrictions at Community airports. Official Journal of the European Communities 28/3/2002 L 85/40, pp. 40–6.

EC (2002b) Directive 2002/49/EC of the European Parliament and of the Council of 25 June 2002 relating to the assessment and management of environmental noise. Official Journal of the European Communities 18/7/2002 L 189/12, pp. 12–25.

European Environment Agency (2002) Children's Health and Environment: A review of evidence. EEA and the WHO Regional Office for Europe. Available on 13 July 2002 at http://org.eea.eu.int/documents/newsreleases/eip_29.pdf.

Federal Ministry for Environment, Youth and Family (1999) Towards Sustainable Transport in the CEI Countries. Vienna: FMEYF; Paris: Organization for Economic Co-operation and Development; Nairobi: United Nations Environment Programme.

International Civil Aviation Organization (1993) International Standards and Recommended Practices: Environmental Protection. Annex 16, Vol. I: 'Aircraft Noise'. Annex 16 (Chapter 2 and 3) to the Convention on International Civil Aviation. ICAO, [Air Navigation (Noise Certification) Order 1990 – Statutory Instrument 1514]. Montreal.

International Civil Aviation Organization (2001) Aircraft Noise. Available on 24/8/2005 at http://www.icao.int/icao/en/env/noise.htm

International Commission on Biological Effects of Noise (2002) ICBEN: www.icben.org.

International Comission on Biological Effects of Noise (2004) Ninth Congress on Noise as a Public Health Problem: www.icben.org.

International Institute of Noise Control Engineering (1997) Technical Assessment of Upper Limits on Noise in the Workplace. Final Report 97-1. I-INCE, Heverlee-Leuven, Belgium: www.i-ince.org.

International Institute of Noise Control Engineering (1999) Technical Assessment of the Effectiveness of Noise Walls. Final Report 99-1. I-INCE, Heverlee-Leuven, Belgium: www.i-ince.org.

International Institute of Noise Control Engineering (2001) Noise Emissions of Road Vehicle – Effect of Regulations. Final Report 01-01. I-INCE, Belgium: www.i-ince.org.

International Institute of Noise Control Engineering (2004) International INCE Technical Initiatives. I-INCE, Heverlee-Leuven, Belgium: www.i-ince.org.

International Labour Organization (1977a) C148 Working Environment (Air Pollution, Noise and Vibration) Convention, 1977. Available on 28/4/2004 at www.ilo.org/ilolex/cgi-lex/convde.pl C148.

International Labour Organization (1977b) R156 Working Environment (Air Pollution, Noise and Vibration) Recommendation 1977. Available on 28/4/2004 at www.ilo.org/ilolex/ cgi-lex/convde.plR156.

International Labour Organization (1997) Technical and Ethical Guidelines for Workers' Health Surveillance, ILO, Geneva, 1997. Report available on 21/1/2001 at www.ilo.org/public/english/protection/safework/health/whsguide. htm.

International Labour Organization (1998) Encyclopaedia of Occupational Health and Safety, Fourth Edition. ISBN 92-2-109203-8, ILO, Geneva, 1998. Details of online version by subscription given on 21/1/2001 at www.ilocis.org.

International Labour Organization (2001a) Ambient Factors at the Workplace; Code of Practice. Geneva: ILO. Available on 13/7/2002 at www.ilo.org/public/ english/protection/safework/cops/english/download/e000009.pdf

International Labour Organization (2001b) Draft Code of Practice on Managing Disability in the Workplace. Available on 13/7/2002 at www.ilo.org/public/ english/employment/skills/disability/draftcod.htm#1.

Organization for Economic Co-operation and Development (1978) Recommend-ation of the council on noise abatement policies. Environment Committee, 3/7/1985 – C(78)73. Paris: OECD.

Organization for Economic Co-operation and Development (1985) Recommend-ation of the council on strengthening noise abatement. Environment Committee, 20/6/1985 – C(85)103. Paris: OECD, http://webdomino1.oecd.org/ horizontal/oecdacts.nsf/f5d1a20f4dd3e32cc1256a9b00360e66/ef5db04bd852f d5dc1256ac30053012b?OpenDocument.

Organization for Economic Co-operation and Development (1991a) State of Environment Reports. Third Report. Paris: OECD.

Organization for Economic Co-operation and Development (1991b) Fighting Noise in the 1990s. Paris: OECD.

Organization for Economic Co-operation and Development (2000) Project on Environmentally Sustainable Transport (EST) – The Economic and Social Implications of Sustainable Transportation. Proceedings from the Ottawa Workshop. Report ENV/EPOC/PPC/T(99)3/FINAL/REV1. Paris: OECD.

Organization for Economic Co-operation and Development, European Conference of Ministers of Transport (1995) Urban Travel and Sustainable Development. Paris: OECD-ECMT.

Schwela D (1998) WHO Guidelines on Community Noise. In NL Carter, RFS Job (eds) Noise Effects '98. Seventh International Congress on Noise as a Public Health Problem. Vol. 2. Sydney: Noise Effects '98, pp. 475–80.

ten Wolde T, Ross B (1999) Noise from traffic as a worldwide policy problem. In J Cuschieri, S Glegg, Yan Yong (eds) Internoise 99 – The 1999 International Congress on Noise Control Engineering, 6–8 December 1999, Fort Lauderdale, FL, pp. 1985–8.

United Nations (2000) Organizational Chart. UN Department of Public Information: www.unsystem.org/en/organizational.chart.en.htm.

United Nations Economic Commission for Europe (2001) Report on March, 2001 WP.29 Meeting. UNECE. Geneva, Switzerland: www.UNECE.org/trans/main/welcwp.29.htm.

United Nations Environment Programme (1999) Global Environment Outlook 2000. London: Earthscan.

United Nations Environment Programme (2001) United Nations System-wide Earthwatch. Health. Noise Pollution, http://earthwatch.unep.net/about/about.html; http://earthwatch.unep.net/health/noisepollution.html.

World Bank (1991) Environmental Assessment Sourcebook 1991 and Updates. Available on 17/9/2002 at http://lnweb18.worldbank.org/ESSD/essdext.nsf/47ByDocName/ToolsEnvironmentalAssessmentSourcebookand Updates.

World Bank (1994) Environmental Assessment Sourcebook. Volume 1, Policies, Procedures, and Cross-sectoral Issues, Vol. 2, Sectoral Guidelines. Vol. 3, Guidelines for Environmental Assessment of Energy and Industrial Projects. Washington DC: World Bank.

World Bank (1995a) Environmental Review Summary, available on 26/1/2001 at http://wbln0018.worldbank.org/ifcext/spiwebsite1.nsf/9456cd2430750 aa9852568890061dfd0/a421ba95708a955f852568b00065f7e6.

World Bank (1995b) Environment, Health and Safety Guidelines Mining and Milling – Open Pit, available on 13/7/2002 at www.ifc.org/enviro/enviro/pollution/min_pit.pdf.

World Bank (1997) Roads and the Environment, a Handbook. World Bank Technical Paper no. 376, available on 13/7/2002 at www.worldbank.org/html/fpd/transport/publicat/reh/covertoc.pdf.

World Bank (1998) The Pollution Prevention and Abatement Handbook, available on 13/7/2002 at http://lnweb18.worldbank.org/essd/essd.nsf/Docs/PPAH.

World Bank (1999) Environmental assessment. In Operational Policies, The World Bank Operational Manual, available on 21/1/2001 at http://wbln0018.world-bank.org/institutional/manuals/opmanual.nsf/opolw/ (click on 4.01 Environmental assesment).

World Bank (2002) Environmental Review Summary, available on 13/7/2002 at http://wbln0018.worldbank.org/IFCExt/spiwebsite1.nsf/f451ebbe34a9a8ca852 56a550073ff10/ed7eb3b66f2a4e6c85256bc300690c62?OpenDocument.

World Bank (2002) Urban Poverty: What are the Policy Issues? Environment, available on 13/7/2002 at http://www.worldbank.org/urban/poverty/environment. html.

World Health Organization (1980) Noise. Environmental Health Criteria, Document No. 12. Geneva: WHO.

World Health Organization (1986a) Assessment of Noise Impact on the Urban Environment – A Study on Noise Prediction Models. J Lang on behalf of the

WHO. Environmental Health Series No. 9. Copenhagen: WHO, Regional Office for Europe.

World Health Organization (1986b) Prevention of Deafness and Hearing Impairment. EB79/10, Annex A39/14. Geneva: WHO.

World Health Organization (1991) Report of the Informal Working Group on Prevention of Deafness and Hearing Impairment: Programme Planning. WHO/PDH/91.1. Geneva: WHO.

World Health Organization (1993) Executive Summary of the Environmental Health Criteria Document on Community Noise. Copenhagen: WHO.

World Health Organization (1995a) Noise – Selected Presentations of an Informal Regional Consultation Meeting on Noise Pollution, 2–5 September 1991, Amman, Jordan. Amman, Jordan: Eastern Mediterranean Regional Office, Regional Centre for Environmental Health Activities (CEHA).

World Health Organization (1995b) Concerns for Europe's Tomorrow – Health and the Environment in the WHO European Region, pp. 353–66. WHO European Centre for Environment and Health. Stuttgart: Wissenschaftliche Verlagsgesellschaft.

World Health Organization (1995c) Prevention of Hearing Impairment. Resolution of the 48th World Health Assembly, 12 May 1995. Geneva: WHO.

World Health Organization (1997) Report of the First Informal Consultation on Future Programme Developments for the Prevention of Deafness and Hearing Impairment. World Health Organization. Geneva: WHO.

World Health Organization (1998) Report of an Informal Consultation on Prevention of Noise-Induced Hearing Loss. Geneva: WHO.

World Health Organization (1999a) Charter on Transport, Environment and Health. Copenhagen: WHO Regional Office for Europe.

World Health Organization (1999b) Regional Guidelines for the Development of Healthy Workplaces – Document Series No. 1. Manila: WHO Regional Office for the Western Pacific, Manila, available on 21/1/2001 at www.wpro.who.int/theme_publication/t2f1/Healthy%20Workplaces%20Guidelines.doc.

World Health Organization (2000a) Guidelines for Community Noise. Geneva: World Health Organization, www.who.int/peh/.

World Health Organization (2000b) Transport, Environment and Health WHO Regional Publications, European Series, No. 89. Geneva: WHO.

World Health Organization (2001a) WHO calls on private sector to provide affordable hearing aids in developing world, Press Release WHO/34, 11/7/2001.

World Health Organization (2001b) In B Goelzer, CH Hansen, GA Sehrndt (eds) Occupational Exposure to Noise: Evaluation, Prevention and Control. Publication Series from the Federal Institute for Occupational Safety and Health, Special Report S 64, Dortmung/Berlin, Germany. Geneva: WHO.

World Health Organization (2001c) Environmental Health Indicators System: Report on the WHO Working Group Meeting, Bonn, 28–30 November 2001, available on 13/7/2002 at www.who.dk/EHindicators/Publications/ 20020319_5.

World Health Organization (2002) Transport, environment and health: the results of a Healthy Cities survey in 54 European cities. Available on 24/6/2002 at www.who.dk/ healthy-cities/UrbanHealthTopics/20020128_2.

World Health Organization (2003) Technical Meeting on Exposure-response Relationships of Noise on Health, 19–21 September 2002, Bonn, Germany: Meeting report. Bonn: WHO Regional Office for Europe, European Centre for

Environment and Health, available on 10/6/2004 at www.euro.who.int/ Document/NOH/exposerespnoise.pdf.

World Trade Organization (2000a) Agreement on Technical Barriers to Trade. Overview available on 5/9/2002 at www.wto.org/wto/english/thewto_e/ whatis_e/eol/e/wto09/wto9_14.htm#note1. The agreement itself was available on 23/1/2001 at www.wto.org/english/tratop_e/tbt_e/tbtagr.htm#Agreement.

World Trade Organization (2000b) Notification to Committee on Technical Barriers to Trade G/TBT/Notif.00/153; 29 March 2000. Geneva: WTO.

World Trade Organization (2001) WTO Annual Report 2001, accessed on 5/9/2002 at www.wto.org/english/res_e/booksp_e/anrep_e/ wto_anrep01_e.pdf.

World Trade Organization (2002a) Technical note WT/ACC/10, accessed on 5/9/2002 at www.wto.org/wto/english/thewto_e/acc_e/ tn_a4_specifcommt3_e. htm.

World Trade Organization (2002b) WTO Annual Report 2002, accessed on 5/9/2002 at www.wto.org/english/res_e/booksp_e/anrep_e/ anrep02_e.pdf.

World Trade Organization (2002c) Committee on Trade and Environment, Special Session on Environmental Goods, 6/6/2002, accessed on 5/9/2002 at http://docsonline.wto.org/gen_search.asp.

# Appendix A: EC Council Directives

EC 1970 Council Directive on the approximation of the laws of the Member States relating to the permissible sound level and the exhaust system of motor vehicles. Directive 70/157/EEC of 6/2/1970. Official Journal L 42 (23/2/1970), p. 16. Amended by 73/350/EEC of 7/11/1973; Official Journal L 321 (22/11/1973), p. 33. Amended by 77/212/EEC of 8/3/1977; Official Journal L 66 (12/3/1977), p. 33. Amended by 81/334/EEC of 13/4/1981; Official Journal L 131 (18/5/1981), p. 6. Amended by 84/424/EEC of 3/9/1984; Official Journal L 238 (6/9/1984) p. 31. Amended by 87/354/EEC of 25/6/1987; Official Journal L 192 (11/7/1987) p. 43. Amended by 89/491/EEC of 17/7/1989; Official Journal L 238 (15/8/1989) p. 43. Amended by 92/97/EEC of 10/11/1992; Official Journal L 371 (19/12/1992) p. 1. Amended by 96/20/EEC of 27/3/1996; Official Journal L 92 (13/4/1996) p. 23, Brussels, Belgium.

EC 1973 Commission Directive 73/350/EEC of 7/11/1973 adapting to technical progress the Council Directive of 6/2/1970 on the approximation of the laws of the Member States relating to the permissible sound level and the exhaust system of motor vehicles. Official Journal L 321 (22/11/1973), pp. 33–6.

EC 1978 Council Directive on the approximation of the laws of the Member States on the permissible sound level and exhaust system of motorcycles. Directive 78/1015/EEC of 23/11/1978. Official Journal L 349 (13/12/1978), p. 21, Brussels, Belgium. (Directive 78/1015/EEC is superseded by 97/24/EC, see EC 1997.)

EC 1980 Council Directive on the limitation of noise emissions from subsonic airplanes. Directive 80/51/EEC of 20 December 1979. Official Journal L 18 (24/1/1980) p. 26, Brussels, Belgium.

EC 1984a Council Directive 84/424/EEC of 3/9/1984 amending Directive 70/157/EEC on the approximation of the laws of the Member States relating to the permissible sound level and the exhaust system of motor vehicles. Official Journal L 238 (6/9/1984), pp. 31–3.

EC 1984b Commission Directive 84/372/EEC of 3/7/1984 adapting to technical progress Council Directive 70/157/EEC on the approximation of the laws of the Member States relating to the permissible sound level and the exhaust system of motor vehicles. Official Journal L 196 (26/7/1984), pp. 47–9.

EC 1984c Council Directive on the approximation of the laws of the Member States relating to the permissible sound power level of compressors. Directive 84/533/EEC of 17/9/1984. Official Journal L 300 (19/11/1984), p. 123. Amended by 85/406/EEC of 11/7/1985. Official Journal L 233 (30/8/1985), p. 11, Brussels, Belgium.

EC 1984d Council Directive on the approximation of the laws of the Member States relating to the permissible sound power level of tower cranes. Directive 84/534/EEC of 17/9/1984. Official Journal L 300 (19/11/1984), p. 123. Amended by 87/405/EEC of 25/6/1987. Official Journal L 220 (8/8/1987), p. 60, Brussels, Belgium.

EC 1984e Council Directive on the approximation of the laws of the Member States relating to the permissible sound power level of welding generators. Directive 84/535/EEC of 17/9/1984. Official Journal L 300 (19/11/1984), p. 142. Amended by 85/407/EEC of 11/7/1985. Official Journal L 233 (30/8/1985), p. 16, Brussels, Belgium.

EC 1984f Council Directive on the approximation of the laws of the Member States relating to the permissible sound power level of power generators. Directive 84/536/EEC of 17/9/1984. Official Journal L 300 (19/11/1984), p. 149. Amended by 85/408/EEC of 11/7/1985. Official Journal L 233 (30/8/1985), p. 18, Brussels, Belgium.

EC 1984g Council Directive on the approximation of the laws of the Member States relating to the permissible sound power level of powered hand-held concrete-breakers and picks. Directive 84/537/EEC of 17/9/1984. Official Journal L 300 (19/11/1984), p. 156. Amended by 85/409/EEC of 11/7/1985. Official Journal L 233 (30/8/1985), p. 20, Brussels, Belgium.

EC 1984h Council Directive on the approximation of the laws of the Member States relating to the permissible sound power level of lawnmowers. Directive 84/538/EEC of 17/9/1984. Official Journal L 300 (19/11/1984), p. 171. 87. Amended by 87/ 252/EEC of 7/4/87. Official Journal L 117 (5/5/1987), p. 22. Amended by 88/80/EEC of 22/3/1988. Official Journal L 81 (26/3/1988), p. 69. Amended by 88/181/EEC of 22/3/1988. Official Journal L 81 (26/3/1988), p. 71, Brussels, Belgium.

EC 1986a Council Directive on the protection of workers from the risks related to exposure of noise at work. Directive 86/188/EEC of 12/5/1986. Official Journal L 137 (24/5/1986), p. 28, Brussels, Belgium.

EC 1986b Council Directive on the limitation of noise emitted by hydraulic excavators, rope-operated excavators, dozers, loaders and excavator-loaders. Directive 86/662/EEC of 22/12/1986 as amended by the Directive of 2/8/1989. Official Journal L 384 (31/12/1986), p. 1; L 253 (30/8/1989), p. 35, Brussels, Belgium.

EC 1986c Council Directive on airborne noise emitted by household appliances. Directive 86/594/EEC of 1/12/1986. Official Journal L 344 (6/12/1986), p. 24, Brussels, Belgium.

EC 1989 Council Directive on the limitation of noise emission from civil subsonic jet aeroplanes. Directive 89/629/EEC of 4/12/1989. Official Journal L 363 (12/12/89), p. 27, Brussels, Belgium.

EC 1992 Council Directive 92/14/EEC of 2/3/1992 on the limitation of the operation of aeroplanes covered by Part II, Chapter 2, Vol. 1 of Annex 16 to the Convention on International Civil Aviation, 2nd edn (1988). Official Journal L 076 (23/3/1992) pp. 21–7.

EC 1996 Council Directive to adapt in the light of technical progress Directive 70/157/EEC of 6/2/1970 on the approximation of the laws of the Member States regarding permissible sound levels and exhaust systems of motor vehicles. Directive 96/20/EC of 27/3/1996. Official Journal L 92 (13/4/1996), p. 23, Brussels, Belgium.

EC 1997 Directive on certain components and characteristics of two or three-wheel motor vehicles. Directive 97/24/EC of the European Parliament and of the Council of 17/6/1997. Official Journal L 226 1997, Brussels, Belgium.

# Appendix B: ISO standards

ISO 230-5: 2000 Test code for machine tools – Part 5: Determination of the noise emission.

ISO 362: 1998 Acoustics – Measurement of noise emitted by accelerating road vehicles – Engineering method (available in English only).

ISO 389-4: 1994 Acoustics – Reference zero for the calibration of audiometric equipment – Part 4: Reference levels for narrow-band masking noise.

ISO 1680: 1999 Acoustics – Test code for the measurement of airborne noise emitted by rotating electrical machines.

ISO 1996-1: 1982 Acoustics – Description and measurement of environmental noise – Part 1: Basic quantities and procedures.

ISO 1996-2: 1987 Acoustics – Description and measurement of environmental noise – Part 2: Acquisition of data pertinent to land use.

ISO 1996-3: 1987 Acoustics – Description and measurement of environmental noise – Part 3: Application to noise limits.

ISO 1999: 1990 Acoustics – Determination of occupational noise exposure and estimation of noise-induced hearing impairment.

ISO 2151: 1972 Measurement of airborne noise emitted by compressor/primem-over-units intended for outdoor use.

ISO 2631-1: 1997 Mechanical vibration and shock – Evaluation of human exposure to whole-body vibration – Part 1: General requirements.

ISO 2631-2: 1989 Evaluation of human exposure to whole-body vibration – Part 2: Continuous and shock-induced vibrations in buildings (1 to 80 Hz).

ISO 2922: 1975 Acoustics – Measurement of noise emitted by vessels on inland water-ways and harbours.

ISO 2923: 1996 Acoustics – Measurement of noise on board vessels.

ISO 3095: 1975 Acoustics – Measurement of noise emitted by railbound vehicles.

ISO/TR 3352: 1974 Acoustics – Assessment of noise with respect to its effect on the intelligibility of speech.

ISO 3381: 1976 Acoustics – Measurement of noise inside railbound vehicles.

ISO 3740: 2000 Acoustics – Determination of sound power levels of noise sources – Guidelines for the use of basic standards codes.

ISO 3741: 1999 Acoustics – Determination of sound power levels of noise sources using sound pressure – Precision methods for reverberation rooms.

ISO 3741: 1999/Cor 1: 2001.corrigendum to ISO 3741:1999

ISO 3743-1: 1994 Acoustics – Determination of sound power levels of noise sources – Engineering methods for small, movable sources in reverberant fields – Part 1: Comparison method for hard-walled test rooms.

ISO 3743-2: 1994 Acoustics – Determination of sound power levels of noise sources using sound pressure – Engineering methods for small, movable sources in reverberant fields – Part 2: Methods for special reverberation test rooms.

ISO 3744: 1994 Acoustics – Determination of sound power levels of noise sources using sound pressure – Engineering method in an essentially free field over a reflecting plane.

ISO 3745: 1977 Acoustics – Determination of sound power levels of noise sources – Precision methods for anechoic and semi-anechoic rooms.

ISO 3746: 1995 Acoustics – Determination of sound power levels of noise sources using sound pressure – Survey method using an enveloping measurement surface over a reflecting plane.

ISO 3746: 1995/Cor 1: 1995.

ISO 3747: 2000 Acoustics – Determination of sound power levels of noise sources using sound pressure – Comparison method in situ.

ISO 3822-1: 1999 Acoustics – Laboratory tests on noise emission from appliances and equipment used in water supply installations – Part 1: Method of measurement.

ISO 3822-2: 1995 Acoustics – Laboratory tests on noise emission from appliances and equipment used in water supply installations – Part 2: Mounting and operating conditions for draw-off taps and mixing valves.

ISO 3822-3: 1997 Acoustics – Laboratory tests on noise emission from appliances and equipment used in water supply installations – Part 3: Mounting and operating conditions for in-line valves and appliances.

ISO 3822-4: 1997 Acoustics – Laboratory tests on noise emission from appliances and equipment used in water supply installations – Part 4: Mounting and operating conditions for special appliances.

ISO 3891: 1978 Acoustics – Procedure for describing aircraft noise heard on the ground.

ISO 4412-1: 1991 Hydraulic fluid power – Test code for determination of airborne noise levels – Part 1: Pumps.

ISO 4412-2: 1991 Hydraulic fluid power – Test code for determination of airborne noise levels – Part 2: Motors.

ISO 4412-3: 1991 Hydraulic fluid power – Test code for determination of airborne noise levels – Part 3: Pumps – Method using a parallelepiped microphone array.

ISO 4871: 1996 Acoustics – Declaration and verification of noise emission values of machinery and equipment.

ISO 4872: 1978 Acoustics – Measurement of airborne noise emitted by construction equipment intended for outdoor use – Method for determining compliance with noise limits.

ISO 5128: 1980 Acoustics – Measurement of noise inside motor vehicles.

ISO 5129: 1987 Acoustics – Measurement of noise inside aircraft.

ISO 5130: 1982 Acoustics – Measurement of noise emitted by stationary road vehicles – Survey method.

ISO 5131: 1996 Acoustics – Tractors and machinery for agriculture and forestry – Measurement of noise at the operator's position – Survey method.

ISO 5805: 1997 Mechanical vibration and shock – Human exposure – Vocabulary.

ISO 6190: 1988 Acoustics – Measurement of sound pressure levels of gas turbine installations for evaluating environmental noise – Survey method.

ISO 6393: 1998 Acoustics – Measurement of exterior noise emitted by earth-moving machinery – Stationary test conditions (available in English only).

ISO 6394: 1998 Acoustics – Measurement at the operator's position of noise emitted by earth-moving machinery – Stationary test conditions (available in English only).

ISO 6395: 1988 Acoustics – Measurement of exterior noise emitted by earth-moving machinery – Dynamic test conditions.

ISO 6396: 1992 Acoustics – Measurement at the operator's position of noise emitted by earth-moving machinery – Dynamic test conditions.

ISO 6798: 1995 Reciprocating internal combustion engines – Measurement of emitted airborne noise – Engineering method and survey method.

ISO 6926: 1999 Acoustics – Requirements for the performance and calibration of reference sound sources used for the determination of sound power levels and in situ measurements.

ISO 7182: 1984 Acoustics – Measurement at the operator's position of airborne noise emitted by chain saws.

ISO 7188: 1994 Acoustics – Measurement of noise emitted by passenger cars under conditions representative of urban driving.

ISO 7216: 1992 Acoustics – Agricultural and forestry wheeled tractors and self-propelled machines – Measurement of noise emitted when in motion.

ISO 7235: 1991 Acoustics – Measurement procedures for ducted silencers – Insertion loss, flow noise and total pressure loss.

ISO 7574-1: 1985 Acoustics – Statistical methods for determining and verifying stated noise emission values of machinery and equipment – Part 1: General considerations and definitions.

ISO 7574-2: 1985 Acoustics – Statistical methods for determining and verifying stated noise emission values of machinery and equipment – Part 2: Methods for stated values for individual machines.

ISO 7574-3: 1985 Acoustics – Statistical methods for determining and verifying stated noise emission values of machinery and equipment – Part 3: Simple (transition) method for stated values for batches of machines.

ISO 7574-4: 1985 Acoustics – Statistical methods for determining and verifying stated noise emission values of machinery and equipment – Part 4: Methods for stated values for batches of machines.

ISO 7779: 1999 Acoustics – Measurement of airborne noise emitted by information technology and telecommunications equipment.

ISO/TR 7849: 1987 Acoustics – Estimation of airborne noise emitted by machinery using vibration measurement.

ISO 7917: 1987 Acoustics – Measurement at the operator's position of airborne noise emitted by brush saws.

ISO 7960: 1995 Airborne noise emitted by machine tools – Operating conditions for woodworking machines.

ISO 8041: 1990 Human response to vibration – Measuring instrumentation.

ISO 8528-10: 1998 Reciprocating internal combustion engine driven alternating current generating sets – Part 10: Measurement of airborne noise by the enveloping surface method.

ISO 8687: 1987 Cinematography – Signal-to-noise ratio of 8 mm Type S, 16 mm and 35 mm variable-area photographic sound records – Method of measurement.

ISO 8960: 1991 Refrigerators, frozen-food storage cabinets and food freezers for household and similar use – Measurement of emission of airborne acoustical noise.

ISO 9295: 1988 Acoustics – Measurement of high-frequency noise emitted by computer and business equipment.

ISO 9296: 1988 Acoustics – Declared noise emission values of computer and business equipment.

ISO 9568: 1993 Cinematography – Background acoustic noise levels in theatres, review rooms and dubbing rooms (available in English only).

ISO 9612: 1997 Acoustics – Guidelines for the measurement and assessment of exposure to noise in a working environment.

ISO 9614-1: 1993 Acoustics – Determination of sound power levels of noise sources using sound intensity – Part 1: Measurement at discrete points.

ISO 9614-2: 1996 Acoustics – Determination of sound power levels of noise sources using sound intensity – Part 2: Measurement by scanning.

ISO 9645: 1990 Acoustics – Measurement of noise emitted by two-wheeled mopeds in motion – Engineering method.

ISO 9613-1: 1993 Acoustics – Attenuation of sound during propagation outdoors – Part 1: Calculation of the absorption of sound by the atmosphere.

ISO 9613-2: 1996 Acoustics – Attenuation of sound during propagation outdoors – Part 2: General method of calculation.

ISO 10302: 1996 Acoustics – Method for the measurement of airborne noise emitted by small air-moving devices.

ISO 10494: 1993 Gas turbines and gas turbine sets – Measurement of emitted airborne noise – Engineering/survey method.

ISO 10844: 1994 Acoustics – Specification of test tracks for the purpose of measuring noise emitted by road vehicles.

ISO 10847: 1997 Acoustics – In-situ determination of insertion loss of outdoor noise barriers of all types.

ISO 10996: 1999 Photography – Still-picture projectors – Determination of noise emissions.

ISO 11094: 1991 Acoustics – Test code for the measurement of airborne noise emitted by power lawn mowers, lawn tractors, lawn and garden tractors, professional mowers, and lawn and garden tractors with mowing attachments.

ISO 11200: 1995 Acoustics – Noise emitted by machinery and equipment – Guidelines for the use of basic standards for the determination of emission sound pressure levels at a work station and at other specified positions.

ISO 11201: 1995 Acoustics – Noise emitted by machinery and equipment – Measurement of emission sound pressure levels at a work station and at other specified positions – Engineering method in an essentially free field over a reflecting plane.

ISO 11202: 1995 Acoustics – Noise emitted by machinery and equipment – Measurement of emission sound pressure levels at a work station and at other specified positions – Survey method in situ.

ISO 11203: 1995 Acoustics – Noise emitted by machinery and equipment – Determination of emission sound pressure levels at a work station and at other specified positions from the sound power level.

ISO 11204: 1995 Acoustics – Noise emitted by machinery and equipment – Measurement of emission sound pressure levels at a work station and at other specified positions – Method requiring environmental corrections.

ISO 11546-1: 1995 Acoustics – Determination of sound insulation performances of enclosures – Part 1: Measurements under laboratory conditions (for declaration purposes).

ISO 11546-2: 1995 Acoustics – Determination of sound insulation performances of enclosures – Part 2: Measurements in situ (for acceptance and verification purposes).

ISO/TR 11688-1: 1995 Acoustics – Recommended practice for the design of low-noise machinery and equipment – Part 1: Planning.

ISO/TR 11688-2: 1998 Acoustics – Recommended practice for the design of low-noise machinery and equipment – Part 2: Introduction to the physics of low-noise design.

ISO 11689: 1996 Acoustics – Procedure for the comparison of noise-emission data for machinery and equipment.

ISO 11690-1: 1996 Acoustics – Recommended practice for the design of low-noise workplaces containing machinery – Part 1: Noise control strategies.

ISO 11690-2: 1996 Acoustics – Recommended practice for the design of low-noise workplaces containing machinery – Part 2: Noise control measures.

ISO/TR 11690-3: 1997 Acoustics – Recommended practice for the design of low-noise workplaces containing machinery – Part 3: Sound propagation and noise prediction in workrooms.

ISO 11821: 1997 Acoustics – Measurement of the in situ sound attenuation of a removable screen.

ISO 11957: 1996 Acoustics – Determination of sound insulation performance of cabins – Laboratory.

ISO 12001: 1996 Acoustics – Noise emitted by machinery and equipment – Rules for the drafting and presentation of a noise test code.

ISO 14163: 1998 Acoustics – Guidelines for noise control by silencers.

ISO 15086-2: 2000 Hydraulic fluid power – Determination of the fluid-borne noise characteristics of components and systems – Part 2: Measurement of the speed of sound in a fluid in a pipe.

ISO 15667: 2000 Acoustics – Guidelines for noise control by enclosures and cabins.

# Appendix C: IEC standards

IEC 60034-9 (1997-07) Rotating electrical machines – Part 9: Noise limits.

IEC 60151-18 (1968-01) Measurements of the electrical properties of electronic tubes and valves. Part 18: Methods of measurement of noises due to mechanical or acoustic excitations.

IEC 60195 (1965-01) Method of measurement of current noise generated in fixed resistors.

IEC 60235-1A (1975-01) Measurement of the electrical properties of microwave tubes – Part 1: Terminology – First supplement.

IEC 60235-2A (1974-01) Measurement of the electrical properties of microwave tubes – Part 2: General measurements – First supplement: Chapter V: Methods of measuring parasitic noise.

IEC 60235-2D (1976-01) Measurement of the electrical properties of microwave tubes – Part 2: General measurements – Fourth supplement.

IEC 60244-3B (1972-01) Methods of measurement for radio transmitters – Part 3: Wanted and unwanted modulation – Second supplement: Unwanted modulation, including hum and noise modulation.

IEC 60268-5 (1989-08) Sound system equipment. Part 5: Loudspeakers.

IEC 60487-3-4 (1982-01) Methods of measurement for equipment used in terrestrial radio-relay systems – Part 3: Simulated systems – Section Four: Measurements for f.d.m. transmission.

IEC 60487-3-5 (1982-01) Methods of measurement for equipment used in terrestrial radio-relay systems – Part 3: Simulated systems – Section Five: Measurement of mutual interference.

IEC 60534-8-1 (1986-09) Industrial-process control valves. Part 8: Noise considerations. Section One: Laboratory measurement of noise generated by aerodynamic flow through control valves.

IEC 60534-8-2 (1991-05) Industrial-process control valves – Part 8: Noise considerations – Section 2: Laboratory measurement of noise generated by hydrodynamic flow through control valves.

IEC 60534-8-3 (2000-07) Industrial-process control valves – Part 8: Noise considerations – Section 3: Control valve aerodynamic noise prediction method.

IEC 60534-8-4 (1994-05) Industrial-process control valves – Part 8: Noise considerations – Section 4: Prediction of noise generated by hydrodynamic flow.

IEC 60704-1 (1997-03) Household and similar electrical appliances – Test code for the determination of airborne acoustical noise – Part 1: General requirements.

IEC 60704-2-1 (2000-12) Household and similar electrical appliances – Test code for the determination of airborne acoustical noise – Part 2-1: Particular requirements for vacuum cleaners.

IEC 60704-2-2 (1985-01) Test code for the determination of airborne acoustical noise emitted by household and similar electrical appliances. Part 2: Particular requirements for forced draught convection heaters.

IEC 60704-2-3 (2001-12) Household and similar electrical appliances – Test code for the determination of airborne acoustical noise – Part 2-3: Particular requirements for dishwashers.

IEC 60704-2-4 (2001-07) Household and similar electrical appliances – Test code for the determination of airborne acoustical noise – Part 2-4: Particular requirements for washing machines and spin extractors.

IEC 60704-2-5 (2005-07) Test code for the determination of airborne acoustical noise. Part 2-5: Particular requirements for electric thermal storage room heaters.

IEC 60704-2-6 (2005-02) Test code for the determination of airborne acoustical noise – Part 2-6: Particular requirements for tumble-dryers.

IEC 60704-2-7 (1997-09) Household and similar electrical appliances – Test code for the determination of airborne acoustical noise – Part 2: Particular requirements for fans.

IEC 60704-2-8 (1997-02) Household and similar electrical appliances – Test code for the determination of airborne acoustical noise – Part 2: Particular requirements for electric shavers.

IEC 60704-2-9 (2003-06) Household and similar electrical appliances – Test code for the determination of airborne acoustical noise – Part 2-9: Particular requirements for electric hair care appliances.

IEC 60704-2-10 (2004-04) Household and similar electrical appliances – Test code for the determination of airborne acoustical noise – Part 2-10: Particular requirements for electric cooking ranges, ovens, grills, microwave ovens and combination microwave ovens.

IEC 60704-2-11 (1998-12) Household and similar electrical appliances – Test code for the determination of airborne acoustical noise – Part 2-11: Particular requirements for electrically-operated food preparation appliances.

IEC 60704-2-13 (2000-05) Household and similar electrical appliances – Test code for the determination of airborne acoustical noise – Part 2-13: Particular requirements for range hoods.

IEC 60704-3 (1992-06) Test code for the determination of airborne acoustical noise emitted by household and similar electrical appliances – Part 3: Procedure for determining and verifying declared noise emission values.

IEC 61063 (1991-04) Acoustics – Measurement of airborne noise emitted by steam turbines and driven machinery.

IEC 61265 (1995-04) Electroacoustics – Instruments for measurement of aircraft noise – Performance requirements for systems to measure one-third-octave-band sound pressure levels in noise certification of transport-category aeroplanes.

IEC 61265 Corr.1 (1995-06) Electroacoustics – Instruments for measurement of aircraft noise – Performance requirements for systems to measure one-third-octave-band sound pressure levels in noise certification of transport-category aeroplanes.

IEC 61400-1-Ed. 2.0 (2002-12) Wind turbine generator systems – Part 11: Acoustic noise measurement techniques.

# Index

absorbent material 651–2, 659, 662–5
acetylcholine 93, 100, 466, 642
  tinnitus 259, 270
acoustic ecology 350–1, 352, 366
acoustic neuroma 416, 418, 419–20
acoustic reflex 50, 131–3, 209, 422, 641
  military NIHL 450, 451
  organic solvents 479, 481
  susceptibility 131–3, 143, 209, 467
acoustic trauma 115–17, 190, 192–3,
    499, 637–40
  acute 402–3
  ageing 44, 65, 68, 638
  CAS changes after damage 113,
    115–17, 119, 121
  causes of SNHL 184
  chronic 399, 402–3
  cochlear response 88, 95, 99, 100–2
  conditioning 637–40, 641–5
  diagnosis 190, 192–3, 210, 213,
    214, 217, 220
  glutamate 269
  laws 607
  military 436, 439, 448
  music 455, 467
  occupational noise 399, 402–3,
    419, 424
  susceptibility 132, 135, 137–8,
    140, 141–2, 413, 467
  tinnitus 121, 269–71
ACTH 518–19, 524, 539
actin filaments 89, 90, 97
action levels 335, 494, 667–8, 674
  measurement of noise 14, 16, 28,
    35, 36, 39
  music 454, 455
activation 535, 536
activity limitations 681, 683–7
actomyosin system 90
adaptation 90, 97, 403, 466, 527, 569
  environmental noise 351, 363, 366
  stress 527, 534, 535, 542, 543
  tinnitus 258, 263

additive effect 302–3, 322
  AHL and NIHL 50–3, 67–8, 70,
    79–80, 243, 302–3, 305, 413
  NIHL and hypertension 322
  occupational noise and solvents
    477, 483–4, 491
adrenal cortex 520, 538, 542
adrenal gland 538
adrenal medulla 520
adrenaline 501, 518–25, 529–30, 539–41
  sleep 570
  tinnitus 272
afferent system 260–1
  cochleae and hazardous noise 85,
    92–3, 98, 102
  conditioning 641, 645
  feedback control 259, 260–1, 263
  susceptibility 132, 138, 411
  tinnitus 260–1, 263, 265–7, 268–73
age 2, 134–5, 202–4, 244–5, 250–1,
    299–305, 332, 576–7, 708
  acoustic trauma 44, 65, 68, 638
  babies' reaction to noise 502
  blast effects 282, 284
  cognition and noise 561–2
  conditioning 637
  databases 313, 315–16, 322, 329,
    331, 332
  diagnosis 184, 192–3, 196–7,
    199–206, 213, 215–16, 221
  disability assessment 233, 236–8,
    242–7, 250–1, 254
  environmental noise 354, 356,
    363, 365
  hearing conservation programmes
    333–4, 339
  interaction with NIHL 64–80, 413
  interaction with noise exposure
    44–58
  laws 611
  measurement of hearing
    thresholds 148–9, 162
  military 437–8, 450

music 453, 461–2, 466, 467, 705,
    707–10
NIHL and health 293, 298
occupational noise 399–400, 403,
    407–8, 411–13, 419
occupational noise and solvents
    479–80, 482, 487–8, 492–4
rehabilitation 682, 684, 689,
    692, 700
sleep 576–7, 581
stress 541
susceptibility 129, 134–5, 202–6,
    411–13, 467
tinnitus 270, 700
WHO 717–18
see also age-related hearing loss;
    children; presbyacusis
age-related hearing loss (AHL or
    ARHL) 46–7, 65–7, 71–5, 299–305
age at onset 47
apportionment 67–70
databases 315, 322
definition of NIHL 166
diagnosis of NIHL 185, 215–16, 221
gender 48
genetics 71–5, 137
interaction with NIHL 50–3,
    64–80, 243, 302–3, 305, 413
interaction with noise exposure
    44–9, 50–2, 58
predictive factors 302
PTA 215–16
rate and pattern 45, 46–7, 50, 77–9
SNHL 184–5
susceptibility 137
see also presbyacusis
Agenda 21, 714
agriculture 183
air–bone gap 209, 234–5, 241, 419
airborne stimulation deafness 281
aircraft noise 524–6, 726
agencies 720–1, 726, 728–31, 736
children 165, 552–7
cognition 552–8
environment 345, 347, 350, 352,
    355
laws 606, 614
measurement 15, 18, 21, 24, 27, 40
medical environments 502
night–time 539–40
occupational HL 498

sleep 567, 572–5, 578–81, 583
stress 517–18, 520–1, 523, 524–6,
    529, 539–42
see also helicopters
air pollution 718, 728
environmental noise 346, 348,
    352–3, 357, 361
road traffic 528–9
stress 346, 352
surgery 505
air pressure 2, 4, 7, 11–12, 32–3
alarm phase 527
alcohol 76, 209, 242, 296, 414
sleep 571
stress 525
aliphatic solvents 479, 485
allergies 528–9, 530
allopurinol 138, 425
alternative dispute resolution 615–16
ambient noise 15–16, 25, 31, 117,
    718, 727
cognition 556–9, 561
health 355, 356, 358
measurement of hearing
    thresholds 150, 153–5, 160
see also background noise;
    environmental noise
ambulances 501–2, 503, 510
aminoglycoside antibiotics 184, 321,
    207, 210, 508
amplifiers and amplification 130,
    138, 150–1, 259
music 455, 470, 473
amplitude 4–5, 8, 10, 16, 112–14,
    116, 139
medical environment noise 499,
    503
military NIHL 439
music 466
amygdale 519, 526
analgesics 314, 322
anechoic areas 16, 37, 41
angina pectoris 292
angiotensins 133, 425
angle of sound incidence 381–2, 384,
    390, 392
animal experiments 188, 194–6
ageing 44–58, 68,71–6
babies' reaction to noise 502
biochemical mechanisms 118–20
blast effects 284, 285, 288

cochleae and hazardous noise
  94–5, 97, 98–100, 102
  conditioning 639–43
  databases 321, 322, 324–5
  impulse noise 393
  music 458, 468
  neural hyperactivity 113–14
  NIHL and AHL 302–5
  noise and health 291, 293–5, 298
  organic solvents 477–8, 485–6,
    488–9
  sleep 501
  susceptibility 128, 131, 133, 135,
    137–41, 203–8, 411–15
  tinnitus 269–71
  tonotopic reorganization 111
  vibration 321
annoyance 212, 294, 355
  cognition and noise 557, 559
  environmental noise 346–8,
    350–1, 354, 355, 356–8
  laws 613–14
  measurement of noise 15, 21,
    23, 39
  medical environment noise 498,
    500–1, 503
  night-time 23
  occupational noise 397–8
  rehabilitation 684, 699
  sleep 567, 570–2, 579, 584
  stress 516–17, 522–3, 530
  tinnitus 699, 701
  WHO 721, 722–4
anteroventral cochlear nucleus
  (AVCN) 54–6
antibiotics 289, 411
  aminoglycoside 184, 321, 207,
    210, 508
antinodes 8, 10
antioxidants 65, 76, 321
  occupational noise 424, 425
  susceptibility 133, 137–8, 141, 204
anxiety 183, 212, 222, 705
  medical environment noise 506–7,
    510
  rehabilitation 684, 698–701
  sleep 577, 584
  stress 520, 526
  tinnitus 176, 698–701
aperiodic sounds defined 6
apocrine gland 500

apoptosis 66, 94, 100–1, 137
aromatic solvents 479, 485
arrhythmia 292
arterial hypertension 292, 322
artificial test fixture (ATF) 444, 445
artillery 77
ascending reticular activating system
  (ARAS) 526
aspartate 98
asphyxiants 412
aspirin 207–8, 242, 411
assumed protection values (APVs)
  671–2
asthma 528–9, 530
asymptotic threshold shift (ATS)
  187, 403
atherogenic diet 293
atheromatous disease 205
atherosclerosis 133, 292
attention 551, 553–5
  children 551, 553–5, 557–8, 561
  cognition and noise 549–50, 551,
    553–5, 557–8, 561
  see also concentration
attenuation 25, 26, 51, 442–5, 660, 735
  blast 282
  cognition and noise 552, 559
  conditioning 640–1
  databases 325–6, 327
  hearing conservation programmes
    335–6
  hearing protectors 668–78
  helicopters 502
  impulse noise 386, 388
  music 470–1
  PTA 150–1, 153–4
  sleep 571, 576–9, 584
  susceptibility 131
  tinnitus 259
audiological rehabilitation programmes
  (ARPs) 681–3, 685, 692, 700–1
  group 692–8
  tinnitus 700–1
audiometers 316, 436, 598–600
audiometry 46, 65–7, 328–9, 331, 446
  baseline 166, 174, 240
  children 166, 169–73, 174, 176–7
  classification of NIHL 166–7
  hearing conservation programmes
    334, 336
  impulse noise 384, 394

laws 609, 610, 613
medical environment noise 509
military NIHL 441, 444, 446,
    447, 449
NIHL and ageing 65–7, 69–70,
    74, 78–9
noise exposure and ageing 45,
    46, 49
occupational noise 401, 403, 409
organic solvents 479
speech 235
standards 592
tinnitus 176–7
see also pure–tone audiometry
auditory brain–stem responses
    (ABRs) 102, 297
ageing 45, 48, 52
conditioning 644
music 468
occupational noise 412, 421–3
occupational noise and solvents
    478, 480, 482, 486, 488, 493
susceptibility 135, 412
auditory cortex (AC) 111, 112–13,
    263–5
CAS changes after damage 118, 121
music 466
organic solvents 491
tinnitus 260–1, 262–5, 271
auditory evoked potentials 416, 421,
    423
auditory masking 556–7
auditory nerve (VIIIth cranial)
    111–13, 132, 135–6, 151
conditioning 642–3
organic solvents 489, 493
susceptibility 127, 135–6
tinnitus 121–2, 260, 262, 265, 270
auditory pathway 259–63
auricles 282, 283
automotive component industry 199
autonomic nervous system 208, 570,
    577
sleep 568–71, 574, 576, 577, 579
stress 517, 536
tinnitus 698
awakenings 568, 571–3, 575–6,
    579–82
A–weighting 93, 324, 642
environmental noise 347, 350
hearing protectors 668, 673

impulse noise 384, 386–7, 388–9,
    391–4
measurement of noise 17–18,
    20–4, 27–9, 31–2, 36–7, 185
music 454
occupational noise 407
axodendritic synapses 642
axons 93

background noise 68, 211, 262,
    345–6, 357, 417
databases 314, 330
disability assessment 233, 244,
    246, 248–9, 254
impulsive 379
machinery 37–8
measurement 24, 37–8
medical environment 506, 508
military NIHL 436
rehabilitation 685, 686
sleep 578
see also ambient noise;
    environmental noise
baclofen 270
bandwidth 50, 388
barotraumas 219
basilar membrane 48–9, 86–91,
    94, 303
ageing 48–9, 51
blast 288
conditioning 641
music 466, 473
susceptibility 132
basolateral membranes 90
bass playing 456, 458, 461
bassoons 456, 461
bedrooms 356, 359, 360, 722–3
stress 525, 541
behavioural changes 46, 217, 447, 584
medical environment noise
    499–500, 508, 511
stress 518–19, 535, 544
Békésy audiometry 158–9, 170,
    328, 421
music 464, 467
Bell's palsy 131
benzene 479, 481
benzoic acid 485, 492
best frequency 111–12, 236, 422
bicuculline 118
biochemical mechanisms 118–20

birth 170, 184
  weight 184, 210, 398
*Black Book* 232, 248, 250, 251–2
blast 209, 279–90, 379, 389–94, 402,
  439–41
  diagnosis 192–3
  hearing protection devices 670
  laws 608
  military NIHL 439–41, 444–5
  PTA 216
  *see also* bombs; explosions
Blast Overpressure Project (BOP)
  389–92, 393–4
blood pressure 76, 205, 293–4, 298,
  314, 321–2
  children 165
  medical environment noise
    499–500, 509
  occupational noise 398
  smoking 298
  stress 536, 538
  susceptibility 133, 202, 205
  *see also* hypertension;
    hypotension
blood viscosity 292
*Blue Book* 249, 252
blues music 455, 472
body movements 570
  sleep 568–76, 579–80
boiler makers 609
bombs 192–3, 281, 286, 288
  *see also* blast; explosions
bone conduction 214, 234–5, 328, 507
  hearing protection devices 670–1
  measurement of hearing thresh-
    olds 151, 157, 159
  military NIHL 442, 451
  standards 591, 596
bone vibrators 151, 153
border cells 87
bowel damage from blast 281
brass playing 461, 468, 470–3
breweries 522, 658
broadband noise 6, 52–3, 135, 554
  conditioning 639–40
  diagnosis 187–8, 189
  music 453–4, 470
  occupational 404, 412
bronchitis 528–9, 530
buildings 32, 348, 351–2, 357, 362–3,
  366, 662–5

industrial noise 651, 654, 662–5
  WHO 720, 722
bulges 70, 215
B–weighting 17–18

calcineurin 100, 102
calcitonin–related peptide 643
calcium (Ca) 88, 90, 93, 96–8, 101–2
  magnesium 446
  music 466
  susceptibility 137, 141, 204
  tinnitus 269
calibration 30–1, 151–3, 218–19
  cognition and noise 562
  disability assessment 235, 252,
    239, 241
  headphones 26
  legal metrology 598–600
  measurement of hearing thresh-
    olds 150–3, 160
  measurement of noise 26–7,
    29–31, 33, 38
  medicolegal matters 419
  PTA 215, 218–19, 220
  standards 591–2
calmodulin 102
calpain 100, 102
cAMP 643
canal caps 425
carbogen 424
carbon disulphide 208, 412, 489, 492
carboxyhaemoglobin 134
cardiac disease 205, 208, 242
cardiovascular system 292–5, 296–7,
  302, 352
  medical environment noise 501
  occupational noise 397
  stress 538
  susceptibility 467
  WHO 722
caregiver behaviour 557–8, 561–2
caroverine 102, 269, 424
catecholamines 519, 521, 524–5,
  538, 539–41
cations 88–90
cats 265, 640
cello playing 456, 458, 461, 472
cellular redox status 98
central auditory system (CAS) 53–7,
  258–63
  ageing 44–5, 52, 53–8, 65–6, 76, 80

cochlear damage 110–22
  disability assessment 247
  feedback control 258–63
  hyperacusis 121–2
  noise and health 294
  occupational noise 419, 479
  organic solvents 479, 484–8,
    491, 493
  stress 526
  susceptibility 128–9, 135–6
  tinnitus 121–2, 263–73
central nervous system (CNS) 262, 320
  ageing 71, 244
  feedback control 259, 262, 263
  *n*-hexane 488
  stress 520–1, 523, 526, 536, 538
  styrene 486
  tinnitus 259, 262, 263, 271
  toluene 485
cerebrovascular disease 292, 294–5
cerumen (earwax) 130, 220,
    282, 285
characteristic frequency (CF) 115–18
chemicals 411, 412
chemotherapy 184, 207, 210, 411
children 165–75, 528–9, 551–6,
    708–9, 730
  cognitive performance 549–62
  diagnosis 202–3, 210, 212, 219–20
  environmental noise and health
    349, 354–7, 363–5
  incubator noise 502
  measurement of hearing thresh-
    olds 162
  middle–ear disease 243
  music 464, 707, 708–9
  prevalence of NIHL 172–3, 174
  rehabilitation 700–1
  road traffic 528–9, 530
  sleep 576
  stress 524, 525, 528–30, 540–2
  susceptibility 202–3
  tinnitus 175–7
  UN 714
  WHO 718, 723, 724
  *see also* neonates
chinchillas 50–2, 94, 99, 113–14, 194–5
  ageing 45–54, 75
  conditioning 639–42
  susceptibility 128, 131, 139, 412
  toughening 468

cholesteatoma 193
cholesterol 76, 206, 292, 293–4,
    321–2
cholinergic system 93, 100
chromosomes 58, 72–5, 184, 304
church 211
cinemas 211, 706–7
cisplatin 411
cisternae 90
clarinet playing 456, 458
classical music 168
  *see also* orchestras
Claudius' cells 87
click–evoked OAEs (CEOAEs) 447–8,
    464–5
clicks 6, 149, 217, 267, 421–2
CM amplitude 139
coal mining 399
cochleae 55, 85–103, 132–3, 138–40,
    259
  acoustic trauma 638–9
  anatomy 86–92
  blast effects 281, 283, 288
  CAS changes after damage 110–22
  causes of SNHL 184
  conditioning 637–8, 641–4
  databases 321
  diagnosis 184–6, 188, 192, 194–5
  disability assessment 244
  efferent control 138–40
  feedback control 259, 260–3
  genetics 71–2, 74, 219
  hyperacusis 121
  impedance 7
  innervation 92–3, 98–100, 102
  investigations 217
  laws 609, 611
  length 46
  measurement of hearing
    threshold 149, 151
  medical environment noise 499,
    507
  military NIHL 442, 447
  music 464–8, 470
  NIHL and ageing 66, 71–2, 74,
    75–6, 79–80
  NIHL and AHL 46–8, 303–4, 305
  noise exposure and ageing 45–57
  noise and health 296–7
  occupational noise 402, 410,
    411–12, 414–15, 419–20, 424

organic solvents 477, 484–6,
    488–9, 491
  repair and regeneration 100–3
  susceptibility 127, 129–33,
    136–42, 202–3, 205, 207,
    411–12, 414–15, 467
  tinnitus 121, 263, 265–71, 273, 700
cochlear blood flow (CBF) 101,
    132–3, 424, 638–9
  susceptibility 129, 132–3, 205, 411
cochlear implants 85
cochlear nerve 92–3, 98–100, 102, 151
cochlear nucleus (CN) 53–4, 58
  biochemical mechanisms 118
  dorsal 54–6, 116–17, 270
  neural hyperactivity 113
  susceptibility 127
  tinnitus 260–2, 270
  tonotopic reorganization 111
cochlear sensory epithelium 85–6
cocktail party effect 460, 467
cognitive performance 499, 549–62
Coles–Worgan method 252, 254
collagens 91
comfort index 672
common law 601–3, 605–6, 609
communication see speech and
    communication
Communication Strategies Scale
    (CSS) 691
compensation 162, 397, 402–3
  ageing 44, 64–5, 78
  diagnosis 182, 209, 212, 221, 222
  disability assessment 232, 250,
    253–4
  exaggeration 221
  laws 601, 605–6, 608, 609–10, 612
  medicolegal matters 419, 420–1,
    423
  military NIHL 439
  rehabilitation 683, 685
  WHO 717
compound action potential (CAP)
    112–13, 641, 642
compressors 94, 650, 654–5, 657
computed tomography (CT) 418, 420
concentration 160, 314, 511, 554, 557
  stress 516–17, 538
  surgery 505, 510
  tinnitus 177, 701
  WHO 724
  see also attention

concerts 453, 455, 463–4, 469, 472,
    705–8, 710–12
  agencies 722, 730
  rock–and–roll music 165, 171, 174
condensation of sound waves 7
conditioning 141–2, 143, 188, 195,
    637–46
  cochleae and hazardous noise
    100–1
  susceptibility 129, 414
conductive hearing loss 70, 193, 209,
    214, 328
  disability assessment 238
  impulse noise 393
  occupational noise 402, 414–15,
    419
  tinnitus 700
confounding factors 332–3, 339
construction industry 183, 346, 721
continuous noise 316, 346, 580
  cognition 554
  conditioning 639
  diagnosis 186–8, 194–5, 197–8,
    200, 209
  medical environment 498, 506
  military NIHL 435, 438, 440,
    446, 451
  music 462
  occupational 402–4, 407, 410, 417
  risk of NIHL 378–9, 382–4, 386, 393
  sleep 575, 580
  stress 517–18
contralateral superior olivary com-
    plex 93
Control of Noise at Work Act (2005)
    16–18, 18, 34, 36
Control of Noise at Work Regulations
    (2005) 14–15, 33–4, 36, 39–40
Control of Pollution Act (1974) 604
coping strategies 558, 571, 687–8
  active 687–8, 691, 693–4, 697
  avoiding 687–8, 691, 693, 694–5
  environmental noise and health
    349, 351–2, 355, 357, 364
  rehabilitation 681–4, 686–8,
    691–8, 701
  shifts 558, 560
  sleep 569, 571, 574
  stress 518–19, 523, 535
  tinnitus 698, 701
copper superoxide dismutase 98
coronary heart disease 205, 292, 349

corpus callosum (CC) 261
cortical electric response audiogram
    (CERA) 234, 235–6
cortical evoked potentials 421
cortical evoked response audiometry
    218, 221–2, 481, 484
cortico–releasing factor (CRF) 538
corticosteroids 424, 425
corticosterones 141, 519
corticotrophin (ACTH) 518–19,
    524, 539
cortisol 518, 520–8, 529–30, 538,
    539–44
    children 165
    sleep 570, 581
    tinnitus 272
country and western music 455
couplers 66, 152, 220, 591
creatinine 480, 482, 491–2
crossed olivocochlear bundle 93
customary law 601
cuticular plate 88–9, 97, 102
C–weighting 17–18, 29, 35–6, 529,
    668, 673
cyclohexane 481, 483
cyclosporine 102
cysteine 138
cytochrome *c* 101
cytocochleograms 119, 412
cytokines 501
cytoplasmic structures 127
cytoskeletal proteins 90, 97–8
cytosol 118–20, 137

daily noise exposure level 22–3, 28,
    34–5, 36
damage risk criteria (DRC) 405–10
damages *see* compensation
damping 10
databases 312–39, 347–8, 407–8
    hearing conservation programme
        332–9
    construction of program 317–31
deafness 47, 210, 314, 419
    blast effects 279, 281, 286, 288–90
    disability assessment 254
    magnesium 445
    susceptibility 204, 412
    WHO 717–19
decision trees 338–9
defeat reaction 518–20, 530

defence reaction 518–19
deflections of blast 280, 282, 284
Deiter's cells 87, 95
dendrites 93, 98, 424
    conditioning 642, 643, 645
    susceptibility 135, 136, 138
denial of hearing loss 683–5, 688, 692
depression 183, 272
    tinnitus 177, 272, 698–701
dextran 290
diabetes 184, 202, 206, 292, 295, 418
diagnosis 166–7, 182–223, 294
    children 165–7
    difficulties 218–22
    disability assessment 232–3,
        235–6, 238–9, 245, 252
    laws 610
    medical environment noise 503–4,
        510
    military NIHL 436, 447
    music and musicians 464
    NIHL and ageing 64, 65, 70
    occupational NIHL 415–23
    stress 529
    tinnitus 699
diastolic blood pressure 293–4, 398
diet 44, 73, 332, 293, 295–6
diffraction 11, 26
digital signal processing 25–6, 27
diplacusis 453, 460, 465, 473
direct noise level 651–2, 655, 662, 665
Directives 313–14, 603, 612, 728–30,
    741–3
    79/113/EEC 612
    81/1051/EEC 612
    86/188/EC 23, 39, 335–6, 602, 612,
        667, 678
    89/391/EC 14
    89/392/EC 607, 612
    89/656/EC 667
    89/686/EC 667, 671–2
    2000/14/EC 729
    2002/30/EC 730
    2002/49/EC 729, 347, 355, 364
    2003/10/EC 14, 23, 34–5, 39, 313,
        318–19, 335, 339, 667
    databases 313–14, 318–19, 335,
        339
    hearing protectors 667, 671–2, 679
    laws 602–3, 606–7, 612, 614
    standards 595, 597

directivity 7, 11
disability 247–8, 253, 255, 328
　ageing 44, 80
　assessment 232–55
　history 209, 212
　laws 609
　medicolegal matters 420, 423
　music 456
　otological normality 242–3
　rehabilitation 681, 683, 688–9,
　　692, 700
　susceptibility 134
　tinnitus 700
　UN 714
　WHO 716, 718
disc jockeys 460, 705, 707, 711
discotheques 165, 176, 325, 705–8,
　710–12
　agencies 720, 722, 730
　rehabilitation 700
display outputs 25, 27
distortion product input/output
　function 66
distortion product otoacoustic
　emissions (DPOAEs) 217–18,
　465–6
　ageing 45, 46, 51, 66, 75
　medicolegal matters 422–3
　military NIHL 447–8
　music 464, 465–6
　organic solvents 488
　susceptibility 135, 139, 412
distress 534–5
DNA damage 65, 73–5, 412
Dobie's median–based allocation
　method 245–6, 254
dockyards 477, 482–5, 493
dogs 346, 516, 605
door bells 211, 248
dopamine 269, 272, 642–3
Doppler flowmetry 133
dorsal cochlear nucleus (DCN) 54–6,
　116–17, 270
dorsal periolivary (DPO) nucleus
　644–5
dorsolateral periolivary (DLPO)
　nucleus 644–5
dose–effect relationship 407
dose–response curves 72, 134, 493,
　552, 559, 562, 724
　children 171, 177

environmental noise 347, 348,
　353–5, 361
　sleep 572–4, 580
dosimeters 25, 28–9, 168, 454
drop–forge workers 128
drugs and medication 101–2, 338
　acoustic trauma 638
　ageing 76, 80
　causes of SNHL 184
　conditioning 637
　databases 322, 332
　history 210
　medicolegal matters 416, 418
　ototoxicity 508, 510–11
　sleep 571
　susceptibility 138, 411–12, 467
duration of exposure 216, 380–1,
　393–4, 596
　ageing 45, 50, 53, 55–7, 64–5, 69,
　　76–9
　blast effects 280–2, 440
　children 166–8
　cognition 552–7, 560, 562
　databases 315–16, 323, 324–6, 337
　diagnosis 187, 188–201, 203–10,
　　213, 216, 222
　disability assessment 233, 236–8,
　　243, 245, 253
　environmental noise 32
　hearing conservation programmes
　　337
　hearing protection 678
　hearing thresholds 148, 149, 155
　history 209, 210, 213
　impulse noise 378–94
　industrial noise 34–5
　measurement of noise 15–16,
　　20–2, 28–9, 32, 34–5
　medical environment noise
　　499–500, 502–3, 506, 509–10
　medicolegal matters 415–17
　military NIHL 436, 438, 440, 441
　music 167, 454, 456, 458–9, 468
　NIHL and AHL 299, 301, 303, 305
　occupational noise 399, 401–7,
　　409, 410, 412, 415–17
　sleep 572, 576
　stress 517–18, 520–30, 540, 542
　susceptibility 128, 135–6, 139,
　　203–8, 410, 412
　tinnitus 270

D–weighting 17–18, 40
dynorphins 262, 272, 643
dysacusis 499

ear canal 9, 129–30, 220, 336
    ageing 49
    attention 445
    blast effects 282–5
    hearing protection 669, 678
    hearing thresholds 150, 155, 160
    length 130, 203
    music 470, 471
    susceptibility 129–30, 131, 203, 411
ear disease 300, 302, 318, 320, 328
    see also otitis media
eardrums 160, 242, 402, 414, 470
    disability assessment 238, 241, 243
earmuffs 336, 425, 442, 668–71,
    675, 678
    blast effects 288–9, 390
    military NIHL 442, 445
earphones 66, 150–3, 455–6, 723
    circum–aural 150, 152
    hearing thresholds 148, 150–7,
        159–60
    insert 150–2, 157, 159
    military NIHL 436, 447
    music 453, 455–6, 460, 473
    supra–aural 150–2, 154, 157, 159
    see also headphones
earplugs 442, 605, 668–71, 675–6, 678
    blast effects 288, 390
    hearing conservation programme
        336
    military NIHL 442, 444–5
    music 470–3, 708
    occupational noise 414, 425
    sleep 576, 578
    surgery 506, 510
ear protection 76, 470–1, 707
    medical environment noise 502,
        505, 509–10
    music 469–71, 706, 707
    stress 522, 524
    World Bank 727
    zones 16, 35
    see also earmuffs; earplugs; hear-
        ing protection devices (HPDs);
        protection of hearing
earwax 130, 220
echoing tinnitus 268

economics 359–60
    environmental noise 346–7, 358,
        359–60, 362–3
    military NIHL 439
    occupational noise 397, 398, 409
    see also socioeconomics
Economic and Social Council
    (ECOSOC) 713–14, 715
efferent system 92–3, 99–100,
    138–40, 261–2, 269–70, 294, 466
    ageing 50–1
    conditioning 637, 641–5
    feedback control 259–63
    feedback loop 93
    lateral reflex 637, 639, 641,
        642–5, 638–9
    medial 406, 637–9, 641–2, 645,
    music 466, 467
    stress 537
    susceptibility 129, 132, 136,
        138–43, 411–13, 467
    temperature 297
    tinnitus 259–63, 263, 266, 269–70,
        273
electric response audiometry (ERA)
    235
electrodermal reactions to stress 536
electroencephalograms (EEGs) 569,
    571, 573
electromyograms (EMGs) 569, 641
electro–oculograms (EOGs) 569
emotional factors of music 468
encephalitis 184
endocochlear potential 206
endocrine system 263, 518–21
    stress 518–21, 526–9, 536, 538–40,
        542–4
endolymph 88, 90, 288, 411
    see also fluid in ears
endoplasmic reticulum 90
endorphins 519
enkaphalin 643
environmental health impact assess-
    ment (EHIA) 354, 363, 366
environment 312, 338, 472–3, 578–9,
    686–7
    ageing 65, 74
    agencies 713–16, 726–7, 728, 731,
        736
    cognition 559
    database 322, 323

hearing protection devices 674–7, 679
laws 603, 614
legal metrology 598
music 467, 469, 472–3
refraction 12
rehabilitation 681–2, 684, 685, 686–7
sleep 567, 569–72, 577–9, 582, 584
standards 590
stress 535–6
Environmental Assessment (EA) 727
environmental noise 31–3, 41, 345–66, 522–4
ageing 65
agencies 716–18, 720–5, 728–30, 732–3, 735, 736
assessment of impact 354–60
blast effects 282, 283
children 165, 173
conceptual approaches 346–54
databases 312, 314–15, 321, 329, 332
health 291, 293
hearing thresholds 148, 151, 153–5, 160–1
history 211
industrial 33
integrated management 360–6
laws 603, 606, 607, 614
measurement 13–17, 20, 25, 27–8, 30–3, 38, 41
medical 498
occupational 404–5, 410, 420
rehabilitation 695, 700
stress 518, 522–4, 526, 529
susceptibility 130, 136, 140
tinnitus 258, 268, 700
Environmental Protection Act (1990) 16, 604
enzymes 98, 118, 425, 643
susceptibility 137–8, 204
equal energy principle 68, 194–6
databases 316, 324
diagnosis 194–6, 197, 198–9, 200
impulse noise 378–9, 382–3, 391–2
occupational noise 402, 406
equipment 25–9, 40, 149–63, 589–90
calibration 151–3
checks 153
disability assessment 235

laws 600–16
legal metrology 598–600
measurement of noise 15, 25–9, 31–3, 37–8, 40–1
PTA 149–63, 214
reliability 160–2
standards 590–8
equivalent continuous sound pressure level 20–2
EqTTS–weighting 388–9, 391–3
ethanol 480
ethics of human experiments 44, 187
ethyl acetate 480
ethyl benzene 477, 481, 483, 485, 492
eumelanin 142
European Treaty 602–3
eustress 534–5
evoked potentials 76, 479
recorded from the inferior colliculus (IC–EVPs) 45–6, 51, 54, 75
evoked response audiometry 112–14, 218, 221–2
CAS changes after damage 112–14, 118–19, 121–2
hyperactivity 112–14
medicolegal matters 420–1
exaggeration 218, 221–2, 234, 416, 419–22
exchange rates 459
executive strategies 550
excitation 52–3, 76, 259, 261–3, 265–71
CAS changes after damage 115–17
excitotoxicity 96, 99, 268–9, 424
conditioning 639, 643, 645
susceptibility 135, 136
tinnitus 262, 268–9, 272–3
exercise 296–7, 712
exposure to noise 296–9, 707–8, 712
military NIHL 435
tinnitus 699
exhaustion 527, 535
expert witnesses 611, 613, 615
explicit memory 550–1, 553
explosions 280, 282, 379–80, 384–9, 402, 499, 608
databases 320, 326–7
hearing protection devices 670, 678
large calibre weapons 379, 384–9
susceptibility 414
see also blast; bombs

external (outer) ear 48, 131, 150–1
   difficulties 220–1
   examination 214
   hearing protection devices 670
   susceptibility 411, 414–15
   *see also* ear canal
eye colour 142, 206, 314, 413

facial nerve 131
F–actin 97
factories 318, 498
   hearing conservation programmes
      336–7
   industrial noise 652–3, 655, 660,
      663, 665
fall time 27, 149, 379, 381, 499
fan noise 650, 655, 658, 659
fatty acids 519
feedback control 259–63, 534
   tinnitus 258, 259–63, 270
fences 201, 250, 419
   disability assessment 249–50, 253–4
fight–flight reaction 518–20
fimbrin 89
fire engines 502
firearms *see* guns and gunfire
fire crackers 379, 706
fireworks 723, 730
fixation 131
fluid in ears 7, 87–8, 96
   endolymph 88, 90, 288, 411
   susceptibility 131, 132
flute playing 458
forestry workers 324, 674–5
forges 77, 324
free–field 3, 32–3, 41, 651, 723
   BOP 390
   hearing protection devices 675, 678
   impulse noise 380–1, 386–9, 390
   measurement of noise 15, 26,
      30–3, 37, 41
   microphones 26, 30–1
free oxygen radicals 65, 73–4, 76,
   137–8, 413, 424–5
   outer hair cells 94, 100, 102
   scavengers 98
frequency 2–6, 8–11, 219–20,
   248–50, 293
   ageing 46–51, 54, 66, 69–70, 74,
      76–8
   blast effects 281, 286, 439–40

CAS changes after damage
   111–14, 115–17, 119–21
children 166–7, 169–75
cochleae and hazardous noise 85,
   90, 93–5
conditioning 641, 642, 644
databases 313–14, 322–3, 325–6,
   328, 330, 332
diagnosis 185–92, 198–9, 201,
   209, 215–20, 222
   difficulties 218, 219–20, 222
disability assessment 232–42, 244,
   247–54
environmental noise 350
feedback control 261–2
hearing conservation programmes
   334, 336
hearing thresholds 148–51, 153–8,
   161–2
hearing protection devices 442–5,
   668, 669, 672–3
impulse noise 381, 384, 386–9, 393
industrial noise 658
investigations 215–16, 217, 218
laws 609, 668
measurement of noise 15–18, 26,
   30–1, 185–6
medical environment noise 499,
   500, 503
medicolegal matters 416–19, 421–2
military NIHL 435–7, 439–40,
   442–5, 446–9
music 453–8, 460–1, 463–7, 470–3
neural hyperactivity 113–14
NIHL and AHL 299–300, 303–5
occupational noise 404, 406–9,
   416–19, 421–2
organic solvents 483–4, 487–8, 491
presbyacusis 238–41, 407
PTA 215–16, 218
sleep 572, 581
stress 518, 528
susceptibility 127, 130–2, 134,
   136, 139, 202–3, 205, 207
tinnitus 261–2, 267, 271
tonotopic reorganization 111–12
WHO 721
   *see also* high frequencies; low
      frequencies
frequency–weighting 27, 384, 387–9,
   393–4

impulse noise 384, 386–9, 391–4
measurement of noise 17–18, 20, 25, 27, 31, 36–8, 40
Friedlander waves 380–1, 387–9, 393
functional magnetic resonance imaging (fMRI) 263, 271
fundamental frequency 5, 248–9
fuzzy logic 318, 338

GABA (γ–aminobutyric acid) 118, 269–70, 642
  feedback control 259
  mediated inhibition 118, 120, 121
gadolinium 321
ganglion cells 305, 560
ganglion neurons 110
gear noise 650, 658
gender 48, 202, 576–7
  ageing 46, 48, 49, 64–5, 66, 74, 76–8
  AHL 46, 48, 299–303
  children 169–73, 174–6
  cognition and noise 552
  databases 313–16, 321–2
  diagnosis 183, 189, 202
  disability assessment 236–7, 238, 240–2, 244
  health 293–4, 296, 299–303
  hearing conservation programmes 337
  music 460, 461, 463, 467
  occupational noise 407–8, 411–13
  organic solvents 487
  presbyacusis 240–1, 244, 407
  rehabilitation 682, 683
  sleep 576–7
  stress 525, 541
  susceptibility 202, 411–13, 467
  tinnitus 175–7
general practitioners 609
genes and genetics 71–5, 136–7, 172–3, 204, 304
  acoustic trauma 638
  ageing 44, 47, 50, 58, 65, 71–5, 79–80
  AHL 302–5
  causes of SNHL 184
  children 168–70, 172–8
  cochleae and hazardous noise 97–8, 100–3
  conditioning 637, 639–40
  databases 314, 317–18, 320–1, 339

diagnosis 202, 204, 210, 219
  expert systems 338–9
  health 293, 295
  hearing conservation programmes 312, 333
  medicolegal matters 416, 418, 420
  stress 519
  susceptibility 129, 136–7, 141, 411–12, 467
  tinnitus 269, 273
gerbils 135, 303, 639–41
  ageing 45–7, 50, 52–3, 68
glia–derived neurotrophic factors (GDNFs) 137
glucocorticoids 101, 141, 272
  stress 521, 538, 539
glutamate 93, 268–9, 424–5, 643
  acoustic trauma 639
  cochleae and hazardous noise 93, 96, 98, 100, 102
  feedback control 259, 262
  susceptibility 135, 136
  tinnitus 102, 259, 262, 268–70, 272–3
glutamic acid decarboxylase (GAD) 118–20
glutathione monoethyl ester 133, 138
glycine 270
glycogenolysis 519
glycoproteins 91
gonadotrophins 519
Guide to the Expression of Uncertainty in Measurement (GUM) 589–90
guinea pigs 194, 468, 507
  cochleae and hazardous noise 95, 97–8, 102
  conditioning 639–41, 643
  susceptibility 133, 135, 139, 141, 412, 414
guitar playing 710
guns and gunfire 190, 209, 216, 404, 677–8, 706
  blast effects 279, 281
  children 171
  databases 322, 325, 326–7
  hearing protection devices 678
  hunting 77, 325
  impulse noise 379, 380, 383, 389
  large calibre weapons 384–9
  laws 605, 608

military NIHL 437, 440, 445, 449–51
WHO 722, 723

habenula perforate (HA) 92
habituation 575–6, 579, 698
  sleep 570, 575–6, 579, 581–3
  stress 527, 544
hair cells 94–8, 321, 518
  ageing 46–7, 50–2, 66–7, 72, 75,
    79–80
  blast effects 288
  CAS changes after damage 110,
    111, 119
  conditioning 637, 641
  diagnosis 184, 188, 204
  hearing thresholds 149
  medicolegal matters 415–16
  organic solvents 477, 489
  response to hazardous noise
    85–98, 100–3
  susceptibility 134–9, 141–2, 204,
    411
  see also inner hair cells (IHCs);
    outer hair cells (OHCs)
hammering 324, 650, 654, 721
hand–arm vibration syndrome
  (HAVS) 202, 208
handedness 449–50, 451
handicaps 209, 212, 414
  databases 312–13, 320, 328, 330–1
  disability assessment 247, 254, 255
  medicolegal matters 416, 420, 423
  rehabilitation 683, 688–9, 692,
    698, 700
  tinnitus 698, 700
  WHO 720, 724
harmonics 3, 5, 461, 470–1
harp playing 456, 461
headphones 455–6, 511
  calibration 26
  music 453, 455–6, 460, 708
  PTA 215, 220
  surgery 506, 510
  WHO 723
see also earphones
head shadow 216, 457
head trauma 210, 219, 220, 242, 320
  causes of SNHL 184
  children 170
  medicolegal matters 416, 418
  tinnitus 266

health 291–305, 349–50, 364–6, 584
  ageing 44
  agencies 713–16, 718, 720, 722–4,
    725–7, 730, 732
  databases 313–14
  disability assessment 242
  environmental noise 346, 348,
    349–66
  hearing protection devices 671
  laws 605
  measurement of noise 13
  medical environment noise 498–511
  medicolegal matters 417–18, 423
  music 467, 705–12
  occupational noise 397–8, 402,
    417–18, 423
  rehabilitation 682, 684, 691, 699
  sleep 568–70, 572, 578–80, 583, 584
  stress 526–7, 529, 534–5, 538, 541
  susceptibility 467
  tinnitus 699
Health and Safety Executive (HSE)
  34, 128, 200–1
  diagnosis 196, 198, 200–1
Health and Safety at Work Act (1974)
  608
hearing aids 10, 155, 234, 248, 254
  rehabilitation 425, 681, 693, 694,
    696
hearing conservation programmes
  (HCPs) 312, 314, 317–18, 332–9,
  493–4
  early detection of problems 337–8
  expert systems 338–9
  hearing protection devices 678
  impulse noise 384, 394
  measurement of noise 35
  medical environment noise 502,
    503, 509
  military NIHL 441
  motivation of workers to use 336–7
  music 454
  occupational noise 401, 405, 425–6
  organic solvents 478, 493–4
Hearing Disability and Handicap
  Scale (HDHS) 690–1
Hearing Handicap Inventory for the
  Elderly 689
Hearing Handicap Scale 689
Hearing Handicap and Support Scale
  (HHSS) 690–1

Hearing Measurement Scale 689
hearing protection devices (HPDs)
    325–6, 336–7, 393, 442–5, 667–79
    children 167
    conservation programmes 333–7
    databases 314, 317, 325–6, 330–1
    impulse noise 386–7, 390, 392,
        393, 394
    industrial noise 660, 661
    laws 608
    measurement of noise 14, 28,
        39–40
    military NIHL 435–8, 441, 442–5,
        446, 451
    occupational noise 167, 425–6
    personal protective equipment
        (PPE) 667, 671, 672
    rehabilitation 693, 696–7
    see also earmuffs; earplugs; ear
        protection; protection of
        hearing
hearing thresholds 3–4, 148–63, 185,
    246, 248–50, 295
    ageing 45, 48, 51, 64, 66–72, 74,
        76–80
    blast effects 286
    CAS changes after damage
        113–14, 116–19
    children 166–7, 169–73, 174
    cognition and noise 560
    databases 313, 318, 327, 328–9, 332
    diagnosis 185, 189, 192–3
    disability assessment 232–54
    laws 610–11
    medical environment noise 505, 507
    medicolegal matters 416, 419–23
    military NIHL 436, 444, 447, 449–50
    music 456–7, 460–1, 462–3, 464–6
    NIHL and AHL 299–301
    occupational noise 403, 406–8,
        412–13, 416, 419–23
    organic solvents 479, 481–2, 484,
        487–8, 491, 493–4
    presbyacusis 238–42, 243, 251
    protection devices 678
    sleep 572–3, 577
    standards 591, 596–7
    stress 517–18
    susceptibility 127–31, 134–6,
        139–40, 142, 412–13
    WHO 717–18

see also permanent threshold
    shifts (PTSs); temporary thresh-
    old shifts (TTSs)
heart rate 499, 500, 508–9
    sleep 569, 570
    stress 536, 538
heat shock 638
heat shock proteins (hsps) 97–8,
    137, 298, 638
heat stress 97–8, 101, 298, 640
heavy metals 412
height 321
helicopters 326, 501, 502, 510, 729
helicotrenia 86, 88
helmets 437, 442, 669–72
Hensen's cells 87, 92, 288, 415
hertz defined 2
high frequencies 31, 152, 293, 325,
    685
    ageing 46–8, 66, 70–1, 74, 77–8
    airborne stimulation deafness
        281, 286
    CAS changes after damage 111,
        114, 116, 119, 121, 122
    children 169–75, 177
    cochleae and hazardous noise 86,
        93, 94–5
    diagnosis 185–7, 192, 203, 205,
        207, 215–16
    disability assessment 234–5, 244,
        249, 252
    hearing protection devices 442,
        445, 669–70, 672–3, 676
    impulse noise 386, 387–8, 391, 393–4
    industrial noise 655, 659
    medicolegal matters 416–17, 419
    military NIHL 436–7, 442, 445,
        447–8
    music 460, 462, 470–3
    NIHL and AHL 299–300, 305
    occupational noise 398, 404, 407,
        412–13, 416–17, 419
    organic solvents 480, 484, 487,
        491, 493–4
    PTA 215–16
    rehabilitation 683, 685
    SNHL 165, 167
    susceptibility 131–2, 134, 203,
        205, 207, 412–13
    tinnitus 271
    WHO 717, 721

high–performance liquid chromatography (HPLC) 543–4
hippuric acid 485, 491, 492
history 209–13, 320–5
    ageing 65, 79
    databases 314, 317–35, 331, 333
    diagnosis 185, 197, 204, 209–13, 219–22
    disability assessment 232, 238, 242, 246, 253
    environmental noise 349
    medicolegal matters 416, 418
    music 463
    tinnitus 265
    WHO 717
HL check method 673
HML method 673
hormone replacement therapy 48
hormones 48, 349, 397–8, 570
    stress 517–20, 522–7, 529–30, 536, 538–44, 569–71, 574
horn playing 456, 458, 472
hospitals 503–9, 723
    medical environment noise 498, 501–2, 503–9, 510–11
humidity 32–3
humming 470
hydroxydopamine 643, 644
hydroxyl radicals 137
hyperacusis 121–2, 266, 446, 684
    music 453, 460, 473
hyperbaric oxygen 424–5
hypercholesterolaemia 292
hyperlipidaemia 184, 292
hyperlipoproteinaemia 292–3
hypertension 293–4, 322, 332, 501
    environmental noise 349, 360
    health 291, 292–6
    occupational noise 397–8, 418
    see also blood pressure
hyperthermia 297
hypoacusis 402, 420
hypophyseal (pituitary) gland 534, 538–9
hypothalamus 263, 519, 526, 534
hypothermia 297
hypoxia 101, 184, 210
    susceptibility 132, 138, 141

imaging units 503, 504–5, 510
immune system 397–8, 527–8, 529, 536, 538

impact noise 35, 194, 379, 380
    industrial 650, 655, 658
impedance 7, 9, 131, 217, 423
implicit memory 550–1, 553
impulse (impulsive) noise 49, 68, 94, 96, 378–94
    BOP 389–92, 393–4
    conditioning 640
    databases 324, 327, 339
    diagnosis 188, 190, 192, 194–7, 199, 209
    environmental 31, 347
    exposure 390, 392, 393
    hearing conservation programmes 335
    hearing protection devices 668–9, 677–8
    laws 668
    measurement 15–16, 23, 25, 27, 29, 31
    medical environment 499
    military NIHL 435, 437–9, 445–6, 451
    music 167, 459, 462
    NIHL and AHL 302
    occupational 194–6, 199, 209, 402, 404, 410, 423
    stress 516–17, 518
    susceptibility 128, 141
    WHO 723
    see also blast; gunfire
impulse rate 379, 383
incidental memory 558
incubators 502, 508–9, 511
incus 50, 286
industrial chemicals 202, 208, 209, 412
industrial noise 33–6, 346, 397–9, 401, 425, 650–65
    agencies 720–1, 723, 727, 736
    control 650–65
    databases 315–16, 318, 329
    diagnosis 187, 189
    disability assessment 233, 238, 240, 251
    hearing conservation programmes 333
    hearing protection devices 469, 669, 672
    laws 603, 606, 608
    measurement 14, 27, 33–6, 40
    medicolegal matters 417, 419

music 453, 454, 460, 468
organic solvents 478
propagation paths 650–1, 653
sleep 567
sources 650, 659
susceptibility 128, 467
see also machinery
infections 210, 320, 501, 561
    blast effects 289
    causes of SNHL 184
    conditioning 637
    hearing conservation programmes
        336
inference engine 317
inferior colliculus (IC) 112–14,
        115–17, 118–20
    evoked potentials 45–6, 51, 54, 75
    feedback control 260–3
    tinnitus 260–3, 270–1
inhibition 52, 66, 76, 115–17
    lateral 114, 115–17, 118
    tinnitus 259, 261–3, 266–71
inner ear 87, 100–3, 286–8, 289–90, 295
    acoustic trauma 638
    ageing 50
    blast effects 286–8, 289–90
    CAS changes after damage 122
    causes of SNHL 184
    conditioning 639
    databases 320, 326
    diagnosis 216, 220–1
    disability assessment 233, 243–5,
        247
    hearing protection devices 670
    hearing thresholds 151
    military NIHL 441–2, 442, 446, 451
    NIHL and AHL 304–5
    occupational noise 167, 402, 411,
        413–16, 419, 424
    rehabilitation 684
    stress 517–18
    susceptibility 129, 137, 141, 411,
        413–15
    transmission of sound 129–30
    see also cochleae
inner hair cells (IHCs) 87–95, 97–9
    acoustic trauma 638–9
    ageing 47, 50–1, 67, 75
    blast effects 288
    CAS changes after damage 111, 119
    conditioning 642–5, 638–9
    diagnosis 188

feedback control 259–61
medical environment noise 507
medicolegal matters 416
music 466
NIHL and AHL 304–5
stress 518
susceptibility 127–8, 132, 135–8, 412
therapy 424
tinnitus 259–61, 269, 272
tonotopic reorganization 111
inner phalangeal cells 87
inner pillar cells (IPCs) 87
inner spiral bundle 643
insertion loss (IL) 442–3
instrumentation 15, 25–9
    see also equipment
insulation 24
insurance 162, 232, 610
    rehabilitation 683, 685, 696
intensity see sound intensity
intensive care units 501, 503, 507–9,
        510–22
interdental cells 91
interface 317–19
intermittent (interrupted) noise 346,
        404, 580–1
    conditioning 639
    diagnosis 188, 194–5, 197, 209
    medical environment 498
    music 458–9, 473
    risk of NIHL 378–9, 393
    stress 516, 523, 530
internal auditory meatus 420
International Civil Aviation
        Organization 715, 726, 728
International Commission on
        Biological Effects of Noise 733–4
International Electrotechnical
        Commission 735–6, 747–9
    standards 635–6, 747–9
International Institute of Noise
        Control Engineering 732–3
International Labour Organization
        713–15, 725–6, 736
International Organization for
        Standardization 715, 734–5, 736,
        743–7
    standards 626–35, 636, 680, 743–7
    see also ISO 1999
inverse square law 651
ipsilateral DCN 116
ipsilateral superior olivary complex 93

iron 138
iron and steel industry 134, 399
irrelevant speech effect (ISE) 560
irritation and irritability 212, 557, 685
    medical environment noise 505,
        509, 511
    tinnitus 177
ischaemia 94, 101, 292, 398, 638
    susceptibility 132–3, 205, 411
ISO 1999 198–9, 611
    ageing 65, 67–9, 71, 76–9
    databases 313, 316–17, 318, 331–2
    diagnosis 196, 197–9, 200
    hearing conservation programmes
        337
    impulse noise 378–9
    music 454, 458
    NIHL and AHL 302, 305
    occupational noise 405, 407–8
isobaric oxygen 424
isoprostane 133

jazz 168, 455, 460, 463, 472
jute weavers 78, 167, 189, 197

K complex 571
kanamycin 411
keratin 285
kinase 643
kynurenate 98, 135, 424

labyrinthitis 184, 219
lacquers 477, 481, 483–6
land–use planning 362, 720, 726, 731
    environmental noise 351–2,
        361–4, 366
lateral efferent reflex system 642–5
    acoustic trauma 638–9
    conditioning 637, 639, 641, 642–5
lateral lemniscus (LL) 260, 261, 262
lateral nucleus of trapezoid body
    (LNTB) 644–5
lateral olivocochlear (LOC) system
    93, 642, 644
    feedback control 259, 261, 262
    susceptibility 136, 138, 140
    tinnitus 269, 272
lateral superior olivary (LSO) 138,
    260, 644–5
laterality 447, 449–50
    music 457, 461, 462–4

    see also symmetry
law of delict 600–1
law of torts 601, 609
laws and regulations 600–16, 667–8,
    741–9
    agencies 715, 719–26, 728–30,
        731, 733
    environmental noise 346, 360
    hearing protection devices 667–8
    measurement of noise 13–16,
        33–6, 39–40
    measurements and standards
        588–616
    music 168, 454, 458, 471, 707,
        709–10
    occupational noise 193, 401–3,
        405, 425–6
    rehabilitation 682, 684
    see also Directives
lazaroids 138
learned helplessness 555–6
learning disabilities 554, 560
legal metrology 589, 598–600
leisure noise 165, 209–10, 211, 325,
    410, 418, 721–2
    children 170–1, 174, 177
    databases 317, 322, 325, 339
    environmental 346
    hearing conservation programmes
        335
    hearing protection devices 679
    laws 603
    measurement 14, 36, 39
    music 453, 706, 708
    NIHL and AHL 301–2
    WHO 720, 721–2, 723
leucoderms 467
leupeptin 102
lifestyle 292, 296–9, 330
    environmental noise 348, 352, 365
    rehabilitation 682, 684
limbic system 263, 264, 698
    stress 520, 526, 534, 537
lip reading 234, 247, 681
lipids 206, 292, 293–4, 424, 538
    databases 314, 322
    susceptibility 202, 206
local field potential 112–13
localization of sound 19, 26, 130,
    330, 518, 689
    military NIHL 435–6, 442

longitudinal waves 6–7
loop diuretics 207–8, 210
loss of amenity 609–10
loudness 3–4, 294
  cognition 553, 559
  databases 325, 329
  diagnosis 185–6, 189, 192, 204–5
  disability assessment 232
  environmental noise 350
  measurement of noise 18, 185–6
  medical environment noise 498,
    506–7, 509
  music 455, 465, 470, 707–8
  susceptibility 204, 205
  tinnitus 701
  *see also* sound level; sound pres-
    sure level
loudspeakers 6, 7, 711–12
low density lipoprotein (LDL) 206
low frequencies 86, 93, 94–5, 189,
  325, 393–4, 609
  ageing 46, 47, 66, 74
  blast effect 286
  CAS changes after damage 111,
    115–17, 121
  cognition 551
  disability assessment 234, 239,
    249, 252
  environmental noise 348, 365
  hearing conservation programmes
    336
  hearing protection devices
    669–70, 672–3, 676, 678
  impulse noise 386–7, 393–4
  industrial noise 654
  military NIHL 446–7
  music 455, 458, 471
  occupational noise 404, 411, 416–17
  PTA 216
  stress 521, 522, 525, 538
  susceptibility 130, 131, 132–4, 411
  tinnitus 271
  tonotopic reorganization 111
  WHO 717, 721
lung damage from blast 281
lysosomes 415

machinery 36–8, 209, 347, 397, 399,
  650–61
  agencies 720–1, 729–30, 736
  databases 323

  enclosure 654, 659–61
  hearing protection devices 678
  jute weavers 189
  laws 605, 606–7, 608, 612
  measurement of noise 13–17, 19,
    30, 33–9, 41–3
  rehabilitation 697
  standards 592, 595
  *see also* industrial noise
Machinery Noise Test Codes 16
magnesium 141, 445–6, 451
  susceptibility 129, 133, 141, 143,
    411, 413
magnetic fields 32–3, 271
Magnetic Resonance Imaging (MRI)
  33, 321, 504–5, 510
  medicolegal matters 418, 420
malaria 210
malingering 162, 221
  medicolegal matters 418–19, 420–3
malleus 50, 131
Management of Health and Safety at
  Work Regulations (1999) 609
mandelic acid 486, 492
mannitol 138
masking 66, 157, 159
  hearing thresholds 150–1, 152–3,
    157, 159, 160
  tinnitus 701
mastoid cavity 193
mastoid process 151
mathematics 552
meaning and comprehension 550–1, 552
measurement of noise 589–90, 616,
  688–92
  cognition 559–60
  conditioning 641
  diagnosis 185–6, 197, 209
  hearing protection devices 671
  hearing thresholds 148–63
  laws 606, 608, 610, 613
  legal metrology 598–600
  music 453, 706, 709
  rehabilitation 696
  standards 590–8, 626–36
mechanotransduction 88–90, 97
medial efferent system 466, 638–9,
  641–2
  conditioning 637, 639, 641–2, 645
medial geniculate body (MGB)
  260–1, 262, 270

medial olivocochlear (MOC) system
93, 639, 641
  feedback control 259, 261, 262
  susceptibility 138–40
  temperature 297
medial superior olivary complex
(SOC) 138, 273, 260
medication *see* drugs and medication
medicolegal matters 402,
415–23, 613
  ageing 44, 68, 70, 80
  diagnosis 184, 197, 209
  disability assessment 232–3, 238,
242, 253–4
  hearing thresholds 162
  laws 612, 613, 615
melanin 76, 142
  susceptibility 129, 142, 143, 206,
413
melanocytes 142, 206, 320
melanoderms 467
membrane lipid peroxidation 137
memory 261, 549–53
  cognition 549–56, 558, 560–2
  children 165, 552–6, 561–2
  environmental noise 349
  stress 517, 536
Ménière's disease 140, 184, 416,
418–19
meningitis 184, 210
menstruation 48
metabolites 73–4, 94
metals 138, 207, 293, 399, 499,
481, 482
  impact noise 380, 382, 383
metanephrine 521
methyl ethyl ketone (MEK) 483
methylhippuric acid 485, 492
mice 100, 302, 303–4
  ageing 45–50, 52–8, 71–5
  conditioning 639–40
  genetics 71–5
  susceptibility 137–8, 141,
204, 206
microcirculation 129, 132–3, 411,
415, 446
microphones 26, 31–2, 152
  hearing protection devices 444,
670, 678
  inside real ear (MIRE) 445
  measurement of noise 19, 25–6,
28–34, 38

music 454, 471
  positioning 28–9, 31–2, 34, 38
middle ear 131–2, 209, 220–1, 283–5,
289, 640–1
  ageing 48–9, 66
  blast effects 193, 281, 283–5, 289
  causes of SNHL 184
  conditioning 637, 639, 640–1, 645
  databases 328
  disability assessment 233, 241, 243
  examination 214
  hearing thresholds 151
  impedance 7, 217
  music 470
  occupational noise 404, 411,
414–15, 419, 422
  stress 517
  susceptibility 130, 131–2, 202,
209, 414–15
  *see also* ossicular chain
military 326–7, 402, 418, 435–51, 608
  blast effects 279
  children 169
  databases 318, 326–7
  diagnosis 183, 203, 209, 220
  disability assessment 242
  hearing protection devices 677–8
  low altitude flights 518, 520–1, 523–4
  magnesium 141
  music 461, 464
  susceptibility 203, 412
mines and mining 77, 183
mitochondria 65, 90, 101, 184, 321
  genetics 73–5
  occupational noise 415, 424
mitochrondrial DNA 412
mixed hearing impairment 70, 402,
419
mobile phones 346
mobile sound–attenuated room 436
modiolus 86–7, 89, 92–3
monoamine neurotransmitters 272–3
motivation 336–7, 668, 678, 710
  children 555–6, 561
music 167–8, 209, 302, 453–73,
705–12
  children 171, 176
  conditioning 639–40
  databases 315, 325, 331
  exercise 297
  feedback control 261
  measurement of noise 36

surgery 505, 506, 510
WHO 717, 720, 721, 723
musicians 167–8, 171, 454–5, 461–2,
    710
    damage prevention 707–8, 710, 711
    orchestras 453–62, 468, 472–3
multifrequency acoustic calibrators
    30–1
multiple sclerosis 294
myocardial infarction 292

narrowband noise 151, 152, 159, 404
National Physical Laboratory tables
    236–8
    disability assessment 236–8, 245,
        252
    otological normality 242–3
    presbyacusis 239–42, 252
negative pressure phase 279–80, 285,
    439
negligence 609
neighbours and neighbourhoods
    721, 730
    environmental noise 346, 348,
        352–3, 359, 361–3, 365
    WHO 720, 721, 722
    see also residential noise
neonates 202, 210, 508–9
    medical environment noise 502,
        508–9, 511
    jaundice 184, 210
neoplasia 184
nerve fibres 50, 55, 66–7
neural hyperactivity 110, 112–14
neuritis 184
neuroendocrine system 352, 518–21,
    527, 538
neuroimmune system 527–8, 529
neurons 85, 92–3, 94, 526
    ageing 53–5, 57–8
    CAS changes after damage 110,
        111, 115–17, 118, 122
    conditioning 642–5
    susceptibility 138, 140
    tinnitus 262, 264–5, 270–1
neuropil volume 54, 55
neurotransmitters 71, 93, 96, 98,
    102, 424
    CAS changes after damage 118, 121
    conditioning 642
    feedback control 259
    stress 536

susceptibility 135
    tinnitus 268–70, 272–3
neurotrophic factors 100, 102, 137,
    321, 639
neurotrophins 102
n–hexane 477–8, 488, 490, 492–3
nicotinic acetylcholine 100, 139
nicotinic cholinergic receptor 139,
    269–70
night–time 539–40, 559, 583
    agencies 722–3, 727, 729, 732
    environmental noise 345–6, 352,
        360
    laws 605, 606, 613
    measurement of noise 23–4
    sleep 567, 569–71, 577–8, 582, 583
    stress 524–5, 528–9, 535, 539–40,
        542
NMDA (N–methyl–D–aspartate) 102,
    262, 269, 273
nodes 8
Noise Abatement Act (1960) 604
Noise Act (1966) 602, 604, 613
noise cancellation systems 668–70
Noise Control Act (1972) 607
noise depreciation index (NDI) 359
noise dose 314, 324
    disability assessment 236, 253–4
noise dosimetry 425
noise emissions 36–8, 39, 41–2
noise exposure and health 293–5
noise immisions 70, 194, 236, 734
noise–induced hearing loss (NIHL)
    48–9, 65–7, 71–5, 315–17
    ageing 44–5, 48–53, 57–8, 64–80,
        332, 413
    AHL 64–80, 299–305
    apportionment 67–70
    audiometric classification 166–7
    blast effects 279, 281, 288–90
    cardiovascular disease 292–5
    CAS changes after damage 110–22
    children 165–78
    conditioning 637, 639, 642, 645
    databases 312–32, 337–9
    definitions 174
    diagnosis 182–223, 415–23
    disability assessment 232–55
    early detection 337–8
    expert systems 338–9
    estimation 331
    genetics 71–5

health 291, 292–9
hearing conservation programmes
    333–5
hearing protection devices 668, 677
hearing scales 689–91
hearing thresholds measurement
    149, 161, 163
ICBEN 733
ILO 726
laws 607–12
mechanisms 186–93
medical environment 498–9, 509–11
medicolegal matters 415–23
military 435–51
music 167–8, 454, 460, 464,
    466–8, 472–3, 705, 709–11
occupational noise 167, 397–426
organic solvents 491
otological normality 242–3
presbyacusis 238–42, 243–4, 251
prevalence 182–3, 312
prevention 424–6
progression with age 77–9
rehabilitation 423–6, 681–98, 700
risk factors 202–9, 322–3, 405–10,
    378–94
smoking 298–9
stress 518, 526
susceptibility 127, 131, 133,
    135–8, 140–1, 410–15, 467
tinnitus 175–7, 271, 698, 700
types 402–5
UN 714
WHO 716–20, 722, 724–5
noise maps 559, 614, 730
environmental 31, 347, 348, 362
Noise Pollution Health Effects
    Reduction (NOPHER) project 14
noise refuges 660–1
Noise and Statutory Nuisance Act
    (1993) 16, 604
noise test codes 38, 42–3
Noise at Work Act (1989) 14, 33–6
revocation 35–6
Noise at Work Regulations (1989) 40,
    596, 602, 608
measurement of noise 13–16, 28,
    38, 40
music 454–5
noise zoning 16, 35, 362, 363
NoiseCalc 318
NoiseScan 318–19, 331, 339

non– governmental organizations
    (NGOs) 713, 717–19, 736
non–steroidal anti–inflammatory
    drugs 242
noradrenaline 518–25, 529, 539–41,
    536, 570
tinnitus 272
nortriptyline 699
nosoacusis 65, 315, 333, 403
notches 188, 192, 219–20, 300,
    303, 610
ageing 66, 70, 78–9
children 166, 174–5
disability assessment 237, 242
military NIHL 448
music 460–1, 466, 467
occupational noise 414, 416–17
PTA 214–15, 219–20
susceptibility 127, 130
Nottingham Health Profile (NHP)
    691, 696
nuisance laws 604–6, 613–14

oboe playing 458
obscure auditory dysfunction syn-
    drome 246–7
occupational noise 165, 167, 193–6,
    209, 323–5, 397–426, 524–6
ageing 64, 77
agencies 716–17, 720, 724–7,
    732–3, 735
databases 312–19, 323–5, 327,
    330–1, 336–9
diagnosis 182–3, 188–90, 193–203,
    206–13, 216, 220–1, 415–23
disability assessment 233, 236,
    238, 243
health 293, 294, 296, 298, 350
hearing conservation programmes
    332–5
hearing protection devices 667–8,
    672–4, 675–9
history 209, 210–13
laws 608–12, 667–8
measurement 14–17, 22–3, 25,
    28–9, 33–6, 39–40
medical environment 498–511
military 435–51, 677–8
music 167–8, 453–73, 705–6, 708,
    711
NIHL and AHL 300–2
organic solvents 477–95

rehabilitation 687, 693, 694, 696–7
stress 520–3, 524–6, 529, 540–1
susceptibility 134–6, 201–3,
206–8, 410–15
therapy 424–6
types of NIHL 402–5
see also industrial noise
octave band noise (OBN) 50, 639–40,
668, 672–3
octopus cell area (OCA) 54–6
oestradiol 48–9
oestrogen 48–9
olivocochlear bundle (OCB) 93, 139,
412
music 466, 468, 473
olivocochlear reflex 262
olivocochlear (OC) systems 138–40,
141, 188, 294
feedback control 260–2
conditioning 642, 645
tinnitus 266, 269
one–third octave band 27, 40, 154,
440
ongoing random waveforms defined 6
orchestras 454–5, 461–2
hazardous music 453–62, 468,
472–3
organ of Corti 54, 86–7, 92, 94–8, 415
blast effects 288
feedback control 259–60
medical environment noise 507,
511
response to hazardous noise 85–7,
91–2, 94–8, 102
susceptibility 127, 135
organic solvents 208, 209, 291,
477–95
Organization for Economic Cooperation and Development 731–2
orienting reaction 500, 518, 520
oscillation 259
oscillators 149–50
osseous spiral lamina (osl) 86, 304
ossicular chain 87, 286, 402, 470
blast effects 193, 281, 282, 286, 289
susceptibility 131, 411
otalgia 192, 209
otitis media 217, 302, 418–19
children 168, 170, 172, 174–5
otoacoustic emissions (OAEs)
217–18, 447, 464–6
ageing 66

click–evoked (CEOAEs) 447–8, 464–5
conditioning 641
efferent suppression 466
feedback control 262
medicolegal matters 420, 422
spontaneous (SOAEs) 265–8, 273
susceptibility 138–40, 142–3
temperature 297
tinnitus 267–70
see also distortion product otoacoustic emissions (DPOAEs);
transient evoked
otoacoustic emissions
(TEOAEs)
otolaryngologists 609
otorrhoea 209, 328
otosclerosis 184, 217, 414–15, 418–19
otoscopy 214
ototoxicity 207–8, 210, 291, 424
ageing 44, 65, 71
antibiotics 289
CAS changes after damage 112, 121
causes of SNHL 184
children 170
conditioning 637
databases 321, 332, 339
disability assessment 242
genetics 71
hearing conservation programmes
335
medical environment 508, 510, 511
medicolegal matters 416, 418, 419
organic solvents 477–95
protection 101–2
smoking 134
susceptibility 202–3, 207–8, 411–12
outer ear see external (outer) ear
outer hair cells (OHCs) 87–96, 100
ageing 47, 50–1, 66–7, 72, 75, 79–80
blast effects 288
CAS changes after damage 111, 119
conditioning 638, 641
diagnosis 188, 204, 217–18
disability assessment 244
feedback control 259–60, 262
genetics 72
medical environment noise 507
medicolegal matters 416
military NIHL 447
music 464, 465, 466, 468, 473
NIHL and AHL 304–5
stress 518

susceptibility 127–9, 132, 135–9, 142, 204, 412
tinnitus 269
tonotopic reorganization 111
outer pillar cells 87, 95
outer spiral fibres 92
oval window 87, 131–2, 411
overhangs 472
overstimulation 85, 90–2, 95–7, 102
CAS changes after damage 111–13, 115–17, 118, 120, 122
conditioning 639, 643, 645
NIHL and AHL 303
occupational noise 402, 415
stress 518
susceptibility 127, 135, 137–42
oxidative damage 65, 639
oxygen 129, 133, 411, 424
neonates 508–9, 511
oxypurinol 425
oxytocin 519

Paget's disease 184
pain threshold 3, 185, 402, 517, 518, 707
paint industry 477, 479, 481, 483–6
paper industry 325, 478, 483, 489, 677
participation restrictions 681, 683–7
particle velocity 16, 29
peak levels 326–7, 559
blast effects 280, 282, 439–40
environmental noise 350
hearing conservation programmes 335
hearing protection devices 668, 678
impulse noise 379–82, 384–7, 390, 393
measurement of noise 14, 16, 24, 35–6
medical environment 504, 508
music 455, 459, 464
stress 517, 518, 520
WHO 723
pensions 397, 423
pentoxifylline 133
pepsin 519
peptides 133, 262, 272, 642–3
percussion 456, 459, 462, 471–3
performance test 569, 571
perilymph 88, 90, 98
fistulae 288, 416

susceptibility 137, 141
see also fluid in ears
period defined 2
periolivary nerve cells 93
peripheral auditory system 44–5, 50–3, 57–8, 65
permanent threshold shifts (PTSs) 119, 188–92, 458–9, 461–3
ageing 44–5, 48–9, 52, 67–8, 71–3, 75, 77
children 166, 174
cochleae and hazardous noise 85, 89, 94, 98, 100–1
conditioning 639, 641
databases 315, 316
diagnosis 186–200, 205, 209–14, 218–19
disability assessment 247
genetics 71–3
history 210–13
impulse noise 378–9
measurement of noise 14
medical environment noise 499, 510
music 453–4, 458–9, 460, 461–3, 464, 468
neural hyperactivity 114
NIHL and AHL 302
occupational noise 167, 402–7, 409, 410, 413–15, 491
organic solvents 491
PTA 214, 218
stress 517–18
susceptibility 130–1, 135–7, 139, 141, 205, 209, 410, 413–15
personal cassette players (PCPs) 165, 171, 174
headphones 453, 455–6, 464
personal protective equipment (PPE) 667, 671, 672
see also hearing protection devices
phalangeal processes 87–8, 95
phalangeal scars 95–6
phase defined 4–6
phasic response to noise 500
pheomelanin 142
phons 3, 18
phosphorylation 643
physical fitness 296–9
piano playing 456, 461, 710
piccolo playing 458

pigmentation 75, 206–7, 320
  susceptibility 135, 202, 206–7,
    411, 413, 467
pillar cells 87, 95
pinna 130, 284, 669
pink noise 6
Piribedil 269
pistonphone 30, 33
pitch 2, 5, 127, 155, 416, 560
  music 465, 467
pituitary–adrenal cortical system 519
plane waves 29
planning *see* land–use planning
plasma membrane 90
polluter pays principle 361
polyangliositis 184
polyneuritis 184
polyneuropathy 478
polysomnograms 569–70
popular music 455, 456, 460, 462–4,
  468, 473
  damage prevention 706, 710
  safety limits 167
positive pressure wave 279–80, 281,
  285, 439
positron emission tomography (PET)
  263, 264, 271
posterior fossa meningioma 420
potassium (K) 88, 90, 96
power tools 325
preamplifiers 25, 26, 30
precautionary principle 361
precedent 601, 602
prednisolone 469
pregnancy 170, 184, 210
  susceptibility 202–3, 412–13
prematurity 184, 210, 508, 511
presbyacusis 184, 238–42, 243–4,
  250–1, 299–305, 332
  ageing 47, 51, 52, 65, 67, 73–5
  allocation method 245–6
  cardiovascular disease 292–3
  conductive 67
  databases 315–16, 321, 332
  diagnosis 185, 197, 199, 203–5
  disability assessment 237–42,
    243–6, 250–2, 254
  genetics 73–5
  hyperlipoproteinaemia 292
  music 453, 461
  neural 67
  NPL tables 239–42, 252

occupational noise 403, 407, 413,
  425
  organic solvents 487
  sensorineural 67, 74
  smoking 298
  strial 67, 74
  susceptibility 203–5, 413
presbysocioacusis 403
prescriptive right 606
pressure microphones 26
pressure wave 439, 450, 453, 459
prestin 90
prevalence 64–5, 312–13, 436–9
  databases 312–13, 317
  military NIHL 436–9, 449
  organic solvents 479, 481, 482, 489
  tinnitus 212–13
prevalence rate ratio (PRR) 134
prevention of noise damage 14, 85,
  100–3, 182, 362, 424–6, 420
  agencies 716–19, 725, 734
  blast effects 288–9
  conditioning 637–46
  databases 312, 318
  environmental noise 346–7, 349,
    361–4
  hearing conservation programmes
    333
  hearing protection devices 678
  laws 604, 606, 608
  military NIHL 436, 441, 445
  music 705–12
  NIHL and ageing 64, 80
  organic solvents 493–4
  rehabilitation 688
  sleep disturbance 584
primary auditory dendrites 135
printing industry 478–9, 480, 483,
  485–6, 488, 491
prolactin 519
protection of hearing 441–5, 469–73,
  667–79
  acoustic trauma 638, 639
  blast effects 282, 286, 288–9
  conditioning 639, 641–5
  databases 313, 320, 339
  diagnosis 188, 193, 195, 203–4,
    209
  environmental noise 364
  impulse noise 379, 383, 385–7,
    390, 392–4
  industrial noise 650

laws 612, 616
magnesium 446
military 441–5, 446, 451
music 463, 464, 466, 469–73
occupational noise 404–6, 411, 414–15
sleep 579
smoking 299
susceptibility 129–36, 138, 140–3, 203–4, 411, 414–15
temperature 298
see also hearing conservation programmes; hearing protection devices (HPDs)
Protection Against Noise (PAN) project 14
protective reflex 517
proteins 89–90, 97–8, 101, 119, 424, 643
heat shock 97–8, 137, 298, 638
psychoacoustics 350–1
psychology 498–501, 603–7
environmental noise 349, 351–2, 361, 363–6
occupational noise 397
stress 534–44
tinnitus 698, 701
psychophysical tests 466–7
pyknotic nuclei 94
public health 196, 345–66, 441, 498
agencies 717–18, 732
pure–tone audiometry (PTA) 3, 148–63, 214–17, 218–20, 233–5, 299–301, 460–1
ageing 69
blast effects 287
calibration 151–3
cochleae and hazardous noise 97
databases 313, 318–19
diagnosis 190, 192–3, 214–20, 221–2
disability assessment 232–6, 238–9, 242–4, 246–8, 252–3
equipment 149–53
handicap 689–90
health 298
inconsistency 233–5
laws 609
medicolegal matters 416–17, 419, 420–3
military NIHL 447
music 458, 460–1, 462, 463–6
neural hyperactivity 113

NIHL and AHL 299–301, 303, 304
notches 219–20
occupational noise 405, 425–6, 479, 481–2, 484, 487, 489
organic solvents 493
presbyacusis 239
procedure of tests 155–9
rehabilitation 692–3, 689–90
reliability 160–2
susceptibility 138
symbols 159
test environment 153–5
tinnitus 266, 267

quality of life 328–30, 397, 609–10, 637
databases 312, 314, 315, 320, 328–30
environmental noise 346, 354, 360–1, 363, 365
rehabilitation 682, 687, 690
quarrying 402
questionnaires 74, 168, 365, 528, 538, 571
databases 315, 318
music 460
organic solvent 480, 483–4
rehabilitation 688, 691–2
sleep 569, 571, 584
tinnitus 692, 695–6, 699, 701
quinine 207–8

rabbits 640–1, 501
radial nerve fibre atrophy 67
radios 211
radiotherapy 184
railways and trains 21, 78, 614
agencies 720–1, 730
cognition 553–4, 557
environmental noise 347, 350, 354, 356, 366
sleep 567, 572, 574–5, 578–9, 583
random incidence fields 26, 30–1
range of hearing 2–4, 45–6
rapid eye movement (REM) sleep 567–8, 571, 574, 576–7
rarefaction of sound waves 7
rats 95, 97, 293, 302
CAS changes after damage 118–20
conditioning 639–40
genetics 73–5
oestrogen 48
organic solvents 486

susceptibility 135, 137, 414
Raynaud's phenomenon 295–6, 298
reactive oxygen species (ROS) 424–5
  *see also* free oxygen radicals
reading 549, 551–2, 554, 556–7, 559, 561–2
  children 165, 551–2, 554, 556–7, 561–2
real ear attenuation at threshold (REAT) 444, 445
recreational noise *see* leisure noise
recruitment 113–14, 122
  music 460, 465
  rehabilitation 684, 685
red blood cells 132, 133
redox status 98, 101, 639
redundancy 79–80, 128
reference equivalent threshold sound pressure levels 239
reflections 7, 8–10, 41
  blast effects 280, 282, 283, 284
  environmental noise 32–3
  impulse noise 380–1
  industrial noise 35, 662
  machinery 36
  music 469, 472
refraction 11–12
rehabilitation 332, 420, 424–6, 681–701
  ageing 64, 80
  blast effects 290
Reissner's membrane (rm) 86, 88
renal problems 184, 242, 418
renin 519
residential noise 345–6, 352–3, 355, 357–60, 362–3, 365–6
  cognition 557
  measurement 27, 40
  sleep 576, 578, 583
  *see also* neighbours and neighbourhoods
resistance phase 527
resonance 9–10, 130, 150
respiratory rate 502
response amplitudes 51
response time for stress 527
reticular formation 262
reticular lamina 86–8, 94–6, 288
retrocochlear pathology 216–17, 419–20
  afferent pathway 260–1
  lesions 294
  military NIHL 450

organic solvents 481, 484, 486, 489, 491
tinnitus 700
retrodiction exercise 610–11
reverberation 41, 417, 560
  impulse noise 379, 380, 381
  industrial noise 650–3, 655, 660, 662–3, 665
  machinery 36–7
  music 469
  rooms 330
riluzole 101
rise times 35, 149, 192, 499
  blast effects 282, 284
  impulse noise 379
  sleep 572
  stress 520
risk factors for NIHL 202–9, 405–10, 322–3, 378–94
  children 175
  cognition 552, 559
  databases 312–24, 326–7, 331–3, 335–9
  diagnosis 182–3, 193–4, 196, 200–1, 202–9
  environmental noise 348, 349
  health 291, 292, 298, 302
  hearing conservation programmes 333–4
  hearing protection devices 667–8, 678
  impulse noise 378–94
  laws 608, 609, 612, 613
  military noise 435
  music 456, 458–60, 705–6, 708–9, 710–12
  occupational noise 193–4, 200–1, 405–10, 413
  organic solvents 478, 483–4, 485, 489–90
  sleep 580–1
  susceptibility 129–36, 143, 202–9
  WHO 717, 722
road traffic 524–9
  agencies 714–15, 717–18, 720–1, 728–9, 731–2
  calming 355, 365
  children 165, 528–30, 553, 556–7
  cognition 553, 556–7, 559–60
  databases 325
  environmental noise 345, 347–8, 350, 355–66

laws 603, 606, 614
lorries 21
measurement of noise 24, 27, 40, 42
motorcycles 350, 521, 522, 728
resurfacing 362
sleep 567, 572, 574–5, 578–80, 583–4
speed limits 362
standards 597–8
stress 517, 521–30, 539–41
tyres 362, 715
rock–and–roll music 168, 453, 455, 459–60, 462–3
concerts 165, 171, 174
databases 325
prevention of hearing damage 706, 710
WHO 722
room acoustics 469
rootlets 89, 97–8
round window 87

salicylates 207, 210, 265, 411
sarcoplasmic reticulum 90
sarthran 133, 425
sawmills 478
scala media 86–8, 96, 321
scala tympani 86, 88, 96, 137
scala vestibule 86, 88
scattering of sound 35
screening 158
children 169–73, 176
cognition 556
databases 315–17, 328, 332
diagnosis 199, 200–1, 213, 216–17, 218
disability assessment 242–3, 240–1
military NIHL 436, 447
music 462
NIHL and AHL 299–301
occupational noise 414, 418, 426
organic solvents 495
presbyacusis 240–1
selective membrane permeability 446
selective serotonin re–uptake inhibitor (SSRI) 699
self–recording audiometry 158–9
semi–insert protectors 442
sensitivity 2, 90, 93–4, 100, 244–5, 299, 303

ageing 46, 48, 66, 79
CAS changes after damage 118
cognition 553
conditioning 637–8, 643
databases 314, 317, 328
diagnosis 184, 192
disability assessment 236–7, 238, 244–6, 253
environmental noise 348–9, 355, 357, 360, 363
health 293–4, 296–7
hearing thresholds 148, 150, 151
impulse noise 384
laws 609
music 168, 453, 463, 465
occupational noise 398, 410, 412, 416, 426
sleep 577, 584
susceptibility 127, 132–3, 138, 410, 412
tinnitus 267, 271, 273
sensitization 576
sensorineural hearing loss (SNHL) 151, 204–5
blast effects 286, 289
causes 184, 208, 243
children 165, 170, 173–5, 202
databases 320, 332
diagnosis 184–5, 192, 202–6, 208–10, 213–14, 217, 222
disability ratings 255
health 291, 294
medicolegal matters 416–20
NIHL and AHL 299
occupational noise 402, 412, 416–20
organic solvents 478, 480, 489
rehabilitation 683, 685
surgery 511
susceptibility 202–6, 208, 412
WHO 717
sensorineural high–frequency hearing loss (SHFHL) 165, 167
serotonin 272, 699
serotoninergic system 262, 272
sertraline 699
shadow areas 280
shipyards 77, 324, 467, 673, 696
organic solvents 478, 482, 484, 487
shock waves (shock front) 441, 518
blast effect 279–80, 281, 282, 288–9
shooting see guns and gunfire
shoulder hours 577, 583

signalled awakening 569, 570
signal–to–noise ratio (SNR) 330, 436, 723
  cognition 554, 556, 557
  hearing protection devices 672, 673
silencers 654, 655–7, 659
single–proton emission computer tomography (SPECT) 263, 272
single–unit activity 114, 115–17, 118
sirens 502, 503, 510
skin colour 206–7, 293, 300, 320
  susceptibility 142, 206–7, 413
skin resistance 499
sleep 501, 526–7, 567–84, 605
  depth 568–9, 571–7, 579
  environmental noise 355–6, 363–5, 578–9
  feedback control 262
  function 567–9
  ICBEN 733
  latencies 568, 571, 579
  medical environment noise 499, 501, 503–4, 508–11
  noise disturbance 571–6, 579–82
  occupational noise 397, 421
  personal characteristics 576–8
  recording 569–71
  rehabilitation 691, 699, 701
  stress 516–17, 522, 526–30, 535, 540, 542
  tinnitus 262, 699, 701
  WHO 722–3, 724
smoking 76, 134, 205, 209, 298–9
  databases 314, 322
  disability assessment 242
  health 292–3, 296
  stress 525
  susceptibility 134, 202, 205, 413, 467
smooth endoplasmic reticulum 415
social cost 358–9, 397
  environmental noise 346–7, 349, 352–3, 356, 358–61, 363
Social Hearing Handicap Index 690
social isolation 363, 683–7, 690–1
  databases 312, 315, 328
social noise 209–10, 332, 403, 717
  diagnosis 202, 209–10, 211–12, 220
  susceptibility 202, 209–10
socioacusis 65, 315, 333, 511
socioeconomics 76, 300, 715

cognition 552, 555, 557, 559, 561
  rehabilitation 682, 684, 686
sodium (Na) 88, 90
solvents 314, 325, 412
  organic 208, 209, 291, 477–95
somatic disorders 698–9
somatosensory system 262
sound conduction pathway 49
sound defined 1–2
sound design 350–1
sound engineers 707, 711–12
sound exposure levels (SELs) measurement 21–2
sound intensity 29–30, 188, 572–4
  CAS changes after damage 119
  cochleae and hazardous noise 85–6, 89–90, 93–4, 97–100
  cognition 553, 560
  disability assessment 253
  measurement of noise 16, 17, 19, 29–30
  medical environment 499, 502, 505, 507, 511
  military NIHL 435, 446
  music 458–60, 468–70
  NIHL and AHL 303
  occupational noise 194, 402, 404–7, 409–11, 417, 425–6
  stress 517–18, 520, 522, 529–30, 538
  susceptibility 128–42, 410–11
  temperature 298
  tinnitus 270–2
  see also sound level; sound pressure level
sound intensity analysers 29–30, 41
  measurement of noise 25–31, 34, 36
sound level 491–3
  ageing 45, 51–2, 57–8, 69–77
  agencies 714–15, 717, 722, 728–9
  cognition 557, 560
  environmental noise 345–7, 349–50, 354, 362–3, 365
  hearing protection devices 672–3
  impulse noise 378, 384, 389
  industrial noise 651–9
  laws 606, 607, 613
  medical environment 498, 500–1, 504, 506, 509–10
  military NIHL 435–6
  music 454–6, 458–9, 463–4, 469–70, 472–3, 705–12

organic solvents 478, 491–3
rehabilitation 696–7
sleep 574, 576, 580–2
stress 516–18, 522, 525, 528, 536, 538
*see also* sound intensity; sound pressure level
sound level meters 25–9, 40, 185, 600
measurement of noise 25–33, 34–5, 40
music 454
sound pressure level (SPL) 4, 17–20, 25, 41, 94, 324, 572–4
ageing 49, 68, 73
agencies 720–1, 723, 728–9, 734
diagnosis 185, 187, 189–90, 192, 222–3
difficulties 218–20
genetics 73
hearing conservation programmes 335
hearing protection devices 672, 673–4, 677
hearing thresholds 151, 153–4, 160
history 209–13
impulse noise 382, 387
investigations 215, 217
laws 608, 612
machinery 36–7
measurement of noise 16–25, 27, 29, 32, 35–7, 40–1
medical environment 499, 500, 504
music 455, 456, 459, 466
neural hyperactivity 112–14
occupational noise 193–6, 200–1, 402–3, 406–7
peaks 24, 35–6, 668, 678
PTA 215
sleep 572–5, 577, 580
standards 596
standing waves 8–9
stress 517, 538
susceptibility 130, 203, 208
tinnitus 267
*see also* sound intensity; sound level
sound restoration systems 668–70
sound transfer functions (STFs) 130
sound waves 2–12, 19
types of waveform 6–7
soundscape 350–1, 361, 364

spectacles 155, 670, 675, 678
spectral characteristics of noise 16, 45, 410, 459
music 453, 459, 465, 470
spectral energy distribution 386–7, 391–2, 393–4
spectral smear 149
speech and communication 3, 211, 556–7, 686–7
children 553–4, 556–61
cognition 553–4, 556–62
databases 313–15, 328–31
disability assessment 233, 235, 246, 248–9, 253–4
feedback control 261
hearing conservation programmes 336
hearing protection devices 288, 669–70
hearing thresholds 162
ICBEN 733
medical environmental noise 500
medicolegal matters 416–18, 420–1, 423
military NIHL 436, 442, 446
music 467, 469, 473
organic solvents 479, 480, 484, 488, 491, 493
rehabilitation 682–90, 692–8
stress 516–18, 522, 529
susceptibility 127, 130
WHO 717, 722–3
spiral ganglion cells 54–5, 92–3, 137, 304, 424, 489
spiral ligament 87, 127, 133, 415
spiral limbus 86, 91
spiral modiolar artery 132
spontaneous otoacoustic emissions (SOAEs) 267–8
tinnitus 265–8, 273
squaring and averaging circuits 25, 28
standards 590–8, 615–16, 626–36
hearing protection devices 671–2, 676
standing waves 8–10
stapedial reflex 234, 262, 273, 294, 470, 486
acoustic trauma 638
diagnosis 209, 217, 221, 222
medicolegal matters 419, 420
stapedius muscle 283, 463, 640–1

susceptibility 131, 414–15
stapes 87, 131, 286
startle reflex 518, 500, 506
steel industry 134, 399
stereocilia 67, 88–91, 94–9, 244, 304
    genetics 72
    susceptibility 127, 132, 136, 137,
        204
steroids 289, 290
stick–slip friction 650
stigmatization 314, 684, 686
strategic environment assessment
    (SEA) 354, 363, 366
stress 137–8, 272, 351–4, 516–30,
    534–44, 570
    acoustic trauma 638–9
    acute reaction 535, 538–40, 542–4
    chronic reaction 535, 540–2, 543–4
    cognition 561
    conditioning 642
    diagnosis 183, 212
    environmental noise 346, 349,
        351–4, 357, 363–5
    feedback control 263
    health 291, 294, 296
    hearing conservation programmes
        333
    medical environment noise 501,
        505–6, 510
    music 468
    occupational noise 397
    oxidative 137–8
    rehabilitation 686–7, 697
    sleep 569, 570, 571, 574, 578, 583
    susceptibility 137–8, 141
    tinnitus 272, 517, 699–700
stria vascularis 86, 88, 188, 304–5,
    321, 415
    acoustic trauma 639
    ageing 46, 47, 50, 66, 75
    CAS changes after damage 110
    susceptibility 127, 133, 135, 137,
        142, 206
strychnine 138, 642
stroke 292
styrene 208, 325, 412, 486–8
    occupational noise 412, 477,
        479–82, 486–8, 490–4
subadditivity 303, 305
subsurface cisternae 90, 415
superadditivity 79–80, 303, 305

superior olivary complex (SOC) sys-
    tem 93, 412
    feedback control 260, 261, 262
superoxide 138
superoxide dismutase (SOD) 98,
    137–8, 425
Supply of Machinery (Safety)
    Regulations (1992) 608
supportive environments 365–6
surgery 314, 320, 414–15, 419, 505–7
    blast effects 286, 289
    conditioning 642
    medical environment noise 501,
        505–7, 510–11
susceptibility 127–43, 201–9, 244–5,
    410–15, 467, 578, 583–4
    acoustic trauma 638
    ageing 44–5, 48–52, 58, 75–6, 77,
        79–80
    children 175, 177, 554
    cochleae and hazardous noise 100
    cognition 554
    databases 321, 322, 329, 339
    diagnosis 187–8, 190, 201–9
    disability assessment 236–7, 238,
        244–5
    genetics 71, 73
    health 297
    hearing conservation programmes
        312–13, 335
    impulse noise 383
    medical environment noise 505,
        510
    military NIHL 435–8, 446
    music 168, 467, 468, 470
    NIHL and AHL 302–5
    occupational noise 402, 404–6,
        409–15, 417
    sleep 576–7, 578, 579, 583–4
    stress 539, 542
    toughening 468
symmetry of NIHL 69–70, 209–10,
    216, 251, 419–20
    disability assessment 251, 253
    military 447, 449–50
    music 457, 461, 462–4
sympathetic adrenal medullary sys-
    tem 519, 520
sympathetic nervous system 321, 536
synapses 93, 98, 102
    conditioning 642, 644

feedback control 259
stress 520, 536
susceptibility 135, 136, 138
tinnitus 269, 272
tonotopic reorganization 112, 121
systolic blood pressure 293, 294, 398

Technology and Construction Court
  (TCC) 606
tectorial membrane (tm) 86, 88–9,
  91–2, 411
tectorins 91
telephone use 211–12, 248, 330, 509,
  595
  rehabilitation 684, 690, 694, 696
  surgery 505–7, 510
television 211–12, 248, 331, 356,
  511, 721
  rehabilitation 683, 685, 694
temperature 32, 296, 297–8, 299, 725
  acoustic trauma 638
  hearing protection devices 671,
    674–5
  industrial noise 658
  occupational noise 402, 424
  refraction 11–12
  sleep 578
  speed of sound 2, 11
temporary threshold shifts (TTSs)
  135–6, 186–8, 205, 380–9, 390–2,
  458–9, 463–4
  ageing 52
  blast effects 281
  BOP 389, 390–2
  children 166, 176
  cochleae and hazardous noise 85,
    89, 94, 97, 99–100
  conditioning 639, 641–2
  databases 315, 328
  diagnosis 186–8, 192, 195, 202,
    205–6, 209, 214
  health 296–7, 298
  impulse noise 378–9, 380–9, 393–4
  measurement of noise 14
  medical environment noise 499,
    505, 507, 510
  military NIHL 436, 445, 446
  music 168, 458–9, 463–4, 467–8,
    471
  occupational noise 166, 402–5,
    410–11, 413, 415

physical fitness 296–7
smoking 298–9
stress 517
susceptibility 130–42, 202, 205–6,
  209, 410–11, 413, 415, 467
tensor tympani muscle 131
testosterone 519
textile industry 414
threshold of audibility 3
threshold of feeling 3–4
thyroid 184, 424
time–weighting (T-weighting) 27
  impulse noise 388–9, 391, 392, 393
  measurement of noise 17, 23–4,
    25, 27, 29, 31, 38
tinnitus 121–2, 142, 175–7, 212–13,
  258–73, 328, 695–6, 698–701
  blast effects 281, 288
  BOP 390
  children 165, 175–6
  databases 312, 315, 320, 328, 330
  diagnosis 183, 186, 192, 209,
    212–13, 222
  feedback control 259–63, 270
  gender 176–7
  glutamate 102, 259, 262, 268–70,
    272–3
  laws 609
  medical environment noise 499
  medicolegal matters 416–17, 423
  military NIHL 438, 446
  music 453, 458, 460, 464, 467,
    473, 708–10
  prevalence 175–6, 212–13
  rehabilitation 684, 686, 692,
    695–6, 698–701
  stress 272, 517, 699–700
  susceptibility 127, 133, 139, 140,
    142, 143
Tinnitus Severity Questionnaire
  (TSQ) 692, 696, 701
toluene 208, 412, 485–6
  occupational HL 477–81, 483–6,
    488, 490–2, 494
tonic response to noise 500–1
tonotopic reorganization 111–12,
  270–2
  CAS changes after damage 110,
    111–12, 113, 120–1
  feedback control 261, 263
  tinnitus 263, 270–2, 273

torsional waves 7
toughening 68, 188, 467–8
  susceptibility 135–6, 141, 414
trade unions 232, 610
tragus 150
training 38, 40, 214
  hearing conservation programmes
    336
  hearing protection devices 668, 676
  military NIHL 435–8
  music 705–6, 711
  rehabilitation 681, 686, 692
transducers 390, 419, 592
  measurement of noise 151, 153,
    155, 160
transduction 127–8, 136, 259
transient evoked otoacoustic emissions (TEOAEs) 217–18, 221, 222
  medicolegal matters 422
  music 464, 466
  susceptibility 135, 140
  tinnitus 266, 268
transportation 183, 559, 572, 736
  environmental noise 345–6, 353,
    357, 359, 361–3, 366
  occupational noise 399
  OECD 732
  WHO 718, 720–1
  see also aircraft noise; railways
    and trains; road traffic
transverse waves 6–7
trichloroethylene (TCE) 412, 477,
  488–9, 492
trigeminal nerve 131
trombone playing 456, 458
trumpet playing 456, 472
tuberculosis (TB) 210
tuning 94
tuning out 554, 557, 558
tunnel of Corti 87
tunnel radial fibres 93
tunnel spiral bundles 643
twin studies 74–5
tympanic membrane 87, 328
  attenuation 444–5
  blast effects 193, 279, 281–9
  susceptibility 129–30, 131, 411,
    414
tympanometry 217, 222, 419, 420
tyrosine hydroxylase 142, 643,
    644–5

unemployment 312, 328–9
United Nations 713–15, 725–6, 736
United Nations Environment
  Programme (UNEP) 714, 715

Valsalva effect 470
vascular conductance (VC) 133
vascular problems 184, 205–6, 210,
  242
  susceptibility 202–3, 205–6, 208
vasoconstriction 296, 536, 570
  susceptibility 132–3, 208
vasodilation 290
vegetative–endocrine system 536, 544
vegetative nervous system (VNS) 526
ventilation systems 348, 721
verification of measurements 151–3
vertigo 209, 288, 320, 336, 493
vestibular system 192, 210, 262, 281,
  420
  organic solvents 479, 484, 485,
    487–8, 493
vestibulocochlear nerve 85, 92–3
vibration 32–3, 295–6, 402, 650,
  658–9
  agencies 721, 725, 735
  databases 314, 321
  environmental noise 352, 353–4,
    357
  laws 606, 609
  standards 594, 596, 626–36
vibration–induced white finer
  syndrome 208, 296, 321, 335
viola playing 453, 456–7, 461, 471–2
violin playing 453, 456–8, 460–1, 470–2
viruses 103, 184
vitamins 76

Waardenburg's syndrome 206
Walsh–Healy Act (USA) 378
warning signals 330, 536, 684
  hearing protection devices 669
  sirens 502, 503, 510
  surgery 506, 510
wartime noise exposure 68
wavelength 2, 4, 8–9, 11, 16
weaving mills 77, 378
  jute 78, 167, 189, 197
weight 321
white noise 6, 112
wind 12, 32–3

windows 355, 362, 365, 605, 723
  blast 286
  sleep 571, 574, 576, 578
wood impacts 380, 382, 383
woodwind playing 460, 468, 470–3
World Bank 713, 715, 726–7
World Health Organization 713,
  714–15, 716–25, 730, 736
  Guidelines for Community Noise
    716, 720–5

World Trade Organization 713, 715,
  727–8

xanthine oxidase 425
xylene 208, 412, 485
  occupational HL 477, 479, 481,
    483–6, 488, 492, 494
xylophone playing 458

zinc superoxide dismutase 98